Digital Mammography

Your bonus with the purchase of this book

With the purchase of this book, you can use our "SN Flashcards" app to access questions free of charge in order to test your learning and check your understanding of the contents of the book. To use the app, please follow the instructions below:

1. Go to **https://flashcards.springernature.com/login**
2. Create a user account by entering your e-mail address, assigning a password and inserting the coupon code here below.

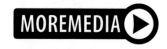

Your personal "SN Flashcards" app code   48341-69945-ABCB1-2A8C7-CE9D2

If the code is missing or does not work, please send an e-mail with the subject "**SN Flashcards**" and the book title to **customerservice@springernature.com**.

Claire Mercer • Peter Hogg
Judith Kelly
Editors

Digital Mammography

A Holistic Approach

Second Edition

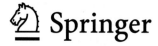 Springer

Editors
Claire Mercer
School of Health and Society
University of Salford
Manchester, UK

Peter Hogg
University of Salford
Manchester, UK

Judith Kelly
The Countess of Chester Hospitals NHS
Foundation Trust
Chester, UK

ISBN 978-3-031-10900-3   ISBN 978-3-031-10898-3   (eBook)
https://doi.org/10.1007/978-3-031-10898-3

This Springer imprint is published by the registered company Springer Nature Switzerland AG
The registered company address is: Gewerbestrasse 11, 6330 Cham, Switzerland

This book is dedicated to a dear friend and colleague, Jo Coward. Jo volunteered to write the Patient Diary for this book at a time when she was terminally ill due to breast cancer secondary disease. Written at the most challenging time of her life, within the chapter she expresses her innermost thoughts and feelings to the world. Jo, we are eternally grateful for your contribution to the development of education in this area. You remain to be an inspiration to your profession, your friends, and to those who matter the most to you—your five children.

Foreword

Breast cancer remains a common disease, and mammography continues to play an essential role in its detection within screening and symptomatic populations. To achieve this, mammography services should provide imaging in a timely fashion, producing accurate results delivered by caring and competent professionals.

Digital Mammography: A Holistic Approach was first published in 2015. It comprised an international line up of authors; and the wide-ranging content addressed a broad spectrum of relevant issues which mammography practitioners needed to understand and apply within clinical practice. Not surprisingly, it was exceptionally popular amongst students and qualified practitioners and has been used in numerous countries; sales of the first edition reflected the value it served.

However, over the last 7 years many changes have occurred in mammography services, including equipment changes, imaging technique modifications and enhanced understanding of breast cancer risk factors which impact into screening regimes and how imaging might be conducted. It is therefore timely that a second edition of *Digital Mammography: A Holistic Approach* is published.

The second edition builds directly on the solid foundation provided by the first edition. The Editors reflected critically on the contents of the first edition and advised authors to update existing chapters where relevant and introduced new chapters to reflect the emerging requirements upon current practitioners today. The inclusion of a patient diary from a patient who is a radiographer and academic is both innovative and extremely moving. Understanding this patient perspective will assist breast professionals in their work, and the author has provided great insight into many areas of practice often neglected. The new chapter on managing anxiety builds upon the 'caring for clients and staff section' of this book, and the author highlights common causes of anxiety in both clients and practitioners whilst exploring solutions and techniques to help reduce anxiety levels; certainly an essential requirement for all staff in today's society. A further chapter provides evidence-based guidance for practitioners when imaging persons living with dementia; detailing the main symptoms, stages, and types of dementia and discussing how these issues can influence care, this chapter will prove essential to support future practitioners. All in all, this book really does prove to be a holistic approach to mammography.

   As immediate past President of the European Federation of Radiographer Societies (EFRS), I wholeheartedly recommend this second edition as a valued addition to a mammography imaging facility, for qualified staff to use as a reference during imaging procedures and for continual professional updating. Equally, I recommend it to students—for those entering the profession through a pre-registration (undergraduate or postgraduate degree), where mammography might be introduced as a specialist field; or as a qualified practitioner studying a post qualification/postgraduate award in which they are specialising into mammography with a view to advancing their skills in this field.

Charlotte Beardmore
Director of Professional Policy
The Society and College of Radiographers
London, UK

Preface

The first edition of this book was used across the world to educate students, inform practice, and assist in formulating healthcare policy. Sales statistics of the first edition reflected the value it has served in many countries. Since the first edition, many changes to practice, education, professional standards, policy, and guidelines have occurred and it is therefore timely that a second edition is published. This second edition revisits the first edition content; that process involved removal of some chapters, introduction of new ones, and updating of all chapters which were present in the first edition. In addition, we would invite readers to explore the Springer Nature Flashcards available with individual chapters. The cards are intended to help with consolidating knowledge from the text. Download the Springer Nature Flashcards app for free (*https://flashcards.springernature.com/login*) and use this exclusive additional material to consolidate your knowledge.

This book has a multinational and multiprofessional authorship, and it is intended to appeal to an international readership. Whilst it is recognised that aspects of mammographic practice vary considerably across different regions and countries, many issues and principles within healthcare remain generic and are transferable across populations.

An important issue to address for a wide readership is the terminology used in clinical practice. For example, the individual performing the mammogram is described variously as radiographer, mammographer, (mammography) practitioner, and radiologic technologist—all performing similar roles. In this book we generally describe the person performing the imaging as the practitioner. Similar differences exist in naming the subject of the mammography procedure as woman/man, client, service user, and patient and this may also vary according to whether the individual is undergoing a screening or symptomatic mammogram. Within this book the term 'client' is often used for screening purposes; similarly patient is often used for symptomatic purposes, and 'service user' is also used.

The editors would like to express their sincere gratitude to all the authors of this book; production of this edition during a global pandemic was indeed challenging and each and every one of the authors and co-authors went above and beyond to enable production of this edition.

Manchester, UK	Claire Mercer
Manchester, UK	Peter Hogg
Chester, UK	Judith Kelly

Terminology

Client/service-user/patients	The representative terms used within this book for all those who have mammography to include those non-identifying, men and women
Practitioner	This term is used to encompass assistant practitioners, associate practitioners, those undertaking mammography apprenticeships, mammographers, practitioners and advanced practitioners and others who specialise in mammography This term is also used to encompass those who are radiographer who undertake mammography and technicians/technologists who undertake mammography
Image receptor	This term is used to represent the image platform to which the breast is placed upon

Acknowledgements

We wish to express our sincere gratitude and appreciation to the book Copy Editor, Johanna Mercer. Johanna worked tirelessly to improve the quality of the book, improving its value and usability. She corrected grammatical and spelling errors within the chapters as part of the chapter review process, additionally making proposals to content and literature where supporting information could be beneficial. Johanna formatted all chapters into the correct style and updated learning objectives to guarantee a consistent style with good accuracy, additionally ensuring chapter references complied with the referencing style.

Claire Mercer
Peter Hogg
Judith Kelly

Contents

Editors and Contributors

About the Editors

Claire Mercer has an academic work focus with several research interests. She joined the University of Salford in 2015 and is currently the Head of Radiography in the School of Health and Society at the University of Salford, UK. A radiographer by background, specialising in mammography she has 10 years' experience in NHS management, with an MSc in Advanced Medical Imaging and a PhD by published works in mammography. Claire is passionate about workforce and research development across her field. Her focused research interests lie within digital mentorship in radiography, breast imaging and quality metrics such as compression force and positioning technique. Claire is passionate about workforce development across Medical Imaging.

Peter Hogg holds professional qualifications in Diagnostic Radiography, Nuclear Medicine, and Radiation Protection. He also holds computer science and teaching qualifications. He became a Professor of Radiography in 2002 at the University of Salford and held a range of senior academic positions there, including Research Dean. He holds several Visiting and Honorary academic positions around the world, including Visiting Professorship (Chair) in the Netherlands. He is currently an Emeritus Professor at the University of Salford.

Judith Kelly has worked in Breast Imaging as a Consultant Radiographer since 2004 and undertakes all aspects of breast imaging interpretation and interventional work. Currently, she is the clinical lead for breast screening at a local hospital trust. She is also a member of the Advisory Committee on Breast Cancer Screening to the Department of Health.

Contributors

Raed Mohammed Kadhim M. Ali Faculty of Medicine, University of Kufa, Najaf, Iraq

University of Kufa, Najaf, Iraq

Clare S. Alison Breast Imaging, Thirlestaine Breast Centre, Cheltenham, UK

Sue M. Astley Division of Informatics, Imaging and Data Sciences, Faculty of Biology, Medicine and Health, The University of Manchester, Manchester, UK

Rebecca Berry Breast Radiology Department, Tameside and Glossop Integrated Care NHS Foundation Trust, Ashton-under-Lyne, UK

Bernadette Bickley Dudley, Wolverhampton and South West Staffordshire Breast Screening Service, Russells Hall Hospital, Dudley, West Midlands, UK

Lisa Bisset Dorset Breast Screening Unit, Poole General Hospital, Dorset, UK

Marcela Böhm-Vélez Weinstein Imaging Associates, Pittsburgh, PA, USA

Rita M. Borgen Breast Screening Service, East Lancashire Hospitals NHS Trust, Burnley General Hospital, Burnley, UK

Breast Screening Service, East Lancashire Hospitals NHS Trust, Burnley, UK

Claire Borrelli St George's National Breast Education Centre, St George's University Hospital NHS Foundation Trust, London, UK

Woutjan Branderhorst Sigmascreening B.V. Enschede, Amsterdam, The Netherlands

Patrick C. Brennan Discipline of Medical Imaging Sciences, Faculty of Medicine and Health, Sydney School of Health Sciences, The University of Sydney, Sydney, NSW, Australia

Mireille J. M. Broeders LRCB Dutch Expert Centre for Screening, Nijmegen, The Netherlands

Ariane Chan Volpara Health Technologies, Wellington, New Zealand

Volpara Health Technologies Ltd, Wellington, New Zealand

Amanda Coates Breast Imaging, Mid Yorkshire Hospitals Trust, Pinderfields Hospital, Wakefield, UK

Joanne Coward University of Salford, Manchester, UK

Alison Darlington Department of Breast Imaging, North Manchester General Hospital, Manchester, UK

Jerry E. de Groot Sigmascreening B.V. Enschede, Amsterdam, The Netherlands

Gerard J. den Heeten Sigmascreening B.V. Enschede, Amsterdam, The Netherlands

Department of Radiology and Nuclear Medicine, University of Amsterdam, Amsterdam, The Netherlands

Caroline J. Dobson Breast Imaging, Thirlestaine Breast Centre, Cheltenham, UK

Fiona Dobson Medicines Support Team, Burnley General Teaching Hospital, Burnley, UK

Victoria L. Ebanks Breast Imaging, Whipps Cross Hospital, Barts Health NHS Trust, London, UK

Joleen K. Eden Breast Screening Service, East Lancashire Hospitals NHS Trust, Burnley General Hospital, Burnley, UK

Eva Maria Fallenberg Klinikum rechts der Isar, TU München, Institut für diagnostische und interventionelle Radiologie, München, Germany

Sue Garnett Breast Unit, University Hospital, Coventry, UK

Susan E. Garnett Breast Unit, University Hospital, Coventry, UK

Rosalind Given-Wilson St Georges Healthcare NHS Foundation Trust, Tooting, London, UK

Marie Griffiths Salford Business School, University of Salford, Manchester, UK

Cornelis A. Grimbergen Sigmascreening B.V. Enschede, Amsterdam, The Netherlands

Lisa Hackney New Alderley House, Macclesfield District General Hospital, Macclesfield, Cheshire, UK

East Cheshire NHS Trust, Macclesfield, UK

Elaine F. Harkness Division of Informatics, Imaging and Data Sciences, Faculty of Biology, Medicine and Health, The University of Manchester, Manchester, UK

Elizabeth G. Harrison Nightingale Centre, Wythenshawe Hospital, Manchester University NHS Foundation Trust, Manchester, UK

Rob Higgins School of Health and Society, University of Salford, Manchester, UK

Ralph Highnam Volpara Health Technologies, Wellington, New Zealand

Catherine Hill DetectedX, The University of Sydney, Sydney, NSW, Australia

Catherine A. Hill DetectEd-X, Sydney, NSW, Australia

Peter Hogg University of Salford, Manchester, UK

Sahand Hooshmand Discipline of Medical Imaging Sciences, Faculty of Medicine and Health, Sydney School of Health Sciences, The University of Sydney, Sydney, NSW, Australia

Jaimee Howes Volpara Health Technologies, Wellington, New Zealand

Hannah Kearsley School of Health and Society, University of Salford, Manchester, UK

Allison Kelly Nightingale Centre, Wythenshawe Hospital, Manchester University NHS Foundation Trust, Manchester, UK

Judith Kelly The Countess of Chester Hospitals NHS Foundation Trust, Chester, UK

Lyndsay A. Kinnear Nightingale Centre, Wythenshawe Hospital, Manchester University NHS Foundation Trust, Manchester, UK

Iain Lyburn Thirlestaine Breast Centre, Gloucester Hospitals NHS Foundation Trust, Cheltenham, UK

Dawn McDonald Breast Unit, Broomfield Hospital, Chelmsford, Essex, UK

Mark F. McEntee University College Cork, UGF 12 ASSERT, Brookfield Health Sciences, Cork, UK

Claire Mercer School of Health and Society, University of Salford, Manchester, UK

Johanna E. Mercer Health in Mind, Halisham, East Sussex, UK

Deborah Nelson Breast Radiology Department, Tameside and Glossop Integrated Care NHS Foundation Trust, Ashton-under-Lyne, UK

Cherish B. Parham Department of Radiation Science, Virginia Commonwealth University, Richmond, VA, USA

Anne Pearson Directorate of Psychology, School of Health and Society, University of Salford, Manchester, UK

Sheba Pradeep School of Health and Society, University of Salford, Manchester, UK

Warren M. Reed Discipline of Medical Imaging Sciences, Faculty of Medicine and Health, Sydney School of Health Sciences, The University of Sydney, Sydney, NSW, Australia

Zebby Rees Bronglais Hospital, Hywel Dda Health Board, Carmarthen, West Wales, UK

Bronglais and Singleton Hospitals, Aberystwyth, West Wales, UK

Rachel Reilly Breast Imaging, Mid Yorkshire Hospitals Trust, Pinderfields Hospital, Wakefield, UK

Cláudia Sá dos Reis Escola Superior de Tecnologia da Saúde de Lisboa, Lisbon School of Health Technology, Lisbon, Portugal

School of Health Sciences (HESAV), University of Applied Sciences and Arts Western Switzerland (HES-SO), Lausanne, Switzerland

Sheetal Ruparelia Credit Valley Hospital, Mississauga, ON, Canada

Beverley Scragg School of Health and Society, University of Salford, Manchester, UK

Ioannis Sechopoulos Department of Medical Imaging, Radboud University Medical Center, Nijmegen, The Netherlands

Technical Medical Centre, University of Twente, Enschede, The Netherlands

Dutch Expert Centre for Screening (LRCB), Nijmegen, The Netherlands

Richard Sidebottom Thirlestaine Breast Centre, Gloucester Hospitals NHS Foundation Trust, Cheltenham, UK

AI Imaging Hub, The Royal Marsden NHS Foundation Trust, London, UK

Helen L. Smith Breast Care Unit, Royal Lancaster Infirmary, University Hospitals of Morecambe Bay NHS Foundation Trust, Lancaster, UK

Adam Spacey School of Health and Society, University of Salford, Manchester, UK

Julie R. Stein-Hodgins Pennine Breast Unit, Bradford, UK

Melanie Stephens School of Health and Society, University of Salford, Manchester, UK

Mo'ayyad E. Suleiman Discipline of Medical Imaging Sciences, Faculty of Medicine and Health, Sydney School of Health Sciences, The University of Sydney, Sydney, NSW, Australia

Katy Szczepura School of Health and Society, University of Salford, Manchester, UK

Kathryn Taylor Cambridge Breast Unit, Cambridge, Cambridge University Hospitals NHS Foundation Trust, Cambridge, UK

Cathy Ure School of Health and Society, University of Salford, Manchester, UK

Monique G. J. T. B. van Lier Sigmascreening B.V. Enschede, Amsterdam, The Netherlands

Sarah Vinnicombe Thirlestaine Breast Centre, Gloucester Hospitals NHS Foundation Trust, Cheltenham, UK

Ashley Weinberg Directorate of Psychology, School of Health and Society, University of Salford, Manchester, UK

Samantha West Breast Screening Service, East Lancashire Hospitals NHS Trust, Burnley, UK

Patsy Whelehan Breast Screening and Imaging Department, NHS Tayside, Ninewells Hospital and Medical School, Dundee, UK

Susan Williams Shrewsbury and Telford Hospital NHS Trust, The Royal Shrewsbury Hospital, Shrewsbury, UK

Abbreviations

A	Area
AAFP	American Academy of Family Physicians
AB-MRI	Abbreviated Breast MRI
ABUS	Automated Breast Ultrasound
ACS	American Cancer Society
ADH	Atypical Ductal Hyperplasia
AEC	Automatic Exposure Control
AGD	Average Glandular Dose
AI	Artificial Intelligence
AIHW	Australian Institute of Health and Welfare
ALARA	As Low as Reasonably Achievable
ALH	Atypical Lobular Hyperplasia
AUC	Area Under the (ROC) Curve
BBC	Benign Breast Change
BCa	Breast Cancer
BCD	Breast Cancer Detection
BCT	Breast Computed Tomography
BI-RADS	Breast Imaging Reporting and Data System
BMI	Body Mass Index
BRAID	Breast Screening—Risk Adaptive Imaging for Density
BRCA	Breast Cancer Gene
BREAST	Breast Screen Reader Assessment Strategy
BSE	Breast Self-Examination
BSP	Breast Screening Programme
BSU	Breast Screening Unit
BTWSP	Breast Test Wales Screening Programme
CAD	Computer-Aided Detection
CC	Cranio-Caudal
CDMAM	Contrast Detail (CD) phantom for mammography
CEM	Contrast-Enhanced Digital Mammography
CESM	Contrast-Enhanced Spectral Mammography
CI	Confidence Interval
cnn	Convolutional neural networks
CNR	Contrast to Noise Ratio
COVID 19	Coronavirus Disease of 2019
CPD	Continuing Professional Development

CR	Computerised Radiography
CT	Computed Tomography
daN	DecaNewton
DBT	Digital Breast Tomosynthesis
DCIS	Ductal Carcinoma In Situ
DICOM	Digital Imaging and Communications in Medicine
DM2D	Digital Mammography 2-Dimensional
DNAs	Did Not Attend
DoC	Duty of Candour
DR	Digital Radiography
DVDs	Digital Video Disc/Digital Versatile Disc
EAR	Excellent/Acceptable/Repeat
EDCs	Endocrine-Disrupting Chemicals
EFOMP	European Federation of Organisations in Medical Physics
EP	European Protocol
EPUAP	European Pressure Ulcer Advisory Panel
EQUIP	Enhancing Quality Using the Inspection Program
ER	Oestrogen Receptor
EUREF	European Federation of Organisations in Medical Physics
EUREF	European Reference Organisation for Quality Assured Breast Screening and Diagnostic Services
F	Force
FAQs	Frequently Asked Questions
FDA	Food and Drug Administration
FFDM	Full-Field Digital Mammography
FPR	False Positive Rate
GP	General Practitioner
GPS	Global Positioning System
HCAIs	Healthcare Associated Infections
HCP	Healthcare Practitioners
HCPC	Health Care Professions Council
HRT	Hormone Replacement Therapy
HSE	Health and Safety Executive
HVL	Half Value Layer
IAEA	International Atomic Energy Agency
IARC	International Agency for Research on Cancer
IASP	International Association for the Study of Pain
IMF	Inframammary Fold
IoMT	Internet of Medical Things
IPC	Infection Prevention and Control
IPEM	Institute of Physics and Engineering in Medicine
IQ	Image Quality
IR	Image Receptor
kVp	Kilovoltage Peak
LCIS	Lobular Carcinoma In Situ
MCA	Mental Capacity Act

MD	Mammographic Density
MDT	Multi-disciplinary Team
MGD	Mean Glandular Dose
MLO	Mediolateral Oblique
MPE	Medical Physics Expert
MQAP	Mammography Quality Assurance Program
MQSA	Mammography Quality and Standards Act
MRI	Magnetic Resonance Imaging
MRSA	Methicillin Resistant Staphylococcus Aureus
MSKD	Musculoskeletal Disorders
NCI	National Cancer Institute
NHS	National Health Service
NHSBSP	National Health Service Breast Screening Programme
NICE	National Institute of Clinical Excellence
NKCs	Natural Killer Cells
NPUAP	National Pressure Ulcer Advisory Panel
NRS	Numerical Rating Scale
Pa	Pressure
PACS	Picture Archive Communication Systems
PASH	Pseudoangiomatous Stromal Hyperplasia
PERFORMS	Personal Performance in Mammographic Screening
PET CT	Positron Emission Tomography–Computed Tomography
PGMI	Perfect/Good/Moderate/Inadequate
PHE	Public Health England
PIQR	Periodic Image Quality Review
PLWD	Persons Living with Dementia
PNL	Posterior Nipple Line
PROCAS	Predicting Risk of Cancer at Screening
QA	Quality Assurance
QC	Quality Control
RCTs	Randomised Control Trials
ROC	Receiver Operating Characteristic
ROI	Region of Interest
RSI	Repetitive Strain Injury
SA	Staphylococcus aureus
SCB	Stereotactic Biopsy
SdNR	Signal Difference to Noise Ratio
SEER	Surveillance, Epidemiology, and End Results
SHIM	Screening History Information Management System
SI	Synthetic 2D Image
SICPs	Standard Infection Control Precautions
SNR	Signal to Noise Ratio
SoR	Society of Radiographers
STAR	Skin Tear Audit Research
T/F	Target Filter
TDLU	Terminal Ductal Lobular Unit

TMI	Traumatic Mammography Injury
TPR	True Positive Rate
UK	United Kingdom
USA	United States of America
VAS	Visual Analogue Scale
VRS	Verbal Rating Scale
WHO	World Health Organization
WoMMeN	Word of Mouth Mammography e-Network
www	World Wide Web

Part I

Optimising Breast Screen Reading Efficacy

Mo'ayyad E. Suleiman, Sahand Hooshmand, Warren M. Reed, and Patrick C. Brennan

Learning Objectives
- Understand how breast cancer outcomes vary among and within population
- Appreciate why mortality rates provide a good measure of breast cancer outcomes
- Discuss how image reader expertise varies and affects diagnostic efficacy and mammography screening outcomes
- Evaluate the importance of minimum annual case readings, double reading, artificial intelligence, and test set based training on mitigating the effect of inconsistent diagnostic efficacy in mammography

Note for readers:

In the majority of countries radiologists interpret mammograms. However, in some countries breast physicians and others medically qualified do so. In the UK, and in some other countries, radiographers are additionally trained to interpret and report mammograms. Due to these differences, within this chapter, we have used a generic term 'image reader' to refer to all of these professionals. On occasion, we have used the term 'radiologist', in instances where we are referring to a country that only has these interpreting images or where a journal article has investigated only this professional group.

M. E. Suleiman (✉) · S. Hooshmand · W. M. Reed ·
P. C. Brennan
Discipline of Medical Imaging Sciences, Faculty of Medicine and Health, Sydney School of Health Sciences, The University of Sydney, Sydney, NSW, Australia
e-mail: Moe.suleiman@sydney.edu.au

Introduction

The aim of early detection of disease is to facilitate the delivery of a treatment to those with no or minor symptoms whilst avoiding harm to those who do not need treatment [1]. Screening programmes are focussed at implementing that aim, with certain principles applied to ensure the value of such programmes. Such principles are relevant to breast cancer screening and include ensuring that disease is recognisable at an early stage, those who undergo early treatments have higher survival rates, diagnostic techniques used can be repeated at regular intervals and adequate facilities are available to treat breast cancer once diagnosis is made. Although breast cancer screening has been known as a vital tool in reducing mortality rate, its overall value has been subject to major debates for decades, and its efficacy and associated risks remain a concern around the world. On the one hand with screening, a pattern of increased detection of breast cancer has been seen in the past few decades, which has been attributed to longer life expectancy [2]; On the other, concerns have been expressed on issues that affect the efficacy of mammography screening, such as high recall rates and overdiagnosis.

Since breast cancer accounts for 15% of all female cancers worldwide, 6.6% of all cancer deaths and is the 5th leading cause of cancer death globally [3], we must have a good understanding of the implications of screening programs. This chapter will examine some of the benefits and harms of screening mammography, discuss human errors that can lead to reduced efficacy in screening mammography and consider strategies to mitigate those errors.

Impact of Screening on Survival and Mortality Rates

Ultimately, the purpose of breast cancer screening is to save lives, however, breast cancer outcomes and the effect of breast cancer screening varies among and within populations, due to differences in geography, ethnicity, socioeconomic status and the presence of comorbidities. Youlden et al. [4] investigated, on an international scale, the 5-year relative survival rate of breast cancer and found substantial differences between countries ranging from 12% in parts of Africa (The Gambia) to 89.2%, 88.3% and 88.0%, in the U.S., Australia and Canada respectively. Nonetheless, it is undisputed that early detection of breast cancer will lead to better treatment, increased survival and reduced mortality rates.

Significant improvements in survival rates have been seen with the addition of screening mammography. The Australian Institute of Health and Welfare (AIHW) reported a relative increase in the 5-year survival rate, since the introduction of the breast screening program in 1991, for women of all ages from 76.1% to 81.5% for the periods between 1988–1992 and 1993–1997, and further increasing to 91.5% for the period between 2013–2017 [5]. This is comparable to the Surveillance, Epidemiology, and End Results (SEER) Program survival rate of 85.0% and 90.3% reported for women in the U.S. for the periods 1989–1996 and 2011–2017, respectively [6, 7].

Table 1.1 AIHW 5-year relative survival rates and confidence intervals, 2013–2017 [5], and SEER 5 Year Relative Survival Rates and confidence intervals, 2011–2017 [8]

AIHW/Australia		SEER/US	
Age group (years)	% Survival (C.I. low–C.I. high)	Age group (years)	% Survival (C.I. low–C.I. high)
All ages combined	91.5% (91.2–91.8)	All ages combined	90.3 (90.1–90.5)
20–39	89.6 (88.6–90.6)	15–39	85.9 (85.3–86.5)
40–59	93.4% (93.1–93.7)	40–64	91.0 (90.8–91.2)
60–79	92.5% (92.1–92.9)	65–74	92.3 (92.0–92.6)
80+	78.7% (77.0–80.5)	75+	86.3 (85.6–87.0)

These rates, however, vary depending on the woman's age, where women of the eligible age for screening had the highest survival rates (Table 1.1). Furthermore, the stage at which the cancer is diagnosed is a major factor that affects survival: the results from a study by the American Cancer Society show that 99% of women with stage-I breast cancer survive for 5 or more years after diagnosis compared with 93% for stage-II and 72% for stage-III [8]. However, it is argued that such improvements in survival rates are methodologically biased due to lead time bias. This is where the outcome of a disease is the same if detected by screening compared to being detected from symptoms, but survival time from the time of diagnosis is longer in the screened patient because the disease was detected earlier [9]. This increased time gives the impression of improved outcome, where in fact no benefit has been accrued.

In terms of mortality, after the introduction of breast cancer screening in Australia in 1991, rates decreased [10]. The latest national data show mortality rates from the disease decreasing from 31.2% in 1991 to 18.2% in 2020 [11, 12]. In 2012, a review of 20 cohort and 20 case-controlled studies in developed countries in Europe, as well as Australia and the US, concluded that there was sufficient evidence indicating that mammography screening is an effective tool in breast cancer mortality reduction for women aged 50–74. The review also revealed that women aged 50–69 years, who were invited to attend screening but did not comply, had a less substantial reduction in mortality risk of 23% compared to 40% for women who attended screening [13]. Furthermore, in 2013, Marmot et al. [14] estimated a 20% mortality risk reduction for women invited to screening, with an absolute risk reduction of 0.43% for women aged 55–79 years in the UK compared with women not offered screening.

Tabár et al. [15] highlighted that mortality data includes women who were diagnosed in the previous years, however, incidence data includes women who may die of breast cancer in the future. Hence, incidence and mortality data for a given year are based on different cancer cases. To address this issue, the authors suggested measuring cancer incidences that lead to fatal outcomes as a more accurate statistic. In particular, they investigated annual incidence rates of breast cancer that led to death within 10 years and up to 20 years from diagnosis for women aged 40–69 years, concluding that women who participate in breast cancer screening gain significantly better benefits from therapy than those who do not, resulting in reduced mortality rates [15].

Diagnostic Efficacy

To achieve low mortality rates through mammography screening and the early detection of malignancies, it is vital to maintain high quality breast imaging, accurate image assessment, treatment and management of women with breast cancer. A vital measure of the performance of mammography screening is the image readers' ability to distinguish between positive and negative cases. It is however reported that up to 30% of cancers are missed, 80% of recalled cases receive disease-free diagnoses and 40% of biopsies report benign findings [16]. High speed in reporting, due to large women throughputs and excellent accuracy in identifying the presence of an abnormality on a mammogram, are required of image readers. Such experts' skills include: effective visual search, precise object and pattern recognition,

and accurate decision making. Errors made in mammography relate to deficiencies in one or more of these forementioned skills. Visual search-based perception error, which is the failure to identify an abnormality in mammograms, are scanning errors which occur if the pathology in question is not seen, resulting in termination of search before a target is found [17]. Recognition errors occur when the pathology is focussed upon only for a very brief time and not recognised as an abnormal finding. Decision-making errors occur where the pathology is fixated upon and identified as a potential abnormality, however it is then falsely rejected, leading to a false negative outcome [18].

A study by Suleiman and colleagues in 2014 reported that high quality readers' experience can minimise errors in mammography interpretation, leading to much activity attempting to identify the types of experiences that are most closely associated with the required diagnostic skills. The study also indicates the number of years certified and the number of years reading mammograms have been found to have no significant effect on performance [19]. However, the number of mammograms read per year has been shown to significantly improve cancer detection rates. For example, those who perform ≥2000 annual mammographic readings outperform those with <1000 reads per year, with receiver operating characteristic scores (ROC) of = 0.83 and 0.75, respectively [20]. Interestingly however, those who report ≥5000 annually demonstrate little additional ability to detect cancer compared to those with ≥2000 annual reads (ROC = 0.85 and 0.83, respectively), the former group is better at recognising normal images than the latter [20]. On that basis, this implies that through high numbers, readers become perceptually tuned to recognising familiar breast structures and identifying any unusual deviations.

It is not a surprise therefore that minimum annual case numbers are used as a surrogate for desired experience, however these vary significantly between countries: 960 cases per 2 years in the United States [21]; 5000 cases per year in the United Kingdom [22]; 2000 cases per year for BreastScreen Australia [19] and 1000 per year for Canada [23]. These case numbers do not however take into consideration varying exposure to abnormalities due to the prevalence of breast cancer. For example, in the westernised world, an image reader may see only one cancer case for every 200 cases read, which means that for 2000 annual reads, they may only see 10 cancer cases and in other parts of the world the prevalence can be even lower. This highlights that image readers who work in small practices may not accrue adequate expert skills to recognise the different varieties of breast cancer appearances. Furthermore, an over-reliance on annual reads as a measure for learning-experience ignores the educational need for immediate feedback, which is vital for perceptual learning but is typically absent in clinical practice.

Several methods can offer this immediate feedback to the image readers:

- **Double reading**—This refers to the interpretation of images by two image readers and is standard practice in many screening programs worldwide [24–26]. It has been proven to improve sensitivity by 14% [27], increase cancer detection rates by 7.3% [25], and improve recall rates by 25–32% [28, 29]. Nonetheless, single reading is still common practice in the US.

- **Computer-Aided Detection (CAD)**—This computer-based technique recognises suspicious patterns and features, which are then marked to undergo further investigation by an image reader [30, 31]. To date, CAD has been shown to particularly benefit those with less experience and lower annual volumes of reading compared with high-volume readers [32], when compared to single reading.

- **Artificial Intelligence (AI)**—One may say that AI is the next generation of CAD, though it is important to acknowledge that AI is more robust, accurate, scalable, and more efficient than its predecessor. It often works on deeplearning technologies, involving artificial neural networks (algorithms) inspired by the human brain and learns from large amounts of data, increasingly recognising mistakes, and improving over time. However, in mammography, AI has not yet replaced human image readers, and in fact may not do so anytime soon, although, in current studies, AI's performance detecting cancers in screening mammograms has matched or outperformed that of radiologists [33, 34]. It has also been found that combining an AI algorithm with a reader can result in more cancers being detected than having two readers, whilst offering high specificity (ability to detect normal cases), thus importantly reducing recall rates [34]. Nonetheless, the ideal application of an AI system in the clinical setting and workflow is yet to be determined and one should keep an eye on this exciting space as AI technology is rapidly evolving. *Please refer to Chap. 21 for a wider discussion on AI.*

- **Test set-based training programs**—These are self-assessment modules that provide instant feedback and performance scores to the image readers. The idea is to provide a mix of normal and abnormal cases (with known truths) with more cancer cases than usually found in the clinical environment. The image readers will read these cases and mark any suspicious areas on the mammograms, and once the test set is completed, the image reader is presented with performance scores and can go back and review the cases with marked truths. Whilst this approach can be used as a performance measure to assess image readers' performance by clinic or institution, more importantly it encourages a process of self-reflection on performance, and a chance to compare one's judgements against that of experts, with this type of feedback being immediately available. Test sets have been utilised around the world, including the Breast Screen Reader Assessment Strategy (BREAST) [35] and DetectED-X system [36] from Australia and New Zealand, and the Personal Performance in Mammographic Screening (PERFORMS) [37] from the UK: these platforms have been designed to provide image readers with test sets containing challenging screening cases [37, 38]. A study examining the impact of BREAST over a 3-year period demonstrated a 34.4% statistically significant improvement in readers' performance scores. The increase in diagnostic performance through such training programs was not limited to experience and/or performance, demonstrating the power and potential of these educational strategies [39].

Conclusion

Although the principles of health screening have been rigorously applied to breast cancer, debates on the benefits versus risks of screening mammography have continued for decades and is still a major subject for research worldwide. Nonetheless, since the introduction of screening, survival rates have increased and mortality rates have fallen, with the extent of these changes varying between and within different populations.

To maintain and improve mortality rates, accurate diagnosis of screening mammograms is vital, hence, policies have been implemented worldwide such as minimum annual read numbers and double reading, to ensure image readers operate at the highest performance levels. However, it is understandable that some image readers do not have access to the high number of cases required to obtain the desired experience and achieve the expertise levels required to perform at the highest levels. It is important therefore that image readers contribute to, evaluate and adopt promising new diagnostic and educational technologies. In particular, and with specific reference to AI, this promising innovation will only be as good as the data it is trained upon, and therefore image readers, scientists and vendors must work together to achieve that optimal level of human-machine harmony.

Chapter Review Questions
Review Questions

1. How have mortality risk been affected for women invited to breast screening compared to women not offered screening in the UK?
2. Name three experts' skills that are required of image readers to achieve high speed in reporting

and excellent accuracy in identifying the presence of an abnormality on a mammogram?
3. Name three methods that can offer immediate feedback to image readers.

Answers

1. About 20% mortality risk reduction for women invited to screening, with an absolute risk reduction of 0.43% for women aged 55–79 years in the UK compared with women not offered screening.
2. effective visual search, precise object and pattern recognition, and accurate decision making.
3. Double reading, CAD, AI and Test set based training programmes

Appendix

Test your learning and check your understanding of this book's contents: use the "Springer Nature Flashcards" app to access questions.

To use the app, please follow the instructions below:

1. Go to https://flashcards.springernature.com/login.
2. Create a user account by entering your e-mail address and assigning a password.
3. Use the following link to access your SN Flashcards set: https://sn.pub/dcAnWL.

If the link is missing or does not work, please send an e-mail with the subject "SN Flashcards" and the book title to customerservice@springernature.com.

Flashcard code: 48341-69945-ABCB1-2A8C7-CE9D2.

Short URL: https://sn.pub/dcAnWL.

References

1. Wilson JM, Jungner G. Principles and practice of screening for disease. Geneva: World Health Organization; 1968.
2. Surveillance Epidemiology and End Results (SEER) Program. SEER Cancer Statistics Review

(CSR), 1975–2017. https://seer.cancer.gov/archive/csr/1975_2010/. Accessed 1 Sept 2021.

3. International Agency for Research on Cancer. Cancer Today GLOBOCAN. https://gco.iarc.fr/today/online-analysis-table?v=2020&mode=population&mode_population=countries&population=900&populations=900&key=asr&sex=2&cancer=20&type=1&statistic=5&prevalence=0&population_group=0&ages_group%5B%5D=0&ages_group%5B%5D=17&group_cancer=1&include_nmsc=1&include_nmsc_other=1.

4. Youlden DR, Cramb SM, Dunn NA, Muller JM, Pyke CM, Baade PD. The descriptive epidemiology of female breast cancer: an international comparison of screening, incidence, survival and mortality. Cancer Epidemiol. 2012;36(3):237–48.

5. Australian Insitute of Health and Welfare (AIHW). Cancer data in Australia. 2021. https://www.aihw.gov.au/reports/cancer/cancer-data-in-australia/data?page=4. Accessed 1 Sept 2021.

6. Surveillance Epidemiology and End Results (SEER) Program. SEER Cancer Statistics Review (CSR), 1975–2017. https://seer.cancer.gov/archive/csr/1975_2010/. Accessed 21 Apr 2020.

7. Surveillance Epidemiology and End Results (SEER) Program. SEER*Explorer: An interactive website for SEER cancer statistics. Surveillance Research Program. https://seer.cancer.gov/explorer/. Accessed 1 Sept 2021.

8. The American Cancer Society. Breast cancer: survival by stage. http://www.cancer.org/cancer/breastcancer/detailedguide/breast-cancer-survival-by-stage. Accessed 1 Sept 2021.

9. Dewar JA. Mammography screening: philosophy–evidence for and against. In: Hogg P, Kelly J, Mercer C, editors. Digital mammography. Berlin: Springer; 2015. p. 59–65.

10. Australian Insitute of Health and Welfare. BreastScreen Australia monitoring report 2004–2005. https://www.aihw.gov.au/getmedia/003aa9ad-bbd4-4e0e-aaeb-c2b0c9baedac/bsamr04-05.pdf.aspx?inline=true. Accessed 29 Mar 2019.

11. Australian Insitute of Health and Welfare. BreastScreen Australia monitoring report. https://www.aihw.gov.au/getmedia/e414a344-ab3d-4a35-a79b-a29723f22939/aihw-can-135.pdf.aspx?inline=true. Accessed 21 Apr 2020.

12. Australian Institute of Health and Welfare (AIHW). Australian cancer incidence and mortality (ACIM) books. Breast cancer. Canberra: AIHW; 2021.

13. Lauby-Secretan B, Scoccianti C, Loomis D, Benbrahim-Tallaa L, Bouvard V, Bianchini F, Straif K. Breast-cancer screening—viewpoint of the IARC working group. N Engl J Med. 2015;372(24):2353–8.

14. Marmot MG, Altman DG, Cameron DA, Dewar JA, Thompson SG, Wilcox M. The benefits and harms of breast cancer screening: an independent review. Br J Cancer. 2013;108(11):2205–40.

15. Tabár L, Dean PB, Chen TH, Yen AM, Chen SL, Fann JC, Chiu SY, Ku MM, Wu WY, Hsu CY, Chen YC. The incidence of fatal breast cancer measures the increased effectiveness of therapy in women participating in mammography screening. Cancer. 2019;125(4):515–23.

16. Ekpo EU, Alakhras M, Brennan P. Errors in mammography cannot be solved through technology alone. Asian Pac J Cancer Prev. 2018;19(2):291–301.

17. Palazzetti V, Guidi F, Ottaviani L, Valeri G, Baldassarre S, Giuseppetti GM. Analysis of mammographic diagnostic errors in breast clinic. Radiol Med. 2016;121(11):828–33.

18. Kundel HL, Nodine CF, Carmody D. Visual scanning, pattern recognition and decision-making in pulmonary nodule detection. Invest Radiol. 1978;13(3):175–81.

19. Suleiman WI, Lewis S, Georgian-Smith D, Evanoff MG, McEntee MF. Number of mammography cases read per year is a strong predictor of sensitivity. J Med Imaging. 2014;1(1):015503.

20. Rawashdeh MA, Lee WB, Bourne RM, Ryan EA, Pietrzyk MW, Reed WM, Heard RC, Black DA, Brennan PC. Markers of good performance in mammography depend on number of annual readings. Radiology. 2013;269(1):61–7.

21. Houn F, Elliott ML, McCrohan JL. The mammography quality standards act of 1992. History and philosophy. Radiol Clin North Am. 1995;33(6):1059–65.

22. Liston J, Wilson R, Cooke J. Quality assurance guidelines for breast cancer screening radiology. NHS breast screening programmes publication no. 59; 2005.

23. CAR—Canadian Association of Radiologists. Mammography Accreditation Program (MAP). https://car.ca/patient-care/map/. Accessed 1 Oct 2021.

24. Perry N, Broeders M, de Wolf C, Törnberg S, Holland R, von Karsa L. European guidelines for quality assurance in breast cancer screening and diagnosis—summary document. Oncol Clin Pract. 2008;4(2):74–86.

25. Duijm LE, Louwman MW, Groenewoud JH, Van De Poll-Franse LV, Fracheboud J, Coebergh JW. Interobserver variability in mammography screening and effect of type and number of readers on screening outcome. Br J Cancer. 2009;100(6):901–7.

26. Houssami N, Bernardi D, Pellegrini M, Valentini M, Fantò C, Ostillio L, Tuttobene P, Luparia A, Macaskill P. Breast cancer detection using single-reading of breast tomosynthesis (3D-mammography) compared to double-reading of 2D-mammography: evidence from a population-based trial. Cancer Epidemiol. 2017;47:94–9.

27. Klompenhouwer EG, Voogd AC, den Heeten GJ, Strobbe LJ, de Haan AF, Wauters CA, Broeders MJ, Duijm LE. Blinded double reading yields a higher programme sensitivity than non-blinded double reading at digital screening mammography: a prospected population based study in the south of the Netherlands. Eur J Cancer. 2015;51(3):391–9.

28. Duijm LE, Groenewoud JH, Hendriks JH, de Koning HJ. Independent double reading of screening mammograms in the Netherlands: effect of arbitration following reader disagreements. Radiology. 2004;231(2):564–70.

29. Ciatto S, Ambrogetti D, Bonardi R, Catarzi S, Risso G, Rosselli Del Turco M, Mantellini P. Second reading of screening mammograms increases cancer detection and recall rates. Results in the Florence screening programme. J Med Screen. 2005;12(2):103–6.
30. Castellino RA. Computer aided detection (CAD): an overview. Cancer Imaging. 2005;5(1):17.
31. Katzen J, Dodelzon K. A review of computer aided detection in mammography. Clin Imaging. 2018;52:305–9.
32. Gur D, Sumkin JH, Rockette HE, Ganott M, Hakim C, Hardesty L, Poller WR, Shah R, Wallace L. Changes in breast cancer detection and mammography recall rates after the introduction of a computer-aided detection system. J Natl Cancer Inst. 2004;96(3):185–90.
33. McKinney SM, Sieniek M, Godbole V, Godwin J, Antropova N, Ashrafian H, Back T, Chesus M, Corrado GS, Darzi A, Etemadi M. International evaluation of an AI system for breast cancer screening. Nature. 2020;577(7788):89–94.
34. Salim M, Wåhlin E, Dembrower K, Azavedo E, Foukakis T, Liu Y, Smith K, Eklund M, Strand F. External evaluation of 3 commercial artificial intelligence algorithms for independent assessment of screening mammograms. JAMA Oncol. 2020;6(10):1581–8.
35. Tapia K, Lee W, Brennan P. Breast screen reader assessment strategy: transforming breast cancer diagnosis globally: a mini review. Int J Radiol Radiat Ther. 2017;4(1):00088.
36. Suleiman ME, Rickard M, Brennan PC. Perfecting detection through education. Radiography. 2020;1(26): S49–53.
37. Scott HJ, Gale AG. Breast screening: PERFORMS identifies key mammographic training needs. Br J Radiol. 2006;79(special_issue_2):S127–33.
38. Brennan PC, et al. BREAST: a novel method to improve the diagnostic efficacy of mammography. In: Proceedings of SPIE—The International Society for Optical Engineering; 2013.
39. Suleiman WI, Rawashdeh MA, Lewis SJ, McEntee MF, Lee W, Tapia K, Brennan PC. Impact of breast reader assessment strategy on mammographic radiologists' test reading performance. J Med Imaging Radiat Oncol. 2016 Jun;60(3):352–8.

Screening Programmes for Breast Cancer

2

Raed Mohammed Kadhim M. Ali,
Mark F. McEntee, and Peter Hogg

Learning Objectives

- State reasons why screening programmes are beneficial
- Explain why mammography is considered to be a valuable tool for use in breast cancer screening
- Summarise the evidence which supports the use of mammography in breast cancer screening
- Outline limitations of mammography in breast cancer screening

Introduction

Screening identifies people who are at higher risk of a health problem, in order that early treatment (or intervention) can be offered to reduce incidence, morbidity and/or mortality.

Modern screening began in 1968 with a seminal publication by Wilson et al. [1], in which ten principles of screening were highlighted (Fig. 2.1).

R. M. K. M. Ali
University of Kufa, Najaf, Iraq
e-mail: Raedm.kadhim@uokufa.edu.iq;
r.m.k.mali@edu.salford.ac.uk

M. F. McEntee (✉)
University College Cork, UGF 12 ASSERT,
Brookfield Health Sciences, Cork, UK
e-mail: mark.mcentee@ucc.ie

P. Hogg
University of Salford, Manchester, UK
e-mail: p.hogg@salford.ac.uk

Fig. 2.1 Ten principles
of screening

1. The condition should be an important health problem.
2. There should be an accepted treatment for patients with recognized disease.
3. Facilities for diagnosis and treatment should be available.
4. There should be a recognizable latent or early symptomatic phase.
5. There should be a suitable test or examination.
6. The test should be acceptable to the population.
7. The natural history of the condition, including development from latent to declared disease, should be adequately understood.
8. There should be an agreed policy on whom to treat as patients.
9. The cost of case-finding (including a diagnosis and treatment of patients diagnosed) should be economically balanced in relation to possible expenditure on medical care as a whole.
10. Case-finding should be a continuous process and not a "once and for all" project.

Mammography Screening

For breast cancer, screening programmes aim to reduce mortality by the early detection and early treatment of asymptomatic cancers. Mammography is the most important breast cancer screening modality and is recommended in more than 35 countries worldwide. Screening programme differences exist between countries and these are attributed to the socio-economic differences [2], age of breast cancer incidence in each population and to the results of screening trials upon which the programmes recommendations are designed.

Mammography is considered to be a cost-effective technique for the early detection of breast cancer and for many years it has remained the recommended modality for both diagnosis and screening. Screening mammography involves the evaluation of asymptomatic women with the intention of detecting impalpable breast cancer early in its growth, when recovery is still possible. The first attempt to use X-ray breast imaging as a tool for the early detection of breast cancer was in 1960 by Robert Egan [3].

A suitable measure to assess for screening mammography benefit is its contribution to the reduction in breast cancer mortality. The first screening mammography trial to show a reduction in breast cancer mortality, by using mammography only, was the Swedish two-county trial which demonstrated a reduction of 30% in breast cancer mortality among women aged between 40 and 74 years [4].

The most reliable information about screening mammography is provided by systematic review, meta-analyses and randomised control trials (RCTs). Breast cancer mortality reduction with screening mammography was 15–25% in trials and 28–56% in observational studies in all age groups [5].

Table 2.1 summarises several mammographic breast cancer screening RCTs and meta-analyses. Since a very long time is required for follow up in these trials, most of the RCTs are from the 1980s or earlier. Given the length of time needed to assess the effect of screening mammography, there is a continuous need to update the data.

Recurrent evaluations of the Swedish two-county trial outcome data demonstrated that the relative breast cancer mortality remained constant, despite the continuous increase in breast screening invitations. However, the absolute number of lives saved due to screening has increased with time. This is because long screening time is required to reduce the breast cancer mortality. Accordingly, long-term follow up is necessary to prove the benefit effect (or otherwise) from screening on breast cancer deaths. Overall, a substantial reduction in breast cancer mortality due to screening mammography has been reported by the Swedish two-county trial [4]. These results are consistent with outcome data of other screening trials [9–11, 13–15]. Interestingly, a Canadian screening trial was the only one which documented that screening mammography does not affect breast cancer mortality [12].

Table 2.1 Summary of several mammographic breast cancer screening RCTs and meta analyses

Study type	Study	Study start date	Participant age range (year)	Breast cancer mortality reduction
Meta-analysis	Nelson et al. [6]	2016	39–49 50–59 60–60 70–74	Breast cancer mortality was generally reduced with mammography screening, although estimates were not statistically significant at all ages and the magnitudes of effect were small. Advanced cancer was reduced with screening for women aged 50 years or older
Meta-analysis	Fletcher et al. [7]	1993	40–49 50–56 70+	For women aged 40–49, randomized controlled trials of breast cancer screening showed no benefit 5–7 years after entry. At 10–12 years, benefit was uncertain and, if present, marginal; thereafter, it is unknown. For women aged 50–69, screening reduced breast cancer mortality by about a third. Currently available data for women age 70 or older are inadequate to judge the effectiveness of screening
Meta-analysis	Kerlikowske et al. [8]	1995	40–49 50–56 70+	Significantly reduced breast cancer mortality in women aged 50 to 74 years after 7 to 9 years of follow-up. No reduction in breast cancer mortality in women aged 40 to 49 years after 7 to 9 years of follow-up. Screening mammography may be effective in reducing mortality in women aged 40 to 49 years after 10 to 12 years of follow-up, but the same benefit could probably be achieved by beginning screening at menopause or 50 years of age
RCT	New York Health Insurance Plan (HIP) [9]	1963	40–69	25% reduction in breast cancer mortality for women aged 40–49 and 50–59 at time of entry
RCT	Malmö trial [10]	1976	44–68	Mortality reduction was age dependent; no overall reduction but 20% reduction for women aged 55 year and older
RCT	Swedish Two-County trial [4]	1977	40–74	30% reduction in breast cancer mortality resulted from screening mammography
RCT	Edinburgh trial [11]	1978	45–64	20% reduction in breast cancer mortality resulted from screening mammography for women 50 years and older
RCT	Canada trial [12]	1980	40–59	No resulted reduction in breast cancer mortality due to screening mammography
RCT	Stockholm trial [13]	1981	40–64	In women 40–49 year there was tendency for mortality reduction, 50–64 year women showed better survival with screening mammography
RCT	Göteborg trial [14]	1982	39–59	20–30% reduction in breast cancer mortality and this reduction may be achieved for younger than 50 year old women by short screening interval
RCT	UK Age trial [15]	1990	39–41	Annual screening mammography for women 40–49 year results in mortality reduction

Discussion of the risks and benefits of mammography often compare screening to no screening. However, there are other alternatives to screening mammography such as breast self-examination (BSE) and detecting cancer symptomatically (no screening, but diagnostic services, and screening using other modalities). None of these have been shown to be better than screening mammography at detection of early breast cancer. Early detection, results in earlier starts to effective treatment, often before the manifestation of clinical disease [16].

BSE and alternative methods of imaging detect the cancer later and have been shown to be less effective than mammography as a screening tool. 'compared with clinical breast examination and mammography, the estimated sensitivity of BSE is low (20% to 30%) and is lower among older women' ([17], p. 2196).

In the UK, Marmot et al. [18] assessed the performance of the UK mammography screening programme by reviewing the results of 11 relevant RCTs. Marmot concluded that the UK mammography screening programme should continue, as it resulted in approximately 20% reduction in breast cancer mortality. In the US, the American Cancer Society (ACS) [19] reviewed evidence too, along with the International Agency for Research on Cancer (IARC) [20] and the US Preventive Services Task Force [6]. They illustrated that screening mammography significantly reduces breast cancer mortality for women aged 50–69 years.

The Norwegian mammography screening programme invites women aged 50–69 years for biennial screening mammography. The effect of this on breast cancer mortality was studied on four groups of women by Kalager et al. [21]. They reported that only one third of the reduction in breast cancer mortality was due to screening mammography, with the other two thirds being attributed to the improvement in breast cancer management and treatment. Consequently, the absolute reduction in breast cancer deaths resulting from the Norwegian mammography screening programme was attributed as 10%.

Gotzsche et al. [22] reviewed data from mammography RCTs and meta-analysis studies; they suggested that breast cancer mortality reduction is mainly due to the improvement in breast cancer awareness and treatment and a minor reduction was brought about by mammography. They also reported that breast cancer mortality reduction is not a reliable measure for screening mammography performance because of overdiagnosis and overtreatment which may result in unnecessary mastectomies and deaths. Accordingly, they recommended the reassessment of screening mammography because of the errors associated with published screening trials and overdiagnosis.

Similarly, work by Harding et al. [23], who investigated the breast cancer incidence and mortality in the US counties over 10 years (2000–2010), reported that the prominent effect of screening mammography in US population was overdiagnosis and the breast cancer mortality reduction was not significant. Harding et al. [23] built their conclusions on the fact that there was no reduction in the rate of large breast cancers detection. Likewise, Welch et al. ([24], p. 1438) attributed 'the reduction in breast cancer mortality after the implementation of screening mammography' to be 'predominantly the result of improved systemic therapy'. Esserman et al. [25], recognizing this problem nearly a decade ago, asserted that this is an 'opportunity for improvement' ([25], p. 797).

To this day, breast cancer screening remains a controversial area [26, 27]. Since the introduction of screening mammography, there have been debates about its harms and benefits, and several disadvantages have been identified. Firstly, its false negative rate, which is its inability to detect all breast cancers. Secondly, its false positive rate (wrong diagnosis), which results in time wasted in extra examinations and undesired anxiety. Finally, overdiagnosis, which results in the treatment of low-risk breast cancers that may not always cause health problems [28].

The performance of any screening programme should be assessed by three important parameters: sensitivity, specificity, and the positive predictive value. Programme sensitivity is the proportion of truly diagnosed cancer cases to the total number of actual cancer cases in the participants. Programme specificity is defined as the ratio of women truly identified without cancer. Positive predictive value is the ratio of the actual number of cancer cases against the number of abnormal cases detected by the programme. These parameters can be calculated using the following equations [28]:

$$Sensitivity = \frac{number\ of\ true\ positive\ cases}{true\ positive\ cases + false\ negative\ cases}$$

$$Specificity = \frac{true\ negative\ cases}{true\ negative\ casese + false\ positive\ cases}$$

$$Positive\ Predictive\ value = \frac{true\ positive\ cases}{true\ positive\ cases + false\ positive\ cases}$$

The performance of any screening programme depends on the participant's age [28]. It has been found that annual screenings from 20–29 years of age may result in more radiation-induced cancer deaths than it prevents [29]. This may be an underestimate of radiation risk, given the ICRP increased the tissue weighting factor of the breast from 0.05 in 1991 to 0.12 in 2007 [30]. For women aged under 39, screening mammography is not recommended due to the low breast cancer incidence rate within this age group and the lack of evidence of cancer death reduction [31]. A reduction in breast cancer mortality of 3 deaths per 10,000 screened women is achieved for women aged 39–49 years and 5–8 per 10,000 women for the 50–59 years age group. The highest reduction, 12–21 cases per 10,000 screened women, occurs in women aged 60–69 years [6]. The importance of screening mammography in breast cancer death reduction extends to women aged 70–74 years [20]. The net benefit of screening mammography is also related to lifetime risk of radiation-induced cancer, which is an age dependent factor, because younger tissues are more radiosensitive. According to Public Health England (PHE) [32], the risk of radiation-induced breast cancer reduces from 13.8 per million per mGy to 2.1 per million per mGy as women's age increase from 48 to 72 years.

Some researchers consider that the reduction in breast cancer mortality of less than 10%, by screening mammography has no net benefit because of the radiation risk. Consequently, they do not recommend screening mammography before the age of 50 years [29, 33]. This has added another controversial point of screening mammography. Estimation of radiation risk is complex. Observing cancer development directly resulting from diagnostic exposures is not possible because the radiation effect cannot be isolated from the effect of the other carcinogens the patient will be exposed to in a life time. However, it is possible to directly measure the damage to genes in the cells as a result of diagnostic doses. Likewise, it is possible to directly measure the repair (and failure to repair) of radiation damage [34, 35].

Hendrick et al. [36] investigated the radiation risk with screening at various ages. They assumed an MGD of 3.7 mGy and estimated lifetime risk of radiation-induced breast cancer incidence of 72 and 31 cases per 100,000 women, and a mortality of 20 and 10 deaths per 100,000 women for an annual screening regimen from 40–80 and 50–80 years. Given that the average mammographic examination for both breasts (4 projections) is dropping with digital mammography and is now closer to 2.78 mGy [37]. While the diagnoses of a 10 biennial screens are 13 per 1000 more breast cancers than with no screening [38], a factorially higher saving of life than loss of life.

In the context of this small radiation risk, the recommendations of the Swedish mammography screening programme were changed twice by the National Board of Health and Welfare in Sweden [39]. The first change was in 1987 to exclude women aged 40–49 years from screening mammography and the second, in 1998, re-included them in the screening programme [40]. Malmgren et al. [41] studied the screening outcomes of 1162 women aged 75 years and older, finding for this age group the obvious mammographic cancer detectability is comparable to that of younger women (younger than 75 years). Beyond the age of 50 years the risk of radiation induced cancer is considered acceptable, due to the reported benefits of screening mammography [42, 43]. Overall screening trials demonstrated a 10%–30% reduction in breast cancer mortality due to screening mammography. Consequently, the risk of radiation-induced cancer from screening mammography is considered small and acceptable when compared to this mortality reduction.

The above risk-benefit argument resulted in the introduction of organised mammography screening programmes in many countries. It must also be noted that the recommendations for screening mammography differs between countries. These differences are related to the age of screening commencement, cessation age of the screens, and the time interval between screens. Table 2.2 provides a summary of such data. The majority of mammography screening programmes (e.g. Belgium, Croatia, Cyprus, Denmark, Finland, Germany, Italy, Latvia, Lithuania, Luxembourg, Norway, Poland, Slovenia, Spain / Catalonia, Switzerland) include women aged 50–69 years. However, other countries (e.g. Australia, Canada, Iceland, India, Japan, Korea, Nigeria, Sweden, United States, and Uruguay) extend screening mammography to those at 40 years and may continue after 70 years. The New Zealand, Portuguese, and Spine (Navarra) mammography screening programmes cover women aged 45–69 years. Because of the early incident breast cancer in China, women aged 40–59 are invited for screening mammography. Biennial screening mammography is recommended by most of the mammography screening programmes except in the United States, United Kingdom, Malta and China. The US recommends annual screening and the others recommend triennial screening [44, 45].

The effect of the screening frequency change from annual to biennial was studied by Coldman et al. [46]. They used the data from the mammography screening programme of British Columbia (SMPBC) between 1988 and 2005. In the first decade of SMPBC (1988–1997) annual screening was recommended. However, after July 1997 SMPBC had started to invite women for biennial screenings. Coldman et al. [46] analysed the data of 658,151 women to compare breast cancer detectability and mortality during these two periods. They

Table 2.2 Recommendations of mammography screening programmes in several countries for women with an average risk of developing breast cancer [45, 46]

Country(s)	Age of screening	Time interval between screens	Number of screens
Australia, Japan, Korea, United State (AAFP, NCI, and USPSTF)	40–75	2 years	18
Belgium, Croatia, Cyprus, Denmark, Finland, Germany, Italy, Latvia, Lithuania, Luxembourg, Norway, Poland, Slovenia, Spain (Catalonia), Switzerland	50–69	2 years	10
Canada, France, Israel, Netherlands	50–74	2 years	13
China	40–59	3 years	7
Czech	44–75	2 years	16
Estonia	50–62	2 years	7
Hungary	45–65	2 years	11
Iceland	40–69	2 years	15
India	40–74	1 year (40–49) 2 years (50–74)	23
Ireland	50–64	2 years	8
Malta	50–60	3 years	4
New Zealand, Portugal, Spain (Navarra)	45–69	2 years	13
Nigeria	40–70	2 years	16
Sweden	40–74	18 months (40–49) 2 years (50–74)	19
United Kingdom	47–73[a]	3 years	9
United State (ACOG)	40–75	2 years (40–49) 1 year (50–75)	31
United State (ACS, ACR, and NCCN)	40–75	1 year	36
Uruguay	40–69	2 years (40–49) 1 year (50–69)	25

[a]NHSBSP offers screening mammography for women aged 50–70 and the lower and higher age groups are still part of a trial

found that this alteration in mammographic screening frequency affected neither the breast cancer detection rate nor the mortality rate.

Some mammography screening programmes exclude high risk women, considering them as special cases, while other programmes have a specially designed screening category for them. Table 2.3 summarises screening programme details for high risk women.

In the UK, the Forrest report (1986) recommended the introduction of single view (MLO) screening mammography for women aged 50–65 years with an interval of 3 years [50]. In 1988, the NHSBSP started to invite women aged 50–64 years for MLO, triennial screening mammography. In 2000, the NHS Cancer Plan proposed additional expansion in NHSBSP by using two views (MLO and CC) in screening mammography and extending the screening age to include women aged 64–70 years [51]. The latest age extension in NHSBSP commenced in 2012 to include women aged 47–73. However, until now the NHSBSP offers screening mammography for women aged 50–70 and the lower and higher age groups are still part of a trial. These extensions approximately duplicated the number of screens within a woman's lifetime and hence the cumulative Mean Glandular Dose is duplicated also. The consequent increase in risk of radiation-induced cancer is mainly attributed to earlier screening commencement, since breast tissue radio-sensitivity decreases with age [32]. According to Public Health England (PHE) [49], high risk women should be invited for annual screening mammography from 40 years old or may be earlier.

Table 2.3 Recommendations of mammography screening programmes in several countries for women with a high risk of breast cancer [44, 47–49]

Country(s)	Age of screening	Time interval between screens	Number of screens
Canada	40–74	1 year (40–49) 2 years (50–74)	23
United Kingdom	40–73	1 year	34
United State (ACS)	30–75	1 year	46
United State (NCCN)	25–75	1 year	51

In 2009, the US Preventive Services Task Force changed their recommendation of screening mammography to be biennial for women aged 50–74 years [47]. However, the American Medical Association, American College of Radiology, American Cancer Society, and National Comprehensive Cancer Network have considered the annual screening mammography starting from 40 years old to be superior [6]. For high risk women, such as those with a family history of cancer, the American Cancer Society stated that annual screening mammography should start at 30 years old and continue as long as the women were in good health [48].

Nevertheless, the National Comprehensive Cancer Network (NCCN) and the American Academy of Family Physicians (AAFP) recommended that the annual screening mammography for high risk women should commence either at 25 years old or from the earliest age of cancer onset in the client's family (5–10 years before the youngest breast cancer case in the family) [52, 53]. Screening frequency recommendation is critical as it directly related to the mammographic radiation risk; the radiation risk of annual is twice that of biennial screening. Since breast tissues younger than 40 years are very radio-sensitive, mammographic radiation of early high risk women screening should be considered carefully. Early screening mammography radiation risk causes an additional breast cancer lifetime risk for women younger than 40 years.

As can be seen from the above, screening programmes typically exclude women older than 75. Screening mammography is significantly more accurate in older women. Sinclair et al. [54] found positive predictive value (PPV) of 22.2% for younger women while this increase significantly in the 90–101 year old group to 55.6%. Despite this increased accuracy, screening beyond 75 is not done given life expectancies and the probability of dying with the cancer rather than of the cancer. However, given current life expectancy in the OECD of 79.3 and the associates 6 year increase on average life expectancy between 1983 and 2008 [55], the upper age limit for screening may needed to be reconsidered in future years.

In spite of the controversies, there is currently no strong evidence against screening mammography.

Other Imaging Modalities That May Have Value in Screening for Breast Cancer

Magnetic Resonance Imaging (MRI) Screening

In some countries MRI screening is recommended annually, along with mammography, for high breast cancer risk women because it has higher sensitivity for cancer detection than mammography [56]. Nevertheless, it cannot replace mammography screening because of the lack of standards for MRI screening imaging procedures, interpretation and performance (whether it is cost-effective or not). Also, it is a very high cost procedure and requires a long examination time [53].

Ultrasound Screening

Despite the high sensitivity of ultrasound for breast cancer detection, it is not recommended as a screening tool. This is because of the long examination time, its high false-positive rate and its image quality, which is variable depending on the examiner's skill [6, 56]. The feasibility of using ultrasound for breast cancer screenings was investigated by Wang et al. [57] in a rural area of China. They concluded that ultrasound is more sensitive than mammography for breast cancer detection in Chinese women younger than 55 years old, with lower cost and more convenience for breast screening in such areas [57].

Clinical Pearls

- Breast screening programmes need to be justified before being implemented
- Breast screening programmes should be population specific, thus legitimate differences can exist between countries
- Research data from RCTs should be continually updated and then used to justify, modify or even revoke breast screening programmes as needed

Chapter Review Questions
Review Questions

1. State the ten principles of screening
2. What kind of research study provides the best evidence on the success or otherwise of a screening programme
3. State the limitations / disadvantages of breast screening programmes

Answers

1. The condition should be an important health problem.

   There should be an accepted treatment for patients with recognized disease.

   Facilities for diagnosis and treatment should be available.

   There should be a recognizable latent or early symptomatic phase.

   There should be a suitable test or examination.

   The test should be acceptable to the population.

   The natural history of the condition, including development from latent to declared disease, should be adequately understood.

   There should be an agreed policy on whom to treat as patients.

   The cost of case-finding (including a diagnosis and treatment of patients diagnosed) should be economically balanced in relation to possible expenditure on medical care as a whole.

   Case-finding should be a continuous process and not a "once and for all" project.
2. Randomised Control Trial (RCT)
3. False negatives, false positives, overdiagnosis and radiation risk

---

Appendix

Test your learning and check your understanding of this book's contents: use the "Springer Nature Flashcards" app to access questions using https://sn.pub/dcAnWL.

To use the app, please follow the instructions in Chap. 1.

Flashcardcode:48341-69945-ABCB1-2A8C7-CE9D2.

Short URL: https://sn.pub/dcAnWL.

References

1. Wilson JMG, Jungner G. Principles and practice of screening for disease. Geneva: World Health Organisation; 1968.
2. Akinyemiju TF. Socio-economic and health access determinants of breast and cervical cancer screening in low-income countries: analysis of the World Health Survey. PLoS One. 2012;7(11):e48834.
3. Egan RL. Experience with mammography in Tumour institution : evaluation of 1000 studies. Radiology. 1960;75(6):894–900.
4. Tabár L, Vitak B, Chen TH-H, Yen AM-F, Cohen A, Tot T, Chiu SY, Chen SL, Fann JC, Rosell J, Fohlin H. Swedish two-county trial: impact of mammographic screening on breast cancer mortality during 3 decades. Radiology. 2011;260(3):658–63.
5. Mandrik O, Zielonke N, Meheus F, Severens JLH, Guha N, Herrero Acosta R, Murillo R. Systematic reviews as a 'lens of evidence': determinants of benefits and harms of breast cancer screening. Int J Cancer. 2019;145(4):994–1006.
6. Nelson HD, Fu R, Cantor A, Pappas M, Daeges M, Humphrey L. Effectiveness of breast cancer screening: systematic review and meta-analysis to update the 2009 U.S. Preventive services task force recommendation. Ann Intern Med. 2016;164(4):244–55.
7. Fletcher SW, Black W, Harris R, Rimer BK, Shapiro S. Report of the International workshop on screening for breast cancer. J Natl Cancer Inst. 1993;85(20):1644–56.
8. Kerlikowske K, Grady D, Rubin SM, Sandrock C, Ernster VL. Efficacy of screening mammography. A meta-analysis. JAMA. 1995;273(2):149–54.
9. Shapiro S. Periodic screening for breast cancer: the HIP randomized controlled trial. Health Insurance Plan. J Natl Cancer Inst Monogr. 1997;1997(22):27–30.
10. Andersson I, Aspegren K, Janzon L, Landberg T, Lindholm K, Linell F, Ljungberg O, Ranstam J, Sigfusson B. Mammographic screening and mortality from breast cancer: the Malmö mammographic screening trial. Br Med J. 1988;297(6654):943–8.
11. Alexander FE, Anderson TJ, Brown HK, Forrest AP, Hepburn W, Kirkpatrick AE, McDonald C, Muir BB, Prescott RJ, Shepherd SM, Smith A. The Edinburgh randomised trial of breast cancer screening: results after 10 years of follow-up. Br J Cancer. 1994;70(3):542–8.
12. Miller AB, Wall C, Baines CJ, Sun P, To T, Narod SA. Twenty five year follow-up for breast cancer incidence and mortality of the Canadian National Breast Screening Study: randomised screening trial. BMJ. 2014;348:g366.
13. Frisell J, Lidbrink E, Hellstrom L, Rutqvist LE. Followup after 11 years—update of mortality results in the Stockholm mammographic screening trial. Breast Cancer Res Treat. 1997;45(3):263–70.
14. Bjurstam N, Bjorneld L, Warwick J, Sala E, Duffy SW, Nystrom L, Walker N, Cahlin E, Eriksson O, Hafstrom LO, Lingaas H. The Gothenburg breast screening trial. Cancer. 2003;97(10):2387–96.
15. Moss SM, Wale C, Smith R, Evans A, Cuckle H, Duffy SW. Effect of mammographic screening from age 40 years on breast cancer mortality in the UK Age trial at 17 years' follow-up: a randomised controlled trial. Lancet Oncol. 2015;16(9):1123–32.
16. Foxhall LE, Rodriguez MA. Advances in cancer survivorship management. New York: Springer; 2015.
17. O'Malley MS, Fletcher SW. Screening for breast cancer with breast self-examination: a critical review. JAMA. 1987;257(16):2196–203.
18. Marmot MG, Altman DG, Cameron DA, Dewar JA, Thompson SG, Wilcox M. The benefits and harms of breast cancer screening: an independent review. Lancet. 2012;380(9855):1778–86.
19. Alteri R, Barnes C, Burke A, Gansler T, Gapstur S, Gaudet M, Kramer J, Newman LA, Niemeyer D, Richards C, Runowicz C. Breast cancer facts & figures 2013–2014. Atlanta: American Cancer Society; 2013.
20. International Agency for Research on Cancer (IARC). IARC Handbooks of Cancer Prevention: benefits of mammography screening outweigh adverse effects for women aged 50–69 years. http://www.iarc.fr/en/media-centre/pr/2015/pdfs/pr234_E.pdf.
21. Kalager M, Zelen M, Langmark F, Adami HO. Effect of screening mammography on breast-cancer mortality in Norway. N Engl J Med. 2010;363(13):1203–10.
22. Gotzsche PC, Jorgensen KJ. Screening for breast cancer with mammography. Cochrane Database Syst Rev. 2013;6:CD001877.
23. Harding C, Pompei F, Burmistrov D, Welch HG, Abebe R, Wilson R. Breast cancer screening, incidence, and mortality across US Counties. JAMA Intern Med. 2015;175(9):1483–9.
24. Welch HG, Prorok PC, O'Malley AJ, Kramer BS. Breast-cancer tumor size, overdiagnosis, and mammography screening effectiveness. N Engl J Med. 2016;375(15):1438–47.
25. Esserman LJ, Thompson IM, Reid B. Overdiagnosis and overtreatment in cancer: an opportunity for improvement. JAMA. 2013;310(8):797–8.
26. Independent UK Panel on Breast Cancer Screening. The benefits and harms of breast cancer screening—Authors' reply. Lancet. 2013;381(9869):803–4.
27. Gøtzsche PC, Jørgensen KJ. The benefits and harms of breast cancer screening. Lancet. 2013;381(9869):799.
28. Jin J. Breast cancer screening: benefits and harms. JAMA. 2014;312(23):2585.
29. de Gonzalez AB, Reeves G. Mammographic screening before age 50 years in the UK: comparison of the radiation risks with the mortality benefits. Br J Cancer. 2005;93(5):590–6.

30. ICRP. The 2007 Recommendations of the International Commission on Radiological Protection (Publication 103). Ann ICRP. 2007;37(2–4):1–332.
31. Toward Optimized Practice [TOP] Working Group for Breast Cancer Screening. Breast cancer screening: clinical practice guideline. 2013. https://actt.albertadoctors.org/CPGs/Lists/CPGDocumentList/Breast-Cancer-Screening-CPG.pdf.
32. Warren LM, Dance DR, Young K. Radiation risk with digital mammography in breast screening. London: Public Health England; 2017. www.gov.uk/government/publications/breast-screening-radiation-risk-with-digital-mammography/radiation-risk-with-digital-mammography-in-breast-screening.
33. Djulbegovic B, Lyman GH. Screening mammography at 40–49 years: regret or no regret? Lancet. 2006;368(9552):2035–7.
34. Nguyen PK, Lee WH, Li YF, Hong WX, Hu S, Chan C, Liang G, Nguyen I, Ong SG, Churko J, Wang J. Assessment of the radiation effects of cardiac CT angiography using protein and genetic biomarkers. J Am Coll Cardiol Img. 2015;8(8):873–84.
35. Lee WH, Nguyen PK, Fleischmann D, Wu JC. DNA damage-associated biomarkers in studying individual sensitivity to low-dose radiation from cardiovascular imaging. Eur Heart J. 2016;37(40):3075–80.
36. Hendrick RE. Radiation doses and cancer risks from breast imaging studies. Radiology. 2010;257(1):246–53.
37. Suleiman ME, McEntee MF, Cartwright L, Diffey J, Brennan PC. Diagnostic reference levels for digital mammography in New South Wales. J Med Imaging Radiat Oncol. 2017;61(1):48–57.
38. Barratt A, Howard K, Irwig L, Salkeld G, Houssami N. Model of outcomes of screening mammography: information to support informed choices. BMJ. 2005;330(7497):936.
39. Olsson S, Andersson I, Karlberg I, Bjurstam N, Frodis E, Hakansson S. Implementation of service screening with mammography in Sweden: from pilot study to nationwide programme. J Med Screen. 2000;7(1):14–8.
40. Lind H, Svane G, Kemetli L, Tornberg S. Breast Cancer Screening Program in Stockholm County, Sweden—Aspects of Organization and Quality Assurance. Breast Care. 2010;5(5):353–7.
41. Malmgren JA, Parikh J, Atwood MK, Kaplan HG. Improved prognosis of women aged 75 and older with mammography-detected breast cancer. Radiology. 2014;273(3):686–94.
42. van Agt H, Fracheboud J, van der Steen A, de Koning H. Do women make an informed choice about participating in breast cancer screening? A survey among women invited for a first mammography screening examination. Patient Educ Couns. 2012;89(2):353–9.
43. Dellie ST, Rao ADP, Admassie D, Meshesha AZ. Evaluation of mean glandular dose during diagnostic mammography examination for detection of breast pathology, in Ethiopia. OMICS J Radiol. 2013;1(109):2.
44. Internation Cancer Screening Network (ICSN). Breast Cancer Screening Programs in 26 ICSN Countries, 2012: Organization, Policies, and Program Reach. 2015. http://healthcaredelivery.cancer.gov/icsn/breast/screening.html.
45. Lerda D, Deandrea S, Freeman C, López-Alcalde J, Neamtiu L, Nicholl C, Nicholson N, Ulutuck A, Villanueva S. Report of a European survey on the organisation of breast cancer care services. Luxembourg: Publications Office of the European Union; 2014. http://publications.jrc.ec.europa.eu/repository/bitstream/JRC89731/lbna26593enn_002.pdf.
46. Coldman AJ, Phillips N, Olivotto IA, Gordon P, Warren L, Kan L. Impact of changing from annual to biennial mammographic screening on breast cancer outcomes in women aged 50-79 in British Columbia. J Med Screen. 2008;15(4):182–7.
47. US Preventive Services Task Force. Screening for breast cancer: US Preventive Services Task Force recommendation statement. Ann Intern Med. 2009;151(10):716–1236.
48. American Cancer Society (ACS). Mammograms and other breast imaging tests. http://www.cancer.org/healthy/findcancerearly/examandtestdescriptions/mammogramsandotherbreastimagingprocedures/mammograms-and-other-breast-imaging-procedures-toc.
49. Public Health England (PHE). Protocols for surveillance of women at very high risk of developing breast cancer; 2021. www.gov.uk/government/publications/breast-screening-higher-risk-women-surveillance-protocols/protocols-for-surveillance-of-women-at-higher-risk-of-developing-breast-cancer.
50. Forrest SP. Breast cancer screening: report to the health ministers of England, Wales, Scotland, and Northern Ireland. London: Her Majesty's Stationery Office; 1986.
51. Advisory Committee on Breast Cancer Screening. Screening for breast cancer in England: past and future. J Med Screen. 2006;13(2):59–61.
52. Vetto JT, Luoh SW, Naik A. Breast cancer in premenopausal women. Curr Probl Surg. 2009;46(12):944–1004.
53. Tirona MT. Breast cancer screening update. Am Fam Physician. 2013;87(4):274–8.
54. Sinclair N, Littenberg B, Geller B, Muss H. Accuracy of screening mammography in older women. Am J Roentgenol. 2011;197(5):1268–73.
55. Organisation for Economic Co-operation and Development (OECD). Society at a Glance 2011—OECD Social Indicators. 2011. www.oecd.org/social/societyataglance2011.htm.
56. American Cancer Society (ACS). Breast cancer early detection and diagnosis. Atlanta: American Cancer Society; 2021. https://www.cancer.org/cancer/breast-cancer/screening-tests-and-early-detection.html.
57. Wang FL, Chen F, Yin H, Xu N, Wu XX, Ma JJ, Gao S, Tang JH, Lu C. Effects of age, breast density and volume on breast cancer diagnosis: a retrospective comparison of sensitivity of mammography and ultra-sonography in China's rural areas. Asian Pac J Cancer Prev. 2013;14(4):2277–82.

Breast Anatomy

Alison Darlington

Learning Objectives
- Identify breast anatomical structures
- Recognise the stages of breast development and understand the visual impact of these changes on the resultant mammography image

Introduction

Breasts are made up of fat and glandular tissue, with nerves, arteries, veins, and connective tissue that provides the support structure. Breast anatomy is such that the internal and external support structures enable the breast to be mobile inferiorly and at the lateral border. The superior and medial aspects are relatively fixed. This allows the breast to be positioned for mammography [1–7].

The breast is a modified apocrine sweat gland. It develops at puberty and is sited on the anterior chest wall overlying the pectoralis major muscle between the 2nd to 6th ribs vertically and from the sternum medially to the mid axillary line laterally. Various physiological changes occur throughout life in response to hormonal stimulation, pregnancy and lactation and eventually a process of involution takes place. These changes are apparent on mammography and should be understood in order to appreciate the visual impact on mammograms [1–7].

Embryology and Development

The breast is composed of a collection of glands arising from the epidermis during foetal development. They are sited between the deep and superficial fascia of the anterior thorax which is derived from the dermis. The nipple is a local proliferation of the stratum spinosum of the epidermis. Breast development begins during the second month of gestation, two lines of thickened ectoderm form on the ventral body wall of the foetus; these extend from the axilla to the groin (Fig. 3.1) and are called the milk lines. Mammary glands can develop at any point along these. By the ninth week of foetal development this ridge regresses: usually leaving a single functional bud in the pectoral region which persists and, at puberty, develops into an adult mammary gland. However, in 2–6% of the population ectopic or accessory breast tissue may be present along the milk line which may or may not have a visible nipple. This should be considered during breast imaging as breast disease can develop wherever breast tissue is present [1–7].

The glandular component of the breast develops from the ectoderm. It arises from local thickening of the epidermis; 15–20 groups of ectodermal cells grow into the underlying mesoderm (dermis) during the 12th week of gestation.

A. Darlington (✉)
Department of Breast Imaging, North Manchester General Hospital, Manchester, UK
e-mail: Alison.darlington@mft.nhs.uk

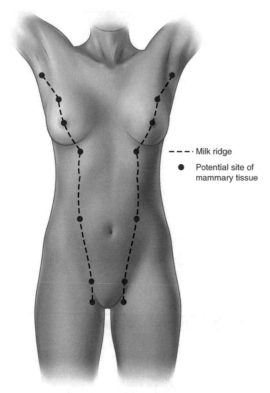

- - - - Milk ridge

● Potential site of mammary tissue

Fig. 3.1 Illustration of milk (ridge) line

These groups of cells then develop spaces that will become the lactiferous ducts. The nipple initially develops as a shallow epidermal indentation which becomes everted near term [1–7].

The connective tissue stroma of the breast forms from the mesoderm, which also forms the dermis of the skin and the superficial fascia. Fibres forming the Cooper's suspensory ligaments develop from both layers. At birth males and females have the same breast anatomy. In the female, at puberty, hormonal stimuli cause the breast to develop; initially oestrogen causes fat to be deposited in the breast, and the lactiferous milk ducts to enlarge.

Following the onset of menstruation, the ovaries begin to produce progesterone and this causes lobules and acini or milk glands to develop at the ends of the lactiferous ducts. The breasts develop from the buds sited bilaterally on the anterior chest wall overlying the pectoralis major muscle and once formed will lie between the 2nd to 6th ribs vertically and from the sternum medially to the mid axillary line laterally. The process of development usually takes about 3–5 years [1–7].

Male breast development, when present, is termed gynaecomastia. This condition arises as a response to hormonal imbalances which can occur at puberty or in later life as a result of disease, medication, recreational drug use or excessive alcohol consumption. The condition is investigated in the same way as female breast disease utilising mammography and ultrasound. Pseudogynecomastia occurs when fat is deposited on the anterior chest wall under the nipple areolar complex and looks very similar outwardly to true gynaecomastia, however, in gynaecomastia proper breast tissue development is evident whereas in pseudogynecomastia the enlargement is purely due to adipose tissue [1–7].

Macroscopic and Microscopic Anatomy

Once fully developed the breast is 'tear drop' shaped. The breast itself can be described in terms of both its external and internal composition and by its macroscopic and microscopic anatomy. Externally the breast comprises of [8]:

- The nipple
- The areolar
- Skin
- Inframammary Fold
- Montgomery's Glands (Tubercles)

Internally the breast comprises of:

- Glandular Tissue—15–20 lobes
- Lactiferous Ducts
- Lactiferous Sinuses (Ampullae)
- Terminal Ductal Lobular Units (TDLU)
- Adipose Tissue
- Superficial Fascia
- Deep Fascia
- Retromammary Space
- Cooper's Ligaments
- Blood vessels

Figure 3.2 illustrates the gross anatomical structures of the breast. It is important to understand the external anatomy when positioning the breast for mammography and the internal anatomy when assessing the mammo-

Fig. 3.2 Overview of external and internal breast anatomy [8]. (*Reprinted with permission from: Shiffman MA, Di Giuseppe A, editors. Cosmetic surgery: art and techniques. Springer Science & Business Media; 2012*)

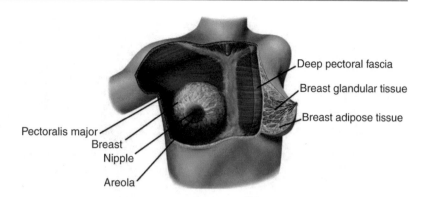

Deep pectoral fascia

Breast glandular tissue

Breast adipose tissue

Pectoralis major

Breast

Nipple

Areola

graphic image. On mammography, the fat contained within the breast is radiolucent whilst the glandular component appears as areas of increased density [8].

Macroscopic Anatomy

The breast can be macroscopically divided into two main parts. The glandular component is the first of these and is concerned with milk production. The second part consists of all the other tissues that make up and support the breast, including: fat, fascia (connective tissue) and muscles.

Breast tissue extends into the low axilla as a triangular shaped projection—this portion of the breast is called the axillary tail or 'Tail of Spence'. The glandular component consists of 15–20 lobes which radiate out from the nipple. Each one of these is made up of 10–100 lobules which contain multiple acini—where milk is produced and stored during lactation [1–7].

These are drained by a network of small ducts (intralobular ducts) which come together to form a single duct draining each lobule (interlobular duct). The interlobular ducts in turn join to form intralobular ducts which jointly form a single lactiferous duct that drains the lobe. The purpose of the ducts is to transport milk; the lactiferous ducts dilate just under the nipple to form the lactiferous sinus or ampulla and then narrow and terminate at the surface of the nipple. The lobes are separated by fibrous septae and connective tissue stroma [1–9].

The skin overlying the breast is typically 0.5–2.0 mm in thickness. Beneath the skin is a superficial layer of fascia that divides into the superficial and deep layers as it reaches the breast. Between these layers the breast proper develops. The deep layer of fascia lies directly on the fascia of the pectoralis major muscle. This allows slight movement of the breast on the chest wall. The breast is supported by the Cooper's ligaments, skin and the deep and superficial layers of the fascia and pectoralis major muscle. The superficial fascia is covered by a layer of adipose tissue 2–2.5 cm thick and is attached to the skin by the Cooper's Ligaments which pierce the fat. The retro mammary space lies between the deep fascia of the breast and the fascia of the pectoralis major muscle and is filled by loose connective tissue [1–9]. The main internal components of the breast and the corresponding mammographic features are demonstrated in Fig. 3.3.

Externally the whole of the breast is covered by skin; the skin of the nipple areolar complex contains sweat glands, sebaceous glands and hair follicles. The nipple promontory is surrounded by a circular area of pigmented skin called the areolar. Montgomery's glands are sited around, but not on, the nipple and are transitional between sweat and lactiferous glands. They lubricate the nipple during lactation and are visible as small bumps on the areolar. The infra mammary fold is the lower border of the breast where the breast tissue meets the chest wall. Most women have a degree of breast asymmetry; that is the size, shape and position on the chest wall differs slightly from right to left. Nipple characteristics also vary greatly [1–9].

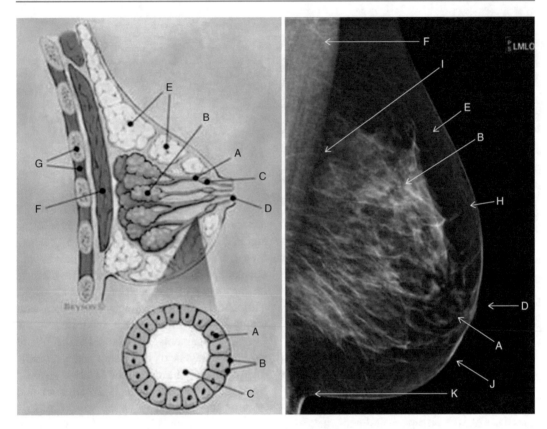

A   Lactiferous duct

B   Lobules

C   Cross section of lactiferous duct

D   Nipple

E   Adipose tissue

F   Pectoralis major muscle

G   Chest wall / ribs

H   Cooper's ligaments

I   Retromammary space

J   Skin

K   Inframammary fold

Fig. 3.3 Internal anatomy of the breast: schematic and mammographic illustrations [9]. (Reprinted with permission from Sun Y, Suri JS, Desautels JE, Rangayyan RM. A new approach for breast skin-line estimation in mammograms. Pattern Analysis and Applications. 2006 May;9(1):34–47)

Microscopic Anatomy

Microscopic description of the breast centres on the TDLU. This is the functional unit of the breast and is composed of acini, an intralobular terminal duct and an extralobular duct. Over 90% of breast carcinomas originate in these units as do many benign breast diseases.

The acini and ducts are made up of three layers:

- Basement Membrane
- Myoepithelial Layer
- Epithelial Lining

The epithelial layer is usually only one cell thick but if this becomes two or three cells thick it is called hyperplasia. Further proliferation is categorised according to how many layers of cells are present and how atypical the cells appear; these conditions range from atypical ductal hyperplasia to ductal carcinoma in situ. The basement membrane acts as a barrier to the spread of a cancer. A carcinoma is termed invasive if this is breached. Figure 3.4 shows a simplified diagram of the structure of a TDLU [1–9].

Fig. 3.4 Illustration of Terminal Ductal Lobular Unit (TDLU)

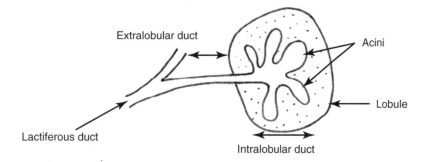

Fig. 3.5 Illustration of vascular supply to the breast

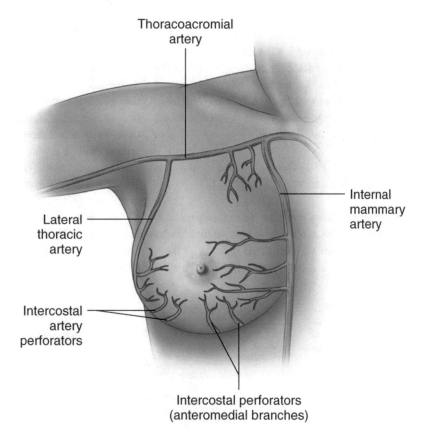

Arterial Supply

The blood supply to the breast skin comes from the subdermal plexus, which is in communication with deeper underlying vessels supplying the breast parenchyma. The main arterial supply is from perforating branches of the internal mammary artery (most notably the 2nd and 5th perforators). The superomedial perforator supply, arising from the internal mammary artery, accounts for around 60% of the total breast arterial blood supply. Additional arterial supply is derived from the thoracoacromial artery, the lateral thoracic artery and the intercostal arteries. Figure 3.5 gives a pictorial representation of the breast arterial vasculature [1–9].

Venous Drainage

Venous drainage of the breast is mainly through the axillary vein, with some through the internal mammary and thoracic veins. In general, the venous drainage system of the breast follows the arterial system. The superficial venous system of the breast drains into the internal thoracic vein. The deep venous system drains into the perforating branches of the internal thoracic vein, lateral thoracic, axillary vein, and upper intercostal veins. A circular venous plexus lies around the areola [1–9].

Innervation

The nerve supply to the breast is from the anterior and lateral branches of the second to sixth intercostal (T2–6) nerves. The nipple supply is complex but is mainly from the anterior branch of the lateral cutaneous ramus of T4. Nerve endings in the nipple are activated during suckling and initiate the 'let down' reflex via the central nervous system [1–9].

Lymphatic Drainage

Lymphatic drainage of the breast begins in a peri-lobular plexus sited in the connective tissue stroma of the breast, lymphatic fluid flows from here alongside the lactiferous ducts into a sub-

areolar plexus; Sappey's Plexus. Internal mammary lymph nodes may be present along these channels. From this plexus the breast drains into the axillary, subscapular, central, pectoral, apical, and clavicular node groups laterally and the para-sternal (internal mammary) nodes medially.

Drainage to the internal mammary nodes means that lymphatic fluid can cross to the contralateral breast. Communication between these groups frequently occurs. Lymphatic fluid may also reach the abdominal nodal groups from the inferomedial breast. Knowledge of these pathways is important in order to understand potential metastatic pathways in breast carcinoma. 67% of the breast lymphatic drainage is to the axillary nodal groups. The sentinel lymph node is the first node to which cancer cells are most likely to spread from a primary tumour; in breast carcinoma this is most likely to lie low in the axilla and is the node removed at surgery in order to assess the spread of disease. This gives prognostic information regarding likelihood of local recurrence [10]. Figure 3.6 illustrates the relative lymph node groups providing the breast lymphatic drainage.

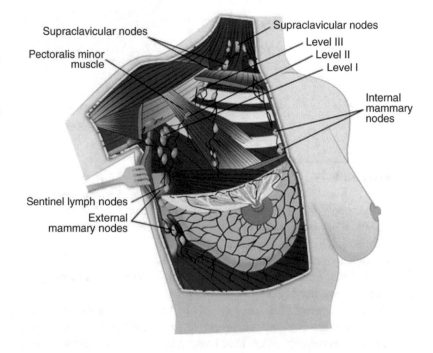

Fig. 3.6 Lymphatic drainage of the breast indicating position of the sentinel lymph node [10]. (Reprinted with permission from Urban C, Rietjens M, Kuroda F, Hurley J. Oncoplastic and Reconstructive Anatomy of the Breast. In Oncoplastic and Reconstructive Breast Surgery 2013 (pp. 13–21). Springer, Milano)

Fig. 3.7 Illustration of Level I, level II and Level III axillary lymph nodes [11]. (Reprinted with permission from Harisinghani MG, O'Shea A, editors. Atlas of lymph node anatomy. New York: Springer; 2013)

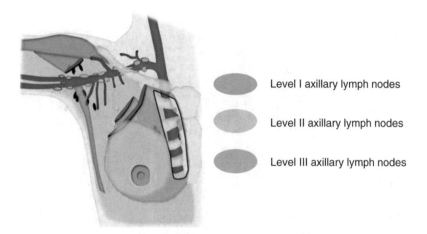

Level I axillary lymph nodes

Level II axillary lymph nodes

Level III axillary lymph nodes

Axillary lymph nodes are divided into three groups: Level I, Level II, and Level III as demonstrated below in Fig. 3.7. Level I nodes lie lateral to the lateral border of the pectoralis major muscle and can extend into the axillary tail, Level II nodes lie beneath the pectoralis minor muscle and Level III nodes lie medially and superiorly to the pectoralis minor muscle up to the clavicle. Level I nodes are often visible on mammogram, as are intramammary nodes when present [11].

Pregnancy and Lactation

During pregnancy, rises in oestrogen, progesterone and prolactin lead to growth of the acini, hyperplasia of the lactogenic (milk producing) epithelium and an increase in myoepithelial cells in preparation for milk production. The lobules enlarge until only thin fibrous septations separate them. Once breastfeeding ceases the breasts undergo a degree of involution and may appear less glandular than before pregnancy. This return to a new baseline takes around 3 months to complete [12].

Involution

The female breast undergoes gradual regression, called involution, starting at the end of the fourth decade. The function of the ovaries declines which causes the supporting connective tissues in the breast to be replaced by adipose tissue. Changes are also seen in the TDLU; the epithelium shrinks to one layer and there is progressive lobular atrophy. There is a reduction in glandular component with an increase in fatty tissue. The regressive process continues until and after menopause [13].

The breasts of post-menopausal women may be entirely fatty on mammogram, however, most post-menopausal women produce enough endogenous oestrogen to maintain some glandular component. As the woman ages the support structures of the breast weaken causing corresponding 'sag' of the breast tissue—this is called ptosis [13]. A mammographic image of an involuted breast is shown in Fig. 3.8b; note that the glandular component seen in Fig. 3.8a has been almost entirely replaced by fatty tissue.

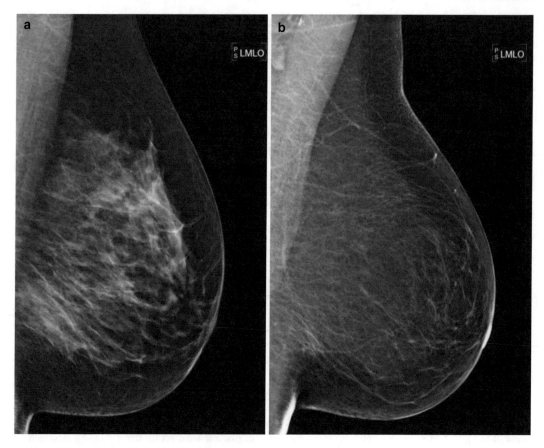

Fig. 3.8 Mammographic illustration of (**a**) Mature female breast, (**b**) Involuted breast

Clinical Pearls
- Breast cancer can develop wherever there is breast tissue – bear in mind accessory axillary tissue and the embryonic milk line. A nipple is not always present.
- Use both the CC and MLO projections to determine lesion position within the breast.

Chapter Review Questions
Review Questions

1. What is the medical term for enlargement of breast tissue in males?
2. What is the sentinel node?
3. What is ectopic breast tissue?

Answers

1. Gynaecomastia
2. A sentinel lymph node is the first lymph node to which cancer cells are most likely to spread from a primary tumor. Sometimes, there is more than one sentinel lymph node. In breast cancer this node is likely to lie low in the axilla.
3. Ectopic or accessory breast tissue is residual breast tissue persisting from embryologic development, found in up to 6% of the population, most commonly in the axilla, but can occur anywhere along the milk line.

Appendix

Test your learning and check your understanding of this book's contents: use the "Springer Nature Flashcards" app to access questions using https://sn.pub/dcAnWL.

To use the app, please follow the instructions in Chap. 1.

Flashcard code: 48341-69945-ABCB1-2A8C7-CE9D2.

Short URL: https://sn.pub/dcAnWL.

References

1. Kopans DB. Breast imaging. Philadelphia: Lippincott Williams & Wilkins; 2007.
2. Gershon-Cohen J. Atlas of mammography. Berlin: Springer Science & Business Media; 2013.
3. Drake R, Vogl AW, Mitchell AW. Gray's anatomy for students. 3rd ed. London: Churchill Livingstone; 2014.
4. Whitley AS, Jefferson G, Holmes K, Sloane C, Anderson C, Hoadley G. Clark's positioning in radiography. 13th ed. Boca Raton: CRC; 2015.
5. Moore KL, Persaud TV, Torchia MG. The developing human-e-book: clinically oriented embryology. Amsterdam: Elsevier Health Sciences; 2018.
6. Lampignano J, Kendrick LE. Bontrager's textbook of radiographic positioning and related anatomy-E-book. 10th ed. Amsterdam: Elsevier Health Sciences; 2020.
7. Williams S, Taylor K, Campbell S. Fundamentals of mammography-E-book. Amsterdam: Elsevier Health Sciences; 2021.
8. Shiffman MA, Di Giuseppe A. Cosmetic surgery: art and techniques. Berlin: Springer Science & Business Media; 2012.
9. Sun Y, Suri JS, Desautels JE, Rangayyan RM. A new approach for breast skin-line estimation in mammograms. Pattern Anal Applic. 2006;9(1):34–47.
10. Urban C, Rietjens M, Kuroda F, Hurley J. Oncoplastic and reconstructive anatomy of the breast. In: Urban C, Rietjens M, editors. Oncoplastic and reconstructive breast surgery. Milan: Springer; 2013. p. 13–21.
11. Harisinghani MG, O'Shea A. Atlas of lymph node anatomy. New York: Springer; 2013.
12. Alex A, Bhandary E, McGuire KP. Anatomy and physiology of the breast during pregnancy and lactation. In: Alipour S, Omranipour R, editors. Diseases of the breast during pregnancy and lactation. Cham: Springer; 2020. p. 3–7.
13. Watson CJ. Key stages in mammary gland development-involution: apoptosis and tissue remodelling that convert the mammary gland from milk factory to a quiescent organ. Breast Cancer Res. 2006;8(2):1–5.

Breast Density and Influencing Factors

4

Dawn McDonald

Learning Objectives
- Demonstrate knowledge of breast anatomy
- Identify and state the factors which influence breast density
- Demonstrate knowledge of the different types of breast density

Breast Structure

Breast parenchyma consists of three types of tissue: skin, subcutaneous adipose tissue and functional glandular tissue. The breast itself is divided into approximately 15–18 lobes. Lobes consist of branching ductal systems which lead from the collecting ducts to the terminal ductal lobular units (TDLU). Most breast diseases, with the exception of papillomas in major ducts, arise in the TDLU. The TDLU normally regresses at menopause [1]. The main duct within each lobe has an opening, draining 20–40 lobules. The acini, consisting of a number of lobules, are the site of milk production in the lactating breast [1]. The number of lobules per lobe varies according to age, lactation, parity, and hormonal status. Towards the end of the reproductive life there is an increase in the amount of adipose tissue, and a considerable loss of lobular units, although the main ductal system is preserved. This process, in which there is a reduction in the number, and size, of the acini per lobule, and replaced by fatty tissue, is known as age-related lobular involution, or physiologic atrophy of the breast [2–4].

The changes in breast composition can be demonstrated by variations in breast density on mammography. Usually, younger women tend to have more dense glandular tissue. In older women, the mammographic density tends to decrease with the replacement of glandular tissue by fatty tissue [5]. Figures 4.1 and 4.2 illustrate this.

D. McDonald (✉)
Breast Unit, Broomfield Hospital,
Chelmsford, Essex, UK
e-mail: dawn.mcdonald1@nhs.net

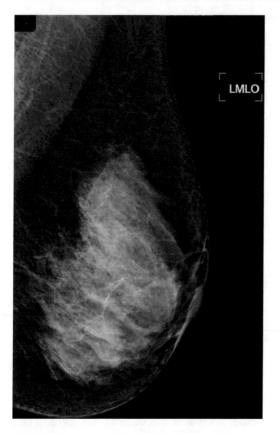

Fig. 4.1 Example of a 40-year-old with dense breast tissue pattern

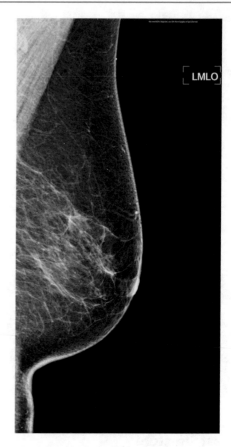

Fig. 4.2 Example of a 65-year-old with fatty tissue pattern

Breast Density Classification

Before we discuss breast density classification, we need to understand what breast density is. Simply put, breast density is the proportional amount of glandular breast tissue, relative to the amount of fatty tissue. It is mainly identifiable by a mammogram, and the proportionate amounts can vary significantly within women (and some men).

Over the passage of time several methods have evolved to aid in the classification of breast density, for example classification of breast composition by Wolfe [6] explains that in 'fatty breasts' almost all of the tissue appears to be fat, and less than 25% will be fibro-glandular tissues. If a breast has scattered fibro-glandular tissue, 26–50% volume of the breast is visible as

fibro-glandular tissue. Heterogeneously dense tissue will have 51–75% tissue. Extremely dense breasts will have more than 75% of fibrous connective tissue [6]. 10% of postmenopausal and 20% of premenopausal women have a breast density of above 50%. It is estimated that one in three women have a high mammographic density [7]. Further classifications of breast composition include Boyd's [8], in which mammographic density is divided into six categories:

A	0%
B	>0–10%
C	>10–25%
D	>25–50%
E	>50–75%
F	>75%

and Tabar [9], which classifies the mammograms into five patterns:

I	Balanced proportion of all components of breast tissue with a slight predominance of fibrous tissue
II	Predominance of fat tissue (fatty breast)
III	Predominance of fat tissue with retro-areolar residual fibrous tissue
IV	Predominantly nodular densities
V	Predominantly fibrous tissue (dense breast)

The commonly known American BI-RADS system (Breast Imaging Reporting and Data System) [10] used to categorise breast density and mammographic abnormalities, since 2013, is based on the following definitions:

(a)	The breasts are almost entirely fatty
(b)	There are scattered areas of fibro glandular density
(c)	The breasts are heterogeneously dense
(d)	The breasts are extremely dense

The system has been recently updated [11] to further classify breast density by incorporating mammography, alongside other imaging modalities such as ultrasound and MRI, to work as a more effective diagnostic tool to help in the evaluation of breast lesions. This more comprehensive seven assessment category is defined as follows:

- **BI-RADS 0**: incomplete: need additional imaging evaluation (additional mammographic views or ultrasound) and/or
  - for mammography, obtaining previous images not available at the time of reading
- **BI-RADS 1**: negative symmetrical and no masses, architectural distortion, or suspicious calcifications
- **BI-RADS 2**: benign 0% probability of malignancy
- **BI-RADS 3**: probably benign<2% probability of malignancy
  - short interval follow-up suggested
- **BI-RADS 4**: suspicious for malignancy
  - 2–94% probability of malignancy

- For mammography and ultrasound, these can be further divided [11]:
  BI-RADS 4A: low suspicion for malignancy (2–9%)
  BI-RADS 4B: moderate suspicion for malignancy (10–49%)
  BI-RADS 4C: high suspicion for malignancy (50–94%) biopsy should be considered
- **BI-RADS 5**: highly suggestive of malignancy
  - >95% probability of malignancy
  - appropriate action should be taken
- **BI-RADS 6**: known biopsy-proven malignancy

The use of other imaging modalities to further classify breast density is also becoming prevalent in the UK. An on-going, randomised multi-centre trial is currently in the process of recruiting and assessing high risk women of screening age, for example, 50–70 years, to investigate further the risks of dense breast tissue. High risk women could be those women, for example, who are at higher risk due to gene mutation. A dense breast pattern is a concern because it leads to an increasing risk of breast cancer, this is because the tissue could mask small lesions within the breast. This trial—BRAID—(Breast Screening—Risk Adaptive Imaging for Density) is aiming to investigate the use of supplementary imaging techniques (similarly to the above BIRADS) such as automated breast ultrasound (ABUS), contrast enhanced spectral mammography (CESM), or abbreviated breast MRI(AB-MRI) [12].

While breast MRI is well known, and often used in the diagnosis of breast cancer, *Abbreviated Breast MRI* is a faster, targeted MRI scan. It can be used for screening of women at average risk of breast cancer. The use of a contrast injection as part of the examination process enables better visualisation of small lesions, even in dense breasts; but this will be further discussed in Chap. 10. However, the significance of AB-MRI is it should help to detect the smaller cancers not easily identified, or in fact missed, in those women with dense breasts.

Drawbacks of Categorisations

Despite the extra categories described in the fore-going to further classify the density of the breast, it is thought that a potential drawback of this is that this has introduced more disparity between (and within) the film readers in gaining consensus. One of the reasons for this is thought to be because the sensitivity of mammography decreases with this increased categorisation due to the lesions being hidden in the dense breast tissue. The suggestion is that film readers may find it more difficult to agree on the mammographic features and presenting abnormalities depending on the category of the breast tissue [13]; there appears to be more inter and intra-observer variation between, and within, film readers as the categories increase [13]. However, despite this perceived drawback, BIRADS is still widely used to classify breast density in mammograms.

The Significance of Sensitivity

The sensitivity of mammography in the detection of breast cancer is the number of true positives as a proportion of all those with breast cancer [14] and is directly related to the density of the breast tissue. Generally, mammographic sensitivity is higher in older, post-menopausal women because the breast tends to be composed of greater proportions of fatty tissue.

A high mammographic density is thought to be associated with an increased risk of breast cancer and is estimated to account for 16% of all breast cancers [15]. The screening population is also deemed to be at higher risk if breast density is high [16]. However, what is less clearly understood is the breast cancer risk associated with the change in breast density over time; we understand that risk increases with age and breast density, but density decreases with age, which seems almost contradictory.

To investigate this further, one study [17] has suggested that the evolution of the density of the breast (as a function of time) may be significant for the risk of developing breast cancer—the faster the changes that occur, the higher the risk. This study does however acknowledge a small sample size and that the cases were not randomly selected. It suggests further research into this with speculation that women would like to know their risk factor of developing breast cancer. This seems to be proven in a more recent study, the PROCAS 1 study [18]. The study aimed to recruit 60,000 women to investigate the risk of breast cancer developing over time—this was achieved by using density measurements between routine breast screening and using these to analyse any risk factors in the screening population. Over a 6-year recruitment span, the study was seen as a great success, with over 94% of women wanting to know their risk score of developing breast cancer. Even though full results are still not available for this study, what has been so far established is that it appears to add weight to the notion that women want to know their risk factors and how the breast density can affect this, as speculated in the earlier study. A woman may receive a negative mammogram, but she may still be at risk of a higher risk of developing BCa. This could be due to the density of the breast. PROCAS 2, the next stage of the project, aims to provide women of their risk factor within 6 weeks; as opposed to between 1 and 3 years [19]. Nonetheless, regardless of the rate at which breast density changes, sensitivity is reduced in the dense breast [4, 5]. Figures 4.3, 4.4 and 4.5 illustrate a focal lesion which is barely visible in a dense breast, more easily seen in a mixed breast, and clearly seen in a fatty area of the breast.

The images illustrate how the detection of breast cancer through mammography is highly dependent on breast tissue characteristics. A dense breast structure will significantly reduce the detection sensitivity [20].

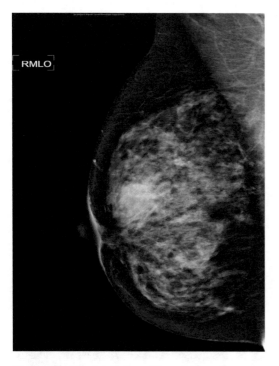

Fig. 4.3 Focal lesion in 'dense' breast

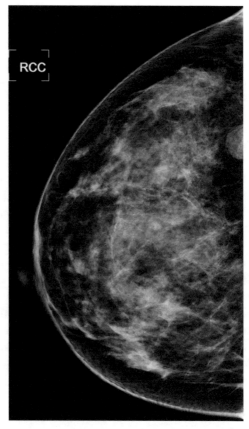

Fig. 4.5 Focal lesion in 'fatty' area of breast

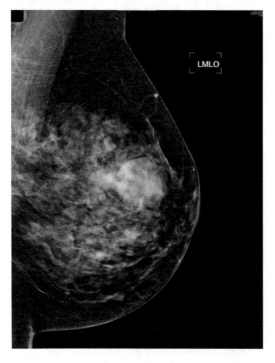

Fig. 4.4 Focal lesion in 'mixed' breast

Factors Influencing Breast Density

Age

Age is a common factor that influences breast density (Fig. 4.1). A high percentage of women under the age of 30 tend to have dense breasts; approximately 90% dense versus 10% fatty. The density rate decreases steadily at approximately 1–2% per year. At 40 years, the ratio is 80/10; 50 years 70/30. It is approximately 50/50 at 65 years [21]. Older women tend to have more of a fatty breast tissue type.

Pregnancy and Lactation

Women with fewer than two pregnancies usually have denser breast types. During pregnancy and breast feeding, the number of acini increase with glandular tissue predominating. When lactation ceases, the glandular tissue involutes. The significance of this is that the breast of a woman who has given birth is less glandular than that of a woman of the same age who has not [22].

Hormonal Status

Pre and post hormonal status and reproductive factors have an effect on the density of the breast. Oestrogen levels, which decline with age and menopausal status, can lead to a decline in mammographic density. Oestrogen, post menopause, is positively associated with Body Mass Index (BMI). Tamoxifen, a selective oestrogen receptor modulator, is used to prevent breast cancer in women and treat breast cancer in women and men. Tamoxifen is typically taken daily by mouth for 5 years for breast cancer [23] and is also said to reduce density in premenopausal women [7].

Body Mass Index

Women with a large BMI tend to have large breasts with significant fatty tissue and an associated loss in breast density. The breast is a store for fat and as a woman gains or loses weight, this will have an effect in the percentage of dense breast tissue [21]. Consequently, weight gain/loss is associated with significant change in breast density. An increase in weight, and a corresponding increase in fat in the breast, leads to an increase in fat cells. Fat cells make oestrogen, and an increase in fat cells means an increase in oestrogen. This in turn can make hormone-receptor-positive breast cancers develop and grow [24].

There has been further study into the significance of a high BMI and the possibility that this risk may be further increased with a higher risk of ER-negative cancers, compared with ER-positive cancers, in women with a high BMI. This could be another reason to suggest that these women may benefit with weight loss and a more active lifestyle [25].

A large BMI could almost be thought of as a paradox, because being overweight usually means fatty breast tissue which would mean any changes in the breast are more able to be diagnosed easier. However, as seen above, being overweight also leads to an increase in the risk of developing breast cancer.

Lifestyle Factors

Physical Activity

Literature in 2006 suggests that physical activity is associated with the reduction of the incidence of breast cancer, quoting a 20–30% reduction in women who are active in comparison to their non-active colleagues [26]. This is in contradiction to more recent data which suggests that whilst increasing alcohol consumption is thought to be associated with an increase in density, smoking and physical activity are thought not to be associated [27]. Despite the more recent data, it is widely seen that weight loss is likely to be reflected in a reduced breast density. The health benefits of physical activity are commonly considered to be beneficial.

Alcohol

Alcohol is increasingly becoming known as a risk factor for BCa; alcohol can lead to an increase in the levels of hormones such as oestrogen and insulin. A higher level of hormones can lead to cell division more often, and this in turn increases the risk that cancer cells can divide more frequently [28].

Malignant and Benign Breast Change

The skin in the breast can sometimes appear to be thickened, manifesting as increased density on the mammogram [1]. This inflammation, or oedema, can be caused by primary breast cancer, axillary lymph node metastases, abscesses, congestive heart failure, or radiotherapy [29]. Diffuse increase in the density of breast tissue is caused by oedema, or an increase in glandular and/or fibrous tissue. This is also commonly seen in benign breast changes (BBC).

Benign breast change may be accompanied by evidence of cysts, and women taking hormone replacement therapy (HRT) for menopausal symptoms. Benign breast change and high breast density are thought to constitute a risk factor for the future development of breast cancer. A low breast density appears to reduce this risk [30].

Summary

We have seen that several methods exist for classifying breast density. Recent developments show that the use of supplementary imaging is acting as an aid for this. The significance of breast density and related factors such as categorisation of the breast shows that the accuracy of mammography is variable according to the nature of the underlying breast tissue. Dense breast tissue may obscure a focal abnormality, fatty breast tissue is less likely to do so. The risk of breast cancer is therefore higher in women who have dense breast tissue, and anything that reduces this risk is clearly beneficial.

HRT, alcohol consumption, pregnancy, lactation and inflammation are among the factors that appear to be significant in increasing the density of breast tissue. Ageing, some medications (e.g. Tamoxifen), and a decrease in oestrogen levels, are among the factors thought to be significant in reducing the density of the breast. It is well documented that there appears to be a correlation between fatty breast tissue and the prevalence of cancer. This may be indicated by older women who demonstrate a tendency towards fatty breasts and experience an increased risk of breast cancer. However, it is also well documented that those women with a dense breast pattern also have a higher risk.

Clinical Pearls

- Breast density is dependent on a number of factors, some hereditary, some lifestyle dependent.
- Breast density classification is dependent on the proportion of fatty tissue in relation to glandular tissue.
- The denser the breast, the higher the risk of a breast cancer diagnosis.

Chapter Review Questions
Review Questions

1. Breast parenchyma consists of how many layers of breast tissue?
2. What is a high breast density associated with, and why is this significant?
3. Why is mammographic sensitivity increased in older women?

Answers

1. Three layers; skin, subcutaneous adipose tissue, functional glandular tissue.
2. It is associated with an increased risk of breast cancer, because this type of breast pattern can obscure small malignant lesions.
3. Older, post-menopausal women, generally have a greater amount of fatty breast tissue compared to younger women who have a more glandular dense breast pattern.

Appendix

Test your learning and check your understanding of this book's contents: use the "Springer Nature Flashcards" app to access questions using https://sn.pub/dcAnWL.

To use the app, please follow the instructions in Chap. 1.

Flashcard code: 48341-69945-ABCB1-2A8C7-CE9D2.

Short URL: https://sn.pub/dcAnWL.

References

1. Tabar L. Teaching course in diagnostic breast imaging, multimodality approach to the detection and diagnosis of occult breast cancer. Cave Creek, AZ: Mammography Education; 2008.
2. Hughes LE, Mansel RE. Breast anatomy and physiology. In: Hughes LE, Mansel RE, Webster DJT, editors. Benign disorders and diseases of the breast: concepts and clinical management. London: W.B. Saunders; 2000. p. 7–20.
3. Vorrherr H. The breast: morphology, physiology, and lactation. New York: Academic; 1974.
4. Ghosh K, Hartmann LC, Reynolds C, Visscher DW, Brandt KR, Vierkant RA, Scott CG, Radisky DC, Sellers TA, Pankratz VS, Vachon CM. Association between mammographic density and age-related lobular involution of the breast. J Clin Oncol. 2009;28(13):2207–12.
5. Grainger RG, Allison DJ, Adam A, Dixon AK. Grainger and Allison's diagnostic radiology, a textbook of medical imaging, vol. 2. 5th ed. Philadelphia: Churchill Livingstone; 2008.
6. Wolfe JN. A study of breast parenchyma by mammography in the normal woman and those with benign and malignant disease of the breast. Radiology. 1967;89(2):201.
7. Ursin G, Qureshi S. Mammographic density—a useful biomark for breast cancer risk in epidemiologic studies. Norsk Epidemiologi. 2009;19(1):59–68.
8. Boyd NF, O'Sullivan B, Campbell JE, Fishell E, Simor I, Cooke G, Germanson T. Mammographic signs as risk factors for breast cancer. Br J Cancer. 1982;45(2):185–93.
9. Gram IT, Funkhouse E, Tabar L. The Tabar classification of mammographic parenchymal patterns. Eur J Radiol. 1997;24(2):131–6.
10. Sickles EA, D'Orsi CJ, Bassett LW, et al. ACR BI-RADS® mammography. In: ACR BI-RADS® atlas, breast imaging reporting and data system. American College of Radiology: Reston; 2013.
11. Weerakkody Y, Niknejad M. Breast imaging-reporting and data system (BI-RADS). https://radiopaedia.org/articles/breast-imaging-reporting-and-data-system-bi-rads?lang=us.
12. Vinnicombe S, Harvey H, Healy NA, Papalouka V, Schiller A, Moyle P, Kilburn-Toppin F, Allajbeu I, Sharma N, Maxwell AJ, Payne N, Graves M, Gilbert FJ. Introduction of an abbreviated breast MRI service in the UK as part of the BRAID trial: practicalities, challenges, and future directions. Clin Radiol. 2021;76(6):427–33.
13. Kerlikowske K, Grady D, Barclay J, Frankel SD, Ominsky SH, Sickles EA. Variability and accuracy in mammographic interpretation using the American College of Radiology breast imaging reporting and data system. J Natl Cancer Inst. 1998;90(23):1801–9.
14. Forrest P. Breast cancer screening: report to the health ministers of England, Wales, Scotland and Northern Ireland. London: Her Majesty's Stationery Office; 1986.
15. Assi V, Warwick J, Cuzick J, Duffy S. Clinical and epidemiological issues in mammographic density. Clin Oncol. 2012;9(1):33–40.
16. Boyd NF, Guo H, Martin LJ, Sun L, Stone J, Fishell E, Jong RA, Hislop G, Chiarelli A, Minkin S, Yaffe MJ. Mammographic density and the risk and detection of breast cancer. N Engl J Med. 2007;356(3):227–36.
17. Ting C, Astley SM, Morris J, Stavrinos P, Wilson M, Barr N, Boggis C, Sergeant JC. Longitudinal change in mammographic density and association with breast cancer risk: a case-control study. In: Maidment ADA, Bakic PR, Gavenonis S, editors. Breast imaging: international workshop on digital mammography. Lecture notes in computer science, vol. 7361. Berlin: Springer; 2012. p. 205–11.
18. Sergeant JC, Warwick J, Evans G, Howell A, Berks M, Stavrinos P, Sahin S, Wilson M, Hufton A, Buchan I, Astley SM. Volumetric and area based breast density measurement in the predicting risk of cancer at screening (PROCAS) study. In: Maidment ADA, Bakic PR, Gavenonis S, editors. Breast imaging: international workshop on digital mammography, lecture notes in computer science, vol. 7361. Berlin: Springer; 2012. p. 228–35.
19. Prevent Breast Cancer. Working towards a new screening process for breast cancer. https://preventbreastcancer.org.uk/breast-cancer-research/research-projects/early-detection-screening/procas/.
20. Oliver A. A novel breast tissue density classification methodology. Inf Technol Biomed. 2008;12(1):55–65.
21. Kopans DB. Breast imaging. 2nd ed. Philadelphia: Lippincott Williams and Wilkins; 1998.
22. Ryan S, McNicholas M, Eustace S. Anatomy for diagnostic imaging. 2nd ed. London: WB Saunders; 2007.
23. Wikipedia. Tamoxifen. https://en.wikipedia.org/wiki/Tamoxifen. Accessed 12 Aug 2021.
24. Breast Cancer Now. Hormone receptors and breast cancer. https://breastcancernow.org/information-support/facing-breast-cancer/diagnosed-breast-cancer/hormone-receptors-breast-cancer.
25. Shieh Y, Scott CG, Jensen MR, Norman AD, Bertrand KA, Pankratz VS, Brandt KR, Visscher DW, Shepherd JA, Tamimi RM, Vachon CM. Body mass index, mammographic density, and breast cancer risk by oestrogen receptor sub type. Breast Cancer Res. 2019;21(1):1–9.

26. Warburton ER, Nicol CW, Bredin SSD. Health benefits of physical activity: the evidence. CMAJ. 2006;174(6):801–9.
27. Brand JS, Czene K, Eriksson L, Trinh T, Bhoo-Pathy N, Hall P, Celebioglu F. Influence of lifestyle factors on mammographic density in postmenopausal women. PLoS One. 2013;8(12):e81876.
28. Cancer Research UK. Alcohol and cancer. https://www.cancerresearchuk.org/about-cancer/causes-of-cancer/alcohol-and-cancer.
29. Sutton D. Textbook of radiology and imaging, vol. 2. 7th ed. New York: Churchill Livingstone; 2003.
30. Tice JA, O'Meara ES, Weaver DL, Vachon C, Ballard-Barbash R, Kerlikowsk EK. Benign breast disease, mammographic breast density, and the risk of breast cancer. J Cancer Inst. 2013;105(14):1043–9.

Mammographic Density

5

Elaine F. Harkness and Sue M. Astley

Learning Objectives
- Develop an understanding of mammographic density
- Demonstrate knowledge of subjective, semi-automated and automated measures of mammographic density
- Demonstrate knowledge of artificial intelligence and mammographic density measurement

Introduction

We developed an understanding in the previous chapter (Chap. 4) of breast density. Within this chapter we will now refer to this as mammographic density and develop a deeper understanding of this area.

Mammographic density (MD) refers to the radiographic density of the breast [1]; the amount of parenchymal and connective tissue which appears white on the mammogram [1–7]. Cancerous tissue also appears white on a mammogram. Tumours can be difficult to perceive amongst dense tissue, thus lowering the sensitiv-

ity of mammography in dense versus fatty breasts. As a woman ages, particularly after the menopause, the breast tissue usually involutes, becoming more fatty, and the sensitivity of mammography typically increases. The risk of developing breast cancer is 4–5 times higher for women with the highest MD (>75% parenchyma) compared to women with the lowest MD (<25% parenchyma) or fatty breasts [8–10]. The increased risk is related to biological mechanisms [11–14] and decreased sensitivity of mammography (tumour masking effect) [15–17].

Until now, MD has mainly been used for risk estimation using an epidemiological approach [18–21]. However, in 2019 in the United States, it was proposed by the Food and Drug Administration (FDA) that all women attending for breast screening should receive information about their breast density together with their screening results [22]. Nevertheless, clinical application has been hampered by the inability to automatically and objectively measure MD, lack of MD incorporated in risk estimation models (however, this is becoming more commonplace) and limited options for additional or other screening tests for women with dense breasts. A wider understanding of the sensitivity of mammography in dense breasts is emerging, and supplementary imaging techniques such as digital breast tomosynthesis (DBT), whole breast ultrasound, contrast-enhanced mammography and magnetic resonance imaging (MRI) are considered important adjuncts [23–27]. Stratifying women for additional imaging and/or increased or

E. F. Harkness (✉) · S. M. Astley
Division of Informatics, Imaging and Data Sciences,
Faculty of Biology, Medicine and Health,
The University of Manchester, Manchester, UK
e-mail: Elaine.F.Harkness@manchester.ac.uk;
Sue.Astley@manchester.ac.uk

decreased screening intervals based on their MD might therefore be the future of breast screening programmes. Currently a number of clinical trials are underway to assess the impact of risk-stratified screening based on MD [28, 29] and MD in combination with other risk factors [30, 31].

Measuring Mammographic Density

MD can be measured subjectively [5, 32–41], semi-automatically [42, 43] or automatically [44–59]. Subjective measurement is usually performed by an image reader's visual assessment of the mammogram. Semi-automated measurement is performed by a reader and computer, while automated measurement is performed objectively, solely by computer, and requires a digital mammogram.

Subjective Classification

The first classification system for mammographic patterns was developed in 1967 by Wolfe [32]. The pattern was divided into four categories; N1, P1, P2, and DY depending on the predominant tissue composition: N1 indicates mammographic lucent tissue with no visible ducts and a low risk of breast cancer, P1 and P2 refer to linear densities associated with an intermediate degree of risk, P1 has mostly fatty tissue with ducts occupying up to a quarter of the breast volume, while P2 has ducts occupying more than a quarter of the breast volume. DY describes a breast with diffuse densities and represents a high risk of developing breast cancer.

Boyd described a six-class system (0%, 1 < 10%, 10 < 25%, 25 < 50%, 50 < 75% and >75%) for subjectively quantifying breast density; based purely on amount of dense tissue and containing no descriptors of distribution or pattern [2]. The method has been used widely and is related to breast cancer risk. Boyd demonstrated the potential for measures purely based on quantity of dense tissue and paved the way for later automated methods. The proportion of the breast area occupied by dense tissue has also been measured using subjective assessment with Visual

Analogue Scales (VAS): image readers mark the percent of dense tissue for each mammographic view on a VAS marked with 0 and 100% at each end of the scale. An average is then taken across all four mammographic views and across readers. This method has been used in several research studies and is related to risk of developing cancer, especially where both views are assessed, and for interval cancers [33, 60, 61].

In 1997, Laszlo Tabár introduced a five-point classification system [34] based on density and pattern. Mammograms were classified according to the proportion of four components: nodular density, linear density, homogeneous fibrous tissue, and radiolucent adipose tissue. Density I included mammograms with a balanced proportion of all components of breast tissue with a slight predominance of fibrous tissue; density II comprised predominantly fatty breasts; density III fatty tissue with retroareolar residual fibrous tissue; density IV nodular and fibrous tissue (dense breast) and density V included extensive homogeneous fibrosis. Patterns I, II and III were considered as low-risk, while patterns IV and V were considered as high-risk.

Today the 5th edition of the BI-RADS (Breast Imaging Reporting and Data System) of the American College of Radiology (ACR) is the most commonly used system for classification of MD [5]. BI-RADS 5th edition is based on subjective visual assessment of the breast composition of the mammogram. Category A refers to almost entirely fatty tissue; B to scattered areas of fibroglandular density; C to heterogeneously dense breast tissue, which could obscure detection of small masses, and D to extremely dense breast tissue, which lowers the sensitivity of mammography. Categories A and B are considered as non-dense, while categories C and D are considered dense. Despite the quantitative and objective definitions, these measurements and assessments are highly subjective and show significant intra (within) and inter (between) observer variability [35–41, 62–65]. Due to the subjectivity and labour-intensive nature of these methods, semi-automated and automated objective techniques have been developed.

Semi-Automated Methods

Developing semi-automated methods, also known as computer-assisted methods, was a natural progression to decrease the subjective nature of visual assessment of MD. Computer-assisted methods require mammograms in a digital form. Since most computer-assisted measurement predated the widespread use of Full Field Digital Mammography (FFDM), such methods involved a digitisation step, where film images were scanned and converted to pixels, each of which has an associated grey level. The most widely used computer assisted methods are Madena [42] and Cumulus [43]. Semi-automated methods require the operator to delineate the breast by applying a threshold to the pixel values, allowing correction and removal of the pectoral muscle area where necessary, and then selecting a further threshold to separate dense fibroglandular areas from fatty regions. The output gives the percentage density based on the relative proportion of the breast area occupied by dense tissue, and an absolute area of density.

Cumulus has been widely used and was regarded as the gold standard for density assessment for many years due to its unequivocal relationship with breast cancer risk. Despite this, it suffers from the limitations of being subjective (since the user defines the threshold for each image), labour intensive and area-based. Mammograms are projection images, and the area of density depends on the compression of the breast. More recent versions of Cumulus using increasingly higher thresholds (Altocumulus and Cirrocumulus) have been developed for FFDM [66] but are still operator dependent.

Automated Methods

The introduction of FFDM brought the opportunity to compute breast density directly from images without human intervention. The appearance of a mammogram depends on the physical properties of the breast tissue, the X-ray spectrum and exposure factors, properties of the detector and any image processing that has been applied. Automated methods aim to eliminate variability in mammographic appearance attributable to the imaging process and thus measure the fatty and dense tissue (including glandular tissue, the acinar and ductal epithelium and associated stroma, all of which have similar X-ray attenuation properties) in the breast.

More recent automated methods have been based on artificial intelligence (AI) applications. AI applications are computer-based methods used to mimic human behavior, which may include machine and deep learning techniques, and may incorporate additional mammographic features. Automated methods can be 'area' or 'volume' based and generally output a relative measure (the proportion of the breast area/volume occupied by dense tissue) as well as absolute area/volume of dense and/or fatty tissue. A number of automated methods also produce BI-RADS like categories. Several methods are available commercially and have been approved by the US Food and Drug Administration (FDA) whilst others are available for research purposes only.

Area-Based Measures

Several fully automated area-based measures have been developed since the introduction of FFDM. These methods use the 2D area-based image from the mammogram. The algorithms work in different ways with the majority of area-based methods using processed or 'for presentation' images. The most commonly used, and commercially available, area-based methods include Densitas®densitasai™ [54, 67] and DenSeeMammo® [57]. Both use an AI-based approach with DenSeeMammo® using a "nearest neighbor" imaging comparison method based on a large reference database of images assessed by radiologists, to classify mammograms into BIRADS fifth edition categories [57]. DM-Densitas ™ is an area-based approach that has recently been replaced by Densitas®Densityai™ that uses a deep learning approach based on image features to output a percentage density as well as a qualitative assessment based on BI-RADS categories [67]. PowerLook® [68] (previously iReveal®) is also a commercially available and FDA approved software that uses deep learning for assessing synthetic 2D mammograms from digital breast tomosynthesis (DBT) and providing a BI-RADS category.

Area based measures predominantly used in research include AutoDensity [69], an Image-J based method [70], Stratus [59] and LIBRA [55, 71]. All methods produce a continuous measure of percentage density and use the 'for presentation' images, with the exception of LIBRA, which can estimate breast density from both the 'for presentation' or 'for processing' images and is freely available [71]. Stratus produces BI-RADS like categories and includes an alignment protocol to improve the assessment of change in density over time. Some methods provide output across single vendors whilst others have been validated across multiple vendor types. Several area-based methods work in the same way as Cumulus, segmenting fibroglandular from fatty tissue (e.g. AutoDensity, Image-J, LIBRA), whilst others project the 2D information into 3D space and others are based on machine learning approaches [72]. In addition, some algorithms incorporate other aspects of the mammogram, such as texture.

Volumetric Measures

Volumetric methods generally use the raw 'for processing' FFDM using either calibration or physics-based approaches. In calibration-based methods (Cumulus V [44, 45], Single X-ray Absorptiometry [46], and the Manchester Method [47]) an object such as a stepwedge calibration using tissue-equivalent material is imaged. The calibration enables accurate density measurement, but the requirement of imaging a calibration object and the inability to retrospectively analyse images acquired without one, represent disadvantages. In the physics-based methods (e.g. Quantra™ [48], Volpara™ [49] and Insight BD [56]) knowledge about tissue attenuation

coefficients and the physics of the imaging process are used. All methods require knowledge of compressed breast thickness; whilst this is relatively straightforward in the region where the breast is in contact with the compression plate, it is much more difficult to accurately measure the uncompressed breast edge. However, since this region mainly comprises skin and subcutaneous structures with little dense tissue, such inaccuracies do not usually have a great impact on overall density measures.

All three physics-based methods are fully automatic and can be used prospectively or retrospectively, provided that raw ('for processing') mammogram data are available. Insight BD has been specifically developed for the Siemens MAMMOMAT Revelation mammography machine, with breast density results available immediately. Volpara™ and Quantra™ can be used with multiple vendors. They all produce BI-RADS categories as well as volume of fibroglandular (dense) tissue, total breast area and a continuous measure of percent density. The methods have been validated and are currently in use both clinically and for research purposes. Volpara™ and Insight BD use a relative physics model, similar to that described by van Engeland et al. in 2006 [53]. This has the advantage of reducing the need for accurate imaging physics data, but depends on identifying a suitable fatty reference area within the image [52, 53]. Volumetric measures of breast density such as these are intuitively better at describing breast composition than area-based methods (which are susceptible to variation depending on the positioning and compression of the breast) or subjective techniques, which demonstrate significant inter-observer variability.

Additional artificial intelligence, including machine and deep learning techniques, have been developed more recently to assess MD. Models are trained to learn variability in appearance of mammogram images and a particular outcome (e.g. percent MD or BI-RADS classification). Machine learning techniques require large datasets for model training and testing. There are currently several FDA approved applications for assessing MD that incorporate an AI approach [73] including Quantra™, DM-Densitas and DenSeeMammo® as described above, which were all approved pre-2019. More recent AI applications include Densitas®densityai™ (which has replaced DM-Densitas) [67], WRDensity (Whiterabbit AI) [58, 74], Visage Breast Density (Visage Imaging) [75], PowerLook (iCAD) [68], and Volpara TruDensity™ (Volpara Health) [49]. The majority of AI applications have been trained to produce BI-RADS like categories since reporting MD has become particularly important in the United States where all states have mandatory breast density notification for patients [22]. Densitas®densityai™ and Volpara TruDensity™ also produce a continuous percentage density measure.

Other AI methods have been used in research studies to estimate MD [76–78]. Deep-LIBRA uses convolutional neural networks to segment the breast area and to further differentiate dense and non-dense tissue in the breast [76]. Kallenberg et al. segmented the MD but also incorporated mammographic texture [77] and Ionescu used convolutional neural networks to mimic reader VAS (predicted VAS or PVAS) to estimate MD [78]. Many other researchers have developed AI methods to predict breast cancer risk directly using features from mammographic images [79–82].

Validation data linking increased density to risk of developing cancer has used all types of methods (subjective, semi-automated and auto-mated). Availability of longitudinal data sets using FFDM images is becoming more widely available and the use of cancer-free prior mammograms enables researchers to establish the temporal relationship. However, measurement of change in mammographic images is difficult due to differences in breast positioning and imaging parameters. Stratus, developed by the Karolinska Institutet, has decreased the variability in density change from repeated mammograms over time using an image alignment protocol [59].

The majority of breast density methods (subjective, area, volumetric) tend to demonstrate an increased risk of developing breast cancer with increased MD, demonstrating both a clear dose-response and temporal relationship [60, 83, 84]. However, there is significant disagreement between automated methods and human readers, and even between automated measures themselves [85, 86]. Thus, identifying women with the highest breast density and consequently the highest risk of breast cancer varies according to the measurement method used [87]. Machine learning techniques also demonstrate promise, in terms of their relationship to the risk of developing breast cancer, indeed many machine learning techniques incorporating mammographic images for risk prediction show improved performance compared to non-AI approaches [77, 78, 88]. These methods are likely to be an additional viable option for risk-based stratification in the future.

Increasingly, MD is used in breast cancer risk prediction models. For example, the Tyrer-Cuzick risk assessment model can incorporate MD based on BI-RADS, VAS and Volpara™ [89], while the Breast Cancer Surveilllance Consortium (BCSC) [90] and CanRisk [91] risk models incorporate MD based on BI-RADS assessment. Results from current clinical trials stratifying women to different screening protocols based on their MD (and MD plus other classical risk factors) will be important in determining the benefit of a personalised screening approach.

Acknowledgments The authors would like to acknowledge the two previous authors of this chapter from the first edition: Solveig S.H. Hofvind and Gunvor Gipling Waade. This research was supported by the Manchester National Institute for Health Research (NIHR) Biomedical Research Centre (IS-BRC-1215-20007).

Appendix

Test your learning and check your understanding of this book's contents: use the "Springer Nature Flashcards" app to access questions using https://sn.pub/dcAnWL.

To use the app, please follow the instructions in Chap. 1.

Flashcard code: 48341-69945-ABCB1-2A8C7-CE9D2.

Short URL: https://sn.pub/dcAnWL.

References

1. Kopans D. Breast imaging. 3rd ed. London: Lippincott Williams & Wilkins; 2007.
2. Boyd NF, Byng JW, Jong RA, Fishell EK, Little LE, Miller AB, Lockwood GA, Tritchler DL, Yaffe MJ. Quantitative classification of mammographic densities and breast cancer risk: results from the Canadian National Breast Screening Study. J Natl Cancer Inst. 1995;87(9):670–5.
3. Ginsburg OM, Martin LJ, Boyd NF. Mammographic density, lobular involution, and risk of breast cancer. Br J Cancer. 2008;99(9):1369–74.
4. Vachon CM, van Gils CH, Sellers TA, Ghosh K, Pruthi S, Brandt KR, Pankratz VS. Mammographic density, breast cancer risk and risk prediction. Breast Cancer Res. 2007;9(6):1–9.
5. Sickles EA, D'Orsi CJ, Bassett LW. American College of Radiology, et al. ACR BI-RADS® mammography. In: ACR BI-RADS® atlas, breast imaging reporting and data system. Reston: American College of Radiology; 2013.
6. White J. Breast density and cancer risk: what is the relationship? J Natl Cancer Inst. 2000;92(6):443.
7. Alonzo-Proulx O, Jong R, Yaffe MJ. Volumetric breast density characteristics as determined from digital mammograms. Phys Med Biol. 2012;57(22):7443–57.
8. McCormack V, dos Santos SI. Breast density and parenchymal patterns as markers of breast cancer risk: a meta-analysis. Cancer Epidemiol Biomarkers Prev. 2006;15(6):1159–69.
9. Ursin G, Ma H, Wu AH, et al. Mammographic density and breast cancer in three ethnic groups. Cancer Epidemiol Biomarkers Prev. 2003;12(4):332–8.
10. Shepherd JA, Kerlikowske K, Ma L, Duewer F, Fan B, Wang J, Malkov S, Vittinghoff E, Cummings SR. Volume of mammographic density and risk of breast cancer. Cancer Epidemiol Biomarkers Prev. 2011;20(7):1473–82.
11. Lisanti MP, Reeves K, Peiris-Pagès M, Chadwick AL, Sanchez-Alvarez R, Howell A, Martinez-Outschoorn UE, Sotgia F. JNK1 stress signaling is hyper-activated in high breast density and the tumor stroma: connecting fibrosis, inflammation, and stemness for cancer prevention. Cell Cycle. 2014;13(4):580–99.
12. Sherratt MJ, McConnell JC, Streuli CH. Raised mammographic density: causative mechanisms and biological consequences. Breast Cancer Res. 2016;18(1):1–9.
13. Archer M, Dasari P, Evdokiou A, Ingman WV. Biological mechanisms and therapeutic opportunities in mammographic density and breast cancer risk. Cancer. 2021;13(21):5391.
14. Ironside AJ, Jones J. Stromal characteristics may hold the key to mammographic density: the evidence to date. Oncotarget. 2016;7:31550–62.
15. Checka CM, Chun JE, Schnabel FR, Lee J, Toth H. The relationship of mammographic density and age: implications for breast cancer screening. AJR Am J Roentgenol. 2012;198(3):W292–5.
16. Destounis S, Johnston L, Highnam R, Arieno A, Morgan R, Chan A. Using volumetric breast density to quantify the potential masking risk of mammographic density. Am J Roentgenol. 2017 Jan;208(1):222–7.
17. Rossi P, Djuric O, Hélin V, Astley S, Mantellini P, Nitrosi A, Harkness EF, Gauthier E, Puliti D, Balleyguier C, Baron C. Validation of a new fully automated software for 2D digital mammographic breast density evaluation in predicting breast cancer risk. Sci Rep. 2021;11(1):1–8.
18. Boyd NF, Martin LJ, Bronskill M, Yaffe MJ, Duric N, Minkin S. Breast tissue composition and susceptibility to breast cancer. J Natl Cancer Inst. 2010;102(16):1224–37.
19. Highnam R, Sauber N, Destounis S, Harvey J, McDonald D. In: Maidment A, Bakic P, Gavenonis S, editors. Breast density into clinical practice in breast imaging. Berlin/Heidelberg: Springer; 2012. p. 466–73.
20. Evans DG, Astley S, Stavrinos P, Harkness E, Donnelly LS, Dawe S, Jacob I, Harvie M, Cuzick J, Brentnall A, Wilson M. Improvement in risk prediction, early detection and prevention of breast cancer in the NHS Breast Screening Programme and family history clinics: a dual cohort study. Southampton: NIHR Journals Library; 2016.
21. Gabrielson M, Eriksson M, Hammarström M, Borgquist S, Leifland K, Czene K, Hall P. Cohort profile: the Karolinska mammography project for risk prediction of breast cancer (KARMA). Int J Epidemiol. 2017;46(6):1740–1.
22. Are You Dense Advocacy, Inc. http://www.areyoudenseadvocacy.org/.
23. Rebolj M, Assi V, Brentnall A, Parmar D, Duffy SW. Addition of ultrasound to mammography in the case of dense breast tissue: systematic review and meta-analysis. Br J Cancer. 2018;118(12):1559–70.
24. Yuan WH, Hsu HC, Chen YY, Wu CH. Supplemental breast cancer-screening ultrasonography in women with dense breasts: a systematic review and meta-analysis. Br J Cancer. 2020;123:673–88.
25. Phi XA, Tagliafico A, Houssami N, Greuter MJW, de Bock GH. Digital breast tomosynthesis for breast cancer screening and diagnosis in women with dense breasts—a systematic review and meta-analysis. BMC Cancer. 2018;18(1):1–9.
26. Melnikow J, Fenton JJ, Whitlock EP, Miglioretti DL, Weyrich MS, Thompson JH, Shah K. Supplemental screening for breast cancer in women with dense breasts: a systematic review for the U.S. preventive services task force. Ann Intern Med. 2016;164(4):268–78.
27. Hadadi I, Rae W, Clarke J, McEntee M, Ekpo E. Diagnostic performance of adjunctive imaging modalities compared to mammography alone in women with non-dense and dense breasts: a systematic review and meta-analysis. Clin Breast Cancer. 2021;21:278–91.
28. Vinnicombe S, Harvey H, Healy NA, Papalouka V, Schiller A, Moyle P, Kilburn-Toppin F, Allajbeu I,

Sharma N, Maxwell AJ, Payne N. Introduction of an abbreviated breast MRI service in the UK as part of the BRAID trial: practicalities, challenges, and future directions. Clin Radiol. 2021;76(6):427–33.

29. Bakker MF, de Lange SV, Pijnappel RM, Mann RM, Peeters PH, Monninkhof EM, Emaus MJ, Loo CE, Bisschops RH, Lobbes MB, de Jong MD. Supplemental MRI screening for women with extremely dense breast tissue. N Engl J Med. 2019;381(22):2091–102.

30. Shieh Y, Eklund M, Madlensky L, Sawyer SD, Thompson CK, Stover Fiscalini A, Ziv E, van't Veer LJ, Esserman LJ, Tice JA, Athena Breast Health Network Investigators. Breast cancer screening in the precision medicine era: risk-based screening in a population-based trial. J Natl Cancer Inst. 2017;109(5):djw290.

31. ClinicalTrials.gov. My Personalized Breast Screening (MyPeBS). https://clinicaltrials.gov/ct2/show/NCT 03672331?term=mypebs&rank=1. Accessed 30 Jan 2022.

32. Wolfe JN. Breast patterns as an index of risk for developing breast cancer. AJR Am J Roentgenol. 1976;126(6):1130–7.

33. Duffy SW, Nagtegaal ID, Astley SM, Gillan MG, McGee MA, Boggis CR, Wilson M, Beetles UM, Griffiths MA, Jain AK, Johnson J. Visually assessed breast density, breast cancer risk and the importance of the craniocaudal view. Breast Cancer Res. 2008;10(4):1–7.

34. Gram IT, Funkhouser E, Tabár L. The Tabár classification of mammographic parenchymal patterns. Eur J Radiol. 1997;24(2):131–6.

35. Gram IT, Bremnes Y, Ursin G, Maskarinec G, Bjurstam N, Lund E. Percentage density, Wolfe's and Tabár's mammographic patterns: agreement and association with risk factors for breast cancer. Breast Cancer Res. 2005;7(5):54–61.

36. Berg WA, Campassi C, Langenberg P, Sexton MJ. Breast imaging reporting and data system: inter and intra observer variability in feature analysis and final assessment. Am J Roentgenol. 2000;174(6):1769–77.

37. Weigert J, Steenbergen S. The Connecticut experiment: the role of ultrasound in the screening of women with dense breasts. Breast J. 2012;18(6):517–22.

38. Harvey JA, Bovbjerg VE. Quantitative assessment of mammographic breast density: relationship with breast cancer risk. Radiology. 2004;230(1):29–41.

39. Ciatto S, Visioli C, Paci E, Zappa M. Breast density as a determinant of interval cancer at mammographic screening. Br J Cancer. 2004;90(2):393–6.

40. Martin KE, Helvie MA, Zhou C, Roubidoux MA, Bailey JE, Paramagul C, Blane CE, Klein KA, Sonnad SS, Chan HP. Mammographic density measured with quantitative computer-aided method: comparison with radiologists' estimates and BI-RADS categories. Radiology. 2006;240(3):656–65.

41. Ren B, Smith AP, Marshall J. Investigation of practical scoring methods for breast density in digital mammography. In: Martí J, Oliver A, Freixenet J, Martí R, editors. 10th international workshop, IWDM 2010, Girona, Catalonia, 2010 June 16–18. Berlin/Heidelberg: Springer; 2010. p. 651–8.

42. Ursin G, Astrahan MA, Salane M, Parisky YR, Pearce JG, Daniels JR, Pike MC, Spicer DV. The detection of changes in mammographic densities. Cancer Epidemiol Prev Biomarkers. 1998;7(1):43–7.

43. Byng JW, Boyd NF, Fishell E, Jong RA, Yaffe MJ. The quantitative analysis of mammographic densities. Phys Med Biol. 1994;39:1629–38.

44. Pawluczyk O, Augustine BJ, Yaffe MJ, Rico D, Yang J, Mawdsley GE, Boyd NF. A volumetric method for estimation of breast density on digitized screen-film mammograms. Med Phys. 2003;30(3):352–64.

45. Yaffe MJ, Boone JM, Packard N, Alonzo-Proulx O, Huang SY, Peressotti CL, Al-Mayah A, Brock K. The myth of the 50–50 breast. Med Phys. 2009;36(12):5437–43.

46. Malkov S, Wang J, Kerlikowske K, Cummings SR, Shepherd JA. Single x-ray absorptiometry method for the quantitative mammographic measure of fibroglandular tissue volume. Med Phys. 2009;36(12):5525–36.

47. Diffey J, Hufton A, Astley S. A new step-wedge for the volumetric measurement of mammographic density. In: Astley SM, Brady M, Rose C, Zwiggelaar R, editors. Digital mammography. IWDM 2006, LNCS 4046. Berlin: Springer; 2006. p. 1–9.

48. Hologic, Inc. Hologic-Quantra 2.2 Breast Density Assessment. https://healthcare-in-europe.com/en/radbook/it/1808-hologic-quantra-2-2-breast-density-assessment.html. Accessed 30 Jan 2022.

49. Volpara Health. TruDensity™. https://www.volpara-health.com/science/algorithms/density/. Accessed 30 Jan 2022.

50. Highnam RP, Brady M. Mammographic image analysis. Dordrecht: Academic; 1999.

51. Hartman K, Highnam R, Warren R, Jackson V. Volumetric assessment of breast tissue composition from FFDM images. In: Proceedings of IWDM 2008, LNCS 5116. Berlin: Springer; 2008. p. 33–9.

52. Highnam R, Brady M, Yaffe MJ, Karssemeijer N, Harvey J. Robust breast composition measurement—VolparaTM. In: Proceedings of IWDM 2010, LNCS 6136. Berlin: Springer; 2010. p. 342–9.

53. Van Engeland S, Snoeren PR, Huisman H, Boetes C, Karssemeijer N. Volumetric breast density estimation from full field digital mammograms. IEEE Trans Med Imaging. 2006;25(3):273–82.

54. Abdolell M, Tsuruda K, Schaller G, Caines J. Statistical evaluation of a fully automated mammographic breast density algorithm. Comput Math Methods Med. 2013;2013:651091.

55. Keller BM, Nathan DL, Wang Y, Zheng Y, Gee JC, Conant EF, Kontos D. Estimation of breast percent density in raw and processed full field digital mammography images via adaptive fuzzy c-means clustering and support vector machine segmentation. Med Phys. 2012;39(8):4903–17.

56. Fieselmann A, Jerebko A, Mertelmeier T. Volumetric breast density combined with masking risk: enhanced characterization of breast density from mammography images. In: Tingberg A, Lång K, Timberg P, editors. Breast imaging IWDM 2016, LNCS 9699. Cham: Springer International; 2016. p. 486–92.

57. Balleyguier C, Arfi-Rouche J, Boyer B, Gauthier E, Helin V, Loshkajian A, Ragusa S, Delaloge S. A new automated method to evaluate 2D mammographic breast density according to BI-RADS® atlas fifth edition recommendations. Eur Radiol. 2019;29(7):3830–8.

58. Matthews TP, Singh S, Mombourquette B, Su J, Shah MP, Pedemonte S, Long A, Maffit D, Gurney J, Hoil RM, Ghare N. A multisite study of a breast density deep learning model for full-field digital mammography and synthetic mammography. Radiology. 2020;3(1):e200015.

59. Eriksson M, Li J, Leifland K, Czene K, Hall P. A comprehensive tool for measuring mammographic density changes over time. Breast Cancer Res Treat. 2018;169(2):371–9.

60. Astley SM, Harkness EF, Sergeant JC, Warwick J, Stavrinos P, Warren R, Wilson M, Beetles U, Gadde S, Lim Y, Jain A. A comparison of five methods of measuring mammographic density: a case-control study. Breast Cancer Res. 2018;20(1):1–3.

61. Burnside ES, Warren LM, Myles J, Wilkinson LS, Wallis MG, Patel M, Smith RA, Young KC, Massat NJ, Duffy SW. Quantitative breast density analysis to predict interval and node-positive cancers in pursuit of improved screening protocols: a case–control study. Br J Cancer. 2021;125(6):884–92.

62. Portnow LH, Georgian-Smith D, Haider I, Barrios M, Bay CP, Nelson KP, Raza S. Persistent inter-observer variability of breast density assessment using BI-RADS® 5th edition guidelines. Clin Imaging. 2021;83:21–7.

63. Pesce K, Tajerian M, Chico MJ, Swiecicki MP, Boietti B, Frangella MJ, Benitez S. Interobserver and intraobserver variability in determining breast density according to the fifth edition of the BI-RADS® atlas. Radiologia. 2020;62(6):481–6.

64. Alomaim W, O'Leary D, Ryan J, Rainford L, Evanoff M, Foley S. Variability of breast density classification between US and UK radiologists. J Med Imaging Radiat Sci. 2019;50(1):53–61.

65. Ang T, Harkness EF, Maxwell AJ, Lim YY, Emsley R, Howell A, Evans DG, Astley S, Gadde S. Visual assessment of breast density using Visual Analogue Scales: observer variability, reader attributes and reading time. [Lecture] SPIE. Accessed 10 Mar 2017.

66. Nguyen TL, Aung YK, Evans CF, Dite GS, Stone J, MacInnis RJ, Dowty JG, Bickerstaffe A, Aujard K, Rommens JM, Song YM. Mammographic density defined by higher than conventional brightness thresholds better predicts breast cancer risk. Int J Epidemiol. 2017;46(2):652–61.

67. Densitas. Align with ACR BI-RADS Atlas breast density scales. https://densitas.health/solutions/density/. Accessed 30 Jan 2022.

68. iCAD. The Power of Deep Learning. https://www.icadmed.com/powerlook-density-assessment.html. Accessed 30 Jan 2022.

69. Nickson C, Arzhaeva Y, Aitken Z, Elgindy T, Buckley M, Li M, English DR, Kavanagh AM. AutoDensity: an automated method to measure mammographic breast density that predicts breast cancer risk and screening outcomes. Breast Cancer Res. 2013;15(5):1–2.

70. Li J, Szekely L, Eriksson L, Heddson B, Sundbom A, Czene K, Hall P, Humphreys K. High-throughput mammographic-density measurement: a tool for risk prediction of breast cancer. Breast Cancer Res. 2012;14(4):1–2.

71. Perelman. Laboratory for individualized breast radiodensity assessment. https://www.med.upenn.edu/sbia/libra.html. Accessed 30 Jan 2022.

72. Destounis S, Arieno A, Morgan R, Roberts C, Chan A. Qualitative versus quantitative mammographic breast density assessment: applications for the US and abroad. Diagnostics. 2017;7(2):30.

73. Bahl M. Updates in artificial intelligence for breast imaging. Semin Roentgenol. 2022;57:160–7. https://doi.org/10.1053/j.ro.2021.12.005.

74. Whiterabbit.ai. Artificial intelligence driven breast density software. https://www.whiterabbit.ai/products/wrdensity. Accessed 30 Jan 2022.

75. Mills T. Division Director. Personal communication. https://www.accessdata.fda.gov/cdrh_docs/pdf20/K201411.pdf. Accessed 21 Dec 2020.

76. Maghsoudi OH, Gastounioti A, Christopher Scott C, Pantalone L, Wu FF, Cohen EA, Winham S, Conant EF, Vachon C, Kontos D. Deep-LIBRA: an artificial-intelligence method for robust quantification of breast density with independent validation in breast cancer risk assessment. Med Image Anal. 2021;73:102138.

77. Kallenberg M, Petersen K, Neilson M, Ng AY, Diao P, Igel C, Vachon CM, Holland K, Winkel RR, Karssemeijer N, Lillholm M. Unsupervised deep learning applied to breast density segmentation and mammographic risk scoring. IEEE Trans Med Imaging. 2016;35(5):1322–31.

78. Ionescu GV, Fergie M, Berks M, Harkness EF, Hulleman J, Brentnall AR, Cuzick J, Evans DG, Astley SM. Prediction of reader estimates of mammographic density using convolutional neural networks. J Med Imaging (Bellingham). 2019;6(3):031405. https://doi.org/10.1117/1.JMI.6.3.031405.

79. Dembrower K, Liu Y, Azizpour H, Eklund M, Smith K, Lindholm P, Strand F. Comparison of a deep learning risk score and standard mammographic density score for breast cancer risk prediction. Radiology. 2020;294(2):265–72.

80. Yala A, Lehman C, Schuster T, Portnoi T, Barzilay R. A deep learning mammography-based model for improved breast cancer risk prediction. Radiology. 2019;292(1):60–6.

81. Ha R, Chang P, Karcich J, Mutasa S, Van Sant EP, Liu MZ, Jambawalikar S. Convolutional neural network based breast cancer risk stratification using a mammographic dataset. Acad Radiol. 2019;26(4):544–9.

82. Schmidt DF, Makalic E, Goudey B, Dite GS, Stone J, Nguyen TL, Dowty JG, Baglietto L, Southey MC, Maskarinec G, Giles GG. Cirrus: an automated mammography-based measure of breast cancer risk based on textural features. JNCI Cancer Spectr. 2018;2(4):pky057.

83. Eng A, Gallant Z, Shepherd J, McCormack V, Li J, Dowsett M, Vinnicombe S, Allen S, dos-Santos-Silva I. Digital mammographic density and breast cancer risk: a case–control study of six alternative density assessment methods. Breast Cancer Res. 2014;16(5):1–2.

84. Patterson J, Stinton C, Alkhudairy L, Grove A, Royle P, Fraser H, Mistry H, Senaratne P, Clarke A, Taylor-Phillips S. Additional screening with ultrasound after negative mammography screening in women with dense breasts: a systematic review. https://warwick.ac.uk/fac/sci/med/research/hscience/pet/screening/evidence/breast_ultrasound_and_density_report_2018_-_warwick.pdf. Accessed 30 Jan 2022.

85. Brandt KR, Scott CG, Ma L, Mahmoudzadeh AP, Jensen MR, Whaley DH, Wu FF, Malkov S, Hruska CB, Norman AD, Heine J. Comparison of clinical and automated breast density measurements: implications for risk prediction and supplemental screening. Radiology. 2016;279(3):710–9.

86. Youk JH, Gweon HM, Son EJ, Kim JA. Automated volumetric breast density measurements in the era of the BI-RADS fifth edition: a comparison with visual assessment. AJR Am J Roentgenol. 2016;206(5):1056–62.

87. Hee JRWS, Harkness EF, Gadde S, Lim YY, Maxwell AJ, Evans DG, Howell A, Astley SM. Does the prediction of breast cancer improve using a combination of mammographic density measures compared to individual measures alone? In: Proceedings SPIE 10134 Medical Imaging; 2017.

88. Arefan D, Mohamed AA, Berg WA, Zuley ML, Sumkin JH, Wu S. Deep learning modeling using normal mammograms for predicting breast cancer risk. Med Phys. 2020;47(1):110–8.

89. https://ems-trials.org/riskevaluator/

90. BCSC. Risk Calculator V2. https://tools.bcsc-scc.org/BC5yearRisk/ calculator.htm. Accessed 30 Jan 2022.

91. University of Cambridge. CanRisk. https://www.canrisk.org/. Accessed 30 Jan 2022.

Aetiology and Epidemiology of Breast Cancer

6

Lisa Hackney

Learning Objectives
- Demonstrate an understanding of the variance in incidence rates and mortality rates of breast cancer worldwide
- Identify the risk factors associated with the development of breast cancer
- Explain the relative importance of the various risk factors

Introduction

Multiple risk factors are associated with increasing an individual's probability of developing breast cancer [1–3]. Numerous genes are involved in controlling the process of normal cell division. This process requires an equilibrium of activity between the genes that stimulate and suppress cell proliferation and those that signify when damaged cells should undergo apoptosis, a form of controlled cell death. Cancerous cells develop once mutations accumulate in the genes responsible for cell proliferation [4]. Breast cancer is a heterogeneous disease with multiple subtypes [5]. Changes in risk factors have led to an increase in the incidence of the disease [6].

How Common Is Breast Cancer?

Breast cancer represents the most common female cancer worldwide [7]. Figures from the worldwide cancer data confirm that there were 2,261,419 new cases of breast cancer diagnosed in 2020 (represents 24.5% of all female cancers) and 0.6 million deaths from the disease globally. Although hereditary and genetic factors account for 5% to 10% of breast cancer cases [8], non-hereditary factors are considered the leading cause of the international and interethnic variation in incidence [9]. Higher incidence rates in some countries are attributed to a higher prevalence of established risk factors and increases in breast cancer screening and awareness.

Breast cancer is undoubtedly the commonest female cancer in the UK with 55,545 invasive cancers diagnosed in 2018 [10] and 11,512 related deaths. The International Agency for Research on Cancer [11] predicts a rise in incidence in the UK from 55,439 cases to 66,612 (+20.2%) between 2018 and 2040. However, mortality rates in the UK are estimated to fall by 26% (period 2014–2035) [10], with reductions attributed to improved detection, earlier diagnosis via screening and more effective treatments delivered by specialist multi-disciplinary teams [12, 13].

L. Hackney (✉)
New Alderley House, Macclesfield District General Hospital, Macclesfield, Cheshire, UK
e-mail: Lisa.hackney@nhs.net

Lifetime Risk (Females)

Lifetime risk refers to the chance a person has of developing or dying from cancer over their lifetime (from birth to death). Risk estimates are based upon current incidence and mortality rates, but an individual's risk may be higher or lower than the population risk as genetic and lifestyle factors are influential. Cancer Research UK [10] reported that in 2017, the lifetime risk of developing breast cancer is 1 in 7 for women.

Risk Factors for Breast Cancer

Risk factors are merely an indicator and not a certainty that an individual will develop the disease. Some women may have multiple risk factors and never have breast cancer, whilst many women diagnosed have no attributable risk factors. Some risk factors are unalterable (i.e., gender or age), but others are controllable and linked to the environment and personal lifestyle. Certain risk factors

are more influential than others, and an individual's risk for breast cancer will change over time.

Biological Risk

Gender

Being female is the main risk factor for developing breast cancer. Although men do develop the disease, the incidence rates are very low in comparison, comprising of 0.5–1% of all patients with breast cancer [14]. Cancer Research UK reports that 387 men were diagnosed with breast cancer in the UK in 2017, with rates remaining stable over the last 24 years [10]. As with females, breast cancer incidence is strongly associated with increasing age [15]. The strongest risk factor for this disease in men is a mutation of the *BRCA2* gene [15].

Age

After gender, the most influential risk factor for breast cancer in women is age [16]. Figure 6.1

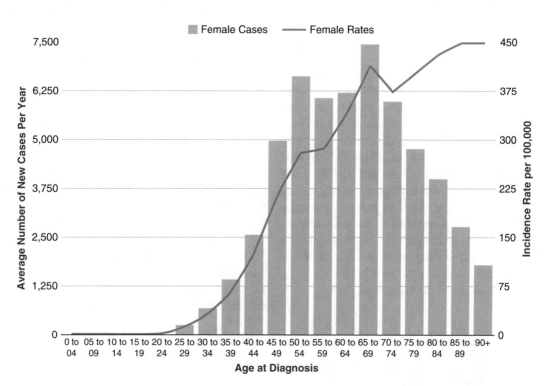

Fig. 6.1 Demonstrating the average number of new cases per year and age-specific incidence rates per 100,000 females, 2016–2018. (*Source: Cancer Research UK,* www.cancerresearchuk.org/health-professional/cancer-statistics/statistics-by-cancer-type/breast-cancer/incidence-invasive#heading-One/Nov2021)

from Cancer Research UK (2016–2018) demonstrates a plateau after 50–54 when breast screening is first routinely offered and relates to detecting prevalent cases.

The data demonstrates that almost half (48%) of female breast cancer cases are diagnosed in women in the 50–69 age group. This contributed to the original rationale underpinning the UK NHS Breast Screening Programme, which invites women in the 50–70 age group for screening every 3 years. The AgeX is a nationwide randomised controlled trial to establish if extending the age range (47–73 years) is beneficial [17]. The trial commenced in 2009, but the information is not expected until the mid-2020s. The trial received ethical approval for three yearly invitations for ages 71–76 or 71–79 to evaluate the effects of continuous screening after 70. However, routine screening was suspended in the UK in March 2020 due to COVID19. Therefore, the trial investigators decided there would be no further randomisation as the pandemic created a considerable backlog on breast screening services.

The incidence of breast cancer in young women (i.e., teenagers until 30 years old) is uncommon [18]. However, it remains the main cancer diagnosed in women under 40 and often presents at an advanced stage [18].

Endogenous Factors

Endogenous sex hormones (oestrogens, androgens and Anti-Mullerian Hormone (AMH) are also considered to influence risk [19]. Studies undertaken in postmenopausal women demonstrate an increased breast cancer risk in those with the highest levels of circulating concentrations of sex hormones compared to those with the lowest levels [19–21]. Less data is available for premenopausal women. A meta-analysis undertaken in 2011 [22] reported no significant association with premenopausal breast cancer risk and oestrogen levels. AMH concentrations were also not found to have a strong correlation [23, 24]. However, measurements of hormones in premenopausal women are complex as there are substantial variations in concentrations through a menstrual cycle.

Breast Density

The Breast Imaging Reporting and Data System (BI-RADS) visually estimates the breast composition. Various studies have established that women with high-density breast tissue (>75% glandular tissue) have a higher risk (4–6 times) of developing a breast carcinoma compared to those with a low breast density (<5% glandular tissue) [25, 26]. A 2017 study [27] affirmed that high breast density was considered the predominant risk factor equally for premenopausal and postmenopausal women representing the main effect on population-attributable risk proportion of breast cancer. Several contributory factors affect breast density, e.g., age, endogenous hormones, menopausal status, body mass index (BMI), parity and genetics [28–30]. The other main problem associated with a high breast density is that the mammographic sensitivity is reduced, as dense glandular tissue conceals the detection of tumours, and therefore the risk of an interval carcinoma is greater [31]. A linear association relating to mammographic sensitivity and breast density is reported, with sensitivity decreasing from 95% in a fatty breast to 65% in an extremely dense breast [32]. This predicament has been a source of much debate [33, 34], with personalised screening based on risk factors and mammographic density assessment considered the future.

Legislation laws have been put into effect in 38 states in the USA so that women who have undergone mammography are informed of their breast density and associated risk [35]. Although capable of measuring breast density, computer software analysis is still being evaluated to assess the consistency of results relative to density changes over time [36]. Therefore, the Australian Standing Committee on Breast Screening states that until more evidence is available on breast density assessment, management and clinical pathways, routine recording of breast density and supplementary screening would not be undertaken. Currently, there is no requirement within the NHSBSP to record breast density. Public Health England is evaluating this issue as there are increasing pressures from clinicians and patients [37].

Reproductive Factors

The link between breast cancer risk and reproductive factors is associated with the influence of ovarian hormones, which are affected by the following factors:

Age at menarche (first menstrual period) has been the subject of many studies. Early menstruation is reported to increase breast cancer risk (5% increase each year younger) [16, 38–40] due to prolonged exposure to oestrogen. However, this association varies depending on the tumour subtype and receptor status (oestrogen and progesterone receptor-positive or negative [39]. Conversely, in other studies, no association was demonstrated between early age menarche and an increased risk of breast cancer [41–43].

Delayed menopause may also prolong the period of oestrogen exposure. Several studies, therefore, report that older age at menopause increases the risk (3% for each year older) [16, 39, 40]. A 2012 meta-analysis [44] stated that post-menopausal women had a lower risk of breast cancer than pre-menopausal women irrespective of age and parity.

Hereditary Factors

Most breast cancers are not hereditary [45]. Increased risk does not mean that an individual will develop the disease as more than 85% of women with a first-degree relative (sister, mother, or daughter) with breast cancer will never develop the disease [46].

Family History

A family history of breast cancer is one of the main risk factors mentioned in various studies [16, 47, 48]. Meta and pooled analysis data demonstrate that having one first–degree relative diagnosed with breast cancer almost doubles a woman's risk of developing the disease compared to an individual with no family history [46, 49]. This risk increases further if two or more women are under 50 years of age or three or more relatives at any age [50, 51].

Genetic Factors

A small percentage of women (0.11%–0.12% of the general population) are identified as having a high risk, a consequence of mutations in the BRCA1 and BRCA2 (breast cancer susceptibility) genes [45, 52]. The estimated prevalence of mutations means this will affect approximately 1 in 450 women who, as a result, have a high (45–65%) chance of developing the disease by the age of 70 [53].

Mutations in BRCA1 and BRCA2 genes are classified as high-penetrance with an average relative risk of 11.4 and 11.7, respectively, along with the rare gene Tumour Protein 53 (TP53) (Li-Fraumeni syndrome) with an age-adjusted relative risk 105 (90% CI 62–165) [54]. Moderate risk genes, for example, Checkpoint kinase 2 (CHEK2), Ataxia Telangiectasia Mutated (ATM), Partner And Localizer of BRCA2 (PALB2) and RECQL, confer average relative risks of 2.26–5.3 [54]. Several low-penetrance gene variants have also been identified [55].

The National Health Service Breast Screening Program (NHSBSP) offer screening for very high-risk women with a proven germline pathogenic variant.

Personal History of Breast Cancer

Women with a prior history of breast cancer have an increased risk of developing a new primary cancer in the contralateral breast. Studies report a variance from a twofold to almost sixfold risk increase relative to the general female population [56, 57]. This risk is not the same as the risk of recurrence (return) from primary cancer.

The risk of contralateral breast cancer is higher for individuals whose primary tumour was hormone-receptor-negative than a hormone-receptor-positive tumour [57]. Some studies state that a younger age at primary diagnosis and older age at menopause are significant factors, but the evidence is variable [56, 57]. Although contralateral breast cancer is reported to be the commonest second cancer amongst breast cancer patients, a decrease in incidence rates is plausibly related to advances in systemic treatments [57].

Previous Benign Breast Disease

Research studies have demonstrated that benign breast diseases (BBDs) are a risk factor for breast cancer [3, 58–60]. BBDs encompasses a broad spectrum of conditions and are divided into three subtypes- non-proliferative disease, proliferative disease without atypia, and proliferative disease with atypia. The degree of risk for each subtype varies with the risk greater for proliferative disease [3].

Proliferative lesions without atypia, e.g., intraductal papilloma, sclerosing adenosis, moderate hyperplasia of usual type, appear to raise (approximately twofold increase) risk slightly [3, 59, 60]. Proliferative lesions with atypia imply a more significant risk (3 1/2- to 5-fold) and include Atypical Ductal Hyperplasia (ADH) and Atypical Lobular Hyperplasia (ALH) [3, 60]. However, it is unclear if non-proliferative diseases (e.g., cysts, apocrine metaplasia, and mild hyperplasia of usual type) affect the risk [60].

Breast Carcinoma In Situ

Ductal carcinoma in situ (DCIS) and lobular carcinoma in situ (LCIS) have the potential to develop into invasive carcinoma [61]. Some studies report that a diagnosis of DCIS results in an increased breast cancer risk of 40–100%. However, the risk is not the same for all DCIS subtypes but appears equal for the ipsilateral and contralateral breast [62–64]. It is currently impossible to distinguish which DCIS lesions will develop to invasive breast cancer, although more probable with high grade rather than a low-grade disease [64]. The development of an IBC appears also to depend on the treatment received, with lower rates reported for those undergoing more intensive treatment [65].

Lobular Carcinoma In Situ (LCIS)is also associated with an increased breast cancer risk (relative risk three to tenfold compared to the general population) [66]. Some studies affirm that LCIS may be a precursor to invasive lobular carcinoma (ILC) [66, 67].

Obesity

Being overweight or obese is one of the few risk factors that is amenable to change. However, the relationship between body weight and breast cancer risk is multifaceted, with substantial heterogeneity between studies [68–70]. An increase in body fat and BMI is associated with higher amounts of sex hormones (oestrogen) which is plausible in justifying the correlation [71, 72].

Post-Menopausal

There is a modest association between an elevated BMI (obesity) and breast cancer risk in postmenopausal women, particularly associated with oestrogen receptor-positive–breast cancer [1, 72, 73]. However, there is stronger evidence from epidemiological studies demonstrating the risk is attributed to higher levels of adulthood weight gain, with an 11% higher risk reported per 5 kg of weight increase [69, 74].

The waist-to-hip (WHR) ratio is also identified as a measure of breast cancer risk among postmenopausal women, with a 50% higher risk stated for women with the highest WHR compared to the lowest [74]. Conversely, it is acknowledged that the risk association may vary according to the tumour's hormone receptor status and non-HRT usage [74, 75].

Importantly, in postmenopausal women, the effectiveness of treatments and hence disease-free and overall survival is reported to be lower in women who were obese at the time of diagnosis [76].

Pre-Menopausal

The evidence in pre-menopausal women is weaker, with epidemiological studies reporting an inverse or no correlation between obesity and breast cancer risk [1]. Converse to postmenopausal women, the risk is reported to have no association with weight gain during adulthood (classified as age 20) [69]. However, the risk may be increased if the weight gain is between the age of 40–50 [77]. Several studies state an 8% lower risk per 5-unit BMI increase [69, 78–80] but, this could differ for ER/PR positive tumours and different ethnicities [78–81].

The evidence indicates that several factors (income, race/ethnicity) are causal to obesity. Obesity increases the incidence of breast cancer through increased resistance to insulin, a decrease in immunity, and increased levels of hormones in postmenopausal women. Large prospective studies will be required to evaluate further the strength of association of body fatness and breast cancer risk, [74, 80, 81] which may inform individuals who are considered high risk, enabling personalised prevention strategies. More recent data proposes that body mass index (BMI) alone is an unreliable predictor of breast cancer risk, and that specific blood and clinical biomarkers should supplement this. Blood biomarkers of chronic inflammation have been linked to increased risk [73, 82].

Vitamin D

The existing data on the relationship between vitamin D and breast cancer risk remains inconsistent, with prospective and case-control studies reporting discrepant findings [83]. Several studies report an inverse correlation between vitamin D levels and breast cancer risk [84–86]. A 2018 meta-analysis [83] reports a protective effect of high vitamin D levels only in premenopausal women. However, further clinical trials are warranted to clarify the correlation between vitamin D levels with menopausal status. Recurrent disease and overall survival will need to be considered with varying factors to include ethnicity, lifestyle, and diet [87].

Medical Conditions

Several medical conditions are also associated with an increased risk of breast cancer, e.g., Graves' Disease (hyperthyroidism), conferring a slight but significant increase of 9% [88–90]. Metabolic syndromes, e.g., hypertension, dyslipidemia, and Type 2 diabetes mellitus, are also independent risk factors for breast cancer [70, 91]. However, this may depend on menopausal status, obesity, and treatment received [92].

Behavioural Risk

Parity

In addition to the number of full-term pregnancies, the maternal age at first live birth has been the subject of many studies.

Having Children

Full-term pregnancies are considered a protective factor [42, 93]. However, the association between parity and breast cancer risk may vary by tumour subtype (receptor status, molecular subtype) [93, 94]. Breast cancer risk is also reported to decrease with multiparity (7% for each live birth) [41, 42]. However, some studies report no association or that high parity is associated with an increased risk of breast cancer dependent on maternal age [16, 95].

Maternal Age

Maternal age is also considered a relevant factor. Numerous studies report that among parous women, an advanced age at first birth increases the risk of breast cancer with a 3% increase for each year older [16, 39, 41, 93] (again, the association between maternal age and breast cancer risk may be limited to receptor status (ER/PR/HER2). Early maternal age is therefore often associated with reducing the risk [16].

Breastfeeding

The protective factor of breastfeeding has been the subject of several studies, again with controversial results. Some studies suggest that breastfeeding can lower breast cancer risk [16, 39, 93, 96] (16% lower), and this was irrespective of menopausal status [97]. ER/PR-positive and triple-negative breast cancer risk are reported to be lower (23% and 21%) in women who have breastfed for any length of time, but there was no association with HER2-positive breast cancers [93].

Various studies report the lactation period as a significant factor in reducing breast cancer risk [41, 96, 98], with one study reporting a decreased rate of recurrent disease, although the effect varied for different ER statuses [41]. However, in other studies, the protective effect of breastfeeding has not been proven [16, 43].

Hormonal Contraceptives

The association of hormonal contraceptives and the risk of breast cancer has been addressed in various studies [16, 41, 99–101]. Some studies have reported that women who currently or recently used oral contraceptives have a slightly greater risk of breast cancer than non-users [102] (7% higher per 5-year increment and 14% higher per 10-year increment) [99]. The risk diminishes over time, and 10 years post-use, there does not appear to be a residual risk [100]. However, other studies report that the use of hormonal contraception was not associated with an increased risk or demonstrated some protective effect [16, 42]. The data relating to the age of first use of oral contraceptives remains controversial and may depend on the breast cancer subtype [41, 103].

The risk associated with hormonal contraceptives may also vary depending upon the differences in formulations used, the method of administration, and frequency of use (continuous/discontinuous) [99, 101].

Hormone Replacement Therapy (HRT)

There are a variety of hormone replacement preparations available. Concerns about the association of HRT and breast cancer risk has brought about a substantial decrease in usage [104]. HRT is comprised of synthetic sex hormones, and greater exposure to oestrogens and androgens could explain the associated higher risk. A 2019 meta-analysis [105] stated that for current users, the risk is raised by 17% for oestrogen-only and 60% for oestrogen-progestogen combinations (1–4 years of use). The risk increases to 33% and 100%, respectively, for more prolonged usage (5–14 years). The study also demonstrated an increased residual risk even after HRT was stopped.

Conversely, although a recent observational study [106] reinforced that most HRT drugs raise the risk of breast cancer, the risk was reported to be lower for long term usage and a more significant decrease in risk once HRT was discontinued. The increased risk was mainly associated with oestrogen-progestogen combinations but was variable depending on the HRT preparation. Duration of use (more prolonged exposure) was also a significant factor.

Alcohol Consumption

Numerous studies have addressed the correlation between alcohol and breast cancer risk [107–112]. In the UK, it is estimated that 8% of breast cancer cases are attributable to drinking alcohol [109]. The association between alcohol consumption and an increased risk of developing breast cancer is relative to the amount. In women, a 9% breast cancer risk is reported for consuming two units of alcohol per day. This risk rises to 60% with 6+ units of alcohol per day, compared to non-drinkers [110, 111]. Over a lifetime, the breast cancer risk is reported to be 28% higher in women consuming a high intake of alcohol compared to those with a low intake [112].

It is hypothesised that multiple factors explain the link between alcohol consumption and breast cancer risk. First, alcohol may increase levels of sex hormones [113], stimulating the proliferation of oestrogen receptor-positive cells [114, 115]. Second, some studies suggest that alcohol metabolism can result in carcinogenic products [116, 117]. Finally, studies reporting an association with binge and heavy drinking imply metabolic processes are insufficient to eliminate the alcohol resulting in raised inflammation and insulin resistance [118, 119].

Coffee Consumption

Overall, the existing literature on coffee consumption and the risk of developing breast cancer is controversial. Most studies state no association or a small negative association [120–122]. However, risk levels may vary when considering menopausal status, genetic mutations, and the hormonal status of the tumour. Further studies are required to evaluate the effects in these subgroups [123].

Diet

Various studies have been undertaken to identify an association between dietary factors and breast cancer risk, but the results remain conflicting [16, 124–126]. Nutritional fibre intake, fruit, vegetables, and meat have been studied [16, 126]. However, the most significant factor is diets containing low polyunsaturated and saturated fatty acids rather than overall fat consumption [127]. Higher intakes of saturated fat appear to correlate with an increased risk [128].

Physical Activity

Evidence supports that a lack of physical exercise increases an individual's breast cancer risk, independent of body weight [129, 130]. It is believed that physical activity is associated with decreased levels of oestrogen and progesterone and hence may partway justify the association [130]. However, the evidence is more controversial as to whether the intensity, duration or frequency of the exercise undertaken lead to a further reduction in the risk. Some studies report improvements in risk reduction associated with high vs low-intensity activity [131, 132], the frequency [131, 133, 134], but not always relating to the intensity [133, 135].

A lack of physical exercise has also been reported to result in inferior outcomes in women who have been diagnosed with early-stage breast cancer [76]. Studies report reduced breast cancer mortality, total mortality, and longer overall survival rates for women with higher physical activity levels than those with the lowest [76, 136, 137]. The beneficial effects are evident even after controlling for health behaviours, comorbidities, and cancer treatment. However, it is acknowledged that observational studies are more prone to bias, confounding, and reverse causation [138].

Smoking

There is some evidence to support a link between cigarette smoking and breast cancer risk. This risk is reported to be higher in those who currently smoke (7–13%) or have formerly smoked (6–9%) compared with non-smokers [139–141]. A long history of smoking is reported to increase an individual's risk by 37% [142]. However, it is acknowledged that results within these studies may be affected by multiple confounding factors, i.e., alcohol consumption [140], obesity, [141], a family history of breast cancer [143] and tumour receptor status [144, 145].

Larger studies undertaken in 2011 [146, 147] demonstrated that long-term heavy smoking is associated with a higher risk of breast cancer, particularly for specific cohorts, i.e., women who started smoking when they were young (under the age of 20) and before their first birth [139]. Smoking tobacco has been linked with higher levels of circulating sex hormones, which could support the association between tobacco and breast cancer risk [71].

Medications

Certain medications have been associated with reducing breast cancer risk, mainly aspirin and non-steroidal anti-inflammatory drugs (NSAID) [148–151]. Although these studies report a protective effect of NSAID usage, there is variance in the dosage, duration of use, and whether this applies to all breast cancer subtypes. However, findings from the recent ASPirin in Reducing Events in the Elderly (ASPREE) trial suggest an adverse effect in those aged 70 and older [152]. The Aspirin for Breast Cancer (ABC) Trial aims to determine if aspirin can prevent a breast cancer recurrence [153]. Other medications, e.g., diethylstilboestrol (synthetic oestrogen), may increase breast cancer risk, but the results are inconsistent [154–156].

Social Risk

Numerous social factors have been researched regarding breast cancer incidence, the stage at diagnosis, and overall survival. They consider socioeconomic status (income, education), employment, occupation, race, neighbourhoods, social support, and networks [157, 158].

Data demonstrates that female breast cancer rates are much higher in developed countries than in developing nations, although the incidence in underdeveloped regions is rising [42, 49]. There are several causative factors for this relating to the ethnicity of the population, environmental and lifestyle factors, e.g., use of hormone replacement therapy (HRT), sedentary lifestyle, high-fat diet, increased alcohol consumption, and increasing body mass index (BMI) [16, 42]. Although economically developing countries have lower incidence rates, the mortality rates are slightly higher than developed regions suggesting later detection and insufficient treatment resources [159].

Socio-Economic Factors

Various studies demonstrate an association between a high socioeconomic status (SES) and breast cancer incidence rates for all racial/ethnic groups [16, 157, 160]. In particular, the education level attained appears to be a socioeconomic variable with a positive correlation [157]. This may partly be due to the educated utilising resources to gain more information on cancer risk and subsequently making improved health choices, for example, undergoing frequent screening mammograms [161]. However, education alone cannot be deemed causal in improved decision making [157]. The association of social factors is multifaceted and may be due to the risk element of nulliparity, older age at first birth, late menopause, together with the lifestyle components mentioned [161].

In addition, the SES is a significant indicator of disease-free and overall survival [162, 163]. Studies report that low SES is associated with poor survival rates, but the influence and magnitude of the individual factors are not yet completely understood [164–166]. Although a late-stage presentation may be more common with social deprivation [165, 167], it is not the sole causal mechanism [168]. Evidence suggests a disparity in the treatment received between low- and high-income patients, reflecting inadequate access to health care and/or health insurance in certain countries [158, 167, 169].

Night Work and Sleep Duration

Night shift work has been believed to increase breast cancer risk. However, the results of epidemiological studies have been conflicting due to the diverse evaluation of exposure to night work, i.e., intensity and duration [170]. Several studies show an increased moderate risk of developing breast cancer in women who work night shifts [171–173]. The hypothesis relates this to a reduction in the hormone melatonin (which has anticarcinogenic effects) and the associated increase in oestrogen [171]. However, a 2018 meta-analysis [170] reported that the risk was only higher in pre-menopausal women who recently (last 2 years) or currently undertake night work.

Data on the duration of sleep and breast cancer risk is also conflicting with studies reporting a possible increased risk with longer sleep duration [174], shorter sleep duration [175, 176], the quality of sleep [177], or no association at all [178].

Physical Risk

Medical Radiation Exposure

Exposure to ionising radiation is a known risk factor associated with carcinoma [179].

Radiotherapy

Hodgkins Lymphoma

It is well established that young women who received supradiaphragmatic radiotherapy as treatment for Hodgkin's Lymphoma have a significantly raised risk for breast cancer [180–184]. However, the level of risk differs significantly between studies, with relative risks for those treated under the age of 15 varying between 8 [185] and 458 [186]. The most significant risk is reported at age 14, which would reasonably correlate to the risk of radiation damage to cells when breast development is occurring [180].

Studies have also reported a variable cumulative breast cancer risk ranging from 12 to 34% at 25–30 years follow-up [183, 185] and 35% by the age of 40 [187]. The variation in risk may depend on various factors such as the age at treatment and duration since the treatment.

Prior Radiotherapy for Breast Cancer

Several studies report a statistically significant increased risk of second contralateral breast cancers developing, attributable to radiotherapy [188–191]. The increased risk was predominantly in younger women [191, 192] and more extended follow-up periods [189, 192]. Conversely, a 2017 study [193] found that only 0.8% of contralateral breast cancers were attributable to radiotherapy.

Diagnostic Radiology

In the UK, it is estimated that 0.1% of the cumulative risk of breast cancer in women under 75 years could be attributable to diagnostic X-rays [194]. The risk of cancer incidence or death associated with radiation exposure from 3 yearly breast screenings is reported to be negligible [195]. In women with a familial or genetic mutation, exposure to low-dose examinations (i.e., screening mammograms, chest X-rays) may be associated with a higher but non-significant risk of breast cancer. However, the risk increased significantly in this cohort in those under twenty or with five or more exposures [196].

Passive Smoking

Passive smoke exposure and breast cancer risk remain controversial as there are only a small number of prospective studies. However, several studies and a 2015 meta-analysis concluded that overall, there was a moderate relative risk of breast cancer associated with passive smoking [141, 197–200].

Endocrine-Disrupting Chemicals (EDCs)

Endocrine-disrupting chemicals (EDCs) are substances present in everyday lives via the environment, food products, water systems, personal care products, and manufactured products. Increasing evidence implies that Xenoestrogens (oestrogen mimicking compounds) may affect the endocrine system, potentially linking the association with breast cancer, particularly when repeated exposure occurs during puberty [201]. However, dose, duration, and genetics are important confounding factors affecting the risk [201]. Furthermore, as multiple EDCs co-exist (some with short half-lives), proving a causal relationship via epidemiologic studies is difficult [1]. Therefore, the variability and heterogeneity of the studies to date mean the evidence of exposure to interdependent EDC's and breast cancer risk are limited.

Clinical Pearls

- The aetiology of breast cancer remains essentially unknown, although various factors have been correlated with an increased risk of developing the disease.
- Breast cancer represents the most common female cancer worldwide. Higher incidence rates in some countries are attributed to a higher prevalence of established risk factors and increases in breast cancer screening and awareness.

- After gender, the most influential risk factor for breast cancer is age; increasing age increases the risk.
- Research evidence implies that breast cancer biology is a complex interaction between biological, behavioural, social, and physical factors.

Chapter Review Questions
Review Questions

1. How is age related to the prevalence of breast cancer?
2. What is the role of hereditary factors in the aetiology of breast cancer?
3. Are benign breast diseases (BBDs) a risk factor for breast cancer?

Answers

1. Breast cancer incidence rates rise steeply with increasing age, continuing throughout life. The incidence of breast cancer in young women (i.e., teenagers until 30 years old) is uncommon. However, it remains the primary cancer diagnosed in women under 40. Cancer Research UK data (2015–2017) demonstrates that almost half (48%) of female breast cancer cases are diagnosed in women in the 50–69 age group. There is a plateau after 50–54 when breast screening is first routinely offered and relates to detecting prevalent cases.
2. Having one first–degree relative (sister, mother, or daughter) diagnosed with breast cancer almost doubles a woman's risk of developing the disease compared to an individual with no family history. This risk increases further if two or more women are under 50 years of age or three or more relatives at any age. However, most breast cancers are not hereditary; more than 85% of women with a first-degree relative with breast cancer will never develop the disease. A small percentage of women (0.11%–0.12% of the general population) are at high risk due to mutations in the BRCA1 and BRCA2 (breast

cancer susceptibility) genes. Mutations in BRCA1 and BRCA2 account for most inherited breast cancers; mutations in the rare gene Tumour Protein 53 (TP53) (Li-Fraumeni syndrome) and further moderate and low-penetrance gene variants account for much smaller numbers.

3. BBDs encompasses a broad spectrum of conditions and are divided into three subtypes-non-proliferative disease, proliferative disease without atypia, and proliferative disease with atypia. Non proliferative lesions (for example, simple cysts) confer no more significant risk. Proliferative lesions without atypia (for example, sclerosing adenosis) appear to raise risk slightly (approximately a twofold increase). Proliferative lesions with atypia signify a more significant risk (3 1/2- to 5-fold) and include Atypical Ductal Hyperplasia (ADH) and Atypical Lobular Hyperplasia (ALH).

Appendix

Test your learning and check your understanding of this book's contents: use the "Springer Nature Flashcards" app to access questions using https://sn.pub/dcAnWL.

To use the app, please follow the instructions in Chap. 1.

Flashcard code: 48341-69945-ABCB1-2A8C7-CE9D2.

Short URL: https://sn.pub/dcAnWL.

References

1. Hiatt RA, Engmann NJ, Balke K, Rehkopf DH. A complex systems model of breast cancer etiology: the paradigm II conceptual model. Cancer Epidemiol Biomarkers. 2020;29:1720–30.
2. Stewart BW, Wild C. World cancer report 2014. Geneva: International Agency for Research on Cancer, World Health Organization; 2014.
3. Zendehdel M, Niakan B, Keshtkar A, Rafiei E, Salamat F. Subtypes of benign breast disease as a risk factor for breast cancer: a systematic review and meta-analysis protocol. Iran J Med Sci. 2018;43(1):1–8.
4. Broustas CG, Lieberman HB. DNA damage response genes and the development of cancer metastasis. Radiat Res. 2014;181(2):111–30.
5. Sinn HP, Kreipe H. A brief overview of the WHO classification of breast tumors, 4th edition, focusing on issues and updates from the 3rd edition. Breast Care. 2013;8(2):149–54.
6. Parkin DM, Fernández LMG. Use of statistics to assess the global burden of breast cancer. Breast J. 2006;12(Suppl 1):70–80.
7. Worldwide cancer data. World Cancer Research Fund. https://www.wcrf.org/dietandcancer/cancer-trends/worldwide-cancer-data. Accessed 12 Jul 2021.
8. Bray F, Ferlay J, Soerjomataram I, Siegel RL, Torre LA, Jemal A. Global cancer statistics 2018: GLOBOCAN estimates of incidence and mortality worldwide for 36 cancers in 185 countries. CA Cancer J Clin. 2018;68(6):394–424.
9. Ziegler RG, Hoover RN, Pike MC, Hildesheim A, Nomura AM, West DW, Wu-Williams AH, Kolonel LN, Horn-Ross PL, Rosenthal JF, Hyer MB. Migration patterns and breast cancer risk in Asian-American women. J Natl Cancer Inst. 1993;85(22):1819–27.
10. Cancer Research UK. Cancer incidence for common cancers. https://www.cancerresearchuk.org/health-professional/cancer-statistics/incidence/common-cancers-compared. Accessed 10 May 2021.
11. World Health Organisation. Cancer tomorrow. https://gco.iarc.fr/tomorrow/graphic. Accessed 10 May 2021.
12. Weedon-Fekjær H, Romundstad PR, Vatten LJ. Modern mammography screening and breast cancer mortality: population study. BMJ. 2014;348:3701.
13. Seely JM, Alhassan T. Screening for breast cancer in 2018—what should we be doing today? Curr Oncol. 2018;25:115–24.
14. Yalaza M, İnan A, Bozer M. Male breast cancer. J Breast Health. 2016;12(1):1–8.
15. Abdelwahab Yousef AJ. Male breast cancer: epidemiology and risk factors. Semin Oncol. 2017;44(4):267–72.
16. Thakur P, Seam RK, Gupta MK, Gupta M, Sharma M, Fotedar V. Breast cancer risk factor evaluation in a Western Himalayan state: a case-control study and comparison with the Western World. South Asian J Cancer. 2017;6(3):106–9.
17. Moser K, Sellars S, Wheaton M, Cooke J, Duncan A, Maxwell A, Michell M, Wilson M, Beral V, Peto R, Richards M. Extending the age range for breast screening in england: pilot study to assess the feasibility and acceptability of randomization. J Med Screen. 2011;18(2):96–102.
18. Assi HA, Khoury KE, Dbouk H, Khalil LE, Mouhieddine TH, El Saghir NS. Epidemiology and prognosis of breast cancer in young women. J Thorac Dis. 2013;5(Suppl 1):2–8.

19. Clendenen TV, Ge W, Koenig KL, Afanasyeva Y, Agnoli C, Brinton LA, Darvishian F, Dorgan JF, Eliassen AH, Falk RT, Hallmans G. Breast cancer risk prediction in women aged 35–50 years: impact of including sex hormone concentrations in the Gail model. Breast Cancer Res. 2019;21(1):1–12.

20. Stapelkamp C, Holmberg L, Tataru D, Møller H, Robinson D. Predictors of early death in female patients with breast cancer in the UK: a cohort study. BMJ Open. 2011;1(2):e000247.

21. Zhang X, Tworoger SS, Eliassen AH, Hankinson SE. Postmenopausal plasma sex hormone levels and breast cancer risk over 20 years of follow-up. Breast Cancer Res Treat. 2013;137(3):883–92.

22. Walker K, Bratton DJ, Frost C. Premenopausal endogenous oestrogen levels and breast cancer risk: a meta-analysis. Br J Cancer. 2011;105(9):1451–7.

23. Dorgan JF, Stanczyk FZ, Egleston BL, Kahle LL, Shaw CM, Spittle CS, Godwin AK, Brinton LA. Prospective case-control study of serum mullerian inhibiting substance and breast cancer risk. J Natl Cancer Inst. 2009;101(21):1501–9.

24. Eliassen AH, Zeleniuch-Jacquotte A, Rosner B, Hankinson SE. Plasma anti-Müllerian hormone concentrations and risk of breast cancer among premenopausal women in the Nurses' Health Studies. Cancer Epidemiol Prev Biomarkers. 2016;25(5): 854–60.

25. Winkel RR, von Euler-Chelpin M, Nielsen M, Petersen K, Lillholm M, Nielsen MB, Lynge E, Uldall WY, Vejborg I. Mammographic density and structural features can individually and jointly contribute to breast cancer risk assessment in mammography screening: a case–control study. BMC Cancer. 2016;16(1):1–2.

26. Zhang X, Rice M, Tworoger SS, Rosner BA, Eliassen AH, Tamimi RM, Joshi AD, Lindstrom S, Qian J, Colditz GA, Willett WC. Addition of a polygenic risk score, mammographic density, and endogenous hormones to existing breast cancer risk prediction models: a nested case–control study. PLoS Med. 2018;15(9):e1002644.

27. Engmann NJ, Golmakani MK, Miglioretti DL, Sprague BL, Kerlikowske K. Breast cancer surveillance consortium. population-attributable risk proportion of clinical risk factors for breast cancer. JAMA Oncol. 2017;3(9):1228–36.

28. Byrne C, Ursin G, Martin CF, Peck JD, Cole EB, Zeng D, Kim E, Yaffe MD, Boyd NF, Heiss G, McTiernan A. Mammographic density change with estrogen and progestin therapy and breast cancer risk. J Natl Cancer Inst. 2017;109(9):djx001.

29. Boyd NF, Dite GS, Stone J, Gunasekara A, English DR, McCredie MR, Giles GG, Tritchler D, Chiarelli A, Yaffe MJ, Hopper JL. Heritability of mammographic density, a risk factor for breast cancer. N Engl J Med. 2002;347(12):886–94.

30. Ursin G, Lillie EO, Lee E, Cockburn M, Schork NJ, Cozen W, Parisky YR, Hamilton AS, Astrahan MA, Mack T. The relative importance of genetics and environment on mammographic density. Cancer Epidemiol Prev Biomarkers. 2009;18(1):102–12.

31. Boyd NF, Guo H, Martin LJ, Sun L, Stone J, Fishell E, Jong RA, Hislop G, Chiarelli A, Minkin S, Yaffe MJ. Mammographic density and the risk and detection of breast cancer. N Engl J Med. 2007;356(3):227–36.

32. Destounis S, Johnston L, Highnam R, Arieno A, Morgan R, Chan A. Using volumetric breast density to quantify the potential masking risk of mammographic density. Am J Roentgenol. 2017;208(1):222–7.

33. Onega T, Beaber EF, Sprague BL, Barlow WE, Haas JS, Tosteson AN, Schnall M, Armstrong K, Schapira MM, Geller B, Weaver DL. Breast cancer screening in an era of personalized regimens: a conceptual model and National Cancer Institute initiative for risk-based and preference-based approaches at a population level. Cancer. 2014;120(19):2955–64.

34. Schousboe JT, Kerlikowske K, Loh A, Cummings SR. Personalizing mammography by breast density and other risk factors for breast cancer: analysis of health benefits and cost-effectiveness. Ann Intern Med. 2011;155(1):10–20.

35. Vinnicombe SJ. Breast density: why all the fuss? Clin Radiol. 2018;73(4):334–57.

36. Oliver A, Tortajada M, Lladó X, Freixenet J, Ganau S, Tortajada L, Vilagran M, Sentís M, Martí R. Breast density analysis using an automatic density segmentation algorithm. J Digit Imaging. 2015;28(5):604–12.

37. Sharma N. Special issue on breast imaging: part 1. Clin Radiol. 2018;73(4):325–6.

38. Bodicoat DH, Schoemaker MJ, Jones ME, McFadden E, Griffin J, Ashworth A, Swerdlow AJ. Timing of pubertal stages and breast cancer risk: the Breakthrough Generations Study. Breast Cancer Res. 2014;16(1):1–8.

39. Li H, Sun X, Miller E, Wang Q, Tao P, Liu L, Zhao Y, Wang M, Qi Y, Li J. BMI, reproductive factors, and breast cancer molecular subtypes: a case-control study and meta-analysis. J Epidemiol. 2017;27(4):143–51.

40. Momenimovahed Z, Salehiniya H. Epidemiological characteristics of and risk factors for breast cancer in the world. Breast Cancer. 2019;11:151–64.

41. Laamiri FZ, Hasswane N, Kerbach A, Aguenaou H, Taboz Y, Benkirane H, Mrabet M, Amina B. Risk factors associated with a breast cancer in a population of Moroccan women whose age is less than 40 years: a case control study. Pan Afr Med J. 2016;24(1):19.

42. Balekouzou A, Yin P, Pamatika CM, Bekolo CE, Nambei SW, Djeintote M, Kota K, Mossoro-Kpinde CD, Shu C, Yin M, Fu Z. Reproductive risk factors associated with breast cancer in women in Bangui: a case–control study. BMC Womens Health. 2017;17(1):1–9.

43. Ozsoy A, Barça N, Dolek BA, Aktaş H, Elverici E, Araz L, Ozkaraoğlu O. The relationship between breast cancer and risk factors: a single-center study. Eur J Breast Health. 2017;13(3):145.

44. Cancer B. Menarche, menopause, and breast cancer risk: individual participant meta-analysis, including 118 964 women with breast cancer from 117 epidemiological studies. Lancet Oncol. 2012;13(11):1141–51.

45. Lichtenstein P, Holm NV, Verkasalo PK, Iliadou A, Kaprio J, Koskenvuo M, Pukkala E, Skytthe A, Hemminki K. Environmental and heritable factors in the causation of cancer—analyses of cohorts of twins from Sweden, Denmark, and Finland. N Engl J Med. 2000;343(2):78–85.

46. Collaborative Group on Hormonal Factors in Breast Cancer. Familial breast cancer: collaborative reanalysis of individual data from 52 epidemiological studies including 58 209 women with breast cancer and 101 986 women without the disease. Lancet. 2001;358(9291):1389–99.

47. Ahern TP, Sprague BL, Bissell MC, Miglioretti DL, Buist DS, Braithwaite D, Kerlikowske K. Family history of breast cancer, breast density, and breast cancer risk in a US breast cancer screening population. Cancer Epidemiol Prev Biomarkers. 2017;26(6):938–44.

48. Bravi F, Decarli A, Russo AG. Risk factors for breast cancer in a cohort of mammographic screening program: a nested case-control study within the FRiCaM study. Cancer Med. 2018;7(5):2145–52.

49. Francies FZ, Hull R, Khanyile R, Dlamini Z. Breast cancer in low-middle income countries: abnormality in splicing and lack of targeted treatment options. Am J Cancer Res. 2020;10(5):1568–91.

50. Metcalfe KA, Finch A, Poll A, Horsman D, Kim-Sing C, Scott J, Royer R, Sun P, Narod SA. Breast cancer risks in women with a family history of breast or ovarian cancer who have tested negative for a BRCA1 or BRCA2 mutation. Br J Cancer. 2009;100(2):421–5.

51. Brewer HR, Jones ME, Schoemaker MJ, Ashworth A, Swerdlow AJ. Family history and risk of breast cancer: an analysis accounting for family structure. Breast Cancer Res Treat. 2017;165(1):193–200.

52. Ford D, Easton DF, Stratton M, Narod S, Goldgar D, Devilee P, Bishop DT, Weber B, Lenoir G, Chang-Claude J, Sobol H. Genetic heterogeneity and penetrance analysis of the BRCA1 and BRCA2 genes in breast cancer families. Am J Hum Genetics. 1998;62(3):676–89.

53. Godet I, Gilkes DM. BRCA1 and BRCA2 mutations and treatment strategies for breast cancer. Integr Cancer Sci Ther. 2017;4(1).

54. Wendt C, Margolin S. Identifying breast cancer susceptibility genes–a review of the genetic background in familial breast cancer. Acta Oncol. 2019;58(2):135–46.

55. Turnbull C, Rahman N. Genetic predisposition to breast cancer: past, present, and future. Annu Rev Genomics Hum Genet. 2008;9(1):321–45.

56. Rubino C, Arriagada R, Delaloge S, Lê MG. Relation of risk of contralateral breast cancer to the interval since the first primary tumour. Br J Cancer. 2010;102(1):213–9.

57. Ramin C, Withrow DR, Davis Lynn BC, Gierach GL, Berrington de González A. Risk of contralateral breast cancer according to first breast cancer characteristics among women in the USA, 1992–2016. Breast Cancer Res. 2021;23(1):24.

58. Stachs A, Stubert J, Reimer T, Hartmann S. Benign breast disease in women. Dtsch Arztebl Int. 2019;116(33–34):565–74.

59. Salamat F, Niakan B, Keshtkar A, Rafiei E, Zendehdel M. Subtypes of benign breast disease as a risk factor of breast cancer: a systematic review and meta analyses. Iran J Med Sci. 2018;43(4):355–64.

60. Johansson A, Christakou AE, Iftimi A, Eriksson M, Tapia J, Skoog L. Characterization of benign breast diseases and association with age , hormonal factors , and family history of breast cancer among women in Sweden. JAMA Netw Open. 2021;4(6):1–12.

61. Lopez-Garcia MA, Geyer FC, Lacroix-Triki M, Marchió C, Reis-Filho JS. Breast cancer precursors revisited: molecular features and progression pathways. Histopathology. 2010;57(2):171–92.

62. Li CI, Malone KE, Saltzman BS, Daling JR. Risk of invasive breast carcinoma among women diagnosed with ductal carcinoma in situ and lobular carcinoma in situ, 1988–2001. Cancer. 2006;106(10):2104–12.

63. Innos K, Horn-Ross PL. Risk of second primary breast cancers among women with ductal carcinoma in situ of the breast. Breast Cancer Res Treat. 2008;111(3):531–40.

64. Visser LL, Elshof LE, Schaapveld M, Van de Vijver K, Groen EJ, Almekinders MM, Bierman C, Van Leeuwen FE, Rutgers EJ, Schmidt MK, Lips EH. Clinicopathological risk factors for an invasive breast cancer recurrence after ductal carcinoma in situ—a nested case–control study. Clin Cancer Res. 2018;24(15):3593–601.

65. Mannu GS, Wang Z, Broggio J, Charman J, Cheung S, Kearins O, Dodwell D, Darby SC. Invasive breast cancer and breast cancer mortality after ductal carcinoma in situ in women attending for breast screening in England, 1988–2014: population based observational cohort study. BMJ. 2020;369:m1570.

66. Wong SM, King T, Boileau J-F, Barry WT, Golshan M. Population-based analysis of breast cancer incidence and survival outcomes in women diagnosed with lobular carcinoma in Situ. Ann Surg Oncol. 2017;24(9):2509–17.

67. Begg CB, Ostrovnaya I, Carniello JV, Sakr RA, Giri D, Towers R, Schizas M, De Brot M, Andrade VP, Mauguen A, Seshan VE. Clonal relationships between lobular carcinoma in situ and other breast malignancies. Breast Cancer Res. 2016;18(1):1–11.

68. Kerlikowske K, Gard CC, Tice JA, Ziv E, Cummings SR, Miglioretti DL. Risk factors that increase risk of estrogen receptor–positive and–negative breast cancer. J Natl Cancer Inst. 2017;109(5):djw276.

69. Kyrgiou M, Kalliala I, Markozannes G, Gunter MJ, Paraskevaidis E, Gabra H, Martin-Hirsch P, Tsilidis KK. Adiposity and cancer at major anatomical sites: umbrella review of the literature. BMJ. 2017;356:j477.

70. Miller B, Chalfant H, Thomas A, Wellberg E, Henson C, McNally MW, Grizzle WE, Jain A, McNally LR. Diabetes, obesity, and inflammation: impact on clinical and radiographic features of breast cancer. Int J Mol Sci. 2021 Jan;22(5):2757.

71. Hormones E, Breast Cancer Collaborative Group. Circulating sex hormones and breast cancer risk factors in postmenopausal women: reanalysis of 13 studies. Br J Cancer. 2011;105(5):709.

72. Samavat H, Kurzer MS. Estrogen metabolism and breast cancer. Cancer Lett. 2015;356(2 Pt A):231–43.

73. Denis GV, Palmer JR. 'Obesity-Associated' breast cancer in lean women: metabolism and inflammation as critical modifiers of risk. Cancer Prev Res (Phila). 2017;10(5):267–9.

74. Suzuki R, Orsini N, Saji S, Key TJ, Wolk A. Body weight and incidence of breast cancer defined by estrogen and progesterone receptor status—a meta-analysis. Int J Cancer. 2009;124(3):698–712.

75. Gaudet MM, Carter BD, Patel AV, Teras LR, Jacobs EJ, Gapstur SM. Waist circumference, body mass index, and postmenopausal breast cancer incidence in the Cancer Prevention Study-II Nutrition Cohort. Cancer Causes Control. 2014;25(6):737–45.

76. Lee K, Kruper L, Dieli-Conwright CM, Mortimer JE. The impact of obesity on breast cancer diagnosis and treatment. Curr Oncol Rep. 2019;21(5):41.

77. Kawai M, Malone KE, Tang M-TC, Li CI. Height, body mass index (BMI), BMI change, and the risk of estrogen receptor-positive, HER2-positive, and triple-negative breast cancer among women ages 20 to 44 years. Cancer. 2014;120(10):1548–56.

78. Yang XR, Chang-Claude J, Goode EL, Couch FJ, Nevanlinna H, Milne RL, et al. Associations of breast cancer risk factors with tumor subtypes: a pooled analysis from the Breast Cancer Association Consortium studies. J Natl Cancer Inst. 2011;103(3):250–63.

79. Amadou A, Ferrari P, Muwonge R, Moskal A, Biessy C, Romieu I, Hainaut P. Overweight, obesity and risk of premenopausal breast cancer according to ethnicity: a systematic review and dose-response meta-analysis. Obes Rev. 2013;14(8):665–78.

80. Munsell MF, Sprague BL, Berry DA, Chisholm G, Trentham-Dietz A. Body mass index and breast cancer risk according to postmenopausal estrogen-progestin use and hormone receptor status. Epidemiol Rev. 2014;36(1):114–36.

81. Cheraghi Z, Poorolajal J, Hashem T, Esmailnasab N, Doosti IA. Effect of body mass index on breast cancer during premenopausal and postmenopausal periods: a meta-analysis. PLoS One. 2012;7(12):e51446.

82. Vrieling A, Buck K, Kaaks R, Chang-Claude J. Adult weight gain in relation to breast cancer risk by estrogen and progesterone receptor status: a meta-analysis. Breast Cancer Res Treat. 2010;123(3):641–9.

83. Estébanez N, Gómez-Acebo I, Palazuelos C, Llorca J, Dierssen-Sotos T. Vitamin D exposure and risk of breast cancer: a meta-analysis. Sci Rep. 2018;8(1):9039.

84. Hatse S, Lambrechts D, Verstuyf A, Smeets A, Brouwers B, Vandorpe T, Brouckaert O, Peuteman G, Laenen A, Verlinden L, Kriebitzsch C. Vitamin D status at breast cancer diagnosis: correlation with tumor characteristics, disease outcome, and genetic determinants of vitamin D insufficiency. Carcinogenesis. 2012;33(7):1319–26.

85. Park S, Lee DH, Jeon JY, Ryu J, Kim S, Kim JY, et al. Serum 25-hydroxyvitamin D deficiency and increased risk of breast cancer among Korean women: a case-control study. Breast Cancer Res Treat. 2015;152(1):147–54.

86. O'Brien KM, Sandler DP, Taylor JA, Weinberg CR. Serum vitamin D and risk of breast cancer within five years. Environ Health Perspect. 2017;125(7):77004.

87. Atoum M, Alzoughool F. Vitamin D and breast cancer: latest evidence and future steps. Breast Cancer. 2017;11:1178223417749816.

88. Khan SR, Chaker L, Ruiter R, Aerts JG, Hofman A, Dehghan A, Franco OH, Stricker BH, Peeters RP. Thyroid function and cancer risk: the Rotterdam study. J Clin Endocrinol Metabol. 2016;101(12):5030–6.

89. Søgaard M, Farkas DK, Ehrenstein V, Jørgensen JOL, Dekkers OM, Sørensen HT. Hypothyroidism and hyperthyroidism and breast cancer risk: a nationwide cohort study. Eur J Endocrinol. 2016;174(4):409–14.

90. Weng C-H, Chen Y-H, Lin C-H, Luo X, Lin T-H. Thyroid disorders and breast cancer risk in Asian population: a nationwide population-based case-control study in Taiwan. BMJ Open. 2018;8(3):e020194.

91. Wani B, Aziz SA, Ganaie MA, Mir MH. Metabolic syndrome and breast cancer risk. Indian J Med Paediatr Oncol. 2017;38(4):434–9.

92. Tabassum I, Mahmood H, Faheem M. Type 2 diabetes mellitus as a risk factor for female breast cancer in the population of Northern Pakistan. Asian Pac J Cancer Prev. 2016;17(7):3255–8.

93. Lambertini M, Santoro L, Del Mastro L, Nguyen B, Livraghi L, Ugolini D, Peccatori FA, Azim HA Jr. Reproductive behaviors and risk of developing breast cancer according to tumor subtype: a systematic review and meta-analysis of epidemiological studies. Cancer Treat Rev. 2016;1(49):65–76.

94. Reeves GK, Pirie K, Green J, Bull D, Beral V. Reproductive factors and specific histological types of breast cancer: prospective study and meta-analysis. Br J Cancer. 2009;100(3):538–44.

95. Innes KE, Byers TE. First pregnancy characteristics and subsequent breast cancer risk among young women. Int J Cancer. 2004;112(2):306–11.

96. Kwan ML, Bernard PS, Kroenke CH, Factor RE, Habel LA, Weltzien EK, Castillo A, Gunderson EP, Maxfield KS, Stijleman IJ, Langholz BM. Breastfeeding, PAM50 tumor subtype, and breast cancer prognosis and survival. J Natl Cancer Inst. 2015;107(7):djv087.

97. Unar-Munguía M, Torres-Mejía G, Colchero MA, González de Cosío T. Breastfeeding mode and risk of breast cancer: a dose-response meta-analysis. J Hum Lact. 2017;33(2):422–34.
98. Nazari SS, Mukherjee P. An overview of mammographic density and its association with breast cancer. Breast Cancer. 2018;25(3):259–67.
99. Zhu H, Lei X, Feng J, Wang Y. Oral contraceptive use and risk of breast cancer: a meta-analysis of prospective cohort studies. Eur J Contracept Reprod Health Care. 2012;17(6):402–14.
100. Gierisch JM, Coeytaux RR, Urrutia RP, Havrilesky LJ, Moorman PG, Lowery WJ, Dinan M, McBroom AJ, Hasselblad V, Sanders GD, Myers ER. Oral contraceptive use and risk of breast, cervical, colorectal, and endometrial cancers: a systematic review. Cancer Epidemiol Prev Biomarkers. 2013;22(11):1931–43.
101. Samson M, Porter N, Orekoya O, Hebert JR, Adams SA, Bennett CL, Steck SE. Progestin and breast cancer risk: a systematic review. Breast Cancer Res Treat. 2016 Jan;155(1):3–12.
102. Hanoch Y, Wallin A. Educating intuition. R. M. Hogarth. University of Chicago Press, Chicago, 2001. Appl Cogn Psychol. 2003;17(1):122–4.
103. Ji L-W, Jing C-X, Zhuang S-L, Pan W-C, Hu X-P. Effect of age at first use of oral contraceptives on breast cancer risk: an updated meta-analysis. Medicine (Baltimore). 2019;98(36):e15719.
104. Parkin DM. 10. Cancers attributable to exposure to hormones in the UK in 2010. Br J Cancer. 2011;105(Suppl 2):42–8.
105. Collaborative Group on Hormonal Factors in Breast Cancer. Type and timing of menopausal hormone therapy and breast cancer risk: individual participant meta-analysis of the worldwide epidemiological evidence. Lancet. 2019;394(10204):1159–68.
106. Vinogradova Y, Coupland C, Hippisley-Cox J. Use of hormone replacement therapy and risk of breast cancer: nested case-control studies using the QResearch and CPRD databases. BMJ. 2020;371:m3873.
107. Miller ER, Wilson C, Chapman J, Flight I, Nguyen AM, Fletcher C, Ramsey I. Connecting the dots between breast cancer, obesity and alcohol consumption in middle-aged women: ecological and case control studies. BMC Public Health. 2018;18(1):1–4.
108. Vieira R, Tobar JSS, Dardes R, Claudio L, Thuler S. Alcohol consumption as a risk factor for breast cancer development: a case-control study in Brazil. Asian Pac J Cancer Prev. 2018;19(3):703–7.
109. Brown KF, Rumgay H, Dunlop C, Ryan M, Quartly F, Cox A, Deas A, Elliss-Brookes L, Gavin A, Hounsome L, Huws D. The fraction of cancer attributable to modifiable risk factors in England, Wales, Scotland, Northern Ireland, and the United Kingdom in 2015. Br J Cancer. 2018;118(8):1130–41.
110. Bagnardi V, Rota M, Botteri E, Tramacere I, Islami F, Fedirko V, Scotti L, Jenab M, Turati F, Pasquali E, Pelucchi C. Alcohol consumption and site-specific cancer risk: a comprehensive dose–response meta-analysis. Br J Cancer. 2015;112(3):580–93.
111. Choi Y-J, Myung S-K, Lee J-H. Light alcohol drinking and risk of cancer: a meta-analysis of cohort studies. Cancer Res Treat. 2018;50(2):474–87.
112. Jayasekara H, MacInnis RJ, Room R, English DR. Long-term alcohol consumption and breast, upper aero-digestive tract and colorectal cancer risk: a systematic review and meta-analysis. Alcohol Alcohol. 2016;51(3):315–30.
113. Rinaldi S, Peeters PH, Bezemer ID, Dossus L, Biessy C, Sacerdote C, Berrino F, Panico S, Palli D, Tumino R, Khaw KT. Relationship of alcohol intake and sex steroid concentrations in blood in pre-and post-menopausal women: the European Prospective Investigation into Cancer and Nutrition. Cancer Causes Control. 2006;17(8):1033–43.
114. Fan S, Meng Q, Gao B, Grossman J, Yadegari M, Goldberg ID, Rosen EM. Alcohol stimulates estrogen receptor signaling in human breast cancer cell lines. Cancer Res. 2000;60(20):5635–9.
115. Singletary KW, Frey RS, Yan W. Effect of ethanol on proliferation and estrogen receptor-alpha expression in human breast cancer cells. Cancer Lett. 2001;165(2):131–7.
116. Tao MH, Marian C, Shields PG, Nie J, McCann SE, Millen A, Ambrosone C, Hutson A, Edge SB, Krishnan SS, Xie B. Alcohol consumption in relation to aberrant DNA methylation in breast tumors. Alcohol. 2011;45(7):689–99.
117. Liu Y, Nguyen N, Colditz GA. Links between alcohol consumption and breast cancer: a look at the evidence. Womens Health (Lond Engl). 2015;11(1):65–77.
118. Ward RJ, Colivicchi MA, Allen R, Schol F, Lallemand F, De Witte P, Ballini C, Corte LD, Dexter D. Neuro-inflammation induced in the hippocampus of 'binge drinking'rats may be mediated by elevated extracellular glutamate content. J Neurochem. 2009;111(5):1119–28.
119. Lindtner C, Scherer T, Zielinski E, Filatova N, Fasshauer M, Tonks NK, Puchowicz M, Buettner C. Binge drinking induces whole-body insulin resistance by impairing hypothalamic insulin action. Sci Transl Med. 2013;5(170):170ra14.
120. Boggs DA, Palmer JR, Stampfer MJ, Spiegelman D, Adams-Campbell LL, Rosenberg L. Tea and coffee intake in relation to risk of breast cancer in the Black Women's Health Study. Cancer Causes Control. 2010;21(11):1941–8.
121. Gierach GL, Freedman ND, Andaya A, Hollenbeck AR, Park Y, Schatzkin A, Brinton LA. Coffee intake and breast cancer risk in the nih-aarp diet and health study cohort. Int J Cancer. 2012;131(2):452–60.
122. Oh J-K, Sandin S, Ström P, Löf M, Adami H-O, Weiderpass E. Prospective study of breast cancer in relation to coffee, tea and caffeine in Sweden. Int J Cancer. 2015;137(8):1979–89.
123. Nehlig A, Reix N, Arbogast P, Mathelin C. Coffee consumption and breast cancer risk: a narrative review in the general population and in different subtypes of breast cancer. Eur J Nutr. 2021;60(3):1197–235.

124. Aune D, Chan DS, Greenwood DC, Vieira AR, Rosenblatt DN, Vieira R, Norat T. Dietary fiber and breast cancer risk: a systematic review and meta-analysis of prospective studies. Ann Oncol. 2012;23(6):1394–402.

125. Aune D, Chan DS, Vieira AR, Rosenblatt DA, Vieira R, Greenwood DC, Norat T. Fruits, vegetables and breast cancer risk: a systematic review and meta-analysis of prospective studies. Breast Cancer Res Treat. 2012;134(2):479–93.

126. Taylor EF, Burley VJ, Greenwood DC, Cade JE. Meat consumption and risk of breast cancer in the UK Women's Cohort Study. Br J Cancer. 2007;96(7):1139–46.

127. Jordan I, Hebestreit A, Swai B, Krawinkel MB. Dietary patterns and breast cancer risk among women in northern Tanzania: a case-control study. Eur J Nutr. 2013;52(3):905–15.

128. Sieri S, Krogh V, Ferrari P, Berrino F, Pala V, Thiébaut AC, Tjønneland A, Olsen A, Overvad K, Jakobsen MU, Clavel-Chapelon F. Dietary fat and breast cancer risk in the European Prospective Investigation into Cancer and Nutrition. Am J Clin Nutr. 2008;88(5):1304–12.

129. Peterson LL, Ligibel JA. Physical activity and breast cancer: an opportunity to improve outcomes. Curr Oncol Rep. 2018;20(7):50.

130. Friedenreich CM, Neilson HK, Lynch BM. State of the epidemiological evidence on physical activity and cancer prevention. Eur J Cancer. 2010;46(14):2593–604.

131. Wu Y, Zhang D, Kang S. Physical activity and risk of breast cancer: a meta-analysis of prospective studies. Breast Cancer Res Treat. 2013;137(3):869–82.

132. Moore SC, Lee IM, Weiderpass E, Campbell PT, Sampson JN, Kitahara CM, Keadle SK, Arem H, De Gonzalez AB, Hartge P, Adami HO. Association of leisure-time physical activity with risk of 26 types of cancer in 1.44 million adults. JAMA Intern Med. 2016;176(6):816–25.

133. McTiernan A, Kooperberg C, White E, Wilcox S, Coates R, Adams-Campbell LL, Woods N, Ockene J. Recreational physical activity and the risk of breast cancer in postmenopausal women: the Women's Health Initiative Cohort Study. JAMA. 2003;290(10):1331–6.

134. Shi Y, Li T, Wang Y, Zhou L, Qin Q, Yin J, Wei S, Liu L, Nie S. Household physical activity and cancer risk: a systematic review and dose-response meta-analysis of epidemiological studies. Sci Rep. 2015;5(1):1–10.

135. Bernstein L, Patel AV, Ursin G, Sullivan-Halley J, Press MF, Deapen D, Berlin JA, Daling JR, McDonald JA, Norman SA, Malone KE. Lifetime recreational exercise activity and breast cancer risk among black women and white women. J Natl Cancer Inst. 2005;97(22):1671–9.

136. Loprinzi PD, Cardinal BJ, Winters-Stone K, Smit E, Loprinzi CL. Physical activity and the risk of breast cancer recurrence: a literature review. Oncol Nurs Forum. 2012;39(3):269–74.

137. Zhong S, Jiang T, Ma T, Zhang X, Tang J, Chen W, Lv M, Zhao J. Association between physical activity and mortality in breast cancer: a meta-analysis of cohort studies. Eur J Epidemiol. 2014;29(6):391–404.

138. Spei M-E, Samoli E, Bravi F, La Vecchia C, Bamia C, Benetou V. Physical activity in breast cancer survivors: a systematic review and meta-analysis on overall and breast cancer survival. Breast. 2019;44:144–52.

139. Gaudet MM, Gapstur SM, Sun J, Diver WR, Hannan LM, Thun MJ. Active smoking and breast cancer risk: original cohort data and meta-analysis. J Natl Cancer Inst. 2013;105(8):515–25.

140. Gaudet MM, Carter BD, Brinton LA, Falk RT, Gram IT, Luo J, Milne RL, Nyante SJ, Weiderpass E, Beane Freeman LE, Sandler DP. Pooled analysis of active cigarette smoking and invasive breast cancer risk in 14 cohort studies. Int J Epidemiol. 2017;46(3):881–93.

141. Macacu A, Autier P, Boniol M, Boyle P. Active and passive smoking and risk of breast cancer: a meta-analysis. Breast Cancer Res Treat. 2015;154(2):213–24.

142. Kispert S, McHowat J. Recent insights into cigarette smoking as a lifestyle risk factor for breast cancer. Breast Cancer. 2017;9:127–32.

143. Luo J, Horn K, Ockene JK, Simon MS, Stefanick ML, Tong E, Margolis KL. Interaction between smoking and obesity and the risk of developing breast cancer among postmenopausal women: the Women's Health Initiative Observational Study. Am J Epidemiol. 2011;174(8):919–28.

144. Kabat GC, Kim M, Phipps AI, Li CI, Messina CR, Wactawski-Wende J, Kuller L, Simon MS, Yasmeen S, Wassertheil-Smoller S, Rohan TE. Smoking and alcohol consumption in relation to risk of triple-negative breast cancer in a cohort of postmenopausal women. Cancer Causes Control. 2011;22(5):775–83.

145. Kawai M, Malone KE, Tang M-TC, Li CI. Active smoking and the risk of estrogen receptor-positive and triple-negative breast cancer among women ages 20 to 44 years. Cancer. 2014;120(7):1026–34.

146. Luo J, Margolis KL, Wactawski-Wende J, Horn K, Messina C, Stefanick ML, Tindle HA, Tong E, Rohan TE. Association of active and passive smoking with risk of breast cancer among postmenopausal women: a prospective cohort study. BMJ. 2011;342:d1016.

147. Xue F, Willett WC, Rosner BA, Hankinson SE, Michels KB. Cigarette smoking and the incidence of breast cancer. Arch Intern Med. 2011;171(2):125–33.

148. Bosco JLF, Palmer JR, Boggs DA, Hatch EE, Rosenberg L. Regular aspirin use and breast cancer risk in US Black women. Cancer Causes Control. 2011;22(11):1553–61.

149. Brasky TM, Bonner MR, Moysich KB, Ambrosone CB, Nie J, Tao MH, Edge SB, Kallakury BV, Marian C, Goerlitz DS, Trevisan M. Non-steroidal anti-inflammatory drugs (NSAIDs) and breast cancer risk: differences by molecular subtype. Cancer Causes Control. 2011;22(7):965–75.

150. Cui Y, Deming-Halverson SL, Shrubsole MJ, Beeghly-Fadiel A, Cai H, Fair AM, Shu XO, Zheng W. Use of nonsteroidal anti-inflammatory drugs and reduced breast cancer risk among overweight women. Breast Cancer Res Treat. 2014;146(2):439–46.

151. Clarke CA, Canchola AJ, Moy LM, Neuhausen SL, Chung NT, Lacey JV, Bernstein L. Regular and low-dose aspirin, other non-steroidal anti-inflammatory medications and prospective risk of HER2-defined breast cancer: the California Teachers Study. Breast Cancer Res. 2017;19(1):1–12.

152. McNeil JJ, Gibbs P, Orchard SG, Lockery JE, Bernstein WB, Cao Y, Ford L, Haydon A, Kirpach B, Macrae F, McLean C. Effect of aspirin on cancer incidence and mortality in older adults. J Natl Cancer Inst. 2021;113(3):258–65.

153. Chen WY, Winer EP, Barry WT, Partridge AH, Carey LA, Carvan M, Matyka C, Visvanathan K, Symington B, Holmes MD. ABC trial (A011502): Randomized phase III double blinded placebo controlled trial of aspirin as adjuvant therapy for breast cancer. J Clin Oncol. 2018;36(15):TPS597.

154. Palmer JR, Wise LA, Hatch EE, Troisi R, Titus-Ernstoff L, Strohsnitter W, Kaufman R, Herbst AL, Noller KL, Hyer M, Hoover RN. Prenatal diethylstilbestrol exposure and risk of breast cancer. Cancer Epidemiol Prev Biomarkers. 2006;15(8):1509–14.

155. Hoover RN, Hyer M, Pfeiffer RM, Adam E, Bond B, Cheville AL, Colton T, Hartge P, Hatch EE, Herbst AL, Karlan BY. Adverse health outcomes in women exposed in utero to diethylstilbestrol. N Engl J Med. 2011;365(14):1304–14.

156. Han H, Guo W, Shi W, Yu Y, Zhang Y, Ye X, He J. Hypertension and breast cancer risk: a systematic review and meta-analysis. Sci Rep. 2017;7(1):1–9.

157. Palme M, Simeonova E. Does women's education affect breast cancer risk and survival? Evidence from a population based social experiment in education. J Health Econ. 2015;42:115–24.

158. Coughlin SS. Social determinants of breast cancer risk, stage, and survival. Breast Cancer Res Treat. 2019;177(3):537–48.

159. Akinyemiju TF, Pisu M, Waterbor JW, Altekruse SF. Socioeconomic status and incidence of breast cancer by hormone receptor subtype. Springerplus. 2015;4:508.

160. Orsini M, Trétarre B, Daurès J-P, Bessaoud F. Individual socioeconomic status and breast cancer diagnostic stages: a French case-control study. Eur J Public Health. 2016;26(3):445–50.

161. Lundqvist A, Andersson E, Ahlberg I, Nilbert M, Gerdtham U. Socioeconomic inequalities in breast cancer incidence and mortality in Europe—a systematic review and meta-analysis. Eur J Public Health. 2016;26(5):804–13.

162. Shariff-Marco S, Yang J, John EM, Sangaramoorthy M, Hertz A, Koo J, Nelson DO, Schupp CW, Shema SJ, Cockburn M, Satariano WA. Impact of neighborhood and individual socioeconomic status on survival after breast cancer varies by race/ethnicity: the Neighborhood and Breast Cancer Study. Cancer Epidemiol Prev Biomarkers. 2014;23(5):793–811.

163. Hastert TA, Beresford SAA, Sheppard L, White E. Disparities in cancer incidence and mortality by area-level socioeconomic status: a multilevel analysis. J Epidemiol Community Health. 2015;69(2):168–76.

164. Booth CM, Li G, Zhang-Salomons J, Mackillop WJ. The impact of socioeconomic status on stage of cancer at diagnosis and survival: a population-based study in Ontario, Canada. Cancer. 2010;116(17):4160–7.

165. Quaglia A, Lillini R, Mamo C, Ivaldi E, Vercelli M. Socio-economic inequalities: a review of methodological issues and the relationships with cancer survival. Crit Rev Oncol Hematol. 2013;85(3):266–77.

166. Singer S, Bartels M, Briest S, Einenkel J, Niederwieser D, Papsdorf K, Stolzenburg JU, Künstler S, Taubenheim S, Krauß O. Socio-economic disparities in long-term cancer survival—10 year follow-up with individual patient data. Support Care Cancer. 2017;25(5):1391–9.

167. O'Malley CD, Le GM, Glaser SL, Shema SJ, West DW. Socioeconomic status and breast carcinoma survival in four racial/ethnic groups: a population-based study. Cancer. 2003;97(5):1303–11.

168. Rutherford MJ, Hinchliffe SR, Abel GA, Lyratzopoulos G, Lambert PC, Greenberg DC. How much of the deprivation gap in cancer survival can be explained by variation in stage at diagnosis: an example from breast cancer in the East of England. Int J Cancer. 2013;133(9):2192–200.

169. Berglund A, Lambe M, Lüchtenborg M, Linklater K, Peake MD, Holmberg L, Møller H. Social differences in lung cancer management and survival in South East England: a cohort study. BMJ Open. 2012;2(3):e001048.

170. Cordina-Duverger E, Menegaux F, Popa A, Rabstein S, Harth V, Pesch B, Brüning T, Fritschi L, Glass DC, Heyworth JS, Erren TC. Night shift work and breast cancer: a pooled analysis of population-based case–control studies with complete work history. Eur J Epidemiol. 2018;33(4):369–79.

171. Stevens RG, Davis S. The melatonin hypothesis: electric power and breast cancer. Environ Health Perspect. 1996;104(Suppl 1):135–40.

172. Megdal SP, Kroenke CH, Laden F, Pukkala E, Schernhammer ES. Night work and breast cancer risk: a systematic review and meta-analysis. Eur J Cancer. 2005;41(13):2023–32.

173. Benabu J-C, Stoll F, Gonzalez M, Mathelin C. Night work, shift work: breast cancer risk factor? Gynecol Obstet Fertil. 2015;43(12):791–9.

174. Lu C, Sun H, Huang J, Yin S, Hou W, Zhang J, Wang Y, Xu Y, Xu H. Long-term sleep duration as a risk factor for breast cancer: evidence from a systematic review and dose-response meta-analysis. Biomed Res Int. 2017;2017:4845059.

175. Xiao Q, Signorello LB, Brinton LA, Cohen SS, Blot WJ, Matthews CE. Sleep duration and breast can-

cer risk among black and white women. Sleep Med. 2016;20:25–9.

176. Chiu H-Y, Huang C-J, Fan Y-C, Tsai P-S. Insomnia but not hypnotics use associates with the risk of breast cancer: a population-based matched cohort study. J Womens Health (Larchmt). 2018;27(10):1250–6.

177. Soucise A, Vaughn C, Thompson CL, Millen AE, Freudenheim JL, Wactawski-Wende J, Phipps AI, Hale L, Qi L, Ochs-Balcom HM. Sleep quality, duration, and breast cancer aggressiveness. Breast Cancer Res Treat. 2017;164(1):169–78.

178. Vogtmann E, Levitan EB, Hale L, Shikany JM, Shah NA, Endeshaw Y, Lewis CE, Manson JE, Chlebowski RT. Association between sleep and breast cancer incidence among postmenopausal women in the Women's Health Initiative. Sleep. 2013;36(10):1437–44.

179. John EM, Phipps AI, Knight JA, Milne RL, Dite GS, Hopper JL, Andrulis IL, Southey M, Giles GG, West DW, Whittemore AS. Medical radiation exposure and breast cancer risk: findings from the Breast Cancer Family Registry. Int J Cancer. 2007;121(2):386–94.

180. Swerdlow AJ, Barber JA, Hudson GV, Cunningham D, Gupta RK, Hancock BW, Horwich A, Lister TA, Linch DC. Risk of second malignancy after Hodgkin's disease in a collaborative British cohort: the relation to age at treatment. J Clin Oncol. 2000;18(3):498.

181. Kenney LB, Yasui Y, Inskip PD, Hammond S, Neglia JP, Mertens AC, Meadows AT, Friedman D, Robison LL, Diller L. Breast cancer after childhood cancer: a report from the Childhood Cancer Survivor Study. Ann Intern Med. 2004;141(8):590–7.

182. Taylor AJ, Winter DL, Stiller CA, Murphy M, Hawkins MM. Risk of breast cancer in female survivors of childhood Hodgkin's disease in Britain: a population-based study. Int J Cancer. 2007;120(2):384–91.

183. De Bruin ML, Sparidans J, van't Veer MB, Noordijk EM, Louwman MW, Zijlstra JM, van den Berg H, Russell NS, Broeks A, Baaijens MH, Aleman BM. Breast cancer risk in female survivors of Hodgkin's lymphoma: lower risk after smaller radiation volumes. J Clin Oncol. 2009;27(26):4239–46.

184. O'Brien MM, Donaldson SS, Balise RR, Whittemore AS, Link MP. Second malignant neoplasms in survivors of pediatric Hodgkin's lymphoma treated with low-dose radiation and chemotherapy. J Clin Oncol. 2010;28(7):1232–9.

185. Green DM, Hyland A, Barcos MP, Reynolds JA, Lee RJ, Hall BC, Zevon MA. Second malignant neoplasms after treatment for Hodgkin's disease in childhood or adolescence. J Clin Oncol. 2000;18(7):1492–9.

186. Mauch PM, Kalish LA, Marcus KC, Coleman CN, Shulman LN, Krill E, Come S, Silver B, Canellos GP, Tarbell NJ. Second malignancies after treatment for laparotomy staged IA-IIIB Hodgkin's disease: long-term analysis of risk factors and outcome. Blood. 1996;87(9):3625–32.

187. Bhatia S, Robison LL, Oberlin O, Greenberg M, Bunin G, Fossati-Bellani F, Meadows AT. Breast cancer and other second neoplasms after childhood Hodgkin's disease. N Engl J Med. 1996;334(12):745–51.

188. Roychoudhuri R, Evans H, Robinson D, Møller H. Radiation-induced malignancies following radiotherapy for breast cancer. Br J Cancer. 2004;91(5):868–72.

189. Early Breast Cancer Trialists' Collaborative Group. Effects of radiotherapy and of differences in the extent of surgery for early breast cancer on local recurrence and 15-year survival: an overview of the randomised trials. Lancet. 2005;366(9503):2087–106.

190. Curtis RE, Freedman DM, Ron E, Ries LAG, Hacker DG, Edwards BK, Tucker MA, Fraumeni JF Jr. New malignancies among cancer survivors: SEER Cancer Registries, 1973-2000. Bethesda: National Cancer Institute (NCI); 2006.

191. Berrington de Gonzalez A, Curtis RE, Gilbert E, Berg CD, Smith SA, Stovall M, Ron E. Second solid cancers after radiotherapy for breast cancer in SEER cancer registries. Br J Cancer. 2010;102(1):220–6.

192. Gao X, Fisher SG, Emami B. Risk of second primary cancer in the contralateral breast in women treated for early-stage breast cancer: a population-based study. Int J Radiat Oncol. 2003;56(4):1038–45.

193. Burt LM, Ying J, Poppe MM, Suneja G, Gaffney DK. Risk of secondary malignancies after radiation therapy for breast cancer: comprehensive results. Breast. 2017;35:122–9.

194. Berrington de González A, Darby S. Risk of cancer from diagnostic X-rays: estimates for the UK and 14 other countries. Lancet. 2004;363(9406):345–51.

195. Hendrick RE. Radiation doses and risks in breast screening. J Breast Imaging. 2020;2(3):188–200.

196. National Institute for Health and Care Excellence (NICE). Familial breast cancer: classification, care and managing breast cancer and related risks in people with a family history of breast cancer. NICE guideline [CG164]. 2019. https://www.nice.org.uk/guidance/cg164/resources/2019-exceptional-surveillance-of-familial-breast-cancer-classification-care-and-managing-breast-cancer-and-related-risks-in-people-with-a-family-history-of-breast-cancer-nice-guideline-cg164-pdf-9029474482885. Accessed 15 Jan 2021.

197. Bjerkaas E, Parajuli R, Engeland A, Maskarinec G, Weiderpass E, Gram IT. Social inequalities and smoking-associated breast cancer—results from a prospective cohort study. Prev Med (Baltim). 2015;73:125–9.

198. Gram IT, Park SY, Kolonel LN, Maskarinec G, Wilkens LR, Henderson BE, Le Marchand L. Smoking and risk of breast cancer in a racially/ethnically diverse population of mainly women who do not drink alcohol: the MEC study. Am J Epidemiol. 2015;182(11):917–25.

199. Li B, Wang L, Lu MS, Mo XF, Lin FY, Ho SC, Zhang CX. Passive smoking and breast cancer risk

among non-smoking women: a case-control study in China. PLoS One. 2015;10(4):e0125894.

200. Strumylaite L, Kregzdyte R, Poskiene L, Bogusevicius A, Pranys D, Norkute R. Association between lifetime exposure to passive smoking and risk of breast cancer subtypes defined by hormone receptor status among non-smoking Caucasian women. PLoS One. 2017;12(2):e0171198.

201. Wan MLY, Co VA, El-Nezami H. Endocrine disrupting chemicals and breast cancer: a systematic review of epidemiological studies. Crit Rev Food Sci Nutr. 2021;1–27.

Breast Diseases

7

Susan Williams and Lisa Hackney

S. Williams (✉)
Shrewsbury and Telford Hospital NHS Trust, The
Royal Shrewsbury Hospital, Shrewsbury, UK
e-mail: susan.williams46@nhs.net

L. Hackney
East Cheshire NHS Trust, Macclesfield, UK
e-mail: Lisa.Hackney@nhs.net

Learning Objectives

- Describe a range of conditions that may affect breast tissue
- Recognise some of the typical mammographic features of breast diseases
- Understand and describe breast lesions that confer an increased risk of developing breast cancer

Introduction

A wide spectrum of breast diseases of varying clinical and prognostic significance can be detected on mammography. The majority (80%) of invasive cancers are from the heterogeneous group of ductal carcinomas (no specific type). The most frequent of the special subtype is lobular carcinoma (10%). The less common subtypes include mucinous, tubular, medullary, cribriform, micropapillary, papillary, metaplastic, and inflammatory carcinomas.

Cysts

Breast cysts are formed when there is an accumulation of fluid within the terminal ductal lobular unit. This distension results in ovoid or circular structures that may be evident on mammography, dependent on their size and background breast density. Cysts are most common in premenopausal women in their 30s or 40s. They are less common after the menopause but may persist or reappear in HRT users [1]. Cysts may be unilateral but are frequently bilateral and multifocal. They can be classified according to size, a microcyst being <3 mm and a macrocyst >3 mm. Simple cysts are benign and do not require any treatment or further diagnostic work-up unless painful when aspiration can relieve symptoms. Complex cysts require aspiration or needle core biopsy to exclude intracystic disease [2] (Fig. 7.1).

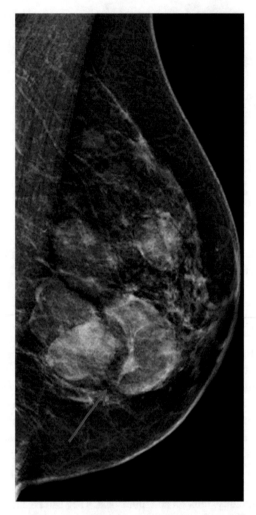

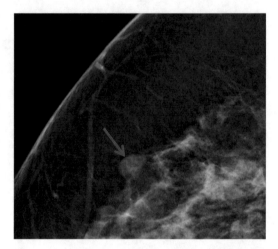

Fig. 7.2 Fibroadenoma. Cranio-caudal (CC) view showing a well-defined lesion (arrow) in the outer aspect of the right breast

Fig. 7.1 Cysts. Medio-Lateral Oblique (MLO) view showing multiple ovoid/lobulated lesions (arrow). Parenchymal structures can be seen through the lesion. The low density, ovoid shape and partial halo suggest a benign lesion, but ultrasound is required to differentiate a cyst from a solid lesion

Fibroadenoma

Fibroadenomas are benign fibroepithelial tumours. They are most common in adolescent girls and young women [3]. Fibroadenomas typically present as smooth, mobile, firm masses but may also be impalpable and detected via mammographic imaging. It is not uncommon for individuals to have multiple fibroadenomata. On mammography, fibroadenomas appear as well-defined round, ovoid, or lobulated masses (Fig. 7.2). However, the masses may calcify over time and develop a typical popcorn-shaped pattern (Figs. 7.3 and 7.4). A typical benign calcified fibroadenoma requires no further work-up. If non-calcified, ultrasound is required to characterise the lesion and dependent upon the age of the patient histological sampling (needle core biopsy) may be performed. There are also special types of fibroadenoma to include: lactating adenomas, tubular adenomas and juvenile fibroadenomas. Occasionally, these masses grow to a large size in adolescent girls and young women and are termed juvenile giant fibroadenomas [3].

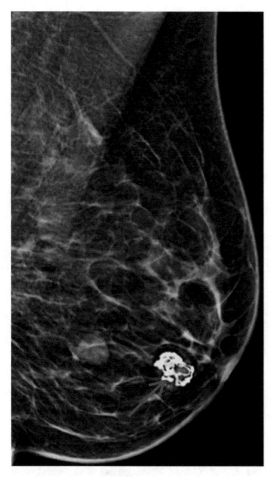

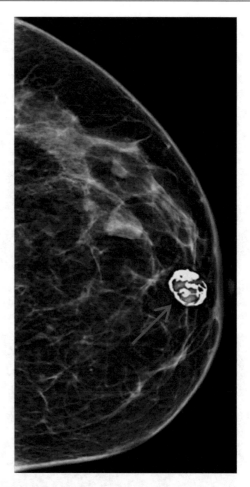

Fig. 7.3 Fibroadenoma: MLO mammogram shows several circumscribed masses. The anterior mass (arrow) contains coarse heterogenous "popcorn" calcifications typical for fibroadenoma

Fig. 7.4 Fibroadenoma: CC mammogram shows several circumscribed masses. The anterior mass (arrow) contains coarse heterogenous "popcorn" calcifications typical for fibroadenoma

Phyllodes Tumours

Phyllodes tumours, also referred to as cystosarcoma phyllodes, are fibroepithelial tumours of the breast which have some similarities to a fibroadenoma but are rare in comparison, accounting for less than 1% of all breast tumours [4]. They most commonly occur between the ages of 40 and 60. Clinically they often present as a large, rapidly growing lump. Mammographically, most phyllodes tumours are large, circumscribed masses that are round, oval, or lobulated (Fig. 7.5). Phyllodes tumours are classified as benign (non-cancerous), borderline or malignant (cancerous). Historically, benign phyllodes tumours required excision with wide histological margins, as some studies reported an increased risk for local recurrence with margins less than 10 mm [5]. However, the evidence for this remains debatable. For large or rapidly growing phyllodes, a mastectomy may be advocated to obtain a negative margin [6]. The role of adjuvant radiotherapy and chemotherapy remains contentious [6].

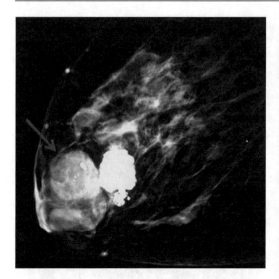

Fig. 7.5 Phyllodes. MLO view shows a heterogeneously dense breast with a rounded, well-circumscribed, 5-cm mass (arrow) in the retro-areolar region of the right breast

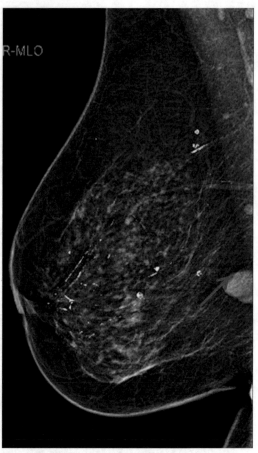

Fig. 7.7 MLO view demonstrating a superficial, well defined ovoid lesion (arrow) in the posterior aspect of the right breast

Haemangioma

Breast haemangiomas are benign vascular tumours, which fall into three categories (capillary, cavernous and venous) dependent upon vessel size [7]. Clinical manifestation is a palpable lump, but they are often incidental findings on screening mammography.

Haemangiomas appear as well-defined, ovoid, or lobulated isodense masses located within the superficial tissues of the breast (Figs. 7.6 and 7.7), and based on mammography alone, can also be difficult to distinguish from fibroadenomas.

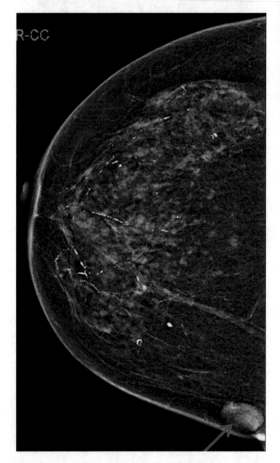

Fig. 7.6 CC view demonstrating a superficial, well defined ovoid lesion (arrow) in the inner aspect of the right breast

Gynaecomastia

Physiological gynaecomastia is the commonest benign male breast condition, with a greater prevalence in neonates, puberty and over 50 years of age. Breast enlargement occurs due to benign ductal and stromal proliferation. There is a wide range of causes, including endogenous hormonal imbalance, systemic disease, hormone-producing tumours, obesity, and some drugs' action. Gynaecomastia usually presents as a firm, palpable subareolar mass that may be tender. It is usually unilateral but may be bilateral. On mammography, gynaecomastia has three typical patterns [8]: nodular, dendritic, and diffuse.

The early florid phase of gynaecomastia (nodular) is associated with a shorter duration of symptoms and is identified on mammography as a large, poorly defined subareolar density (Fig. 7.8). The dendritic growth pattern is observed when symptoms are persistent over a more extended period (more than one year) and mammographically manifests as a smaller, spiculated, subareolar density (Fig. 7.9). The third pattern, diffuse gynaecomastia, is frequently related to oestrogen exposure. Mammographically, this mimics a heterogeneously dense female breast (Fig. 7.10). Psedogynaecomastia is more likely to be bilateral and relates to enlargement of the breast with adipose tissue only (Fig. 7.11).

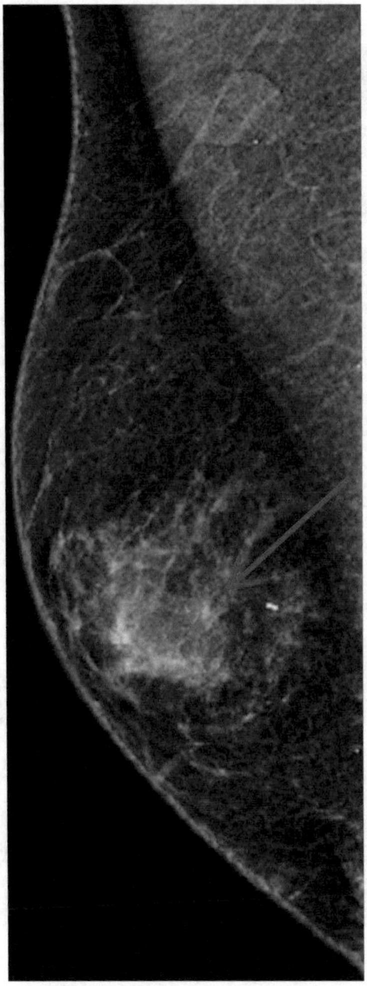

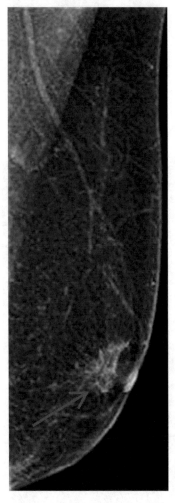

Fig. 7.8 Florid gynaecomastia associated with an acute process

Fig. 7.9 Dendritic gynecomastia representative of a chronic condition

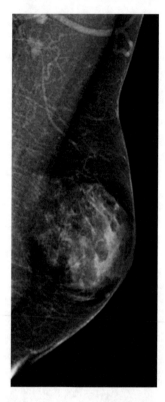

Fig. 7.10 Heterogeneously dense breast tissue

Schwannoma

Most primary tumours of the breast have an epithelial origin. Non-epithelial tumours in the breast are rare [9]. A Schwannoma (Fig. 7.12) develops from 'Schwann' cells of the peripheral nerve sheath and may also be referred to as a neurilemmoma, or peripheral nerve sheath tumour. A Schwannoma may be a spontaneous incidence or occur because of a familial tumour syndrome, i.e., neurofibromatosis Type 2 (NF2) and Carney's complex [9]. For unknown reasons, Schwann cells can occasionally grow in a neoplastic fashion resulting in a benign tumour. However, there is a remote likelihood of a Schwannoma developing malignant cellular

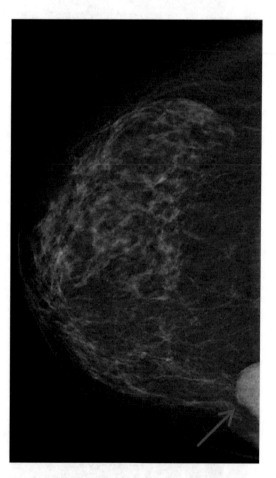

Fig. 7.12 Mammographically schwannomas are most often described as a non-specific well-defined round or oval, high-density lesion. The CC view demonstrates the anterior border of a well-defined dense mass in the inner aspect of the right breast (arrow). The mass is only partially demonstrated due to its posterior and medial location

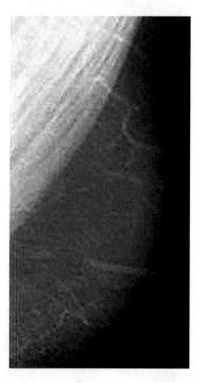

Fig. 7.11 Pseudogynaecomastia, characterised by subcutaneous fat deposition in the breast without a mass or glandular development

characteristics. Malignant peripheral nerve sheath tumours commonly occur in patients with neurofibromatosis Type I (NF 1) [10].

Hamartoma

A breast hamartoma (also referred to as a fibroadenolipoma) is a benign breast lesion resulting from the proliferation of fibrous, glandular, and fatty tissue surrounded by a thin capsule of connective tissue [11]. Lesions can be variable in size and present as painless soft lumps, unilateral breast enlargement without a palpable mass, or can be asymptomatic and an incidental finding on mammography. Multiple hamartomas are associated with Cowden's

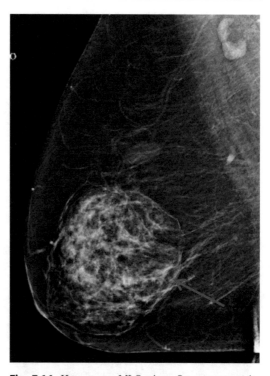

Fig. 7.14 Hamartoma MLO view. On mammography hamartomas have a typical appearance. An encapsulated lucent lesion (arrow) containing varying amounts of fat, fibrous and adenomatous elements

syndrome (a rare autosomal dominant inherited disorder), which carries an increased risk of breast carcinoma [12]. Mammographically, hamartomas are typically seen as well-circumscribed, round, or ovoid masses comprising of both fat and soft-tissue densities (both radiolucent and dense components). Sometimes this is described as a "breast within a breast" appearance [13] (Figs. 7.13 and 7.14).

Lipoma

A lipoma is a benign lesion composed of fat. Generally, breast lipomas present as painless, soft, mobile lumps, which are variable in size (ranging from <1 cm to >6 cm) [14]. Mammographically, lipomas (Figs. 7.15 and 7.16) are identified as radiolucent masses and are often easier to detect in denser breasts.

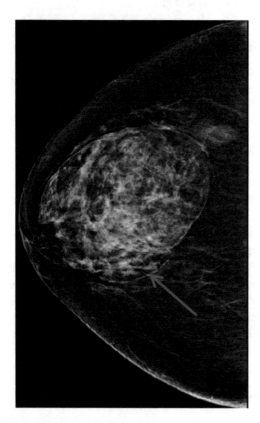

Fig. 7.13 Hamartoma CC view. On mammography hamartomas have a typical appearance. An encapsulated lucent lesion (arrow) containing varying amounts of fat, fibrous and adenomatous elements

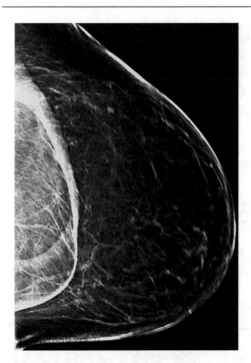

Fig. 7.15 Intra-muscular lipoma visualized as a smooth radiolucent lesion with a surrounding capsule of fibrous tissue (arrow) CC view

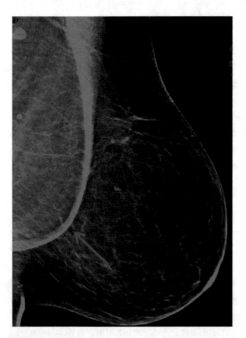

Fig. 7.16 Intra-muscular lipoma visualized as a smooth radiolucent lesion with a surrounding capsule of fibrous tissue (arrow) MLO view

Pseudoangiomatous Stromal Hyperplasia (PASH)

Pseudoangiomatous stromal hyperplasia is a benign, rare form of stromal (mesenchymal) overgrowth within the breast tissue [15]. PASH is typically found in premenopausal women but can be a common incidental finding at breast biopsy. If forming a mass lesion, the presentation is commonly a solitary, circumscribed, firm palpable mass. There is a wide variance of size of PASH mass lesions with the diameter ranging from 1 to 12 cm. PASH is not considered a premalignant lesion [15]. Most frequently, they appear on mammography as a circumscribed/partly circumscribed mass, but variable appearances have also been reported [16].

Galactocele

A galactocele is a benign breast lesion that typically occurs in lactating women or, more commonly, on cessation of lactation [17]. They occur because of ductal obstruction and inspissation of the milk. Galactoceles have differing water, proteins, fat, and lactose proportions, reflecting variable mammographic appearances [18]. Based on this, galactoceles could appear radiolucent, have a fat/fluid level, or appear to have a mixed density. A typical presentation is a painless breast lump that may be solitary and unilateral, but multiple and bilateral nodules have also been reported. Spontaneous resolution occurs in most cases, but if there is diagnostic uncertainty, aspiration can be performed, which will classically yield milky fluid of variable viscosity dependent on how old the liquid is [18].

Haematoma

A haematoma is a blood collection, which usually results from a preceding direct trauma, surgery, or biopsy but can spontaneously occur in those on anticoagulants. Clinical correlation is

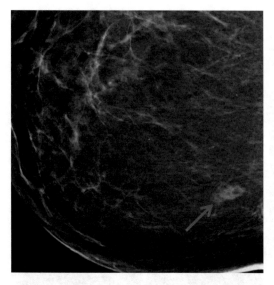

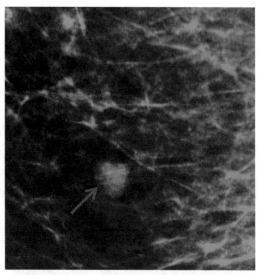

Fig. 7.17 Haematoma. Right CC view shows a relatively well-defined lesion of variable density (arrow)

Fig. 7.18 Papilloma. CC view showing a circumscribed solitary subareolar mass

essential to avoid misinterpretation with breast malignancy. Depending on the stage of haematoma formation, they have variable mammographic appearances, the most common being an area of diffusely increased glandular density [19]. However, if more localised, a relatively well-defined mass may also be seen (Fig. 7.17). Most haematomas resolve within 2–4 weeks, and no further evaluation is required. However, some haematomas may liquefy and develop into a breast seroma or, over time, may evolve into fat necrosis [19].

Papilloma

An intraductal papilloma is a benign tumour that forms within the breast ducts. However, papillomata are heterogeneous lesions with variable pathological features and are subdivided into those without any epithelial atypia, with atypia, and with features of malignancy [20]. Papillomata are also classified based on their location:

- Central—are typically solitary lesions within a large duct in the subareolar region. These may be felt as a small lump and are typically associated with a clear or bloody nipple discharge.

- Peripheral papillomata—are likely to be multiple and located within smaller ducts.

Mammograms are often normal, particularly if the papillomata are small. However, when imaging findings are present, they are identified as a circumscribed subareolar mass, or a solitary dilated retro areolar duct/s, or a cluster of calcifications [21] (Fig. 7.18). Due to intralesional heterogeneity, large volume sampling (Vacuum-Assisted Excision >4 g) or surgical excision is required, depending on whether atypia is present. The probability of malignancy is higher (36–47.8%) when atypia is present in the initial sample [20, 22].

Amyloid Tumour

Amyloidosis results from the abnormal deposition of a protein called amyloid in various body tissues. Breast amyloidosis is rare and can be part of a systemic disease, or it may be localised to the breast [23] (Fig. 7.19). However, the typical clinical presentation is a unilateral, painless, solitary breast mass. Mammographically, they present as diverse masses, often multiple, which may have associated microcalcifications [23].

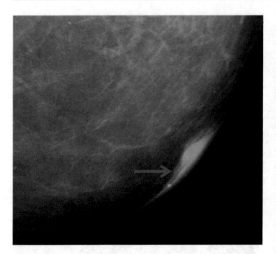

Fig. 7.19 Amyloid tumour. A unilateral, solitary superficial breast mass with associated microcalcification (arrow)

Mastitis/Abscess

Mastitis refers to inflammation of the breast tissue, which may be with or without infection. Early stages of mastitis typically present as localised pain, redness, swelling, and warmth with a rapid onset.

Puerperal

Puerperal mastitis refers to inflammation of the breast in connection with pregnancy, breastfeeding or weaning and is considered a result of blocked milk ducts and stasis [18].

Non-puerperal

The term non-puerperal mastitis refers to inflammation of the breast unrelated to pregnancy and breastfeeding and includes the rarer granulomatous mastitis and iatrogenic inflammation. Later stages of mastitis may have associated systemic symptoms and abscess formation (collection of pus). Abscesses are separated into two groups: (1) Central/subareolar abscesses, which are commonly seen in young women, particularly those who smoke. (2) Peripheral abscesses, which are more frequently observed in older women with

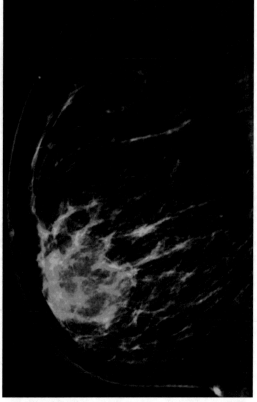

Fig. 7.20 Abscess. Diffuse asymmetric density in the central right breast

underlying medical conditions such as diabetes mellitus, chronic illness, or an impaired immune system making them more susceptible to developing a breast infection [24]. Zuska's disease depicts recurrent non-puerperal abscesses and fistulae formation [25].

Abscesses are managed with antibiotic treatment and percutaneous drainage if amenable. In a certain number of cases, incision and surgical drainage are required. Mammography is rarely indicated but may be undertaken to exclude the possibility of malignancy in non-puerperal abscesses and in puerperal abscesses that are non-responsive to treatment. Inflammatory breast cancer presents with similar symptoms to mastitis and is an aggressive form of the disease. Mammographic appearances of an abscess are often non-specific but include skin thickening, an asymmetric density (Fig. 7.20), distortion, or a focal mass [24, 25].

Breast Metastases

Metastases to the breast are rare. The most frequent source of a metastatic breast lesion is the contralateral breast but it may also arise from: Melanoma [26], sarcomas [27], prostate cancer [28], lung cancer [29], gastric cancer [30], ovarian cancer [31] and renal cell cancer [32]. Metastases in the breast tend to be rounded, well defined, and located in the subcutaneous fat and are much more likely to be multiple and/or bilateral.

Breast Lymphoma

Breast lymphomas can be primary or secondary lesions, but both are uncommon [33]. Secondary breast lymphoma is the most common metastasis to the breast, comprised of lymphoid tissue and breast tissue. The presentation may be a palpable mass or diffused thickening of the breast with enlarged axillary lymph nodes [33]. Lymphomas have variable mammographic appearances but typically manifest with a diffuse increase in parenchymal density (Fig. 7.21).

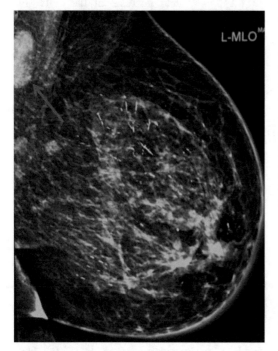

Fig. 7.21 Lymphoma. Diffuse increased reticular pattern with skin thickening and oedema secondary to lymphatic obstruction. Enlarged axillary lymph nodes are evident (arrow)

Breast Sarcoma

A breast sarcoma is a diverse and rare group of cancer that develops from mesenchymal tissue. They can develop as a primary lesion often associated with genetic conditions; radiation therapy of the breast or other intrathoracic malignancies is the most common cause of secondary lesions [34]. Secondary angiosarcoma is the most commonly reported form of sarcoma.

Duct Ectasia

Duct ectasia is an involutionary condition characterised by dilated ducts and chronic inflammation resulting in debris within the duct. Inspissation of the debris and secretions can lead to calcification of the ductal contents. It usually coexists with periductal mastitis as the fluid often sets up an irritant reaction in surrounding tissue leading to periductal mastitis or even abscess and fistula formation. It is more common in females aged 50–60 years. Plasma cell mastitis is often used as an interchangeable term with duct ectasia but tends to refer to a more extreme form of the process [35].

A common mammographic feature is calcification of variable morphology, including calcified ring, oval shapes or elongated, very dense calcification with central lucency. The calcifications are usually higher density and wider calibre than malignant type casting calcification and are directed towards the nipple [36], as shown in Fig. 7.22. The symptomatic features include nipple discharge, nipple retraction, non-cyclical mastalgia and subareolar masses, which all mimic breast cancer. It is a feature commonly seen on screening mammograms [36].

Radial Scar/Complex Sclerosing Lesion

Radial scars and complex sclerosing lesions are the same clinical feature, the differentiation lying in their respective sizes - a radial scar being <10 mm in diameter [37]. A radial scar is a benign lesion but is significant because it can be linked with DCIS and tubular cancers [38]. Histologically

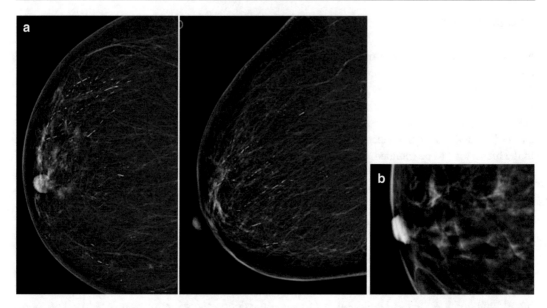

Fig. 7.22 Duct ectasia. Typical mammographic features showing (**a**) thick linear rod-like calcification orientated with the long axes directed towards the nipple, (**b**) dilated ducts in the retroareolar region

mimicking a scar, radial scars are not related to trauma; they are characterised by a central fibro elastotic core with radiating spokes of ducts and lobules.

Mammographically, it is often seen as a stellate lesion (Fig. 7.23) which can mimic an invasive carcinoma, but their appearance often varies on different projections. Typical mammographic features are lesions with a radiolucent centre from which multiple long thin spicules radiate [37–39]. Although they can be palpable, they are more frequently a screen-detected or incidental finding. The mammographic appearances are also similar to a post-surgical breast scar.

Correlation with the clinical breast examination, an ultrasound scan and a needle core biopsy will assist with the differentiation between a radial scar and an invasive carcinoma. Vacuum-assisted biopsies are now routinely used to inform the management of these lesions which are usually removed by vacuum-assisted excision [40].

Fat Necrosis

Fat necrosis is a benign condition resulting from trauma to the breast tissue, however, most cases are diagnosed post-surgery. Following breast trauma, a haemorrhage occurs, which may extravasate into the parenchyma, causing oedema and disruption to the fat cells creating intracellular vacuoles filled with necrotic lipid material [41, 42]. Apoptosis and necrosis of the cells also occur in the tissue, and a greater necrotic component results in changes to the breast, which can mimic more sinister conditions.

Mammographically, fat necrosis can range from clearly benign to malignant appearing masses or calcifications. The most common mammographic finding is dystrophic calcifications followed by a radiolucent oil cyst. An oil cyst is a benign lesion where an area of focal fat necrosis becomes walled by fibrous tissue, which can calcify. On mammography, it is typically seen as a radiolucent rounded mass of fat density with or without wall calcification (Fig. 7.24a, b). Oil cysts are the only mammographic finding that reliably indicates fat necrosis [43].

Suspicious spiculate masses and focal areas of architectural distortion can also occur, resembling carcinoma. The calcification of fat necrosis is typically peripheral with a stippled curvilinear appearance creating the appearance of lucent "bubbles" in the breast parenchyma (Fig. 7.24c). Fat necrosis of the breast can change, regressing, or resolving over time.

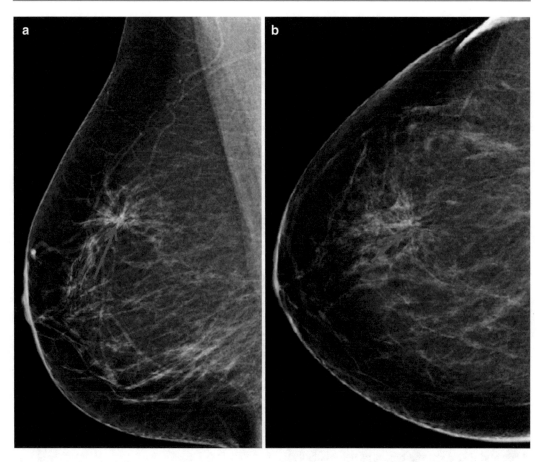

Fig. 7.23 Radial scar with long spicules radiating from a radiolucent centre in (**a**) the MLO and (**b**) the CC views

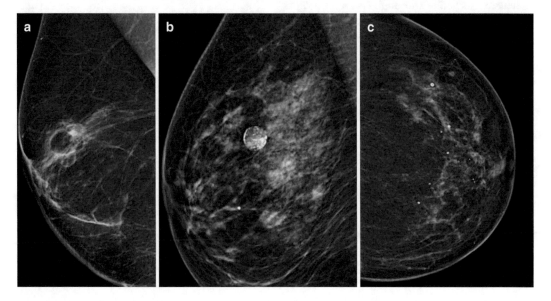

Fig. 7.24 Shows fat necrosis of the breast, shows (**a**) the typical mammographic features of an oil cyst, (**b**) coarse calcifications in peripheral and central portions of mass with lucent centres, (**c**) lucent "bubbles"

Surgical Scar

A benign complication of postsurgical mammography is scar tissue at the site of surgery. The dense fibrous tissue that develops in a postsurgical scar often appears as an irregular mass with spiculate margins, often with retraction of the surrounding tissue (Fig. 7.25). The mammographic appearances are difficult to differentiate from cancer, particularly for the first mammogram after surgery, as distortion and increased density may persist for many months post-surgery [41]. Other mammographic appearances include architectural distortion, a poorly marginated soft-tissue mass with interspersed radiolucent areas, or a spiculate lesion; all of these may have associated calcification. Postsurgical scarring usually relates to the skin scar or site of previous surgery and is either stable or decreases in size over time [41].

Treatment for breast cancer does not necessarily only involve the removal of the tumour. Other interventions such as radiotherapy and axillary surgery will impact on the mammographic appearances (Fig. 7.26), including generalised tissue oedema, skin thickening, and a change in shape and texture of the breast parenchyma [44]. Postsurgical changes can render mammography technically difficult. Thorough history taking is important, including accurate recording of the site of surgery when imaging the client.

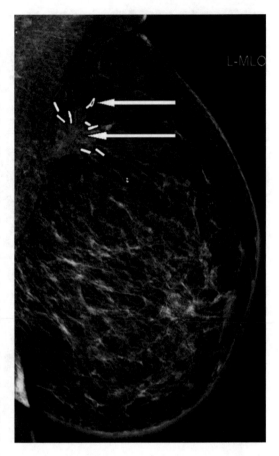

Fig. 7.25 MLO view post-surgery. Although the scarring appears spiculate, there are areas of lucency at the centre. Surgical clips can also be useful to correlate the lesion with the site of surgery

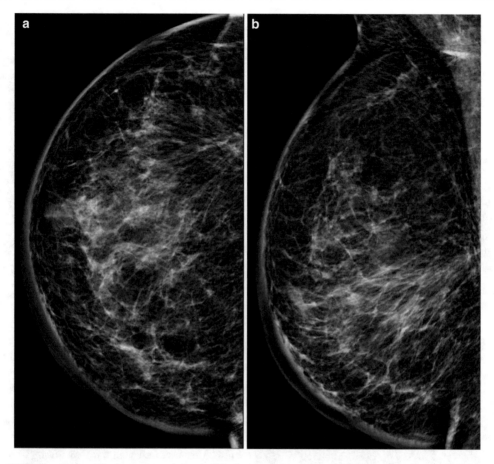

Fig. 7.26 Shows generalised treatment changes of the breast post treatment for breast cancer in the (**a**) CC and (**b**) MLO views. These include skin thickening, tissue oedema and distortion of the breast contour

Calcifications

Microcalcification on a mammogram is an important finding as it can be associated with tumours but is more often seen as part of benign processes. Calcification can be in the breast lobules, ducts, blood vessels, skin, stroma, other breast lesions, or can be artefactual [45, 46]. The distribution of the calcification is important. It can appear scattered (or diffuse), clustered or linear. The number, size, and form the calcification takes is also important and can be rounded/punctate, granular, coarse/popcorn, powderish or linear. All these characteristics inform the underlying biological process and hence the diagnosis [39, 47].

Benign Calcification

Lobular calcifications are usually smooth and round; they may be single, loosely grouped (Fig. 7.27), or scattered widely throughout the breast. They usually form in the acini of microcystic dilated lobules [41]. Ductal calcifications form in the duct lumen (Fig. 7.28) which in benign processes is often caused by the calcification of debris in the duct, and they are usually much larger than suspicious or malignant calcification [41].

Vascular calcifications (Fig. 7.29) in the breast are associated with blood vessels and are most often seen in post-menopausal women with arteriosclerotic heart disease. They are typically seen

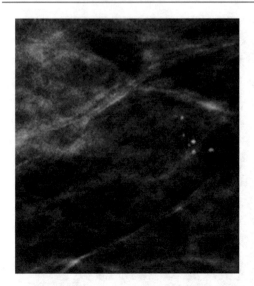

Fig. 7.27 Lobular calcification, the individual flecks are rounded, smooth and loosely grouped together

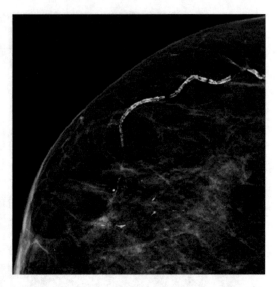

Fig. 7.29 Vascular calcification can be seen to line the blood vessels of the breast and often have a meandering pattern

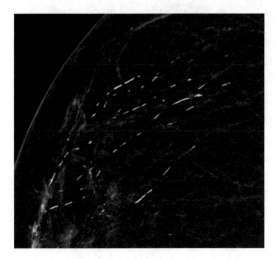

Fig. 7.28 Ductal calcification is linear, large, forms in the ducts, and tends to direct towards the nipple

on mammograms as dense, linear, parallel, circuitous, or tram-track like calcifications and are usually not oriented in the direction of the duct towards the nipple-areolar complex [41].

Skin calcifications (Fig. 7.30) in the breast usually form in dermal sweat glands following processes such as low-grade folliculitis or inspissation of sebaceous material. Often, these calcifications are seen in groups as they extend into small glands in the skin. Skin calcifications are

often round or oval with lucent centres. Calcifications may also form in skin lesions such as moles which can have a lacelike pattern on mammography [46].

Calcification can be associated with other benign breast lesions, and coarse or popcorn calcifications are often seen with involuting fibroadenomas (Fig. 7.31) [46]. The calcifications are usually very dense and much larger than microcalcification. 'Calcification' can also be artefactual from products such as deodorant.

Benign Breast Changes

Benign breast change covers a wide spectrum of conditions. Most benign breast disorders are essentially minor aberrations in the normal development process, hormonal response, and involution of the breast [48]. Processes such as fibrosis, fibrocystic change and sclerosing adenosis are considered disorders of involution. It is less common for post-menopausal women to have benign breast disease [49].

Focal fibrosis of the breast is a benign entity composed of dense collagenous stroma with sparse glandular and vascular elements and presents as localized areas of fibrous tissue. Focal

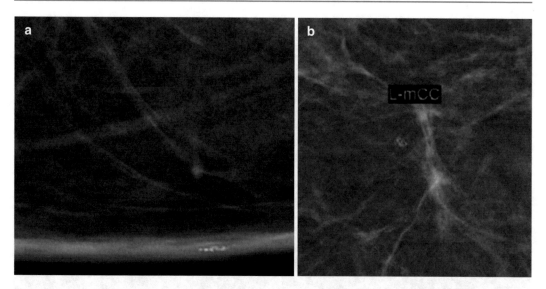

Fig. 7.30 Skin calcification. Tangential view (**a**) and magnification view (**b**) demonstrating skin calcification

fibrosis may appear as either a well-circumscribed mass, an irregular mass, or as focal asymmetry mammographically (Fig. 7.32).

Fibrocystic change is a benign process affecting the terminal duct-lobular unit and is thought to be associated with involution, hormone changes, or related genetic abnormalities. It includes gross and microscopic changes that are often asymptomatic but can present as nodularity and pain. It affects women 20–50 and declines post-menopause. It can be diffuse, patchy, or focal and can form a well or poorly defined mass on mammography as an increased density (Fig. 7.33). It is seen as a wide spectrum of altered morphology from innocuous to those associated with carcinoma risk.

Sclerosing adenosis is usually an incidental finding but may show as a mammographic abnormality such as microcalcification or architectural distortion. It is seen more commonly in a slightly older age group. It is a benign condition in which extra tissue develops within the breast lobules forming multiple small, firm, tender lumps, fibrous tissue, and sometimes small cysts in the breast. Presentation is frequently recurring pain that tends to be linked to the menstrual cycle. Sclerosing adenosis is usually detected during routine mammograms or following breast surgery. A biopsy usually confirms the diagnosis because the condition is otherwise difficult to distinguish from breast cancer.

Atypia

There are two types of atypia, namely atypical ductal hyperplasia (ADH) or atypical lobular hyperplasia (ALH). Neither usually show on a mammogram, and they are often diagnosed as an incidental finding to another mammographic concern following core biopsies. ADH and ALH are controversial due to the poorly understood biology but are considered high-risk premalignant lesions that are bridging between benign and malignant diseases. It is unclear if these lesions are a precursor or histological manifestation of a tissue bed at increased risk. ADH has some, but not all, of the features of ductal carcinoma in situ (DCIS). The distinction between ALH and lobular carcinoma in situ (LCIS) is that ALH occurs in a non-distended lobule or small lobular duct, whereas LCIS is characterised by distension of the lobules [44].

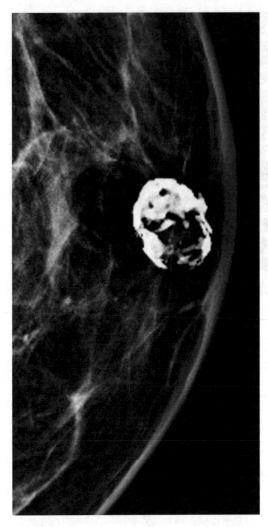

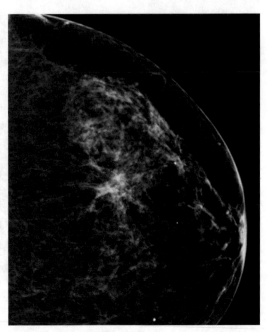

Fig. 7.32 Focal fibrosis showing as an area of possible architectural distortion, a needle core biopsy confirmed this was fibrosis

Fig. 7.31 Popcorn calcification. Very coarse and dense calcification associated with a longstanding fibroadenoma

LCIS

LCIS represents the next step up from ALH along the malignant spectrum of lobular breast carcinoma. LCIS has no macroscopic features, is usually mammographically occult, and the diagnosis is often made as an incidental finding making the true incidence of LCIS in the general population unknown. Characteristically LCIS is both multifocal and bilateral, it originates in the terminal ductal lobular unit but leaves the basement membrane intact [50].

DCIS

Ductal carcinoma in situ (DCIS) is a breast carcinoma limited to the ducts and it does not extend beyond the basement membrane, so cannot metastasise. Although it is often a mammographic finding, some patients present with a palpable abnormality of the breast or nipple changes. DCIS is associated with a spectrum of diseases and has varied mammographic appearances; although calcification is the most common (Fig. 7.34), it may present as a simple mass or asymmetry without calcification [39]. The calcifications may have varied appearances but are often linear or granular. DCIS is likely the precursor of invasive ductal carcinoma.

Paget's

Paget's disease of the nipple is usually a DCIS that initially grows from the terminal ducts and

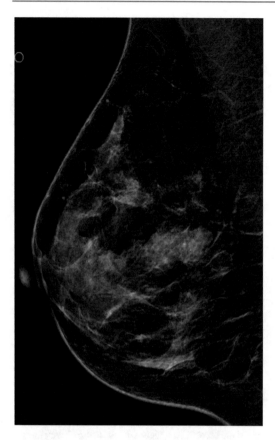

Fig. 7.33 Fibrocystic breast change with multiple well-defined masses (cysts) in a background of fibrous breast tissue. Ultrasound is a good adjunct investigation to confirm the mammographic findings

Fig. 7.34 DCIS presenting as focal calcification on a screening mammogram. The calcification has formed in the ducts in a focal linear pattern

progresses by intraepidermal spread to the nipple skin. It is not demonstrated mammographically, but presentation is often with nipple changes, including redness, itching or a burning sensation.

Clinical Pearls

- Benign breast diseases represent a heterogeneous group of lesions that have variable mammographic appearances. Most are minor aberrations in the normal development process, hormonal response, and involution of the breast.
- Many mammographic findings require further investigations such as Ultrasound, MRI and tissue sampling. Histological confirmation of benignity is often needed as specific lesions cannot reliably be distinguished from malignancy on radiological appearances. However, a comparison of previous mammography images may negate the need for further investigation.
- The implementation of breast screening led to a substantial rise in the incidence of DCIS/LCIS and hence, the concerns of over-diagnosis.
- The incorporation of radiomics (quantitative measures of image texture) could pave the way to personalised precision health. However, research into this will require developing models that link a combination of imaging phenotypes from large mammography datasets and genomic-level variables (radio-genomics). Radio-genomics may uncover specific imaging biomarkers that could potentially help detect tumours that are often missed on mammography.

Chapter Review Questions
Review Questions

1. In what type of patient are you most likely to find a galactocele?
2. Any calcification is a strong indicator of breast cancer. True or False?
3. Name five of the most common types of cancer that may metastasise to the breast.
4. What is the significance of detecting radial scars on mammography?

Answers

1. Lactating women or women who have recently stopped breastfeeding.
2. False. There are many reasons for calcifications in the breast tissue. Most calcifications detected on mammography are benign. However, they may represent initial signs of premalignant/malignant changes. Benign calcifications are typically smooth, round, larger, solitary or scattered widely throughout the breast. Malignant calcifications are typically finer, linear, or granular, and grouped or clustered. Tissue sampling by a needle core biopsy or vacuum assisted biopsy is required for those classified as indeterminate and above.
3. Skin (melanoma), prostate, digestive system (gastric), ovaries (ovarian), kidneys (renal cell).
4. The mammographic features of radial scars cannot dependably be differentiated from low grade cancers. Radial scars require excision or thorough sampling with VAE as the risk of upgrade depends on the presence or absence of epithelial atypia.

Appendix

Test your learning and check your understanding of this book's contents: use the "Springer Nature Flashcards" app to access questions using https://sn.pub/dcAnWL.

To use the app, please follow the instructions in Chap. 1.

Flashcard code: 48341-69945-ABCB1-2A8C7-CE9D2.

Short URL: https://sn.pub/dcAnWL.

References

1. Stachs A, Stubert J, Reimer T, Hartmann S. Benign breast disease in women. Deutsches Arzteblatt Int. 2019;116(33–34):565–74.
2. Athanasiou A, Aubert E, Vincent SA, Tardivon A. Complex cystic breast masses in ultrasound examination. Diagn Interv Imaging. 2014;95(2):169–79.
3. Chung EM, Cube R, Hall GJ, Gonzalez C, Stocker JT, Glassman LM. From the archives of the AFIP: breast masses in children and adolescents: radiologic pathologic correlation. Radiographics. 2009; 29(3):907–31.
4. Tan BY, Acs G, Apple SK, Badve S, Bleiweiss IJ, Brogi E, Calvo JP, Dabbs DJ, Ellis IO, Eusebi V, Farshid G. Phyllodes tumours of the breast: a consensus review. Histopathology. 2016;68(1):5–21.
5. Guillot E, Couturaud B, Reyal F, Curnier A, Ravinet J, Laé M, Bollet M, Pierga JY, Salmon R, Fitoussi A, Breast Cancer Study Group of the Institut Curie. Management of phyllodes breast tumors. Breast J. 2011;17(2):129–37.
6. Li GZ, Raut CP, Hunt KK, Feng M, Chugh R. Breast sarcomas, phyllodes tumors, and desmoid tumors: epidemiology, diagnosis, staging, and histology-specific management considerations. Am Soc Clin Oncol Educ Book. 2021;41:390–404.
7. Aydın OU, Soylu L, Ercan AI, Bilezikçi B, Ozbas S. Cavernous hemangioma in the breast. J Breast Health. 2015;11(4):199–201.
8. Frazier AA. Three patterns of male gynaecomastia. Radiographics. 2013;33(2):460.
9. Ravelomihary TDN, Razafimanjato NNM, Nomenjanahary L, Rakototiana AF, Rakotovao HJL, Rakoto-Ratsimba HN. Schwannoma of the breast: a report of rare location and a brief literature review. Ann Breast Surg. 2019;3:1–5.
10. Yi JM, Moon EJ, Oh SJ, Lee A, Suh YJ, Baek JM, Choi SH, Jung SS. Malignant peripheral nerve sheath tumor of the breast in a patient without neurofibromatosis: a case report. J Breast Cancer. 2009;12(3):223–6.
11. Tse GMK, Law BKB, Ma TKF, Chan ABW, Pang LM, Chu WCW, Cheung HS. Hamartoma of the breast: a clinicopathological review. J Clin Pathol. 2002;55(12):951–4.
12. Ni Y, He X, Chen J, Moline J, Mester J, Orloff MS, Ringel MD, Eng C. Germline SDHx variants modify breast and thyroid cancer risks in Cowden and Cowden-like syndrome via FAD/NAD- dependant destabilization of p53. Hum Mol Genet. 2012;21(2):300–10.
13. Farrokh D, Hashemi J, Ansaripour E. Breast hamartoma: mammographic findings. Iran J Radiol. 2011;8(4):258–60.
14. Lanng C, Erikson BØ, Hoffmann J. Lipoma of the breast: a diagnostic dilemma. Breast. 2004;13(5):408–11.
15. Pash Jones KN, Glazebrook KN, Reynolds C. Pseudoangiomatous stromal hyperplasia: imaging findings with pathologic and clinical correlation. Am J Roentgenol. 2010;195(4):1036–42.
16. Jesinger RA, Johnson T, Demartini S, Dalal K, Evan M. Radiology case (# 53) and image: pseudoangiomatous stromal hyperplasia. Mil Med. 2010;175(11):935–6.
17. Sabate JM, Clotet M, Torrubia S, Gomez A, Guerrero R, de Las HP, Lerma E. Radiologic evaluation of breast disorders related to pregnancy and lactation. Radiographics. 2007;27(Suppl_1):S101–24.

18. Son EJ, Oh KK, Kim EK. Pregnancy-associated breast disease: radiologic features and diagnostic dilemmas. Yonsei Med J. 2006;47(1):34–42.

19. Okcu ÖS, Bilgen IG, Oktay A, İzmir TR. Radiologic appearance of changes in breast after trauma, surgery and radiation therapy: a pictorial review, ECR 2012/C-2145.

20. Rakha EA, Lee AHS, Jenkins JA, Murphy AE, Hamilton LJ, Ellis IO. Characterization and outcome of breast needle core biopsy diagnoses of lesions of uncertain malignant potential (B3) in abnormalities detected by mammographic screening. Int J Cancer. 2011;129(6):1417–24.

21. Eiada R, Chong J, Kulkarni S, Goldberg F, Muradali D. Papillary lesions of the breast: MRI, ultrasound, and mammographic appearances. Am J Roentgenol. 2012;198(2):264–71.

22. Bianchi S, Bendinelli B, Saladino V, Vezzosi V, Brancato B, Nori J, Palli D. Non-malignant breast papillary lesions—B3 diagnosed on ultrasound—guided 14-gauge needle core biopsy: analysis of 114 cases from a single institution and review of the literature. Pathol Oncol Res. 2015;21(3):535–46.

23. Kim B, Kim Y, Hur H, You J. Localized primary breast amyloidosis and 1-year changes in imaging: a case report. Radiol Case Rep. 2020;15(12):2637–40.

24. Klein RL, Brown AR, Gomez-Castro CM, Chambers SK, Cragun JM, Grasso-LeBeau L, Lang JE. Ovarian cancer metastatic to the breast presenting as inflammatory breast cancer: a case report and literature review. J Cancer. 2010;1:27–31.

25. Serrano LF, Rojas-Rojas MM, Machado FA. Zuska's breast disease: breast imaging findings and histopathologic overview. Indian J Radiol Imag. 2020;30(3):327–33.

26. Moschetta M, Telegrafo M, Lucarelli NM, Martino G, Rella L, Ianora AAS, Angelli G. Metastatic breast disease from cutaneous malignant melanoma. Int J Surg Case Rep. 2014;5(1):34–6.

27. Yokouchi M, Nagano S, Kijima Y, Yoshioka T, Tanimoto A, Natsugoe S, Komiya S. Solitary breast metastasis from myxiod liposarcoma. BMC Cancer. 2014;14(1):1–6.

28. Moosavi L, Kim P, Uche A, Cobos E. A synchronous diagnosis of metastatic male breast cancer and prostate cancer. J Investig Med High Impact Case Rep. 2019;7:1–4.

29. Wang L, Wang S-L, Shen H-H, Niu F-T, Niu Y. Breast metastasis from lung cancer: a report of two cases and literature review. Cancer Biol Med. 2014;11(3):208–15.

30. Ma Y, Liu W, Li J, Xu Y, Wang H. Gastric cancer with breast metastasis: clinical features and prognostic factors. Oncol Lett. 2018;16(5):5565–74.

31. Caruso G, Musacchio L, Santangelo G, Palaia I, Tomao F, Di DV, Perniola G, Salutari V, Panici PB. Ovarian cancer metastasis to the breast: a case report and review of the literature. Case Rep Oncol. 2020;13(3):1317–24.

32. Xu Y, Hou R, Lu Q, Deng Y, Hu B. Renal clear cell carcinoma metastasis to the breast ten years aeftr

nephrectomy: a case report and literature review. Diagn Pathol. 2017;12(1):1–7.

33. Raj SD, Shurafa M, Shah Z, Raj KM, Fishman MDC, Dialani VM. Primary and seconadary breast lympoma: clinical, pathologic and multimodality imaging review. Radiographics. 2019;39(3):610–25.

34. Lee JS, Yoon K, Onyshchenko M. Sarcoma of the breast: clinical characteristics and outcomes of 991 patients from the national database. Sarcoma. 2021;2021:8828158.

35. Hoda SA, Rosen PP, Brogi E, Koerner FC. Rosen's breast pathology. 5th ed. Philadelphia: Lippencott Williams & Wilkins; 2020.

36. Chinyama CN. Benign breast disease radiology-pathology-risk assessment. 2nd ed. Berlin: Springer-Verlag; 2013.

37. Cohen MA, Newell MS. Radial scars of the breast encountered at core biopsy: review of histologic, imaging, and management considerartions. Am J Roentgenol. 2017;209(5):1168–77.

38. Quinn EM, Dunne E, Flanagan F, Mahon S, Barry MJ, Kell M, Walsh SM. Radial scars and complex sclerosing lesions on core biopsy of the breast: upgrade rates and long-term outcomes. Breast Cancer Res Treat. 2020;183(3):677–82.

39. Tabar L, Dean DB. Teaching atlas of mammography. 4th ed. New York: Thieme; 2011.

40. Shaaban AM, Sharma N. Management of B3 lesions- practical issues. Curr Breast Cancer Rep. 2019;11(2):83–8.

41. Kopans DB. Breast imaging. 3rd ed. Philadelphia: Lippincott Williams & Wilkins; 2007.

42. Jorge L, Taboada JL, Stephens TW, Krishnamurthy S, Brandt KR, Whitman GJ. The many faces of fat necrosis in the breast. Am J Roetgenol. 2009;192(3):815–25.

43. Harris JR, Lippman ME, Morrow M, Osborne CK. Diseases of the breast. 5th ed. Philadelphia: Lippincott Williams & Wilkins; 2014.

44. Krishnamurthy R, Whitman GJ, Stelling CB, Kushwaha. Mammographic findings after breast conservation therapy. Radiographics. 1999;19(suppl_1):S53–62.

45. Muttarak M, Kongmebhol P, Sukamwang N. Breast calcification: which are malignant? Singap Med J. 2009;50(9):907–14.

46. Nalawade YV. Evaluation of breast calcifications. Indian J Radiol Imag. 2009;19(4):282–6.

47. Pilnik S. Common breast lesions—a photographic guide to diagnosis and treatment. Cambridge: Cambridge University Press; 2003.

48. Hughes LE, Mansel RE, Webster DJT. Benign disorders and disease of breast. 3rd ed. Philadelphia: Saunders Elsevier; 2009.

49. Osuch JR. Breast health and disease over a lifetime. Clin Obstet Gynacol. 2002;45(1):1140–61.

50. Hartmann LC, Radisky DC, Frost MH, Santen RJ, Vierkant RA, Benetti LL, Tarabishy Y, Ghosh K, Visscher DW, Degnim AC. Understanding the premalignant potential of atypical hyperplasia through its natural history: a longitudinal cohort study. Am Assoc Cancer Res. 2014;7(2):211–7.

Signs and Symptoms of Breast Cancer with Management Pathways

8

Sue Garnett and Zebby Rees

Learning Objectives

- State the most common breast symptoms requiring investigation
- Identify the components and grading of triple assessment
- Demonstrate knowledge of the multidisciplinary professionals involved in the patient diagnostic pathway
- Identify and describe the additional imaging modalities that are not part of initial triple assessment, but are vital for further breast lesion evaluation and disease staging

Summary

This chapter will review the most common clinical signs and symptoms associated with breast cancer and will discuss the triple assessment process and the importance of the multi-disciplinary team in decision making processes.

S. Garnett (✉)
Breast Unit, University Hospital, Coventry, UK
e-mail: sue.garnett@uhcw.nhs.uk

Z. Rees
Bronglais Hospital, Hywel Dda Health Board, Carmarthen, West Wales, UK
e-mail: zebby.rees@wales.nhs.uk

Clinical Signs and Symptoms

There is a list of symptoms that present to a breast clinic including a new lump, focal thickening, distortion or dimpling and bloody discharge. The majority of breast cancers are found in the upper outer quadrant, following the pattern of the glandular tissue, although cancer may develop in any part of the breast. Referral to a specialist breast clinic is mainly from general practice within the UK; however incidental findings on CT or MRI scans are now occurring more frequently with improved technology.

Symptoms are investigated within a specific protocol known as triple assessment. This involves clinical examination, history taking, imaging and possible biopsy. Imaging includes mammography for women (age threshold depends on local protocols) and targeted ultrasound. MRI and other imaging modalities, such as CT and PET CT, are not part of triple assessment, but are often necessary for further staging investigations. Other symptomatic work will include post-surgical seroma drainage and infection assessment, neoadjuvant evaluation and surveillance mammography.

The multi-disciplinary team (MDT) uses triple assessment to deliver a patient-centred clinical service to investigate breast symptoms. The MDT includes numerous specialists who combine their expertise to deliver high quality diagnostic treatment and patient care pathways. Team meetings consider holistic needs, discuss patient pathways and ensure triple assessment outcomes are concordant. Patients' needs, anxieties and treatment options are central to breast care services to ensure efficient and effective diagnosis and treatment. The majority of breast cancers are found by clients noticing new symptoms in their breast or axilla, who then visit their general practitioner (GP) [1].

Clients may present with any of the following symptoms which require investigation to rule out or to confirm breast cancer [2]. All the symptoms below require specialist assessment and most of them are clinical indications for mammography and/or ultrasound [3].

- A discrete hard lump with fixation— there may be tethering, dimpling, altered colouration, or contour of the breast
- A lump that has enlarged
- A new discrete mobile lump
- A more focal lump in pre-existing nodularity (more general lumpiness)
- A persistent focal area of lumpiness or a focal change in breast texture
- Progressive change in breast size with signs of oedema and reddening
- Asymmetrical nodularity persisting after menstruation
- Skin puckering
- Previous history of breast cancer with a new lump or suspicious symptoms, as listed above
- Nipple discharge or inversion of the nipple
- Nipple eczema or changes to the nipple that do not respond to topical treatments
- Axillary lymphadenopathy
- Ulceration of the breast skin may indicate locally advanced breast cancer

Locations and Types of Cancers Within the Breast

Research has demonstrated that the majority of breast cancers are found in the upper outer quadrant of the breast. This is the area of the breast that has the greatest volume of glandular breast tissue, but cancer can be found anywhere

within the breast parenchyma [4]. Clients should not be falsely reassured by the location of abnormalities in the breast and seek a referral to a specialist breast centre for any of the aforementioned signs and symptoms. Infiltrating ductal carcinoma is often seen on mammography as a dense spiculate mass [5] and infiltrating lobular carcinomas can be seen as a more subtle density [6]. Calcifications, which may indicate ductal carcinoma in situ [7], architectural distortions, [8] and well-defined lesions [9] are also common appearances.

Breast Density

Breast density on mammography, due to the amount of glandular tissue present in the breast, is seen as a compounding factor for mammography sensitivity to detect breast cancer. Women with extremely dense tissue have a greater risk of developing breast cancer [10, 11] (Chaps. 4 and 5).

The Axilla

Lymph nodes in the axilla are assessed in relation to a suspicious breast lesion. Although there are other lymphatic chains such as the internal thoracic chain and the abdominal nodes, staging of the axillary nodes is the gold standard for a breast cancer treatment pathway [12]. The number of axillary nodes range from 12 to 40. As most breast cancers are located in the lateral half of the breast, axillary nodes are more susceptible to metastatic spread. When breast cancer is suspected, the axillary nodes are assessed with ultrasound for any features suggesting involvement; size, shape and cortical thickness are evaluated. If these features appear abnormal then a core biopsy or fine needle aspiration (FNA) test is performed. Spread to the nodes may have occurred either macroscopically or microscopically even with normal ultrasound findings [13]. For accurate axillary assessment in the presence of normal ultrasound findings, a sentinel lymph node biopsy procedure prior to surgery is performed. If breast cancer spreads to the axillary lymph nodes, staging tests such as CT and bone scans are performed to determine the systemic status of the disease.

Referrals

Referrals to a specialist breast clinic often come from general practitioners. Some breast abnormalities may be identified when patients are in hospital under investigation for other medical conditions. Clients are occasionally referred from Accident and Emergency departments with breast infections, often postnatal breast infections (mastitis) or abscesses [14, 15]. Patients are increasingly being referred with breast related incidental findings during CT and MRI scans to the breast clinic by clinicians from other specialties.

Triple Assessment

Triple assessment by a multidisciplinary team (MDT) includes clinical and radiological examination, supplemented with tissue diagnosis if indicated. This is the gold standard of care for evaluating clients with potential breast cancer in symptomatic and screening clinics in the UK [14–17]. However, it is recognised that breast services are configured differently across countries. Triple assessment consists of:

1. Clinical breast examination and patient medical history
2. Imaging/radiological assessment
3. Pathology assessment—Needle Core Biopsy or FNA.

Each part of the triple assessment process is graded for malignant potential.

Clinical examination and medical history are undertaken to assess the lesion's character and palpability and note any other symptoms. Additionally, the axilla is examined for palpable lymph nodes. The imaging component of the Triple Assessment should include:

Mammography—for women aged 40 or over (but dependent on local protocols)

High frequency ultrasound with probes suitable for breast imaging

Biopsy is undertaken as either a core of tissue (B grading) or as a fine needle aspiration (FNA–C grading) as dictated by local protocol. Studies [14–17] have demonstrated an overall sensitivity for Triple Assessment of 99.6%; Many UK breast units are organised so that all appropriate tests of triple assessment can be carried out on the same visit; the so-called 'Fast Track' or 'One Stop' model.

Triple assessment ensures:

- Efficient service delivery to all clients
- Best use of resources
- Clear communication for clinic scheduling
- Rapid exchange of information and test results
- Effective liaison between all members of the MDT team

This all inclusive clinic method helps to reduce client anxiety and stress due to periods of waiting [14–18] (Chaps. 12 and 13). Symptomatic

Clinical breast examination and medical history	Imaging/radiological assessment	Pathology assessment-needle core biopsy or FNA	
P1—normal	M1/U1/R1—normal	B1—normal/ unrepresentative	C1—acellular aspirate
P2—benign	M2/U2/R2—benign	B2—benign	C2—benign
P3—uncertain/likely benign	M3/U3/R3—uncertain/ likely benign	B3—uncertain malignant potential	C3—uncertain abnormal cells
P4—suspicious of malignancy	M4/U4/R4—suspicious of malignancy	B4—suspicious of malignancy	C4—suspicious of malignancy
P5—malignant	M5/U5/R5—malignant	B5a—in situ carcinoma B5b—invasive carcinoma B5c—microinvasion	C5—malignant cells

clinics and breast screening assessment clinics should be delivered separately. Symptomatic patients are highly anxious and fearful concerning their symptoms. Screening clients have no symptoms, therefore reactions are variable including anger, fear and disbelief. The triple assessment process has a different approach in each scenario. Symptomatic assessment begins with clinical examination and history taking, before imaging is considered; whereas screening assessment is initiated from the routine screening mammogram, which is then followed by clinical assessment and further imaging or biopsy.

Further Imaging

- **Breast Magnetic Resonance Imaging (MRI)** does not form part of the initial imaging assessment but is useful for further investigation of some breast lesions, problem-solving for lesion size, multifocality, multi-centricity or contralateral disease. It is especially useful for the measurement and extent of lobular breast carcinoma [19].

- Neoadjuvant chemotherapy sizing, high-risk screening, pre-operative staging and implant assessment are also important indications for MRI [20–22].
- **Computed Axial Tomography (CT)** is also used in staging of confirmed breast cancers to assess spread of disease to other parts of the body [23].
- **Positron emission tomography–computed tomography (PET CT)** is useful for highlighting occult distant metastases, for systemic treatment planning for advanced disease. It is also efficient for detecting recurrence [24].

The Multi-Disciplinary Team

Multi-disciplinary teams (MDT) need to bring together staff with the necessary knowledge, skills and experience to ensure high quality diagnosis, treatment and care. The MDT meeting discusses the holistic needs of the patient, not just the cancer treatment. To support this, an MDT should take account of the patients' views, preferences and circumstances when considering the care that is most appropriate for the patient's condition. The MDT meeting evaluates each triple assessment result to ensure the case is concordant. Discrepancies and mismatches are highlighted and further investigations agreed. An MDT makes recommendations and decisions which are reliant on the information available to the MDT at the meeting. The final decision on the way forward needs to be made by the patient in conjunction/collaboration with their clinicians. MDTs should be alerted if there are significant changes to their recommendations and the reasons for this, so they have the opportunity to review and learn from these cases. Patient/client communication is at the centre of the MDT process and the care management pathway.

Specialist healthcare professionals in a multi-disciplinary team will usually include the following staff groups [20].

- Consultant Breast Surgeons
- Consultant Clinical Oncologists
- Consultant Radiologists/ Radiographers
- Consultant Histopathologists/ Cytologists
- Advanced Practitioner Radiographers
- Breast Clinicians
- Breast Care Nurses
- Chemotherapy nurses
- Diagnostic Radiographers
- Assistant Practitioner Mammographers
- Therapy Radiographers
- Research Nurses

The initial focus of the MDT is the patient's primary treatment. However, it is for organisations to decide locally if and how patient cases should be reconsidered, in the light of any additional findings. Also taking into account any relevant guidance recommendations by appropriate bodies [15].

Overview

Triple assessment and MDT working are the vital tools used for diagnosis and patient management. Decision making is then agreed in a timely manner. Patient needs, anxieties and treatment options are at the heart of breast care services to ensure an efficient and effective diagnosis and treatment pathway.

Clinical Pearls

- Attend an MDT meeting to review how assessment gradings are managed
- Write your own mini 'report' of a mammogram you have taken
- Compare the ultrasound image of a lesion, with the mammographic appearance

Consider size, shape and position within the breast

Chapter Review Questions
Review Questions

1. A 45 year old female patient has attended the symptomatic clinic with a new breast lump. Can you outline the diagnostic process for this patient?
2. At the MDT meeting, the triple assessment grading was P2 R4 B3. Can you suggest what should be done about this mismatch of grading for this patient?
3. Define the following:
   (a) FNA
   (b) Core biopsy
   (c) IDC
   (d) ILC
   (e) DCIS

4. Can you review the anatomy of a lymph node and explain its importance in breast cancer diagnosis?
5. What is the significance of breast pain?

Answers

1. History taken
   Clinical examination—P grading decision
   Mammogram and ultrasound imaging M + U (R) grading
   Biopsy—B grading
   MDM review, triple assessment and pathway agreed
   Patient consultation
2. Re biopsy of lesion—more cores or a vacuum excision
   MDM review to agree surveillance mammography or lesion excision
3. FNA—fine needle aspiration—21 G needle, aspiration of cells for cytology—C grading
   Core biopsy—different needle sizes for core of tissue, sample for histology—B grading
   IDC—invasive ductal carcinoma
   ILC—invasive lobular carcinoma
   DCIS—ductal carcinoma in situ
4. Macro and micro lymph node anatomy
   Lymph node evaluation is essential for determining breast cancer stage/spread.
   It is the gold standard for local or systemic treatment.
5. Breast pain is commonly seen in the symptomatic clinics. It is contentious as to its relevance for breast cancer diagnosis. Three causes are: hormonal (premenopausal), muscular or trauma.

Appendix

Test your learning and check your understanding of this book's contents: use the "Springer Nature Flashcards" app to access questions using https://sn.pub/dcAnWL.

To use the app, please follow the instructions in Chap. 1.

Flashcard code: 48341-69945-ABCB1-2A8C7-CE9D2.

Short URL: https://sn.pub/dcAnWL.

References

1. Henry N, Shah PD, Haider I, Freer PE, Jagsi R, Sabel MS. Cancer of the breast. In: Niederhuber JE, Armatage JO, Doroshow JH, Kastan MB, Tepper JE, editors. Abeloffs clinical oncology. 6th ed. Philadelphia, PA: Elsevier; 2020. p. 1560–603.
2. National Cancer Institute. Physician Data Query (PDQ). Breast cancer treatment—patient version. https://www.cancer.gov/types/breast/patient/ breast-treatment-pdq. Accessed 9 Nov 2021.
3. Royal College of Radiologists. Guidance on screening and symptomatic breast imaging. 4th ed. London: Royal College of Radiologists; 2019.
4. Rummel S, Huemal M, Constantino N, Shriver C, Ellsworth R. Tumour location within the breast: does tumour site have prognostic ability. 2015. Accessed 9 Nov 2021. https://doi.org/10.3332/ecancer.2015.552.
5. Skandhan A, Niknejad M. Invasive ductal carcinoma. https://doi.org/10.53347/rID-29143. Accessed 23 Nov 2020.
6. Radswiki T, Rasuli B. Invasive lobular carcinoma of the breast. https://doi.org/10.53347/rID-13169. Accessed 13 Nov 2020.
7. Radswiki T, El-Feky M. Breast calcifications. https://doi.org/10.53347/rID-13952. Accessed 13 Nov 2020.
8. Radswiki T, Murphy A. Breast architectural distortion. https://doi.org/10.53347/rID-15462. Accessed 23 Nov 2020.
9. Weerakkody Y, Bell D. Well-defined breast cancers (differential). https://doi.org/10.53347/rID-15777. Accessed 13 Nov 2020.
10. Nickel B, Farber R, Brennan M, Hersch J, McCaffery K, Houssami N. Breast density notification: evidence on whether benefit outweighs harm is required to inform future screening practice. BMJ Evid Based Med. 2021;26(6):309–11.
11. Heine J, Fowler E, Scott CG, Jensen MR, Shepherd J, Hruska CB, Winham SJ, Brandt KR, Wu FF, Norman AD, Pankratz VS, Miglioretti DL, Kerlikowske K, Vachon CM. Mammographic variation measures, breast density and breast cancer risk. Am J Roentgenol. 2021;217:326–35.
12. Kühn T, Classe JM, Gentilini OD, Tinterri C, Peintinger F, De Boniface J. Current status and future perspectives of axillary management in the neoadjuvant setting. Breast Care. 2018;13(5):337–41.
13. Riedel F, Schaefgen B, Sinn HP, Feisst M, Hennigs A, Hug S, Binnig A, Gomez C, Harcos A, Stieber A, Kauczor HU. Diagnostic accuracy of axillary staging by ultrasound in early breast cancer patients. Eur J Radiol. 2021;135:109468.
14. Berg W, Birdwell R, Gombos E, Wang S, Parkinson B, Raza S, Green G, Kennedy A, Kettler M. Diagnostic imaging of the breast. Utah and Canada: AMIRSYS; 2006.
15. National Institute for Health and Care Excellence (NICE). Early and locally advanced breast cancer: diagnosis and management: NICE Guideline [NG101]. 2018. https://www.nice.org.uk/guidance/ ng101. Accessed 13 Nov 2021.
16. Cardoso F, Kyriakides S, Ohno S, Penault-Llorca F, Poortmans P, Rubio IT, Zackrisson S, Senkus E. 2019. Early breast cancer: ESMO clinical practice guidelines for diagnosis, treatment and follow-up. Ann Oncol. 2019;30(8):1194–220.
17. Bray F, Ferlay J, Soerjomataram I, Siegel RL, Torre LA, Jemal A. Global cancer statistics 2018: GLOBOCAN estimates of incidence and mortality worldwide for 36 cancers in 185 countries. CA Cancer J Clin. 2018;68(6):394–424.
18. Wilson R, Asbury D, Cooke J, Michell M, Patnick J. Clinical guidelines for breast cancer screening assessment—NHSBSP Publication No. 49. Sheffield: NHS Cancer Screening Programmes. p. 200. https://www.gov.uk/government/publications/ breast-screening-clinical-guidelines-for-screening-management. Accessed 13 Nov 2021.
19. Ha SM, Chae EY, Cha JH, Kim HH, Shin HJ, Choi WJ. Breast MR imaging before surgery: outcomes in patients with invasive lobular carcinoma by using propensity score matching. Radiology. 2018;287(3):771–7.
20. National Institute for Health and Care Excellence. Breast cancer: recognition and referral. https://www. nice.org.uk/sharedlearning/symptomatic-breast-referral-resource-suite-enhancing-the-suspected-cancer-recognition-and-referral-process. Accessed 9 Nov 2021.
21. Hu K, Ding P, Wu Y, Tian W, Pan T, Zhang S. Global patterns and trends in the breast cancer incidence and mortality according to sociodemographic indices: an observational study based on the global burden of diseases. BMJ Open. 2019;9(10):e028461.
22. Price J. Handbook of breast MRI. Cambridge: Cambridge University Press; 2012.
23. Roszkowski N, Lam SS, Copson E, Cutress RI, Oeppen R. Expanded criteria for pretreatment staging CT in breast cancer. BJS Open. 2021;5(2):zraa006.
24. Groheux D, Moretti JL, Giacchetti S, Hindié E, Teyton P, Cuvier C, Bousquet G, Misset JL, Boin C, Espié M. Différents rôles de la TEP-TDM en sénologie : mise au point. Bull Cancer. 2009;96(11):1053–70.

Disease Progression

9

Susan Williams

Learning Objectives
- To understand the basic processes of breast cancer development
- To develop an understanding of the ways in which cells change from normal to abnormal, advancing to cancerous changes
- To develop knowledge of the different types of breast cancer development and the influences of the biological factors

Introduction

A normal cell has a clearly defined well-regulated life cycle. Chemical and biological mechanisms manage the normal regeneration, life and death (apoptosis) of the cell. This process is required to replace worn out cells. Normal cells communicate with each other and regulate proliferation (division) of cells through chemical signals transmitted by specific proteins [1]. A cancer cell does not respond to this communication or regulation and proliferates without limits. The change from a normal cell to a cancerous cell is complex and involves damage to the genes that regulate the normal cell function. Multiple permanent mutations are needed for cancer to develop and this often occurs over a long period of time [2–5].

The Influence of Genes

At the cellular level, cancer is fundamentally a genetic disease, resulting from a disruption of the normal genetic program. Regulatory genes involved are growth promoting proto-oncogenes, growth inhibiting tumour suppressor genes, genes that regulate apoptosis, and genes involved in gene repair. These genes encode many kinds of proteins that help control cell growth and proliferation; mutations in these genes can contribute to the development of cancer [2–5].

- Oncogenes are a mutation of a proto-oncogene which promote the specialisation and division of normal cells. The resultant oncogenes expressed at abnormally high levels contribute to converting a normal cell to a cancer cell [1].
- Tumour suppressor genes inhibit mitosis of the cell. They regulate uncontrolled cell division by applying the brakes to cell prolifera-

S. Williams (✉)
Shrewsbury and Telford Hospital NHS Trust, The Royal Shrewsbury Hospital, Shrewsbury, UK
e-mail: susan.williams46@nhs.net

tion. Tumour suppressor genes cause cancer when they are inactive [1].

- Neoplastic cells form from mutation in genes controlling apoptosis, initiated through either extrinsic or intrinsic factors [2–5].

The Mutated Cell

The formation of a cancer is a complex process. A mutated cell is normally destroyed by a process called apoptosis meaning it cannot reproduce and pass the mutation onto a daughter cell. However, if the original mutated cell is able to evade this process, they can pass the mutation onto daughter cells and the future cell line, which can then undergo further mutations. Once the cell is a cancer cell its behaviour is altered in five main areas [2–5]:

- Cell Reproduction: The normal reproductive process is disrupted resulting in unchecked growth and reproduction.
- Cell Communication: Cancer cells lose the ability to communicate with other cells and do not respond to chemical signals telling them when to reproduce or stop reproducing.
- Cell Adhesion: Cells have adhesion molecules on their surface allowing them to stick to neighbouring cells and keep them in their proper place. Cell to cell contact is required to suppress proliferation. Loss of the adhesion molecules allows the cells to spread to distant areas of the body through the lymphatic and blood circulatory systems.
- Cell Specialization: Normal cells have the ability to differentiate or develop into specialized cells. Cancer cells are unspecialized and do not develop into cells of a specific type.
- Cell Death: Cell damage goes undetected, and the cell will not undergo programmed cell death.

Hallmarks of Cancer

All of the cells produced by division of the first mutated, ancestral cell will display inappropriate proliferation. This uncontrolled altered cell behaviour results in a primary tumour. The fundamental changes in cell physiology dictate the malignant phenotype but the resultant cancer cells display hallmark features. Mutation of genes that regulate some or all of these cellular traits are seen in every cancer [2–5]:

- The growth pattern is unregulated by physiological cues—cancer cells ignore signals telling them how to behave.
- Lack response to growth inhibitory signals—cancer cells do not respond to signals instructing them to stop their inappropriate behaviour.
- The avoidance of cell death—the gateway in the normal cell cycle inducing apoptosis is missed.
- Immortality—cancer cells will continue to divide indefinitely.
- Development of angiogenesis to sustain the growth of cancer cells—tumour cells develop their own blood supply.
- The ability to invade local and distant sites—they have the capacity to infiltrate, invade, or metastasize to distant sites.
- Programming pathways—tumour cells undergo reprogramming of energy metabolisms marking them as superior in the survival game as they become more resilient in their local environment.
- Ability to avoid the immune system—tumours may avoid the immune system by mechanisms that allow them to go undetected.

Establishing the Tumour

Tumours are made up of 2 basic components:

- The parenchyma—made up of neoplastic cells, this determines the tumors biology
- The supporting host–derived non-neoplastic stroma comprising of connective tissue, blood supply, and host derived inflammatory cells [2–5].

The differentiation of parenchymal tumour cells is the extent to which they resemble their equivalent normal cells morphologically and functionally. Poorly differentiated cells lose the functional capabilities of their normal counterparts and tend to grow more rapidly. The site of the primary tumour will dictate the biology of the tumour. The tumour may remain within the originating tissue, invade nearby tissues or travel to distant tissue sites. Most cancers begin as localised proliferation confined to the epithelium in which they arise. As long as the tumour does not penetrate the basement membrane on which the epithelium rests, they are termed carcinoma in situ [2–5].

The proliferating cancer cells are supported by a stroma of connective tissue and a blood supply influencing the growth pattern, differentiation, and biological behaviour of the developing tumour, promoting or preventing tumorigenesis (the production or formation of a tumour/tumours) [6]. Two theories of tumour progression include: (1) Predisposition of the tumour to progress, where the cancer cells are 'out of control' and mutation continues in the absence of 'regulation' and (2) Where the interaction of the tumour cells and the surrounding stroma nurtures the developing tumour. The microenvironment is composed of the extracellular matrix, numerous types of stromal cells including endothelial and immune cells, fibroblasts and adipocytes, and is an important participant of tumour progression [7] it seems likely both occur.

Tumour cells need oxygen, nutrients, and removal of waste products. Tumours cannot grow beyond 1–2 mm without vascularisation. Cancer cells can stimulate angiogenesis, during which new vessels sprout from previously existing capillaries and these abnormal vessels are leaky and dilated, with a haphazard pattern of connection. Angiogenesis is required for the cancer to grow and metastasize [2–5].

Lymphangiogenesis, the growth of new lymphatic vessels, can be induced in pathological process such as cancer. These lymphatic vessels will transport cancer cells to the lymphatic system [8]. The lymph members of the vascular endothelial growth factor family play major roles in both lymphangiogenesis and angiogenesis.

The vascular and lymphatic anatomy influences the pattern of metastatic spread.

Local Invasion

Tumours exert local effects including compression and displacement of adjacent tissues to effect invasion. Malignant tumour growth pattern is often disorganised and random. Malignant tumours enlarge and infiltrate the normal tissues of their origin but may extend directly beyond the confines of that organ to involve adjacent tissues [2–5].

At the molecular level, continued mutations cause heterogeneity in the tumour, generating subclones with different characteristics. Thus, although cancer origins are monoclonal, by the time they are clinically detectable they can be extremely heterogeneous. During progression, the tumour cells are subject to selection processes, with the more resilient subclones being selected for survival. The genetic evolution and selection processes make tumours become more aggressive and acquire greater malignant potential—tumour progression [2–5].

Metastasizing

Metastasis is the migration of malignant cells from one site to another remote site. Metastasis tend to resemble the primary tumour histologically. Tumour spread is a complex process involving a series of sequential steps which can be interrupted at any stage by host or tumour related factors [2–5]. Figure 9.1 shows a summary of the metastasis cascade.

A lack of adhesion between cells facilitates loosening of the tumour cells, allowing them to move away from the tumour body. Enzymes secreted by the tumour cells cause local degradation of the basement membrane and interstitial connective tissue. Breach of the basement membrane is the first event in cell invasion. The tumour cells attach to the extracellular matrix proteins causing modification to the matrix that

Fig. 9.1 The mechanism of tumour invasion and metastasis

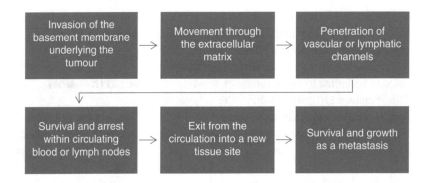

promotes invasion and metastasis and allows the tumour cells to enter the circulatory system. Tumour cells are quite inefficient at colonising distant organs and most cells circulate as micrometastases undetected in the system for prolonged periods of time [2–5].

Extravasation of the tumour cells involves adhesion to the vascular endothelium followed by egression through the basement membrane into the organ parenchyma by mechanisms similar to those involved in invasion [2–5].

The site of extravasation and the organ distribution of metastases can be predicted by the site of the primary tumour and its vascular or lymphatic drainage. This may be the first capillary bed they encounter. Other influences may include expression of adhesion molecules by tumour cells whose ligands are expressed preferentially on the endothelium of the target organ. They are also influenced by the expression of proteins that direct movement. Once the cancer cells reach a target the tumour cells must be able to colonise to continue growth. Tumour cells appear to secrete cytokines, growth factors and proteases that act on the resident stromal cells to make the site habitable [2–5].

Tumour cells arising in tissue with a rich lymphatic network, such as the breast, often metastasize by this route. Invasive tumours may penetrate lymphatic channels more readily than blood vessels. Lymph formation occurs at the microscopic level. During the exchange of fluid and molecules between the blood circulation and body tissues, blood capillaries may not reabsorb all of the fluid; surrounding lymphatic channels absorb the excess fluid and cancer cells. This is then filtered and carried to the sentinel lymph node and from there to distal nodes and other organs [8].

Breast Cancer

The biology of breast cancer is complicated, making it difficult to predict and manage [9–14]. Breast cancer is a heterogeneous process with very variable appearances, biology and clinical behaviour. However, the cancer cells develop from the epithelium of lobules and ducts. There are many ways that breast cancer can develop [11] and a theoretical typical progression may be [2–5]:

- Atypical and in situ disease
- Invasive tumour
- Regional metastases to sentinel lymph nodes
- Involvement of other regional lymph nodes
- Metastatic spread to distant sites

Atypia and In Situ Disease

During this phase, tumour growth is restricted to the lobules and ducts which are delineated by a continuous basal membrane and are therefore non-invasive [15]. Although controversial, atypical ductal and lobular hyperplasia are often considered to be a precursor or risk indicator for subsequent breast cancers [9]. Lobular carcinoma in situ (LCIS) has cells with the morphology of invasive lobular carcinoma, but is contained within the basement membrane. Ductal carcinoma in situ (DCIS) grows within the duct system of the breast and can vary in size and extent. High grade DCIS is a more inherently high-risk disease in terms of progression into invasive breast cancer [10]. All of these conditions are confined within the boundaries of the normal structures of the breast and therefore cannot metastasise at this point.

Invasive Tumour

The transition from in-situ to invasive disease of the breast is poorly understood but is defined by the loss of the myoepithelial cell layer and basement membrane of the terminal ductal lobular units [7]. The infiltration of the surrounding stromal tissue means there is the potential to spread to lympho-vascular spaces and to metastasise. Some invasive breast cancers are more aggressive and may spread earlier to distant sites. There are a variety of methods for classifying invasive breast cancer; most are based on the architectural microscopic pattern and nature of the cancerous cells and indicate differing clinical behaviours and prognoses. The combination of the physical and physiological properties of the tumour such as size, grade, location, and histological features will give an indication of predicted disease progression and prognosis [2–5].

In addition to the more traditional classifications of breast cancer, molecular classification is now widely used to inform the prognostic and risk stratification of individual tumours, promoting targeted treatment options. This includes immunophenotyping and intrinsic subtyping [16, 17].

Although the growth pattern of the breast tumour is influenced by the biology of the tumour, as the cancer starts to grow it takes up more space and forces itself through the normal tissue, often taking the path of least resistance. The space occupying lesion will block small blood vessels causing death of the normal cells, making it easier for the tumour to continue growing. The cancer cells invade the nearby surrounding breast tissue or nearby structures such as the pectoral muscle and ribs [2–5].

Regional Nodes

Breast cancer spread occurs through lymphatic and haematogenous channels. The lymphatic system collects excess fluid in the body's tissues and returns it to the bloodstream. The breast has a rich lymphatic network, and the initial metastases are almost always lymphatic. Tumours located laterally and centrally typically spread first to the axillary nodes. Those in the medial inner quadrants often travel first to the lymph nodes along the internal mammary arteries. The assessment of lymph nodes in the axilla is crucial to staging and prognosis of patients with operable breast cancer. The sentinel lymph node(s) are the primary nodes that drain the breast parenchyma. A sentinel lymph node free of cancer is highly predictive of absence of cancer in the remaining nodes [2–5].

Metastatic Spread

More distant dissemination eventually ensues and can involve virtually any organ or tissue. Common sites for metastases of the breast are lungs, skeleton, liver, adrenals, and (less commonly) brain, but can involve virtually any organ or body tissue. Metastases have histological properties similar to the primary tumour. Metastases may come to clinical attention many years after the apparent control of the primary tumour [2–5].

Clinical Pearls

- There is a wide range of different types of breast cancer ranging from insignificant to highly aggressive rapidly growing cancers that will significantly shorten life expectancy
- More than one type of breast cancer can be present at any given time
- The rapid evolution of genetic medicine is likely to significantly change both our understanding of breast cancer and disease management in the future

Chapter Review Questions
Review Questions

1. Do all breast cancers follow the same development process?
2. How the breast cancer develops and spreads to the rest of the body is determined by both the physiological and physical properties of the tumour? True or False
3. What is the name of the process of supplying blood to the growing tumour?

Answers

1. No. Any one of the regulator mechanisms for cell management could cause cell mutation and abnormal behavior resulting in a cancer formation.
2. True. Increasingly detailed profiles of the physical and physiological properties of tumours resulting in much more individual treatment plans targeting specific tumour behaviours.
3. Angiogenesis

Appendix

Test your learning and check your understanding of this book's contents: use the "Springer Nature Flashcards" app to access questions using https://sn.pub/dcAnWL.

To use the app, please follow the instructions in Chap. 1.

Flashcard code: 48341-69945-ABCB1-2A8C7-CE9D2.

Short URL: https://sn.pub/dcAnWL.

References

1. Lodish H, Berk A, Zipursky SL, Matsudaira P, Baltimore D, Darnell J. Molecular cell biology. 4th ed. New York: WH Freeman; 2000.
2. Cross SS. Underwood's pathology—a clinical approach. 6th ed. Edinburgh: Churchill Livingstone; 2013.
3. Kumar V, Abbas AK, Aster JC. Robbins basic pathology. 9th ed. Philadelphia: Elsevier; 2013.
4. Rosen PP. Rosen's breast pathology. 3rd ed. Philadelphia: Lippincott Williams & Wilkins; 2009.
5. Rubin E, Reisner HM. Essentials of Rubin's pathology. 6th ed. Philadelphia: Lippincott, Williams & Wilkins; 2014.
6. Tot T, Tabar L, Dean PB. Practical breast pathology. 2nd ed. New York: Thieme; 2014.
7. Place AE, Jin Huh S, Polyak K. The microenvironment in breast cancer progression: biology and implications for treatment. Breast Cancer Res. 2011;13(6):1–1.
8. Alitalo A, Detmar M. Interaction of tumor cells and lymphatic vessels in cancer progression. Oncogene. 2012;31(42):4499–508.
9. Hartmann LC, Radisky DC, Frost MH, Santen RJ, Vierkant RA, Benetti LL, Tarabishy Y, Ghosh K, Visscher DW, Degnim AC. Understanding the premalignant potential of atypical hyperplasia through its natural history: a longitudinal cohort study. Am Assoc Cancer Res. 2014;7(2):211–7.
10. Obeng-Gyasi OC, Hwang ES. Contemporary manageamnety of ductal carcinoma in situ and lobular carcinoma in situ. Chin Clin Oncol. 2016;5(3):32.
11. Bombonati A, Sgroi DC. The molecular pathology of breast cancer progression. J Pathol. 2011;223:307–17.
12. Heimann R, Hellman S. Clinical progression of breast cancer malignant behaviour: what to expect and when to expect it. J Clin Oncol. 2000;18(3):591–9.
13. Soyal SD, Tzankov A, Muenst SE. Role of the tumor microenvironment in breast cancer. Pathobiology. 2015;82(3–4):142–52.
14. Rosa M. Advances in the molecular analysis of breast cancer: pathway toward personalized medicine. Cancer Control. 2015;22(2):211–9.
15. Ellis IO. Intraductal proliferative lesions of the breast: morphology, associated risk and molecular biology. Mod Pathol. 2010;23(2):S1–7.
16. Eliatkin N, Yalcin E, Zengel B, Aktas S, Vardar E. Molecular classification of breast carcinoma: from traditional, old-fashioned way to a new age, and a new way. J Breast Health. 2015;11(2):59–66.
17. Tsang J, Tse GM. Molecular classification of breast cancer. Adv Anat Pathol. 2020;27(1):27–35.

Interval Cancers

10

Rosalind Given-Wilson

Learning Objectives
- Understand the frequency of interval cancers in breast screening and the factors associated with them
- Describe the classification system for interval cancers in the NHSBSP
- Recognise and understand how information about interval cancers is offered to those affected by them

2. To provide feedback and learning for services and individuals to improve the quality of image reading and assessment.
3. To enable feedback to those who have had an interval cancer, so that if they wish to receive the information, they can understand if an abnormality was present on their previous images.

Each of these topics will be explored in more detail throughout the chapter.

Why and How Are Interval Cancers Reviewed?

Interval breast cancers are those that are diagnosed in between screening episodes. In the UK the NHSBSP classifies them as invasive breast cancer presenting within 36 months of a negative screen [1]. Interval cancers are audited for 3 main reasons:

1. To monitor the rates of interval cancers as well as screen detected cancers, and thus the performance of screening.

How Common Are Interval Cancers?

Interval cancers are inevitable in a population screening program which cannot be 100% sensitive. Some cancers will develop between screens and some will be present, but not detected at the time of screening. Screening programs should aim, however, to minimise the number of intervals as higher than expected levels indicate reduced sensitivity and less likelihood of reducing mortality. The expected numbers of intervals will be partly determined by the time interval between screens. In the UK, with 3 yearly screening, the rate of intervals will be approximately one third the rate of screen detected breast cancers. In England, 18,000 breast cancers are detected annually on screening and a further 6000 present as interval cancers. In countries with 2 yearly screening, the proportion of interval cancers will be about a quarter and in those

R. Given-Wilson (✉)
St Georges Healthcare NHS Foundation Trust, Tooting, London, UK
e-mail: Rosalind.Given-Wilson@stgeorges.nhs.uk

© The Author(s), under exclusive license to Springer Nature Switzerland AG 2022
C. Mercer et al. (eds.), *Digital Mammography*, https://doi.org/10.1007/978-3-031-10898-3_10

105

countries with annual screening programs about 15% [2].

In the UK NHSBSP the number of interval cancers is measured and monitored to ensure the number is as low as possible. The acceptable level of interval cancers is set at <2.7 per 1000 women screened over 36 months [3]. This standard is subdivided by the level each year following screening, with more cancers expecting to present as the time since the last screen increases:

- <0.65 per 1000 diagnosed <12 months of the previous screen
- <1.40 per 1000 diagnosed between 12 and <24 months of the previous screen
- <1.65 per 1000 diagnosed between 24 and <36 months of the previous screen

It can be challenging to accurately record the numbers of interval cancers (ascertainment) Women may present with their interval cancer in a different hospital or geographical area from the place where they have been screened. In England, however, timely recording of interval cancer numbers has become more accurate in the last few years with the introduction of SHIM (Screening History Information Management system). This allows alignment of information between cancer registries and the NHSBSP. The data allows sensitivity and specificity for the screening program to be calculated. The most recently published rates of English interval cancers are 3.1 per 1000 women screened compared with a screening cancer detection rate of 8.1 per 1000 women [4].

Mammographic Review and Classification of Interval Cancers

Review and classification of interval cancer images is a valuable tool for improving the skills of image readers. Classification and the method of review of intervals is variable in different countries and health systems, but most published reviews will include categories which equate to true intervals (normal prior screening images) and false negative intervals (abnormality missed on prior screening images).

In the NHSBSP, once an interval cancer is identified, review is undertaken within the screening service. This involves at least two readers reading the images from the screening episode prior to the interval cancer diagnosis. They have access to all images prior to that screen but should not have seen the subsequent interval presentation images taken at diagnosis. Any suspicious appearances are recorded and then the diagnostic images viewed to confirm whether possible abnormalities recorded on the screening images did represent the developing cancer [1].

In the majority of cases (around 80%) no abnormality will be found on prior screening images and these are classified as satisfactory (normal). In a minority of cases there will be a subtle abnormality seen on review on the previous screening images by some readers, classified as satisfactory with learning points (uncertain). In the very small number of cases classified as unsatisfactory, clear signs of malignancy will have been missed (suspicious). Cases of interval cancers in the uncertain or suspicious category are usually reviewed at screening unit meetings so that all image readers within a unit can learn from them.

Interval cancers may also arise after a client recall, following assessment and discharge. If the assessed abnormality is in a different breast from the subsequent interval cancer the images should undergo standard interval cancer review. If the subsequent interval cancer is the same side as the previously assessed abnormality the quality of assessment should be reviewed. Interval cancers occurring at the same site as the previous assessment do not necessarily indicate problems with assessment. In most of these cases, on review, the previous assessment was adequate but sometimes there are learning points that can be used to improve assessment. Occasionally the assessment is found to have been unsatisfactory.

Feedback to Women with Interval Cancers and Duty of Candour

The NHSBSP has guidance encouraging transparency in sharing results of review of interval cancers with affected women since 2006: Disclosure of Audit Guidance [5]. In 2015, Duty of Candour (DoC) became law for the NHS within England, requiring health care providers to apologise and be open and transparent when something has gone wrong with healthcare and an individual has been harmed.

Guidance on applying DoC in the breast screening program aligns with the classification of review of interval cancers. Interval cancers that are satisfactory or satisfactory with learning points are inevitable in cancer screening. Those affected should be offered the opportunity to be given the results of audit of their images and discuss them, but no error has been made in their care and the Duty of Candour process should not be triggered. Duty of Candour applies in the rare cases where screening image interpretation or assessment is felt to have been unsatisfactory and thus something has gone wrong. Those should receive a formal apology from the hospital trust as well as openness and an opportunity to discuss their images and findings.

Interviews with those affected by interval cancers can be a stressful experience for all those involved (Chap. 13 can provide some supporting mechanisms). Careful preparation, clear explanation and kindness are essential. Training, guidance and a toolkit [6] are available for staff undertaking these discussions. Information for those being offered screening should include information on all the main harms and benefits of screening. This allows them to make an informed choice about whether to be screened. This should include information about the limits of screening sensitivity and interval cancers. Following a diagnosis of an interval cancer, further information should be offered about interval cancers and how to access the results of review of previous screens.

Factors Associated with Higher Rates of Interval Cancers

Those at higher risk of interval cancers, following a screen, include those with dense breasts on mammography and those currently taking hormone replacement therapy. Interval cancers linked to higher breast density tend to be associated with screening images which are normal on review, rather than missed abnormalities, suggesting a masking effect from dense tissue. Younger women are also at more relative risk than older women which is partially linked to higher breast density.

Despite the relative increased risk of intervals in younger women, the absolute level of interval cancers is higher in older women because the overall rate of breast cancer increases with age. Other factors increasing the risk of developing an interval cancer are a history of previous false positive mammography (recall for assessment with a benign/normal outcome) and a family history of breast cancer [2].

Mammographic Features of Interval Cancers

Published international radiological reviews of interval cancers show that the majority are reported as true or occult intervals. In true intervals the previous screens are normal (40–77%). In occult intervals both the previous screens and the images at diagnosis of the interval cancer are normal (7 to 32%) [2]. Both these categories would be classed as satisfactory on NHSBSP review where 80% of prior screens of intervals are found to be normal on review.

In the 20% of interval reviews where an abnormality is seen on the prior screens, the majority are reported as being masses, followed by asymmetries and distortions. Granular micro calcification has also been reported as being misinterpreted [7]. Missed calcification is a less common feature following the introduction of digital mammography [8].

Biology and Prognosis of Interval Cancers

Interval cancers show poorer prognostic features compared to screen detected cancers. They are larger, have more nodal metastases, are more commonly grade 3, triple negative or Her2 positive and present with more advanced disease. Biological features and prognosis of interval cancers are more similar to cancers occurring in non-screened women than screen detected cancers. Interval cancers where an abnormality is visible on the prior screening images (false negative or missed) show worse prognostic features with larger tumor size and more advanced nodal status than true interval cancers. This is despite true interval cancers being of higher grade than those which are missed. Interval cancers occurring in women with very dense breasts show better prognostic features than those occurring in fatty breasts [2].

Clinical Pearls
- Interval cancers are common and inevitable in breast screening
- Monitoring of interval cancer rates and radiological review of intervals helps quality assure screening and provides education for image readers
- Most interval cancer cases are true intervals with no abnormality seen on review on prior screening images
- Information for women screened should include the possibility of interval cancers and signpost how to access the results of review if they suffer an interval

Chapter Review Questions
Review Questions

1. 18,000 breast cancers are screen detected each year in England. How many interval cancers occur annually?
2. What are the classification categories of interval cancers on radiological review in the NHSBSP?
3. Do interval cancers have a better or worse prognosis than screen detected cancers?

Answers

1. 6000.
2. Satisfactory, Satisfactory with learning points, Unsatisfactory.
3. Worse.

Appendix

Test your learning and check your understanding of this book's contents: use the "Springer Nature Flashcards" app to access questions using https://sn.pub/dcAnWL.

To use the app, please follow the instructions in Chap. 1.

Flashcard code: 48341-69945-ABCB1-2A8C7-CE9D2.

Short URL: https://sn.pub/dcAnWL.

References

1. England PH. Guidance: NHS BSP reporting, classification and monitoring of interval cancers and cancers following previous assessment. https://www.gov.uk/government/publications/breast-screening-interval-cancers.
2. Houssami N, Hunter K. The epidemiology, radiology and biological characteristics of interval breast cancers in population mammography screening. NPJ Breast Cancer. 2017;3(1):1–3.
3. England PH. Guidance: NHS breast screening programme screening standards valid for data collected from 1 April 2017. https://www.gov.uk/government/publications/breast-screening-consolidated-programme-standards/nhs-breast-screening-programme-screening-standards-valid-for-data-collected-from-1-april-2021. Accessed 31 Mar 2021.
4. Burnside ES, Vulkan D, Blanks RG, Duffy SW. Association between screening mammography recall rate and interval cancers in the UK breast cancer service screening program: a cohort study. Radiology. 2018 Jul;288(1):47–54.

5. Given-Wilson R. Commentary on duty of candour and cancer screening. Br J Radiol. 2018;91(1090):20170451.
6. England PH. Guidance: NHS screening programmes: duty of candour. https://www.gov.uk/government/publications/nhs-screening-programmes-duty-of-candour. Accessed 5 Oct 2020.
7. Evans AJ, Kutt E, Record C, Waller M, Bobrow L, Moss S. Radiological and pathological findings of interval cancers in a multi-Centre, randomized, controlled trial of mammographic screening in women from age 40–41 years. Clin Radiol. 2007;62(4):348–52.
8. Blanks RG, Wallis MG, Alison R, Kearins O, Jenkins J, Patnick J, Given-Wilson RM. Impact of digital mammography on cancer detection and recall rates: 11.3 million screening episodes in the English National Health Service Breast Cancer Screening Program. Radiology. 2019;290(3):629–37.

Part II

Patient Diary

11

Joanne Coward

Learning Objectives

- With an emphasis on social and emotional considerations, to provide practitioners with a comprehensive real-life story about a patient's journey from initial diagnosis of breast cancer to the later stages of terminal illness
- To give practitioners insights into the kinds of concerns and pressures their clients might be experiencing when they are having mammography examinations
- To help student and qualified practitioners improve their communication and care skills when performing imaging in screening and symptomatic settings

Background: Professional and Family Context

On Friday 25th November 2016, I was diagnosed with breast cancer. The day was Black Friday, a notorious shopping day before Christmas; it certainly lived up to its name. It was the day that changed my life forever; strange as it might sound, not all for the worst. But, on that day, it was overwhelming, I knew that I had to break the news to my five daughters and my family. I

needed to stay strong and rational for their sakes, but I think I gained the look of a rabbit in headlights. Although I had a diagnosis of invasive ducal breast cancer, I did not have any idea of the extent to which it had spread until 6 months later after further imaging and treatment, which also involved surgical clearance of the axillary nodes on my left side.

At the time of my diagnosis, I was a lecturer at a University in the United Kingdom, where I had worked for 8 years. I lectured in radiography, which was the profession for which I qualified in 1996. As a newly qualified radiographer, I started work at a District General Hospital in the UK, where I trained, and remained there until 2008. During the first few years, I worked as a general radiographer working in different areas of the department, gaining a varied experience. My real passion, however, was CT, which was still very much an evolving technology.

I went on to specialise in cross-sectional imaging and took postgraduate courses in CT and CT reporting that enabled me to report CT brain scans. I went on to become the lead radiographer in the CT department. My background in radiography and specialisation in CT gave me some knowledge of my situation when I was diagnosed with breast cancer; enough to scare me but not enough to reassure me. The phrase 'a little knowledge is a bad thing,' certainly rang true. Whenever I have a CT scan, I can still picture in my mind, some of the pathology I have seen when working as a radiographer. It's taken a lot for me not to

J. Coward (✉)
University of Salford, Manchester, UK

have images in my mind of chest and liver metastases that I have seen other stage 4 breast cancer patients present with. Needless to say, and perhaps in common with other people in my situation, I always think the worst until I hear otherwise. Around the time I have scans, it is very difficult to remain positive and keep an open mind; the common term used by patients about this is 'scanxiety'.

Whilst I said that a little knowledge can be a bad thing, I did actually develop some useful coping strategies working in CT, which helped me greatly in the coming years. The pathology that was demonstrated in CT was fascinating, but it was always displayed on a computer monitor, remote from the patient in the room. Because of this, it became easy to separate the patient from their disease; the disease was displayed on the monitor and the patient was the person that I interacted with. I used this technique almost without realising so that I could talk to the patient as a 'person' and dissociate them from the disease. I was always able to see the patient for the individual they were and maintain their identity rather than seeing them as the disease they were living with. I realise now just how important this is. I found this technique really helped when my mum was diagnosed with ovarian cancer in 2009. I knew that I could do nothing to help with the cancer, but I could help her as a person and give her support with her emotional health and wellbeing. It helped me when I was diagnosed and is possibly one of the most important techniques I have learnt from a personal coping point of view, and also as a professional.

Maintaining your identity when you have been diagnosed with a life-changing illness is paramount. When I was first diagnosed, and at times after my secondary diagnosis, I have wanted to hide away, worried that people would see me differently and feel sorry for me. Of course, how people see you is really down to you more than the disease. Cancer or not, I was still the same person and I wanted people to see that, so I held my head up and braved going out.

My career as a university lecturer still had a strong focus on CT: I taught the principles and practice of CT to undergraduate radiography stu-

dents and, for postgraduate students, I ran a CT head reporting course. As a university academic, it seemed a natural choice that my research work would also be grounded in CT. Consequently, I became involved in a research project investigating incidental findings on low-resolution CT images of the chest. At the time I started my research this area was significantly under-reported within the literature. For the type of CT scanning I investigated the acquisition had not been performed for diagnostic purposes but instead to correct images from nuclear medicine single-photon emission computed tomography scans that had been degraded by radiation attenuation. The CT acquisition was therefore performed for attenuation correction purposes only; the low-quality CT images being a by-product. I embarked upon a PhD by published works and progressed well, but sadly, due to ongoing ill-health, I was unable to complete this. It is worth mentioning here, there was some irony in my research focus on incidental findings, in that when I was diagnosed with breast cancer, it too was an incidental finding.

I mentioned earlier that I have 5 daughters; at the time of writing this chapter their ages are: Emma (age 23), Zoe (age 21), Milly (age 18), Naomi (age 11) and Natalie (age 10). When I was initially diagnosed, they were 18, 16, 14, 6 and 5 years old. Emma had just started her first year at University, studying maths and Zoe was studying towards A-levels.

The day that I received my diagnosis, I had arranged to meet Zoe at the Manchester markets with Milly. It was all a bit of a blur. We met Zoe for something to eat before we walked round the markets and I told them both that I had been diagnosed with breast cancer. Although the thought of having cancer terrified me, I took a positive approach when I gave the news. After all, I was being treated with curative intent, so hopefully would receive a good outcome. Although the breast cancer was invasive, it didn't seem to have spread to the axillary lymph nodes. I was reassured that this was very positive. I later learnt that there was spread to the left axillary lymph nodes and that I was stage 3 at definitive diagnosis.

It seems strange, but I don't remember either of their reactions, other than them being concerned. This led to reassurance from me that it was something that they didn't need to worry about; it was my place to deal with the cancer and everything that went with it; I wanted the girls to carry on leading their lives as normal. That was my intent, but it was inevitably impossible to fully achieve this.

I knew that I needed to speak to Emma as soon as possible because I was scheduled to have a mastectomy in 6 days time. I arranged to visit her at university on the Sunday and confirmed that her boyfriend was with her at the time; I didn't want to break the news and then leave her on her own. When I told her, we both cried and hugged each other. It was such a shock to her. Unlike Zoe and Milly, who were living at home and knew that I was undergoing diagnostic procedures, I had told Emma nothing prior to this, hoping that I wouldn't have to. Again, I tried to be positive and reiterated to Emma what I had said to Zoe and Milly, that I didn't want this to affect her life and that she must carry on as normal and not to worry about me. We went out for the afternoon and visited the local Christmas markets and the cinema, before I returned home.

I told Naomi and Natalie that I had to go to hospital for an operation, but I didn't mention cancer or give them much detail. They were still very young and I felt it was better to protect them as much as I could. If they asked questions, I answered them truthfully but at a level that I felt was suitable. Natalie, the younger of the two, seemed to accept my hair loss, scars and drains more easily than Naomi. After my mastectomy, Natalie looked down my jumper and asked, "What's that plaster where your boob used to be?" She wasn't phased at all. Naomi hated the drain that came home from hospital with me after my mastectomy and hated even more the fact that I was bald because of chemotherapy treatment. I felt that I had to keep my head covered at all times, even when sleeping, in case Naomi caught sight of me.

Milly was almost 15 years old, and thankfully, not fully aware of the implications of a cancer diagnosis. We were able to keep quite upbeat and share a bit of humour. Milly's main worry was how I was going to be able to apply mascara when I lost my eyelashes to chemotherapy. This conversation happened in the car, whilst we were on a camping holiday in Wales, and it still makes me smile today. This contrasts very much to how she was when I received my secondary diagnosis. She was much more informed and had a good understanding of what stage 4 meant. She decided to raise money for MacMillan by doing a sponsored head shave; raising just over £8000. I was so proud of her for doing this and proud of all the girls for how they coped and supported me in those first few months of my stage 4 journey. They are, as they always have been, my raison d'etre.

Wig shopping was another story. A friend took me to a salon in Manchester, just before I started chemotherapy after primary diagnosis. I had my hair cut short and wouldn't need a wig for a few more weeks. However, after hours of trying on different styles and then rushing back to do the school run, my own hair was a real mess. I decided to keep my wig on and try it out. It was short and dark, like my natural hair, but completely devoid of my usual unruly curls. I got so many compliments when I arrived in the school playground and asked how long it had taken to straighten my hair that I couldn't help but smile. Nobody knew, and that's just what I wanted. At that moment in time, I was scared of losing my identity and being seen as a cancer patient. Naomi's and Natalie's reactions were a little bit different. I was greeted by, "You're not my mummy! What have you done to your hair?" I knew that the way they felt about my hair wouldn't last long, and it didn't. It wasn't long before they knew the truth and that my new hairdo was actually a wig. After all, it was better than having a bald mummy.

Finding a Lump

During the summer of 2016, I occasionally thought I could feel a lump in my left breast. The first time was in the shower, but when I tried to locate it later, I couldn't. Perhaps I had imagined it? Then at other times, I thought I could feel something but wasn't really convinced. It niggled at me but the fact that I couldn't always feel a lump and when I did, it seemed mobile, led me to believe I potentially had a benign cyst; mobile, soft lumps are typically benign, I had read.

In July, 2016, whilst away on holiday visiting Disneyland, Florida with the girls, I again thought I noticed a lump whilst I was showering. I was on holiday, so tried to dismiss it, again thinking it was probably nothing. I would enjoy my holiday and then deal with it when I got home. I wasn't really convinced I could feel a lump anyway but there did seem to be an indent along the outside of my breast which I put down to where my bra digged into my skin. I decided to keep an eye on this but, again, managed to convince myself that it was nothing.

In October, the lump/non-lump had niggled at me enough that I eventually made an appointment at the GP practice. I saw one of the practice nurses, who confirmed that she could also feel a lump. At this point, I fell apart and became an emotional wreck. If someone else could feel it too, then I must have cancer. I could not get this thought out of my head. I was referred to a breast clinic on a 2 week wait cancer pathway. I struggled to get through those 2 weeks with my thoughts and emotions making my life a misery. When I attended the breast clinic, the doctor I saw did a physical examination and stated that the lump was soft tissue and nothing to worry about. I broke down with tears of relief. He said that he would need to have a mammogram and ultrasound and sent me across the corridor to the radiology department.

As I sat waiting for the imaging, I felt quite relaxed; it was, as I had thought, simply a benign lump. I had the mammogram first and then a radiologist performed an ultrasound scan. He asked me a few questions whilst he was scanning, one of which was whether I had been having discharge from my nipple. I told him that I hadn't. I was a bit unsure why he was questioning me. When he had completed the examination, he told me that he could not identify a tumour but that the mammogram had revealed a lot of calcification and he would like me to have a biopsy. I asked whether he thought it was malignant and whether it was invasive. I naively thought that because there wasn't an obvious tumour that if cancer was present, it would not have become invasive. I was wrong!

I had to wait for a biopsy appointment, and again, the wait was awful. I imagined all sorts, but I was convinced that if I did have cancer, it was not invasive because there was no tumour to be seen. I had to have two areas of my breast biopsied, which involved a rotating needle being placed into the identified areas and several biopsy samples being taken. I wasn't particularly worried about the examination itself, just the results. The biopsy was performed by two radiographers: I had done my training with one radiographer and the other was the friend of a colleague. I felt in good hands and the atmosphere was light and chatty.

The room was decorated in pleasant light colours and the lighting was relaxing, all of which helped to put me at ease. It is strange how surroundings can change your mood and feelings; I doubt that I would have been quite so relaxed in a dark, gloomy room. The pain with the first biopsied area was so intense that I fainted. I held on for as long as I could and then told the radiographers performing the biopsy that I was going to faint. They quickly brought me out of the mammography machine and removed the needle just before I fainted. They managed to revive me with a drink of water and several biscuits before continuing to biopsy the second area. This was not painful at all.

The wait began again: I would be rung with an appointment to attend clinic to get the biopsy results. On results day, I was called from the waiting room into a small clinic room, where I waited with the door closed until the breast surgeon and breast nurse entered. To this day, this is one of the worst experiences I have had. Waiting with the door closed in that room induces a disproportionate amount of panic and I have come to dread it with every visit to clinic. The breast surgeon asked me what I knew so far and listened to my answer. He then told me, "It's bad news I'm afraid. It's invasive." The room started to spin and I became very faint. How could it be invasive? I didn't understand. There wasn't a tumour. Surely it was still carcinoma in situ? My throat was so dry and the room still spinning. I asked for a glass of water; feeling terrified but also ashamed for being so close to fainting again. The surgeon examined me and pointed out that there was tissue distortion of my left breast. This was the skin crease that I had noticed a few months earlier, but which had not been identified on my first visit to clinic.

I was told that I would need a mastectomy. I had already made this decision for myself, so the news wasn't too much of a shock. I had, in fact, got widespread ductal carcinoma in situ (DCIS) but this had become invasive in several areas. During surgery, this was determined to be 7 cm of invasive cancer in total. Having an immediate reconstruction at the time of mastectomy was discussed but I opted to go for mastectomy without reconstruction as soon as possible; wanting to just get rid of the cancer. My operation was scheduled for 6 days hence. I was to have a mastectomy with sentinel node dissection to check whether the cancer had spread to the lymph nodes in my axilla. The ultrasound of my axillary lymph nodes appeared normal, so it was expected that there hadn't been any spread. This was proven not to be the case, post operatively.

I returned to the ward after surgery and soon needed to pay a visit to the toilet. I made a point of looking in the mirror so that I could see my flat chest on the left and get it out of the way as soon as I could. It didn't bother me as much as I thought; I felt relief. What did shock me was the blue tone my skin had taken on because of the blue dye that had been injected into the lymph system to detect the lymph nodes in my axilla during surgery. I looked like a pale smurf! My urine was blue too, but I was expecting that.

Following surgery, I had a staging CT scan to see whether there had been any spread of the cancer to the rest of my body. This showed a lesion in my liver which had been reported as benign by the radiologist. He had, however, requested a liver MR scan to classify this. Again, I went to pieces. The breast surgeon put his arm round me and reassured me that the lesion had benign appearances and the only reason I was having an

MR was because of my history. I wouldn't be followed up on a regular basis, this was a one off to confirm that it was a benign finding.

The plan was for me to have 4 months chemotherapy starting at the end of January and finishing at the end of May. I would then have a surgical procedure to remove the lymph nodes from my axilla, followed by radiotherapy. I would have two different regimes of chemotherapy, Epirubicin and Cyclophosphamide for 3 cycles with a 3 week break between cycles and then weekly Paclitaxel for 9 weeks. I would lose my hair and have other side effects that would become known during treatment. I had a long mop of curls at this point and didn't relish the thought of finding clumps of them all over the house. I had lost hair after Emma was born, and so, had some insight into the situation. I decided to embrace the situation and take some control; I cut my hair short just before Christmas and then shaved my head once my hair started to fall out on 13th February, my birthday. Of course, there is a positive side to losing one's hair, I did not have to wax or shave other areas of my body for quite a few months!

At this point, I joined an online breast cancer support group. I chatted online to other ladies about to start chemotherapy and became part of a group who would be starting chemotherapy in February. I figured that this was probably a better fit than joining the January group; January was nearly over. We later formed a Facebook group called 'The Fab Febbers,' and we are still in touch today, although I have yet to meet the group in person. I also made friends with some other ladies online. Again, we formed a Facebook group and became 'Our Gang.' Our Gang planned to meet for fish and chips on the beach once treatment was over. We haven't done this yet, but we have met up for social occasions at Christmas and are still very much in touch. I cannot stress enough how important peer support is a time like this. To have a virtual hand to hold of someone who is going through something similar and understands your anxieties is second to none.

I had a short break after chemotherapy before I had my second round of surgery to remove my axillary lymph nodes. This involved a short overnight stay in hospital and recovery was fairly quick. However, I did develop a seroma at the surgical site and had to have this drained weekly for several months. In fact, it didn't resolve completely until I had a hydrocortisone injection for a frozen shoulder which I acquired during radiotherapy. I further complicated things by having a weeks holiday in Corfu, shortly after surgery. Here, I had to have the seroma drained again part way through the holiday. It was a bit disconcerting to have to explain to a Greek-speaking consultant via an English-speaking nurse, how the procedure should be performed. I ended up leaving Corfu, not with a seroma but a large haematoma. Still, I would not have missed that holiday for the world. It was a much-needed tonic after months of treatment.

I returned to work in September. I had worked from home during some of my treatment but had mixed this with sick leave and annual leave. At the end of September, I started radiotherapy at the Christie Hospital, Manchester. During radiotherapy, it became increasingly difficult to get me in the correct position for treatment. The radiographer would ask me to relax my shoulder, and although I felt that I was doing this, it became clear that this wasn't the case. My left shoulder seemed to be getting closer and closer to my left ear! It wasn't really until after treatment, when I began to feel considerable pain, that I was diagnosed with adhesive capsulitis; more commonly known as frozen shoulder.

The pain was excruciating, affecting my sleep and daily activities. When I went to bed, the only position that I found remotely comfortable was on my front with my left arm hanging off the side of the bed. I was unable to move my hand above waist height, and any attempt by the physiotherapist to move my arm, reduced me to tears. I was given exercises to do, which I found impossible, although I did attempt them. After 3 months without improvement, I was referred for a hydrocortisone injection into my shoulder joint. At this point, I joined a gym with a 3-month medical referral and bought a hybrid pushbike, announcing that I was going to cycle from London to Paris. A little ambitious perhaps, but I needed a goal to aim for. Cycling,

combined with gentle exercise at the gym, saw a return of the full range of movement to my left shoulder.

I started to cycle from about the end of February 2018. It was freezing cold some days, so I was limited at first. I was also very weak after treatment and ended up in a ditch on one of my earlier rides. At first, I was glad that nobody had witnessed this, but then quickly realised that I had fallen on my frozen shoulder with the bike on top of me and I could not get up. I then wished that somebody had seen me! After much inelegant struggling, I made my way out of the ditch. Things really could only get better from here. I planned a route, with my friend Hugh, from Windsor Castle to Notre Dame. This partly used the Avenue Verte, which I was hoping would limit the time we had to cycle on the roads. My cousin Debby, Emma and her boyfriend Alex, Zoe and Milly cycled with us. Emma and Alex took turns to drive the accompanying car, and also cycling with the group, for the first 4 days. Hugh drove the last day into Paris and then cycled back out to meet us so that we all cycled into Paris and arrived at Notre Dame together in August 2018.

After this, life carried on as normal. I was back at work and other than regular check-ups, I tried to put cancer to the back of my mind. Of course, it never completely leaves you and there are always those thoughts of 'what if.' I eventually became too busy to go to support groups and focused my time back to everyday life. Though I cycled less, I kept busy and took up gardening and enjoyed time in my greenhouse that my parents had bought me for my 50th birthday. Life, on the whole, was good.

I developed lymphoedema in my left hand and arm during the summer of 2019. The swelling was the result of lymphatic fluid in my tissues that was reluctant to drain following the removal of my axillary lymph nodes. I was referred to a lymphoedema clinic and fitted with a sleeve and glove to wear during the daytime. This miraculously had my arm looking back to normal in no time. However, it has now returned and I'm back to wearing compression garments in a hope that it will again resolve.

In December 2019, I booked a spontaneous holiday to Cyprus over the New Year. The girls would be with their dad and I didn't relish the thought of being home alone. I also felt that I needed some time away to relax and to meditate. As much as I had tried, the thoughts of cancer were never far away. The weather was mixed but nice enough that I could get out and about. I walked a lot and booked myself on a trip around Cyprus, crossing over to the Turkish side in the North. I watched the sun set on New Year's Eve and saw New Year's Day 2020 in Cyprus. I returned home feeling refreshed and grateful to be back with the girls again.

I can't quite pinpoint the exact date, but perhaps sometime in February 2020, I began to get a niggling pain in my right groin, which I noticed more on walking. A couple of ibuprofen and it was gone. I didn't worry too much, it felt like it was soft tissue so I thought I must have injured myself whilst walking. I remembered slipping in my flip flops whilst walking in Cyprus. I would keep an eye on it but mention it at my next meeting with my breast surgeon in March. I was sure that it would have resolved by then. But my appointment was cancelled because we had entered into a pandemic; along with other countries, Covid-19 had put the UK into lockdown.

During lockdown I started to suffer more with pain in my left hip and my lower back had also become painful. Initially, I put this down to poor posture because I was working from home with a laptop balanced on my lap whilst attempting to home school Naomi and Natalie (who were using the available desks and chairs). The pain became so severe that I was unable to walk and I became bed bound. I'm unsure at this point why I didn't realise quite how poorly I was; I still attempted to work from my bed. When I started to get discomfort in my abdomen and started to be sick, I contacted my GP surgery and was prescribed pain relief by the pharmacist. I did not actually have a face-to-face appointment with a GP or healthcare practitioner for 5 weeks because of the Covid-19 pandemic; I was too ill to attend the surgery and a home visit was refused, despite me stating that it was impossible for me to get out of bed.

I struggled to eat and my diet consisted of jelly and ice-cream, which I vomited back soon after I had eaten. I couldn't even keep water down. Eventually, I was admitted to hospital as an emergency. I was critically ill and totally immobile. I was diagnosed with renal failure and quizzed as to whether I had taken an overdose, which, of course, I had not. I had to use a bedpan rather than a commode or toilet because I was unable to get out of bed. By now, I was in considerable pain in my ribs, back and pelvis and had lost over 20 kg in weight. After several days of acute treatment, x-rays, ultrasound, CT and MRI scans, I was told that my cancer had returned. There had been a significant delay in my cancer diagnosis.

Apart from being critically ill, the renal failure had implications in relation to the diagnostic imaging that was required, in particular, the CT scan I had of my chest, abdomen and pelvis. It meant that I was unable to be given the intravenous contrast agent that is normally used to enhance the contrast resolution of the images. As a result, the images of my liver were low-resolution; although my liver appeared abnormal, it was not possible to make an accurate diagnosis. It took 8 months before I had two comparable, diagnostic CT scans that had been performed with intravenous contrast agent.

Further imaging revealed that I had a large metastatic deposit in the neck of my right femur. I was referred to an orthopaedic surgeon, who said that I was not to weight-bear on that leg and was to use a wheelchair. There was concern that the femur could fracture without surgical intervention. However, this would not be possible whilst I was on active treatment for cancer and so had to be deferred until my cancer was considered stable and I could take a break from treatment. This meant that I would be using a wheelchair and unable to stand or walk, indefinitely. Further complications down the line meant that surgery was perhaps no longer an option.

I was desperate to be discharged from hospital because Naomi's birthday was coming up. I had already spent Emma's and Natalie's birthdays in bed, so effectively missed these. Eventually, I was discharged the day after Naomi's birthday and started chemotherapy the following day. I had 16 weekly doses of Paclitaxel; a chemotherapy that I had been treated with as adjuvant therapy after my primary diagnosis. I was quite confident when I started this treatment for a second time because, other than feeling tired and weak, I hadn't had too many side effects the first time around. How different it was after my secondary diagnosis! Looking back, I wasn't really in very good shape to start with. My potassium and magnesium levels were persistently low and meant that as well as supplements, I had to have several infusions which often entailed hospital stays. I also needed blood and plasma transfusions before some of my treatments could go ahead. It certainly wasn't plain sailing, and all credit to my oncologist and oncology team for persevering and making sure treatment went ahead.

I found treatment increasingly gruelling. I went from spending 1 day a week in bed recovering to spending most of the week in bed; it was exhausting. I felt bloated and out of breath all the time and was almost totally immobile. In November, a CT scan revealed that I had large, bilateral pleural effusions and I was told I would need to change treatment. Chemotherapy was stopped immediately. I was left with uncertainty; not knowing what my new treatment would involve. My assumption was that the chemotherapy was responsible for the generalised oedema, which made me feel bloated, and the pleural effusions. On speaking to one of the oncology nurses, I got the impression that the chemotherapy had not been successful. I was in a state of shock and anxiety. After further discussion, it became obvious that we had both jumped to our own conclusions, so I desperately tried to go with my own initial thoughts. I still don't know to this day whether I was right or not; I just didn't have the courage to ask the oncologist.

I was moved onto a recently licensed drug, Abemaciclib along with Fulvestrant, a hormone therapy drug, (my type of breast cancer was oestrogen receptor positive) and Denusomab, a bisphosphonate to strengthen my bones. I was told that the main side effect of this new regime was diarrhoea! There are, of course, a few other side effects, but I have found it much kinder than

the previous treatment. I was sceptical though, convinced that it wouldn't work and feeling that it wasn't as an aggressive approach as chemotherapy. At the time of writing, I have had two stable CT scans and my quality of life has greatly improved.

At the end of December, I was called by an orthopaedic surgeon and told that I could tentatively start to walk again. Although I hadn't had the surgery that was initially thought to be necessary, the lesion in my neck of femur had become less lytic and more sclerotic. It was no longer causing pain, which was considered to be another good sign that weight-bearing was now a possibility. I was told that if I got any pain at all, I had to stop walking immediately and return to my wheelchair. From that day, I have not used a wheelchair in the house. The news was a real lift for me and for my family. I cried happy tears when I was told that I could walk again. It meant so much to the girls as well. I remember getting up the following morning and making Naomi and Natalie pancakes for breakfast. The pain when standing for much more than a minute was immense, so I resorted to sitting on a stool. Naomi's reaction when she saw I had made pancakes made it worth the effort. She ran round the house saying that mum was walking again and making pancakes; a memory to be savoured.

However, increased pleural effusions, partial lung collapse, recurrent pneumonia and further complications meant that I was so breathless, walking became impossible. I was admitted to a local hospital as an emergency in March and remained there for 2 weeks. During this hospital stay, I had imaging for a suspected pulmonary embolism which consisted of an arterial phased CT scan through my thorax followed by portal venous phase CT of my abdomen and pelvis. I was also treated for a chest infection, had a temporary left pleural drain inserted (which fell out) and a right-sided aspiration of part of the right pulmonary effusion.

I had previously had some short hospital stays during which time I had several temporary pleural drains inserted and removed and one permanent drain on the right side. I was told that this would remain in for life. From the very start, I hated this drain with a passion. It was uncomfortable at best, but painful if I put any pressure on it, meaning I could no longer sleep on my right side. This had become my preference as sleeping on my left side was uncomfortable and left me feeling very breathless. I had to resort to sleeping on my back, which again, was uncomfortable. The consequence was that I became quite sleep deprived. It wasn't long before draining ceased. At first it was considered that the effusion might have resolved, whereas it had actually become loculated and the drain had become blocked.

A week after my discharge from hospital, I became increasingly breathless and was admitted to The Christie Hospital. I was told that my cancer was stable; the first time I had heard this since my diagnosis in July the previous year. I was referred to the North West Lung Centre where it was discovered that the permanent chest drain on the right had become infected and, to my great relief, needed to be removed as a priority. This was done the same afternoon and a temporary drain put in. The plan was to let this finish draining, remove it and put a temporary drain in the left side. I was given the option of having a permanent drain in the right but declined this and opted for a pleurodesis procedure instead. The aim of this was to inject liquid talc into the pleural space and irritate the pleura so that they formed a seal. The success rate was approximately 70%. I figured that these were good enough odds to give it a try and resort to a permanent drain only if absolutely necessary. Apart from the discomfort from the previous one I had had, it was also very limiting as I had to keep the drain site dry; showering, soaking in a nice hot bath and relaxing in my hot tub were all out of the question. Swimming was also not a possibility, but at this stage, perhaps a little ambitious.

When I was discharged from hospital, I weighed under 50 kg. I was horrified by this and scared that the weight loss was cancer related. I ate high calorie food and consumed the protein drinks that had been prescribed for me during my hospital stay. I also joined a gym. I was keen to try and strengthen my lungs to compensate for the pleural effusions that seemed to return within a couple of weeks of being drained. I was also hoping that exercise would help my posture, as I was convinced that my loss of height and back pain was partly due to this and muscle spasms, which were almost unbearable by the end of the day I was surprised by how much I could actually achieve at the gym.

At my induction, I tried out the treadmill and the stationary bike but felt most accomplished at being able to do some resistance training that was also shown to me. I built on this and could see improvements each time I went. It gave me such a buzz that at last, I was taking some control back and my body was getting stronger. I was still noticeably stiff when I walked, but I was improving and the pain reduced as I got stronger. Oddly, swimming, the one exercise I thought would be easiest for me to do, turned out to be the most difficult. My posture meant that I was in the wrong position in the water and my breathing was so poor, it was difficult to even complete one length. Over time, this improved so that I could complete multiple lengths. This was really positive, as it reflected the improvement of my breathing and, subsequent reduction in my pleural effusions. So many times, exercise has proved a way of me taking back some control of my body and mind, and has put me in a much better place than I started.

I missed cycling and had given up all hope of getting on a bike again. I was worried about the injuries that might result if I fell, but was also not fit or strong enough to cycle. After a few sessions at the gym and various exercise classes, I was much stronger. I still got breathless walking uphill, but I could see improvements almost every day. I bit the bullet and bought an e-bike. I have never looked back. Imagine going from not being able to walk upstairs (or get out of bed on a bad day) to cycling the hills of the Peak District. I was in my element. My back was still stiff, and this was obvious in my gait, but I could walk and I could ride!

Before my hospital stay, I had been considering buying a camper van so that I could spend some weekends away with Naomi and Natalie. We would lie on my bed watching tv in the evening, pretending that we were in our camper van. That was as close as we got. Even whilst I was doing my research, I realised that I wasn't well enough to follow the plan through. The pain with my back, regular muscle spasms and my posture would just not allow me to make up a bed and do all the necessary lifting, carrying and driving that would be necessary; at best, we would be able to sleep out on the drive at home. I turned my sights to static caravans instead. I saw a caravan I liked on a site in North Wales, and whilst hooked up on oxygen and in a hospital bed, I impulsively paid a deposit. Unfortunately, the caravan was not available, as I'd been led to believe and it seemed like there would be a long wait; in fact, the company were not able to give me a date. We were given a free week stay in another caravan on the site during the Easter holidays and then, after some discussion, I was reimbursed the deposit I had paid. I am so grateful for this now because I went on to buy a caravan, just outside Porthmadog, on the wonderful Aberdunant Hall Holiday Park. I have just spent the most relaxing, yet energetic summer in my beautiful holiday home.

How Do I Feel?

Because of Covid-19 restrictions, I was not allowed visitors during my hospital stays and had to attend all appointments alone. Although sometimes my brother, and occasionally Emma or Zoe, were allowed in to push my wheelchair, this was not always the case. It was a lonely journey and I had no choice but to put my big girl pants on and be strong. I hate that term with a passion; as if any cancer patient chooses to be strong. I know that it is often said in a well-meaning way, and I always take it in the way it is meant, but I don't see myself as stronger than anyone else, I have just found myself in an unfortunate life situation that I have to deal with.

There is a real dichotomy to be had. I am getting fitter and stronger and getting someway back to being my old self. This is what people see. I am getting better, aren't I? No, I am not getting better. Without some miracle, I will never be better. Well, strictly speaking, I will never be cured, though I have to concede that I am much better than I was this time last year. I guess it depends on how you interpret the word 'better.' The can-

cer that lives inside me will always be there. There is no cure. It's what is termed 'treatable but not curable.' Treatable means that I can live with it whilst the treatment works, until cancer decides to pick up its legs and run.

This is a hard concept to grasp, and one that I am still struggling with. It is almost 5 years since my primary diagnosis and just over 1 year since my secondary diagnosis. I am grateful for the treatment and care that I've had that has enabled me to carry on living, but I would dearly like many more years. Some people live for years with secondary cancer, others don't. It's a life of uncertainty, but then, isn't that what life is? Is anybody certain of tomorrow or the day after? I try to think this way when people ask what I have told the children. I feel like asking them what they have told theirs. Have they broached the subject of dying? Because none of us are getting out of here alive. That might sound harsh, but I do struggle with other people's opinions of my illness. There is so much stigma and negative statistics (which are largely outdated), that it is difficult not to be negative some days. It's still the first thing that I think about when I wake up in the morning. The best way to deal with it is to get out of bed and get on with the day; this is often easier than it sounds. Putting one foot in front of the other and getting a few jobs done is very grounding. However, sometimes going to the supermarket is more than I can face.

Having children to look after helps. They give me purpose. They also give me joy and love, which is better than anything else I have known in my life. The cliched term 'making memories' is something that we've always done, sharing precious times, escaping to Anglesey for a short break or getting on a plane to somewhere warm, sitting in the hot tub at home or simply sitting round the table for a Sunday roast. But, now I hate that term, 'making memories.' It makes it sounds so forced, like we are doing something one last time so that we can take a few photos to remind ourselves what we used to have. I much prefer not to label things and just get on with life.

I feel a lot of anxiety and guilt. What will happen if my life is cut short? What upset will it cause to my children and all my family? Of course, this is out of my hands, but those thoughts are always there at the corners of my mind, and on a bad day, they can be all consuming. I do fear dying, although, having been close a few times, I don't think it is the final breath that scares me, more the fear of knowing beforehand, the preempting of it. It's more the fear of not living, of having to face my own mortality. Of course, we all have to face this, so in some ways, it is no different for me. My thoughts are just heightened to the fact because of my condition and that it is likely to be sooner than I had planned. Normally this wouldn't be a consideration numerous times a day.

Support for Breast Cancer

Kris Hallenga was diagnosed with Stage 4 breast cancer in 2009, at the age of 23. Along with her twin sister, Maren, she founded the charity CoppaFeel! with the intention of educating young people and encouraging them to examine their breasts in the hope of detecting cancers at an earlier stage. Some links to CoppaFeel!:

- www.coppafeel.org
- www.facebook.com/coppafeel.org
- www.twitter.com/CoppaFeelPeople
- www.instagram.com/coppafeel

Stage 4 Deserves More (S4DM) is run by Gemma Ellis. Gemma was diagnosed with stage 4 breast cancer in 2017. She is 38 and married with two daughters, Ruby aged 11 and Scarlett aged 9. Gemma founded S4M as a non-profit organisation and is assisted in its running by Ruby and Scarlett. Money raised goes towards providing support packs and a weekly raffle to members of the support group. Gemma is a strong advocate for research into treatment for women who have stage 4 breast cancer, and has been able to raise money through S4DM to help fund research projects at The Christie Hospital in Manchester.

- The link to S4DM charity page is:
- www.stage4deservesmore.com
- The link to the S4DM support group is:
- www.facebook.com/stage4deservesmore/
- Support packs can be requested:

- stage4desevesmore@yahoo.com
- I personally have had the most amazing support from my local Hospice, Blythe House
- https://blythehousehospice.org.uk/our-services/

Sadly, there is still a lot of stigma around hospices, and initially, I refused to go. I was almost dragged by a couple of friends, who told me what an amazing place Blythe House was. Of course, I didn't believe it until I went for the first time and accessed the Living Well Services. I was able to join support groups, take complementary therapies, counselling and physiotherapy to name but a few of the resources available. I learnt mindfulness and meditation which aired such skills to have in your toolbox for times of anxiety and stress. It wasn't a place for the dying but a place for people with life limiting illnesses, like mine, to learn how to live well. I have made so many friends over the years through attending the hospice and of all the therapies I've had, nothing measures up to the peer support of someone riding a similar storm. Living Well services are available at hospices throughout the UK, and I have become a really firm advocate for the support that they give to patients and their families.

Similarly, Maggie's Centres offer support to anyone who has been affected by cancer. Maggie Keswick Jencks was diagnosed with breast cancer when she was 47. After experiencing waits in dull hospital corridors, she decided to design a blueprint for cancer care centres. Having sat in waiting rooms and clinic rooms myself, I can totally relate to negative impact this can have.

Maggie had a passion for gardens and designed the centres so that they were open and light and had access to beautiful gardens. My local centre was in Didsbury, just across the road from The Christie Hospital. It was a place of peace and tranquillity and I used to drop in after appointments for the occasional green tea and to sit in the gardens and gain my composure before driving home. It was also a great place to go for advice or for one of the complementary sessions that were on offer. I attended a 'Look Good Feel Better' session there and learnt how to apply makeup to compensate for lost eyebrows and lashes. I went away with a makeup bag full of amazing products.

- https://www.maggies.org
- https://www.facebook.com/maggiescentres/

After Breast Cancer Diagnosis has been set up by Jo Taylor to support primary and secondary breast cancer patients to make informed choices. Jo's aim was to reduce some of the fear, anxiety and isolation felt by people who had received a breast cancer diagnosis.

- https://www.abcdiagnosis.co.uk/

Jo has also set up a website which is focused to Secondary breast cancer. METUPUK is an advocacy group whose aim is to turn secondary breast cancer into a chronic disease.

- https://metupuk.org.uk/

Appendix

Test your learning and check your understanding of this book's contents: use the "Springer Nature Flashcards" app to access questions using https://sn.pub/dcAnWL.

To use the app, please follow the instructions in Chap. 1.

Flashcard code: 48341-69945-ABCB1-2A8C7-CE9D2.

Short URL: https://sn.pub/dcAnWL.

Psychological Considerations When Attending for Mammography Screening

12

Anne Pearson and Ashley Weinberg

Learning Objectives

- Highlight relevant psychological barriers and facilitators to the uptake of mammography screening
- Raise awareness of behavioural models relevant to screening
- Demonstrate the importance of a sense of agency for those within the screening process and afterwards

Recent Context

Breast cancer is the most common cancer in adult women in the UK [1], with 85% survival 5 years after diagnosis [2], a figure that has doubled over the last 50 years [1, 2]. This figure rises to almost 100% where cases are caught early, indicating clearly that screening can help reduce breast cancer mortality [1]. So why, over the last 10 years, have decreasing proportions (e.g. 74.2% of those aged 53–70 [3]) accepted an invitation for a routine mammogram which may ultimately help to save their lives? This chapter considers a range of psychological considerations and, in light of the Covid-19 pandemic [4], explores issues further

complicating the uptake of breast cancer screening, which in the UK saves 1300 lives each year, equating to 1 in 200 people screened [5, 6].

Statistics are both alluring and perplexing which can make for challenges in understanding healthcare trends. By 2019–2020, breast screening by proportion had declined to 69.1% of six million aged 50–71 in England eligible for a mammogram—and 74.2% of those aged 53–70—from previous highs of around 77% in 2010–2011 [6–8]. Notwithstanding that the inclusion of those in their early 50s appears to influence invitation and recording rates, it seems that geographical as well as operational factors play a role in uptake, which in turn points to the influence of individualised as well as community-related features. Furthermore, the same NHS information provided to those invited for screening makes clear that for each life saved, 3 further women will be found to have a non-life threatening growth for which 'they are offered treatment they did not need'. 1 in 25 women are called back for further screening after initial assessment and of these, 3 in 4 are subsequently given the 'all-clear'. The NHS (2021) [6–8] not only acknowledges the worry caused to those recalled, but also the lack of ability to distinguish between those in danger or not. This underlines concern about additional anxieties surrounding screening, which in the context of Covid-19, was compounded for those who, due to receipt of the vaccine, reported swollen glands in their armpit or neck.

A. Pearson · A. Weinberg (✉)
Directorate of Psychology, School of Health and Society, University of Salford, Manchester, UK
e-mail: a.pearson1@salford.ac.uk; a.weinberg@salford.ac.uk

What Can Psychology Offer?

Psychological models attempt to explain the perceptions and beliefs underlying the decision to attend screening. Research-led efforts to turn these models into predictors of attendance behaviour have met with varying levels of success [9, 10], suggesting that theory is relevant, more so when including additional considerations linked to the following: demographic and socioeconomic factors, external events which cue thoughts about mammography screening, as well as individual differences in psychological attributes and habitual behaviours. In addition, research has highlighted the importance of considering reasons used by those to inform their decisions to avoid, as well as attend for, mammography screening. For example, a Norwegian study found increased capacity for predicting attendance when the following are considered: perceptions of personal risk of having cancer, believing mammography would be beneficial, increased fear and breast-checking behaviour, past attendance and levels of educational attainment [11].

With knowledge of working in a location and its particular mix of client groups, the practitioner is well placed to assess which factors are influential in this process, as geographical variation in uptake of screening would suggest [12]. Whilst no single approach will suit all potential attendees, it is hoped that awareness of a range of factors, such as those discussed in this section, will encourage or confirm practitioners' efforts in understanding what lies behind an individual's decision to attend for a mammogram.

In reviewing the psychological contributors to a decision to attend for screening or not, policy makers are also keen to broaden the focus from 'health-seeking behaviour' to understanding better how we engage with healthcare systems [13]. Adopting this perspective permits a focus not only on individual characteristics, but also on how services interact with those individuals.

The Health Beliefs Model [14] has proved one of the more popular frameworks [15] in aiding understanding of how we assess the threat posed by a specific cause of illness and the use of such

models appears to underpin more successful health education interventions [16]. The COM-B Model has also gained pace in helping explain successful engagement in healthcare, including screening, located within a Behaviour Change Wheel which can act as a vehicle for suggesting potential interventions and guiding implementation [17].

The Health Beliefs Model considers our own susceptibility and perceptions of the severity of a potential health problem—calculations about which may be prompted by a cue, such as the arrival of an invitation for an appointment or seeing an awareness raising advertisement. From this starting point, the model suggests we balance the benefits and barriers provided by the prospect of preventative action. For mammography this means that women are unlikely to come forward when perceiving there is little chance of developing breast cancer but are more likely to attend for screening if there is knowledge about highly increased mortality if the cancer remains undetected [18]. Considerable efforts have been made to raise public awareness of breast cancer in recent years, particularly in the UK, resulting in increased availability of information about both of these aspects of threat [19]. However, the psychological impact of information concerning breast cancer and screening has also been more carefully considered amid calls for even more effective ways in which to understand individual uptake of screening [20].

Perceptions of Risk and Pain

The nature of mammography means that a decision about its personal relevance relies on a combination of physical and psychological considerations. As if to complicate matters, both of these sets of factors are subject to variations in individual perception. Of these, the perception of risk of cancer is viewed as a significant predictor of attendance for screening.

Studies of this individual calculation show wide variation. For example, in a study of women where almost half had first-degree family history and were considered by the researchers to have a

70.6% risk of developing breast cancer, only 24% of women perceived themselves as at high risk [21]. This pattern of inaccurate risk assessment by a majority of those with raised risk is not new [22] or confined to the UK, e.g. two-thirds of women at high risk also underestimated risk in a Turkish study [23].

It is also important to consider the potential role of intersectionality, where multiple factors, such as age and ethnicity, can influence perception of risk. A US study [24] involving White, Black and Hispanic women found lower perceived absolute risk among Black women, although this did not translate into differential uptake of mammography screening. However, in the same study, perceptions of increased risk, as well as more frequent reports of worry about breast cancer, were positively associated with having a mammogram or indeed uptake of one on consecutive occasions; conversely, the effect was reversed among women with decreased perceptions of risk and worry. Orom et al. [25] have previously reported lower perceived risk among ethnic minorities and highlighted factors including the relevance of public health messaging, competing risks, salience of cancer, as well as attributions of risk.

In 2012, the UK's Independent Breast Screening Review Panel [26] indicated a number of policy recommendations to the NHS Breast Screening Programme, one of which concerned the communication of risk and the benefits of routine mammograms. It is important that 'clear communication of the harms and benefits of screening to women is essential. It is at the core of how a modern health system should function' [27]. However, it is also essential to consider the potentially differential impact of this information on the target audience. For example, it may be that as the risks or harms are more effectively communicated, women who already overestimate their risk may tend to utilise this information in a different way from women who do not, with a potential impact on the rate of acceptance of an invitation to attend for routine mammograms. More recent scrutiny in 2019, by the Independent Review of Adult Screening Programmes in England, has also underlined the importance of the practicalities of engaging with service users, as well as the types of message:

> Service organisation has not kept pace with people's expectations for convenience in booking appointments and some groups within society are particularly poorly served [28].

Accordingly, studies in the UK [29] and Germany [30] have highlighted the positive impact of style of presentation of information about colorectal screening; they found that risk information and screening uptake were most effective when presented in a traditional format, offering simple advice and straightforward procedures. Conversely, if risk information was presented as evidence-based information that considered specific criteria, it was more likely to lead to some rationalisation of inaction, i.e. people tended to devalue this information, minimise their perceived risk, and use this as a reason for non-attendance [30]. Perceived risk of breast cancer has been found to predict avoidance of screening too. In Norway—which at 76% has a slightly higher uptake than the UK—a study has revealed how reduced perception of risk, raised fears about cancer and less favourable attitudes to the personal benefit of having a mammogram feed into defensive avoidance of having a mammogram [11].

Anecdotal themes of embarrassment, discomfort and pain [31, 32] indicate that for a significant proportion of women the process itself is physically challenging, in a manner which may well be separate from any consideration about perceptions of the potential benefit of having a mammogram. Certainly, professionals carrying out the screening will do their best to mentally prepare the individual and qualm any concerns, so it is not surprising that attendees are generally positive about the staff working in this field—it has even been noted that satisfaction with the practitioner can actually help to reduce reports of pain and embarrassment [33]. Studies investigating the potentially mitigating effect of a routine painkiller also show beneficial impact [32]. However, and as discussed in the following Chap. 13, the potential for advanced information about the procedure [34] as well as for effective interpersonal skills on the part of the practitioner to impact positively on the experience of having a mammogram is clear: indeed, there are grounds for extending routine professional empathic understanding to training in maintaining this approach when faced with challenging responses from clients [35].

Naturally anyone experiencing serious discomfort or pain is likely to remember that feeling and hold that association with the experience of having a mammogram. It has been suggested that enhancing the levels of control clients have over the mammography procedure could further assist in countering discomfort [36]. Clearly advances in practice are required to minimise the expectation and/or perception of pain or discomfort in the process of deciding whether or not to attend or re-attend; Chap. 16 will discuss this in further detail.

From the Health Beliefs Model to COM-B

The Health Beliefs Model also highlights the cost-benefit analysis made by an individual which determines their next step after assessing their personal risk. For a positive decision to attend screening, it has been suggested that the benefits of the behaviour should outweigh the potential barriers to taking action. For example, this requires confidence in the ability of the mammogram to detect cancer, although painful or otherwise off-putting experiences can over-ride this potential benefit [18].

The Theory of Planned Behaviour [37] goes further to consider judgements of what is the prevalent social expectation when deciding whether to attend or not—in other words do family members, friends and colleagues go for screening? However, there are limitations in the ability of either approach to predict behaviour. For example, studies conducted in different ethnic groups have pointed to the usefulness of the Health Beliefs Model, but additionally suggest the role of culturally distinct factors in determining attendance for mammography [38–40].

It is important to consider that mammography is one of three ways in which the public are encouraged to take preventative action with regard to breast cancer, along with self-examination and a clinical consultation with their doctor if a sign or symptom is noted. Comparisons of perceptions in relation to all three techniques suggest fewer ethnic-group differences in perceived threat or barriers associated with each, but instead differences in the perceptions of the benefits of mammography, along with varying scores for self-efficacy and health motivation [41].

Individual differences due to enduring personal characteristics, such as self-efficacy, have received increasing attention as key factors predicting compliance with health-related behaviours. For example, previous research has documented that uptake by those in some groups may be negatively influenced by such factors as lack of knowledge, language barriers, reduced access to medical services, and unhelpful attitudes of health professionals [42]. However, the role of social support, including a close friendship, supportive relationships with family, or membership of a group (e.g. as a volunteer) can positively predict attendance for a mammogram, whereas isolation from peers—such as indicated by living alone or with children only—or through absence of social participation, significantly increases the likelihood of non-attendance [43].

Accordingly, as part of an overarching approach, the COM-B Model [44] encourages a focus on interacting factors that predict the behaviour (**B**) in question (i.e. attendance for screening), recognising that the individual would need to be physically and psychologically capable (**C**) of taking up the opportunity (**O**) as the environment permits, and that their **m**otivation (**M**) inclines them towards (or away from) screening, based on their knowledge, understanding, emotions and habits.

This combination of features suggests that focusing exclusively on perceptions of risk could omit factors that make vital contributions to uptake of screening. These include the capacity to organise one's own attendance at the appointment, confidence in one's self-efficacy to go through with it, juggling competing demands on one's time and related resources (often financial) and other self-limiting factors [20]. For example, those who reported more confidence about attending for a mammogram were also more likely to declare their intent to accept a screening invitation in the following 2 years [11]. Triggers from the wider social environment shape the opportunity to attend based on what others— from national media to people we know—are doing, recommending and endorsing. Those who believe screening helps reduce the threat of breast cancer and thereby induces feeling safe, are also more likely to show intent to attend [11]. These triggers can extend to physical facilitators of attendance, including invitations, convenience, incentives and guidance through the process [20].

It is therefore instructive that a recent review has highlighted not only the gradual decline in uptake—in the UK and elsewhere—but also underlined the need to update how screening services communicate with those who are eligible for a mammogram: Based on an assessment of interventions, Richards [28] points to more effective use of social media and text message reminders. For example, this includes nationally integrated information technology systems so that medical records follow patients and provision of incentives directly to services, so they offer opportunities for screening out of hours and therefore at more times convenient for potential attendees.

Taken together these approaches highlight the importance of individual perceptions of factors beyond the person's control, making the prospect of having a mammogram—and a preventative approach to ill health generally—easier or harder to follow through. From a positive perspective, efforts to combat weak control beliefs through encouraging those to plan to attend have yielded positive results by increasing attendance for mammography. For example, those who were required to plan their attendance—having previously tended to report reduced confidence in their capacity to overcome difficulties in attending— found the act of planning helped them to problem solve in a way that may have influenced their motivation to take up the screening invitation [45]. Such a focus on implementation intentions,

i.e. helping to link planning and then acting, holds particular promise for those who have intentions to attend but see difficulties in doing so [45].

Joffe [46] points out that 'people are motivated to represent the risks which they face in a way which protects them, and the groups with which they identify, from threat' (p. 10). Consistent with this, it is more likely that women consider mammograms in a manner which strengthens their ability to build psychological defences. This is clearly a phenomenon shared by anyone rationalising a particular course of action and can mean changing one's beliefs (e.g. It is a good idea to attend for a mammogram) to justify one's behaviour (e.g. I did not attend my mammogram appointment), so that one believes differently (e.g. my friends tend not to go for a mammogram and they're fine, so I will be fine too).

This example of cognitive dissonance illustrates how the logic of decision making about attending for a mammogram can be altered. It also highlights the potential risks of relying on theoretical approaches that assume decisions are based on a controlled process free from the influence of negative emotions and from beliefs which disagree with the health promotion literature [47]. It has also been recognised that recent experiences of stress outside of work increase the chances of not attending for a mammogram [43], however, previous research has suggested that psychosocial factors such as fear and fatalism can also negatively influence whether a woman accepts an invitation to attend for routine screening [48]. Chapter 13 expands upon this area.

The Role of Negative Psychological Factors and Practical Barriers

Fear and anxiety can be effective barriers to screening as they have the effect of impairing both judgement and behaviour. Worrying about the possibility of having breast cancer, and agonising over its possible detection by screening, can lead to a decision not to attend for screening [5, 49]. This is further covered within Chap. 13.

This may seem counter-intuitive, but defensive avoidance is the psychological mechanism of rationalising why the individual is not attending for screening by taking steps to reduce their anxiety [11]. Similarly, this cognitive process can also reduce the likelihood of self-examination [50]. Avoidance as a strategy for dealing with fear is readily understandable, but can foster potentially unhelpful psychological defences in a number of ways.

> Cancer fatalism represents a surrender of the human spirit to perceptions of hopelessness, powerlessness, worthlessness and social despair [51] (p. 135).

Those who fear they may have breast cancer and who adopt this way of thinking could view screening as pointless, i.e. the cancer was 'meant' to happen anyway and there is nothing to be done about it, or indeed that if mammography can detect it, then it is already too late. While lower health literacy is linked to lower rates of seeking information about cancer, the belief held by a proportion of people that 'not much can be done to lower chances of getting it' is also a key predictor [52]. Previously attending for a mammogram appears to reduce this type of thinking [53]. This sense of helplessness in contemplating mammography may have echoes in a variety of belief systems, however this does not mean cancer fatalism is limited to certain sections of the population; indeed, it is widespread in many countries [54] and not always in consistent patterns [55].

A potentially surprising finding is that perceptions of low risk can also be associated with defensive avoidance [11]. However, the researchers suggest that this may not necessarily be linked to fear, but to simply perceiving mammography as not relevant to their circumstance. Here, the practice of other health awareness strategies, such as self-examination, may be perceived as protective against cancer. However, the finding that only 60% of those receiving their first invitation for screening actually attend—compared with 86.3% of women who have been screened in the previous 5 years [28]—underlines the possibility that interventions promoting habit-forming

behaviour could yield benefits. Indeed, this figure for first-time attendees had dropped from 68% over a 10-year period [28]. It remains to be seen how the suspension of routine health services during the heights of the pandemic has impacted on numbers of women able to take up the first offer of mammography screening, however if habit-formation is an important factor, then extra efforts may be required to encourage their attendance.

It is perhaps unsurprising that women may experience initial alarm at being invited for screening. It has been argued that this can itself facilitate uptake of a mammogram, unless such levels of anxiety are provoked as to lead an individual to avoid screening for reasons previously discussed [36]. Practical solutions such as increasing regularity of contact with prospective attendees—for example by pre-screening invitations and personalised contact—mean that as well as raising awareness of the screening programme, women can become more habituated to the idea that at some point a screening appointment will be offered [56]. This in-person approach has been extended to effective promotion of screening among religious minorities [57] and indeed the importance of spirituality is already recognised in treatment processes [58].

Community-based communications about mammography can also help address concerns about the perception of screening as a challenge to a female modesty [59] by ensuring accurate information is conveyed in advance of attendance for screening [60]. Similarly, ensuring that information sent out by the UK health service is readily understandable, written in plain language with clear explanations of the terminology, while signposting translation and interpretation services, has reduced potential barriers to screening uptake for women from minoritised groups; previously information circulated in English has risked being ignored and therefore inequalities in access to healthcare deepened [60]. Improving a sense of agency for women of all backgrounds so we can access information about screening without recourse to others, for example for translation or interpretation by family members, is seen as vital.

While the emotional impact of having a mammogram, at least in the short-term, is often palpable, it is also important to highlight the potentially negative psychological effect of being recalled for a further mammogram [28, 61]. During 2020–2021, 7.3% of women who had attended for first time screening were recalled for assessment from the 1.84 million invited [62]. The query triggering recall is satisfied in around 80% of cases and an all-clear result issued [63]. However, stress is caused by receipt of a recall invitation and 40% of those categorised as false-positive cases report extreme anxiety [64], as well as feeling shocked and disempowered as they become 'passive participants' in the next stage of the screening process [61].

In a Norwegian study this increased anxiety state was found to be transient, such that 4 weeks after screening, levels matched those of the general population and initial increases in depressive symptoms had declined. Despite the psychological impact of being recalled, this Norwegian study found 98% of all women stated they would re-attend [65]. Not surprisingly, for women who were diagnosed with cancer, both anxiety and depression levels exceeded the population norms [65].

A major review of the impact of being recalled on psychological well-being found an increase in generalised anxiety together with significant increases in breast cancer specific anxiety, depression, fear and distress [66]. It has been noted that such specific effects may be experienced by women classed as false-positives up to 3 years later [63], which is the point of usual recall in the UK screening programme. The experience of having a false positive result may impact on subsequent attendance with a US study showing average delays of up to 10 months in responding to a subsequent screening invitation [67]. In the UK, double-reading of results has reduced the need for such recalls, where in excess of 90% of such instances women are offered a repeat mammogram within 3 weeks [28].

Qualitative studies of women using UK services highlighted the importance of ensuring recall invitations include the reason for the repeat, as well as practical information and steps that can help address negative emotions and improve a sense of control in an otherwise uncertain environment, e.g. what tests will be done and by whom, who can accompany them, as well as providing a clinical nurse specialist to answer questions before and after the assessment [61, 63]. 'It would be helpful for screening units to be better prepared to deal with the significant distress and uncertainty felt by women' [63] (p. 356) and this could also extend to consideration of the clinic layout so that anxieties experienced by some are less likely to be communicated to others attending. This is further discussed in Chap. 13.

Conclusions

The range of relevant psychological factors in attendance and non-attendance for mammography is broad: beliefs about breast cancer, self-perceptions of control and self-efficacy, social support systems, demography, communications from the mammography service, past physical and/or psychological experience of screening, as well as challenging emotions and symptoms of psychological ill-health. It is likely that psychological models will continue to adapt to take these into account, but the role of the practitioner in knowing their local population and considering which factors may affect them is paramount. In addition, the role of service-related issues—including access and timing of provision as well as user-friendly communications—deserves scrutiny as these can materially impact on how successfully women engage with the offer of breast screening.

Given the influential role that a negative experience can play in future attendance and the identified importance of ensuring a sense of control for clients in their involvement in screening, attention to the psychological aspects of the process warrants careful consideration. With this in mind, the UK's National Institute for Health Research recommends:

> Clear, carefully worded information about the reason for the assessment and process of the assessment (but not in such detail that they become distressed without the support of the screening staff being present), [63].

In response to independent reviews of breast cancer screening [28], there is a growing emphasis on developing 'patient invitation support materials…[to] better support them as they make an informed choice about screening' [26] (p. 5). Marmot et al. [5] have been careful to summarise the impact of screening as follows:

If she chooses to be screened, it should be in the knowledge that she is accepting the chance of benefit, having her life extended, knowing that there is also a risk of overdiagnosis and unnecessary treatment. Similarly, a woman who declines the invitation to screening needs to recognise that she runs a slightly higher risk of dying from breast cancer.

Clinical Pearls

- People are more likely to attend for screening if there is knowledge about highly increased mortality if the cancer remains undetected
- Those who already overestimate their risk may tend to utilise this information in a different way from women who do not
- Defensive avoidance of screening may be an individual's strategy for managing anxiety rather than evidence of disengagement from screening
- Community-based communications about mammography help address concerns about the perception of screening, while provision of translated materials can engender a sense of agency for those of all backgrounds, e.g. bypassing the need for recourse to others to discuss their invitation for a mammogram
- Those who are recalled for follow-up are more likely to be anxious and will benefit from information and support that improves their sense of control in an otherwise uncertain environment, e.g. what tests will be done and by whom, who can accompany, as well as providing a clinical nurse specialist to answer questions before and after the assessment

---

Chapter Review Questions
Review Questions

1. How might psychological considerations impact on the decision to attend mammography screening?
2. What progress has been made by relevant psychological models in advancing understanding of the decision to attend for screening?
3. What can be done to ensure better 'reach' of screening services to those who may otherwise miss out?

Answers

1. It is important to consider a range of factors that influence perceptions of screening. These include, but are not limited to, understanding of the potential risks for the individual as well as associated anxieties they may experience. Perceptions of the relevance of screening are also important in deciding to accept the invitation to attend for screening and it is useful to consider the sources of information women are accessing. Clearly advance communications from the health service are essential and need to consider not only best practice but offer interactions with healthcare professionals where possible. The role of defensive avoidance in negative decisions about attendance should be probed rather than underestimated.
2. The COM-B Model has joined the Health Beliefs Model as a popular driver for understanding contributory factors around healthcare behaviours. Accordingly, relevant theory emphasises capacity, opportunities, and motivations in shaping behaviours linked to uptake of screening. For example, enhancing capacity for individuals to plan their attendance by improving access times as well as locations and ease of booking plays a key role. This links to the key determinant of self-efficacy, whereby individuals feel able to exert control over their own health, not only by being better able to make informed decisions, but also in taking steps to attend. Their experience on attending is naturally important and so healthcare provision that eases physical discomfort

and provides necessary reassurance and advice is vital. The role of both barriers and facilitators is acknowledged in the latest models.

3. The role of a sense of control is vital in determining the decision to attend for screening. Practical barriers that may impede uptake can easily detract from individual agency. For example, invitations and information written in English that require the individual to seek help with translating and understanding may mean postponing or simply never raising the call to attend. Equally, taking steps to make it more possible to attend can be wide-ranging. For example, increasing reliance on electronic communications, means that text messaging can ensure improved reach, while equally, the opportunity to meet and discuss concerns about attending for screening with other women, in the presence of a community-based healthcare professional, can help bolster much-needed social support around this issue.

Appendix

Test your learning and check your understanding of this book's contents: use the "Springer Nature Flashcards" app to access questions using https://sn.pub/dcAnWL.

To use the app, please follow the instructions in Chap. 1.

Flashcard code: 48341-69945-ABCB1-2A8C7-CE9D2.

Short URL: https://sn.pub/dcAnWL.

References

1. Office for National Statistics. Cancer registration statistics, 2017. https://www.ons.gov.uk/peoplepopulationandcommunity/healthandsocialcare/conditionsanddiseases/bulletins/cancerregistrationstatisticsengland/2017#the-three-most-common-cancers-vary-by-sex-and-age-group. Accessed 26 Feb 2022.
2. Office for National Statistics, Cancer survival in England - adults diagnosed 2019. Accessed at: https://www.ons.gov.uk/peoplepopulationandcommunity/healthandsocialcare/conditionsanddiseases/datasets/cancersurvivalratescancersurvivalinenglandadultsdiagnosed.
3. NHS Digital. Breast screening program 2019–20: England. https://files.digital.nhs.uk/F9/98C8E3/breast-screening-programme-eng-2019-20-report.pdf. Accessed 26 Feb 2022.
4. Breast Cancer Now. Almost one million women in UK miss vital breast screening due to COVID-19. https://breastcancernow.org/about-us/media/press-releases/almost-one-million-women-in-uk-miss-vital-breast-screening-due-covid-19. Accessed 26 Feb 2022.
5. Marmot MG, Altman DG, Cameron DA, Dewar JA, Thompson SG, Wilcox M. The benefits and harms of breast cancer screening: an independent review. Br J Cancer. 2013;108(11):2205–40.
6. NHS. Breast cancer screening: benefits and risks. https://www.nhs.uk/conditions/breast-cancer-screening/why-its-offered/. Accessed 26 Feb 2022.
7. NHS. Breast screening program 2019–20: England. https://files.digital.nhs.uk/F9/98C8E3/breast-screening-programme-eng-2019-20-report.pdf. Accessed 26 Feb 2022.
8. NHS. Coronavirus (COVID-19) updates to breast screening. https://www.nhs.uk/conditions/breast-screening-mammogram/coronavirus-covid-19-updates/. Accessed 26 Feb 2022.
9. Carpenter CJ. A meta-analysis of the effectiveness of health belief model variables in predicting behaviour. Health Commun. 2010;25(8):661–9.
10. Lawal O, Murphy F, Hogg P, Nightingale J. Health behavioural theories and their application to women's participation in mammography screening. J Med Imaging Radiat Sci. 2017;48(2):122–7.
11. Ivanova A, Kvalem IL. Psychological predictors of intention and avoidance of attending organized mammography screening in Norway: applying the extended parallel process model. BMC Womens Health. 2021 Dec;21(1):1–4.
12. Nuffield. Cancer screening—quality watch. https://www.nuffieldtrust.org.uk/resource/breast-and-cervical-cancer-screening. Accessed 26 Feb 2022.
13. MacKian S. A review of health seeking behaviour: problems and prospects, HSD/WP/05/03. https://assets.publishing.service.gov.uk/media/57a08d1de5274a27b200163d/05-03_health_seeking_behaviour.pdf. Accessed 26 Feb 2022.
14. Rosenstock IM. Why people use health services. Milbank Mem Fund Q. 1966;44:94–127.
15. Chin JH, Mansori S. Theory of planned behaviour and health belief model: females' intention on breast cancer screening. Cogent Psychol. 2019;6(1):1647927.
16. Naz MSG, Simbar M, Fakari FR, Ghasemi V. Effects of model-based interventions on breast cancer screening behavior of women: a systematic review. Asian Pac J Cancer Prev. 2018;19(8):2031–41.
17. Jatau AI, Peterson GM, Bereznicki L, Dwan C, Black JA, Bezabhe WM, Wimmer BC. Applying the capability, opportunity, and motivation behaviour model

(COM-B) to guide the development of interventions to improve early detection of atrial fibrillation. Clin Med Insights Cardiol. 2019;13:1179546819885134.

18. Hyman RB, Baker S, Ephraim R, Moadel A, Philip J. Health beliefs model variables as predictors of screening mammography utilisation. J Behav Med. 1994;17(4):391–406.

19. Breast Cancer Now. Facts and Statistics 2021. https://breastcancernow.org/about-us/media/facts-statistics. Accessed 26 Feb 2022.

20. Robb KA. The integrated screening action model (I-SAM): a theory-based approach to inform intervention development. Prev Med Rep. 2021;1(23):101427.

21. Rainey L, Jervaeus A, Donnelly LS, Evans DG, Hammarström M, Hall P, Wengström Y, Broeders MJM, van der Waal D. Women's perceptions of personalized risk-based breast cancer screening and prevention: an international focus group study. Psychooncology. 2019;28(5):1056–62.

22. Haas JS, Kaplan CP, Des Jarlais G, Gildengoin V, Pérez-Stable EJ, Kerlikowske K. Perceived risk of breast cancer among women at average and increased risk. J Womens Health. 2005;14(9):845–51.

23. Kartal M, Ozcakar N, Hatipoglu S, Tan MN, Guldal AD. Breast cancer risk perceptions of Turkish women attending primary care: a cross-sectional study. BMC Womens Health. 2014;14(1):1–8.

24. Orom H, Kiviniemi MT, Shavers VL, Ross L, Underwood W. Perceived risk for breast cancer and its relationship to mammography in blacks, hispanics, and whites. J Behav Med. 2013;36(5):466–76.

25. Orom H, Kiviniemi MT, Underwood W, Ross L, Shavers VL. Perceived cancer risk: why is it lower among nonwhites than whites? Cancer Epidemiol Biomarkers Prev. 2010 Mar;19(3):746–54.

26. NHS. NHS breast screening programme: annual review. Sheffield: NHS; 2012.

27. Cameron D. Reviewing the evidence for breast screening, NHS breast screening programme annual review. Sheffield: NHS; 2012.

28. Richards M. Report of the Independent Review of Adult Screening Programmes in England. https://www.england.nhs.uk/wpcontent/uploads/2019/02/report-of-the-independent-review-of-adult-screening-programme-in-england.pdf. Accessed 26 Feb 2022.

29. Robb K, O'Carroll R. Simpler is better—the case of colorectal cancer screening. https://blogs.bmj.com/bmj/2019/10/11/simpler-is-better-the-case-of-colorectal-cancer-screening/. Accessed 26 Feb 2022.

30. Steckelberg A, Kasper J, Redegeld M, Muhlhauser I. Risk information—barrier to informed choice? A focus group study. Soz Preventivmed. 2004;49(6):375–80.

31. Keefe RJ, Hauck ER, Egert J, Rimer B, Kornguth P. Mammography pain and discomfort: a cognitive behavioural perspective. Pain. 1994;56:247–60.

32. Freitas-Junior R, Martins E, Metran-Nascente C, Carvalho AA, Silva MFD, Soares LR, Ximenes CA. Double-blind placebo-controlled randomized clinical trial on the use of paracetamol for per-

forming mammography. Medicine (Baltimore). 2018;97(13):e0261.

33. Hamilton EL, Wallis MG, Barlow J, Cullen L, Wright C. Women's views of a breast cancer service. Health Care Women Int. 2003;24:40–8.

34. Miller D, Livingstone V, Herbison GP. Interventions for relieving the pain and discomfort of screening mammography. Cochrane Database Syst Rev. 2008;(1):CD002942.

35. Whelehan P, Evans A. Client and practitioner perspectives on the screening mammography experience. Eur J Cancer Care. 2017;26(3):e12580.

36. Marks DF, Murray M, Evans B, Willig C, Woodall C, Sykes CM. Health psychology: theory, research and practice. 2nd ed. London: Sage; 2005.

37. Ajzen I. From intention to actions: a theory of planned behaviour. In: Kuhl J, Beckmann J, editors. Action-control: from cognition to behaviour. Heidelberg: Springer; 1985. p. 11–39.

38. Wu TY, West B, Chen YW, Hergert C. Health beliefs and practices related to breast cancer screening in Philippino, Chinese and Asian-Indian women. Cancer Detect Prev. 2006;30(1):58–66.

39. Vadaparampil ST, Champion VL, Miller TK, Menon U, Sugg-Skinner C. Using the health belief model to examine differences in adherence to mammography among African-American and Caucasian women. J Psychosoc Oncol. 2005;21(4):59–79.

40. Consedine NS, Magai C, Horton D, Neugut AI, Gillespie M. Health belief model factors in mammography screening: testing for interactions among subpopulations of Caribbean women. Ethn Dis. 2005;15(3):444–52.

41. Hajian-Tilaki K, Auladi S. Health belief model and practice of breast self-examination and breast cancer screening in Iranian women. Breast Cancer. 2012;21(4):429–34.

42. Thomas VN, Saleem T, Abraham R. Barriers to effective uptake of cancer screening among black and minority ethnic groups. Int J Palliat Nurs. 2005;11(11):562–71.

43. Lagerlund M, Sontrop JM, Zachrisson S. Psychosocial factors and attendance at a population-based mammography screening program in a cohort of Swedish women. BMC Womens Health. 2014;14(1):1–9.

44. Michie S, Van Stralen MM, West R. The behaviour change wheel: a new method for characterising and designing behaviour change interventions. Implement Sci. 2011;6(1):1–2.

45. Rutter D, Quine L, Steadman L, Thompson S. Increasing attendance at breast cancer screening: Field trial. Final Report to NHSBSP. University of Kent. Department of Psychology. Centre for Research in Health Behaviour; 2007.

46. Joffe H. Risk and the 'other'. New York: Cambridge University Press; 1999.

47. Sarafino EP. Health psychology: biopsychosocial interactions. 4th ed. New York: Wiley; 2002.

48. Talbert PV. The relationship of fear and fatalism with breast cancer screening among a selected target popu-

lation of African American middle class women. J Soc Behav Health Sci. 2008;2(1):96–110.

49. Phillips JM, Cohen MZ, Moses G. Breast cancer screening and African American women: fear fatalism and silence. Oncol Nurs Forum. 1999;26(3):561–71.

50. Rippetoe PA, Rogers RW. Effects of components of protection-motivation theory on adaptive and maladaptive coping with a health threat. J Pers Soc Psychol. 1987;52(3):596–604.

51. Powe BD. Cancer fatalism—spiritual perspectives. J Relig Health. 1997;36(2):135–7.

52. Kobayashi LC, Smith SG. Cancer fatalism, literacy, and cancer information seeking in the American public. Health Educ Behav. 2016;43(4):461–70.

53. Molaei-Zardanjani M, Savabi-Esfahani M, Taleghani F. Fatalism in breast cancer and performing mammography on women with or without a family history of breast cancer. BMC Womens Health. 2019;19(1):1–5.

54. Cohen M. Cancer fatalism: attitudes toward screening and care. In: Carr B, Steel J, editors. Psychological aspects of cancer. Boston: Springer; 2013.

55. Emami L, Ghahramanian A, Rahmani A, Mirza Aghazadeh A, Onyeka TC, Nabighadim A. Beliefs, fear and awareness of women about breast cancer: effects on mammography screening practices. Nurs Open. 2021;8(2):890–9.

56. Zelenyanszki C. Maximising screening attendance: a reference guide. London: NHS: North West London Cancer Network; 2009.

57. British Islamic Medical Association. Cancer screening awareness—importance and impact. https://www.britishima.org/cancer-screening-awareness-importance-and-impact/. Accessed 26 Feb 2022.

58. Swenson WT. Survey of spiritual quality of life among survivorship and distress guidelines. J Clin Oncol. 2016;34(15):e21566.

59. Borrayo EA, Jenkins SR. Feeling indecent: breast cancer screening resistance of Mexican-descent women. J Health Psychol. 2001;6(5):537–49.

60. Woof VG, Ruane H, Ulph F, French DP, Quereshi N, Khan N, Evans DG, Donnelly LS. Engagement barriers and service inequities in the NHS breast screening Programme: views from British-Pakistani women. J Med Screen. 2020;27(3):130–7.

61. Long H, Brooks JM, Harvie M, Maxwell A, French DP. How do women experience a false-positive test result from breast screening? A systematic review and thematic synthesis of qualitative studies. Br J Cancer. 2019;121(4):351–8.

62. NHS Digital. Breast Screening Programme: England 2020–21. https://digital.nhs.uk/data-and-information/publications/statistical/breast-screening-programme/england%2D%2D-2020-21/mainreport6. Accessed 27 Feb 2022.

63. Bond M, Pavey T, Welch K, Cooper C, Garside R, Dean S, Hyde C. Systematic review of the psychological consequences of false-positive screening mammograms. Health Technol Assess. 2013;17(13):1–170.

64. Schwartz LM, Woloshin S, Fowler FJ, Welch HG. Enthusiasm for cancer screening in the United States. JAMA. 2004;291:71–8.

65. Bredal S, Kåresen R, Skaane P, Engelstad KS, Ekeberg Ø. Recall mammography and psychological distress. Eur J Cancer. 2013;49(4):805–11.

66. Salz T, Richman AR, Brewer NT. Meta-analyses of the effect of false-positive mammograms on generic and specific psychosocial outcomes. Psychooncology. 2010;19(10):26–34.

67. Dabbous FM, Dolecek TA, Berbaum ML, Friedewald SM, Summerfelt WT, Hoskins K, Rauscher GH. Impact of a false-positive screening mammogram on subsequent screening behavior and stage at breast cancer diagnosis. Cancer Epidemiol Biomarkers Prev. 2017;26(3):397–403.

Managing Anxiety in Mammography: The Client and the Practitioner

13

Johanna E. Mercer

Learning Objectives

- Identify and understand the common causes of anxiety in clients and demonstrate knowledge to implement solutions for reducing client anxiety
- Identify and understand the common causes of anxiety in practitioners and demonstrate knowledge to implement solutions for reducing practitioner anxiety
- Identify resources to support future continued professional development

Introduction

As mammography practitioners, it is important to be responsible for producing high quality images, provide the best possible care to those attending screening and assessment, and encourage clients to attend regular screenings. It is also essential to promote wellbeing and signpost to support if required [1]. Whilst there are a multitude of other factors that must be considered when practising mammography, having a focus on client wellbeing is imperative as it can influence factors such as how likely clients are to attend and then re-attend appointments [2–4] and the level of discomfort or pain experienced during the procedure [5–7]. It is also interesting to note that client wellbeing impacts the effectiveness of treatments in individuals who are diagnosed [8], as both immune function and natural killer cells (NKCs)—lymphocytes produced by the body which help boost the efficacy of anticancer therapy [9]—have been found to be reduced in anxious individuals [10, 11].

The role that wellbeing plays in practitioners is equally as important. Low wellbeing can weaken individual immune systems, which can lead to days off work due to sickness [12], increasing NHS cost and putting a strain on practitioners who pick up their workload. In addition, poor wellbeing is significantly correlated with decreased patient safety, including the increase of medical errors [13].

One of the main contributors to negative wellbeing is anxiety; an emotion which individuals will experience when they are worried, afraid, or tense [14]. This chapter will explore anxiety in more detail, examining this from two different viewpoints: anxiety in the client and in the practitioner.

J. E. Mercer (✉)
Health in Mind, Halisham, East Sussex, UK
e-mail: Johanna.mercer1@nhs.net

Client Anxiety

It is no surprise that many individuals who attend breast cancer screenings, across the globe, experience anxiety during their examination [5, 15, 16]. Anxiety has been demonstrated to reduce the attendance rate of screenings [2], posing a risk to clients with undetected breast cancer, as this increases the chance of the cancer becoming symptomatic and more challenging to treat [17]. Therefore, it is essential that practitioners are aware of how a client presents with anxiety and ways to support them, helping to reduce their anxiety levels.

What Is Anxiety?

Before exploring the causes and reduction strategies for anxiety, we must firstly look at what anxiety is and how best to identify such anxiety in a client. Whilst there are many different types of anxiety, for example social anxiety, agoraphobia, panic disorder, and generalised anxiety disorder, many of them share similar characteristics [18]. Some of the most common symptoms of anxiety which practitioners can look out for are [18]:

• Restlessness	• Rapid breathing
• Fatigue	• Sweating
• Increased heart rate	• Trembling
• Nervousness	• Difficulty concentrating

Practitioners may also identify other signs and symptoms which may not always present themselves, or be harder to identify, for example:

• Expressions of worry/concern from the client	• Client having a panic attack
• Avoidance/ expression of wanting to leave	• Client presenting with anger or being irritable

Precursors for Anxiety

Another aspect which practitioners can consider, prior to seeing the client, is determining if they may be at higher risk for experiencing anxiety.

This can predominantly be done by looking into client history. Whilst practitioners will have brief knowledge over important factors such as previous scans, procedures and family history, it is not typical for practitioners to have extensive knowledge of other history which makes this area challenging.

However, if practitioners were increasingly aware of aspects which could contribute to increased client anxiety, they may be better able to prepare for anxiety reduction strategies to be put in place for such a patient either pre-contact or during initial contact. Examples of aspects which can indicate an increased chance of anxiety occurring with the client are: a previous referral to a GP for anxiety, an indication of high caffeine intake, alcohol consumption, smoking or substance misuse [19–22].

It is also important to consider factors that may not directly be linked to client history or lifestyle which may increase this anxiety. Clark and Reeves [15] conducted a thematic analysis on various experiences of mammography to identify common themes which appeared to impact client experience the most. Five themes were identified which were all linked to an increase in client anxiety levels: staff interactions (1), pain and discomfort (2), waiting (3), fear (4), and the physical environment (5). Whilst it is clear that the quality of staff interaction and experience of pain has an effect on increasing anxiety in clients, other factors such as the physical environment and waiting may be less obvious. It is therefore beneficial to investigate these in more detail to gain a better understanding of both internal and external factors which may increase client anxiety, identifying ways to decrease this, to increase efficiency and effectiveness in practice.

Staff Interactions

Practitioners know that for more senior colleagues, who are expected to engage in communicating difficult news to patients, it is imperative that communication skills are well practised and maintained at a high standard. However, it is also the case that all staff involved with client care should do the same.

When training as a practitioner, all staff members involved in client contact will learn effective communication skills, but may not necessarily understand how great of an impact this communication may have. Strong communication skills have been demonstrated to increase attendance in mammography screening environments [23], whilst staff who are less observant, less sincere, less confident and less empathetic (amongst other aspects) can cause an increase in client anxiety and reluctance to return to future screenings [24].

This is also true when considering client information and how this is communicated; it has been identified that delivering less information and using complicated language can confuse clients and increase their anxiety levels, further reducing re-attendance rates [24, 25]. Whilst this demonstrates how practitioner verbal communication can impact clients, it is important to remember that clients are aware and affected by non-verbal communication styles as well, for example, whether their practitioner is smiling or not [26]. Therefore, looking at ways to improve both non-verbal and verbal communication styles will beneficially help in the reduction of patient anxiety. However, as Agius and Naylor [27] demonstrate, within a 6–10 min session with a client, it may be hard to effectively offer reassurance and an explanation of the full procedure in a clear and empathetic way and so this, in itself, is a barrier that must be considered.

Considerations of other barriers that may contribute to increased client anxiety, such as language barriers, will be considered later in this chapter.

Pain and Discomfort

Whilst it is not certain whether increased pain causes anxiety, anxiety causes increased pain, or both aspects affect each other, it is known that these two factors are linked [5–7]. As such, by targeting the experience of pain and ways to reduce this, whilst introducing anxiety-reducing techniques for clients, both aspects could collectively produce a more pleasant experience for the client and the practitioner.

Waiting

Pre-treatment waiting and post-treatment result waiting times can negatively influence the amount of anxiety individuals experience [16]. In most cases, this may simply be down to the fact that increased waiting allows for increased 'worry time' and overthinking. The Cognitive Avoidance Theory of Worry [28] explains that worrying is a cognitive avoidance response to any perceived threats that may appear, in an attempt to reduce anxiety levels by considering all possible outcomes to prepare for their occurrence. However, rather than reducing the level of anxiety and other negative responses as it should, it instead maintains or worsens such aspects [29]. Through this explanation, it is clear why individuals who experience longer waiting times, pre or post-treatment, may experience increased levels of anxiety. A reduction in waiting times may therefore be beneficial for reducing anxiety.

Fear

If a client experiences fear during any part of their mammogram or investigation, they will more than likely experience some level of anxiety, or symptoms of anxiety. This is because fear is closely linked to the fight or flight response—a natural inbuilt and innate response which helps individuals to escape, or fight, in a situation they perceive to be dangerous or fearful [30]. When the fight or flight response kicks in, various physiological effects will begin to take place to prepare the body to either fight or flee. Many of these physiological effects are the same to what we experience when feeling anxious, as anxiety can both trigger, and be a result of, the fight or flight response. In both cases, an individual will experience symptoms such as an increased heartrate, sweating, rapid breathing, and shakiness.

For individuals who are not educated on the fight or flight response, instead of identifying that what they are experiencing is a natural response to a feared or stressful situation, they can easily misinterpret these symptoms as being harmful, which can increase and worsen symptoms and general feelings of anxiety.

For individuals who perceive these symptoms as harmful, educating them on the role their fight or flight response plays with anxiety may help to reduce this feeling. By identifying that the situation is not stressful or dangerous, the fight or flight response will not kick in and therefore misinterpretations of the symptoms, or the feeling of anxiety, will not occur. However, changing an individual's perception can be hard and take time.

Physical Environment

Out of all five aspects, the physical environment is likely to be the one which is least thought of as an anxiety-inducing factor, and one which is commonly overlooked. There are many parts of the environment which can increase patient anxiety, such as: room/X-ray machine colour, room temperature and light intensity. For example, Simmons [31] reports how the colours brown and red can be associated with unpleasant emotions, with the colour black inducing fear and anxiety in some people. Xu and Labroo [32] investigated the influence of light intensity on mood, finding that increased brightness can exacerbate both positive and negative emotions in individuals, for example if a client is experiencing some anxiety, a brightly lit room may exacerbate this. This may be because cortisol, a stress hormone, is produced at high light levels which can increase individual anxiety [33]. Another factor which can increase anxiety levels in individuals is the temperature of the room. Noelke et al. [34] found that in rooms where temperature levels were above 21 °C, individuals experienced a reduction in positive emotions, such as happiness and joy, and an increase in negative emotions, such as stress and anxiety. Collectively looking into ways clinicians or organisations can adapt the above aspects to help reduce client anxiety is therefore important.

How Practitioners Can Decrease Client Anxiety

Staff Interactions

There are a few things which practitioners can do to help decrease client anxiety levels through the use of effective communication, ranging from facial expressions to delivery of information. When considering one of the most fundamental aspects of best practice, keeping the patient informed, it is vital that this is carried out to a high standard for both informed consent and anxiety-reduction purposes. Though some may

arguably state that providing the client with all the information needed is common sense, it is likely the case that due to time restraints in particular parts of the process [27], practitioners may have to be selective in what information they can provide to clients who have questions. Whilst this is considerably reasonable, it does directly affect the client.

Clients who have extensive knowledge on the procedure/treatment have been found to have reduced anxiety compared to those who do not [35], therefore, it is important to consider how this can be incorporated into the process so clients are less anxious during mammography procedures. Pre-procedural leaflets are regularly sent with appointment letters, but clients may not always read these. A way to tackle this may be to provide information leaflets in the waiting room to explain the procedure and answer common questions. This would keep clients informed, alleviate anxiety levels and ensure that any questions clients may bring into the procedure would be minimal and easily answered within the session time. For those clients who may still have some questions, it is vital that practitioners deliver any additional information in a clear concise way that avoids the use of medical terminology. This is so clients can understand what is being said and also because evidence indicates providing information in this way can reduce anxiety [23].

Alternatively, the introduction of mini-psychoeducational seminars which aim to increase client awareness and knowledge on aspects such as their procedural process, whilst also providing an opportunity for questions to be answered, could also contribute to this reduction of anxiety. This, however, would require funding and may also be operationally difficult to facilitate.

Another factor for practitioners to consider is how their personality comes across. Practitioners who appear less sincere or empathetic can influence clients' perceptions of their practitioner as well as being a contributing factor to increasing anxiety [24]. Practitioners should ensure that they come across as sincere and empathetic, which as investigated by Fogarty et al. [35], can be achieved in around 40 s through the inclusion of aspects such as: expression of support, validation of client emotional state and reassurance. Richards and Whyte [36] discuss communication techniques to improve the therapeutic alliance in PWPs (a positive professional relationship between patient and practitioner in mental health settings), and this discussion is also applicable to practitioners within mammography settings; It is beneficial for practitioners and clients in mammography settings to have a similarly good relationship, to reduce patient anxiety and discomfort and increase attendance rates [24]. Richards and Whyte [36] propose that to have a good quality 'patient-practitioner' relationship, the practitioner must have good verbal and non-verbal skills such as those listed below:

Non-verbal	Verbal
• Good posture • Eye contact with client • Positive facial expressions such as smiling • Awareness of seating/standing position in retrospect to the client e.g. not sitting too high or standing too close	• Use of empathy • Reflection of what the client has said • Using a good tone of voice • Providing factually accurate information • Summarising information • Normalising the experience

It is important for practitioners to be familiar with, and put into practice, the more common communicative styles listed above. Through continuous use of this emotionally supportive and warm communication behaviour, client anxieties will reduce, resulting in a better experience for both practitioner and client [23].

For individuals who require adaptations, such as those whose first language is not English, additional support will be required; a translator for example. In such cases it then becomes more difficult for practitioners to verbally communicate empathetically with the client, therefore, practitioners should focus on making sure their non-verbal behaviour conveys empathy and warmth. Furthermore, it would be beneficial to ensure the translator is educated on the above communication styles and delivers this appropriately.

Pain and Discomfort

Anxiety can be reduced by providing clients with knowledge of the procedure [35]. This is also applicable for reducing pain and discomfort during procedures, as demonstrated in multiple studies [37–39]. Within these cross-cultural studies, explorations of the effects of health education combined with ways to improve relaxation were found to significantly reduce pain and anxiety levels in various radiologic procedures, including mammography. For example, Sharaf and Hafeez [39] gave their study group participants an educational 15-min power point informing them of the mammography exam procedure and related issues. Following this, they were instructed to carry out some deep breathing relaxation exercises in the waiting room and also during the procedure. In the other two studies, the information provided was reduced to 5 min, though still contained all the necessary information surrounding the mammography exam. The same practitioner accompanied individuals to the procedure and provided emotional support throughout. From this research three important factors can be seen to contribute to the reduction of pain, and therefore anxiety, in individuals attending mammography:

1. The inclusion of a practitioner providing health education to individuals pre-procedure, such as what to expect in the procedure and answers to general questions
2. The inclusion of relaxation exercises pre and during procedure
3. The inclusion of emotional support during the procedure

Whilst it may not be necessary, nor possible, to consider the inclusion of all of these aspects, incorporating at least one of these factors would be beneficial for client wellbeing, reducing procedural complications and increasing reattendance. Looking at these options in a practical and realistic manner, it could be considered that point 2 may be more cost effective for a screening service. As such, listed below are some exercises which may be beneficial for clients to undertake pre-procedure, and during procedure (if the procedure allows):

Deep breathing exercise—Wehrenberg [40]	• Place a hand on your chest with the other on your abdomen • Inhale through your nose deeply and slowly before holding your breath for a few seconds • Exhale through pursed lips, trying to spend twice as long exhaling as you did inhaling • Relax your shoulders and chest whilst you are breathing • Repeat for a few minutes
In 2, Out 2-4-6-8-10 Exercise—Wehrenberg [40]	• Inhale for 2 s • Exhale for 2 s • Inhale again for 2 s • Exhale for 4 s • Inhale for 2 s • Exhale for 6 s • Inhale for 2 s • Exhale for 8 s • Inhale for 2 s • Exhale for 10 s
Muscular relaxation—Sambrook [41]	• Whilst sitting in a chair, close your eyes and concentrate on your breathing for a few minutes, ensuring you breathe slowly using one of the above techniques • Begin the muscle exercise remembering to work around the different groups of muscles in your body • Starting with your hands, clench one of your hands tightly for a couple of seconds whilst you breathe in, before relaxing it as you breathe out and repeat with your other hand • Moving to your arms, bend one arms elbow and tense your arms muscles as you breathe in, relaxing on exhaling, then repeat with your other arm • Raising your shoulders, breathe in, ensuring to raise them as high as you can before relaxing as you breathe out • Focusing now on your neck, tilt your head back and slowly roll it side to side for one inhalation and exhalation, before relaxing • For a few seconds, try to frown to lower your eyebrows as hard as you can before raising your eyebrows for a few more seconds. Relax for a couple of seconds before focusing on clenching your jaw whilst you inhale, relaxing as you exhale • Moving to your chest, take a deep breathe before holding your breath for a few seconds, relax whilst you exhale, before going back to normal breathing • Next, try to tense your stomach muscles as tight as you possibly can, holding for a few seconds before relaxing • Whilst inhaling, squeeze your buttocks together and hold in place for a few seconds before relaxing as you exhale • Finally, keeping your legs on the floor, pull your toes and feet towards your face as you inhale, relaxing as you exhale, before bending them in the opposite directions as you inhale again. Relax as you exhale and inhale for a few more seconds, before opening your eyes

These relaxation techniques target the parasympathetic system, increasing its output levels, which in turn helps to reduce sympathetic activity that is involved in anxiety and stress [42]. By encouraging clients to use one of these techniques before carrying out a mammography, or other procedure, individuals will be more likely to be at ease.

Waiting and Fear

Reducing the amount of waiting time will help decrease the levels of anxiety the clients will experience. It is acknowledged that some sessions may overrun due to unforeseen circumstances with which the practitioner has no control of, leading to the client waiting in the waiting room for longer than anticipated, resulting in increased anxiety due to natural worry and fear [16, 30]. Whilst some of the breathing techniques listed above can be useful to help reduce the natural anxiety individuals experience, this may not be enough in cases where clients hyper-fixate on their anxiety symptoms or perceive them to be dangerous.

A beneficial thing to undertake here is to bring in some psychoeducation on the fight or flight response, responsible for the symptoms produced when we experience anxiety, which can often make individuals who are unaware of this response feel fearful and increasingly anxious. By introducing this psychoeducation towards mammography clients, they are provided with a chance to become more informed on the fight or flight response and therefore learn to not incorrectly perceive the symptoms it produces as harmful, helping to reduce their anxiety. This psychoeducation can be achieved by creating a leaflet which explains the response and common symptoms associates with it [30]. Some additional useful tips which can be included in this leaflet to help reduce anxiety are:

5-4-3-2-1 Grounding technique [30]	Take a deep breath and then list 5 things around you that you can see, 4 things around you that you can feel, 3 things you can hear, 2 things you can smell and 1 thing you can taste, finishing with another deep breath. This can help with grounding you back to reality and reduce the amount of fixation you have on your fight or flight symptoms or worrying thoughts. The more detailed you are, the more effective the technique
List the explanations for your symptoms [30]	If you are finding that you are perceiving your physical symptoms caused by the fight or flight response to be dangerous, which is what is leading to your anxiety to be worsened, it may be beneficial to help list the explanations as to why each symptom is occurring. For example, stating 'my heart rate is increasing to pump oxygen infused blood faster around my body in preparation to fight/flee'

Physical Environment

There are many aspects of the physical environment which practitioners can look at to improve anxiety levels in clients. Firstly, colours have been found to influence our emotions [32], therefore, it is imperative to consider colour schemes for mammography rooms and machinery that promote positive emotions rather than anxiety-provoking ones. Researchers have discovered that cooler, paler colours can reduce heart rates in individuals and provide a sense of calmness, with some finding that the colour blue is one of the most likely colours to help decrease anxiety levels by reducing heart rate, decreasing blood pressure and slowing down breathing [43, 44]. Therefore, performing mammograms in a blue room could help promote a reduction of anxiety. Additionally, as blue has also been demonstrated to encourage productiveness, it may also be beneficial for practitioners [44]. It can be seen that manufacturers of mammography equipment are now taking room design into consideration with some manufacturers creating mood lighting around the machines.

Temperature is also a pertinent factor to consider when looking at ways to help improve client anxiety. High temperatures can lead to reduced positive emotions in individuals, whilst increasing more negative emotions such as anxiety [34], and the same can be true for a temperature that is too low [45]. Therefore, it may also be beneficial to consider maintaining a cooler room temperature.

Client anxiety: a summary

For clients attending mammography, anxiety may come about from a variety of different situations including: staff interactions, pain and discomfort, waiting, fear, and the physical environment. To help reduce this anxiety, practitioners can be educated on how best to use verbal and non-verbal communication, and consider altering the mammography environment appropriately. Additionally, providing information on relaxation techniques and psychoeducation on the fight or flight response can also aid in the reduction of client anxiety. The reduction of this anxiety could facilitate increased re-attendance rates, a smoother procedure, more positive reviews, and improved client wellbeing.

Practitioner Anxiety

The Role of Anxiety

Whilst anxiety in practitioners can present in the same way as clients, the role they play can be quite different. For practitioners, anxiety can not only have an impact on themselves, but can impact the people around them as well. If a practitioner experiences short term anxiety, for example in a challenging client case, they may have some difficulty concentrating, as this is a common symptom of anxiety [18]. Naturally, when experiencing this lapse in concentration, there is an increased likelihood that errors are made when carrying out work. This increase in errors may lead to practitioners taking more time when examining clients or requiring repeat imaging, which not only puts additional stress on the client and the practitioner, but leads to financial strain on already stretched services.

One symptom which is linked to anxiety is that of irritability [8], if a practitioner is experiencing irritability, they may find it more difficult to maintain good relationships with their peers and clients. Furthermore, this irritability can make the client themselves more anxious. In practitioners who may experience long-term anxiety, their working memory can negatively be impacted, resulting in aspects such as memory loss, attention deficits and problem-solving abilities [46]. Furthermore, long term anxiety can have an overall effect on the mental health and physical health of the practitioner [47].

As poor mental health and physical illness leads to time off work [48], and irritability can negatively affect relationships within the work environment, it is therefore vital that tactics for anxiety reduction in practitioners are addressed. There are a multitude of factors which can lead to practitioner anxiety occurring, however, the focus in this chapter will be on; burnout, errors, challenging situations, and result disclosure.

Burnout

As previously discussed, practitioner interaction with clients is quite limited due to the short ses-

sion times, typically lasting around 5–6 min [27]. Practitioners are expected to see a large number of clients each day, typically with sessions being back-to-back. In this fast-paced environment, burnout can commonly occur, leading to aspects such as compassion fatigue and anxiety [49]. As both factors can result in practitioners requiring days off work and reducing their performance level within work, looking at ways to reduce burnout will help to reduce practitioner anxiety levels and help prevent re-occurrence. One of the ways that this could be explored is through the use of monthly check-ins from the practitioner's manager. Furthermore, exploring the use of informal debriefing sessions between peers may also be beneficial, along with the inclusion of mindfulness and stress management technique education.

Errors

There are cases where errors are made, during which, reporting of false negatives or false positives can occur [50]. These situations can bring about anxiety in practitioners, an example of which can be considered below:

Imagine you assessed someone a year ago, whether you performed the mammography, interpreted the image, or reported the outcome to the client. Imagine that same client returning, and you find out they had a missed cancer diagnosis. Aside from feeling sadness or guilt, you would also experience some anxiety: You may start worrying if you made that same mistake with other clients, you may worry whether that missed diagnosis had negatively impacted the client, you may worry about a complaint against you. Whilst all of these concerns are completely normal for someone to experience in this situation, looking at ways to decrease this anxiety will help the practitioner to remain calm, not be distracted performing work duties, and be able to rationally come up with a solution to any problems. Furthermore, exploring ways to reduce the likelihood of errors happening will also be beneficial in reducing the chances of practitioner anxiety occurring. These will be discussed later on in the chapter.

Challenging Situations

There will be times when practitioners come across challenging circumstances. This may be different for each practitioner and is subjective in nature. For one practitioner it may mean a client who does not listen to instructions well, for another it may be that they are verbally abusive, excessively tearful or one who asks repeated questions on a day where they may be feeling tired. Regardless of the situation, a range of emotions will be presented on dealing with the specific situation.

It is therefore beneficial for solutions to be in place which act to reduce the anxiety (and other negative emotions) the practitioner experiences at the time. This can be achieved through having managers provide 1-1 slots where practitioners can discuss their experiences, or by providing a specific room where practitioners can go to unwind after this type of contact.

Result Disclosure

Part of a practitioners' role may be to disclose results; another aspect could involve performing images and/or reporting them. It can often be clear that there is an area of concern within an image and often practitioners may have to continue with client interaction and not alert the client to any concern. This can be challenging and can cause stress and anxiety; practitioners will hyper-focus on how they are acting to ensure their emotions remain unchanged which can often take a lot of energy. Additionally, this can lead to practitioners feeling conflicted and increasingly anxious; some clients will ask to have their results as soon as possible or immediately following the procedure which the practitioner is unable to provide [51]. For those in roles where results are disclosed, this can also be an anxiety-provoking experience. For example, the practitioner will have to disclose the results in a way that causes the least amount of stress to the client, whilst also being able to support the client and deal with their response.

Ensuring practitioners are familiar with how to act in these situations, providing them with anxiety-reducing techniques, access to a designated room to relax and refocus, and providing access to a supervisor/manager, can greatly help in reducing anxiety. This will be explored and explained now in more depth.

How to Decrease Anxiety in Mammographers?

Burnout

Thomas and colleagues [51] acquired the views of various sonographers and reported that many participated in informal debriefing sessions with colleagues to assist in reducing their emotional burnout. This study gives insight into the type of support that can be put into place to assist the reduction of burnout and anxiety in practitioners. Though this study did not incorporate informal debrief time within work [51]; providing the opportunity for this within a mammography setting would be beneficial. This could reduce the likelihood of practitioners requiring counselling, which may be required during worktime, as counselling was reported as an alternative source of help when experiencing high levels of burnout [51].

By providing a policy which encourages practitioners to discuss, within a peer setting, any feelings of emotional burnout they are experiencing, and their causes, would allow practitioners to 'offload' some anxieties and help reduce burnout. Extending this, managers can also provide regular check-ins with their team by implementing a designated monthly slot for support. In these sessions, managers can check-in with the practitioner's emotional state, workload, and discuss any solutions to difficulties that may be arising that are causing the practitioner stress. This approach has been found to reduce burnout in other medical areas [52].

Mindfulness and stress management have also been found to reduce burnout, and thus anxiety, in practitioners [52]. Educating practitioners on both of these aspects will be highly beneficial in reducing anxiety levels and decreasing the likelihood of sick-leave. Mindfulness teaches individuals to be more aware of the present, focusing on both internal thoughts and feelings, and on the external environment around them [40]. Stress management works by identifying sources of stress within a person's life, applying techniques to help take positive actions in these areas, and helping individuals to cope better with stress overall [53]. As a practitioner, there are a variety of ways to bring mindfulness and stress management into your life, a few techniques are highlighted below:

Mindfulness Techniques

Wehrenberg [40] identifies six separate aspects which an individual can do to help improve their burnout or anxiety levels:

• Be mindful of your outer world	• Mindfulness with shifting awareness
• Be mindful of your inner world	• Specific mindfulness (for example, mindfulness for panic attacks/social anxiety/generalised anxiety)
• Assess your focus on bodily sensations	
• Assess whether you talk yourself into feeling fear	

Step 1

To develop a solid foundation, focusing on becoming mindful of both your outer and inner world is an essential technique. To begin, you must first learn to be more observing of your surroundings. A good way to do this is to include all five senses in your observations, note what you see, touch, hear, smell and taste. This can help to ground you to the present and allow you to understand situations better before deciding on outcomes. During this, you do not decide what the actions or observations mean, only what they are. For example, you can notice someone is sweating, but until you gather further observational information, you cannot determine if this is due to anxiety or because they are hot.

Next Steps

Following this, you can then become more mindful of your inner world. Set a time every day to stop what you are doing and look within yourself: what are your thoughts, feelings and body sensa-

tions? It can sometimes be helpful to name these things aloud or in your head, for example, saying 'I think I am worried about my appointment' or 'I feel quite anxious'. Through identification, you will learn to be more aware of your own emotions and thoughts. You can then consider if there is anything you would like to change, or if there is anything you can change about this. For example, if you notice you are feeling anxious, you may first consider what is causing that anxiety before thinking up any solutions to the root problem. If you were anxious about a doctor's appointment, you may consider talking to a friend about it, doing some breathing techniques or talking to the doctor about your concerns.

Sometimes you may not be able to identify what is causing your anxiety, in these instances it is better to focus on ways you can reduce the anxiety you are feeling itself, rather than worry about what is causing it. By being more internally mindful, you can notice symptoms of anxiety or burnout earlier.

If you find that you are experiencing physical symptoms such as an increased heart rate, sweating, or shaking for example, you may also want to assess what your focus is on these bodily sensations: Do you think they are dangerous? Do you hyper-focus on them? Do they make you self-conscious? By noticing how focused you are on your physical symptoms and the types of thoughts you are having about them, you can then introduce techniques to reduce or stop any negative thoughts from occurring before they start, which in turn can reduce your symptoms. This can look like:

Negative thought: The person next to me in the waiting room can see me sweat and this worries me	
Evidence for: They are close enough to me to know	**Evidence against**: They are waiting for this appointment too and are probably too focused on themselves to notice They will probably be anxious too and may think I am just hot
New thought: Though I am sweating, the person next to me is likely too focused on themselves to notice or care	

This way of thinking is based on the Cognitive Restructuring model [36] and can be applied to various thoughts and situations. For example, if you find you are more concerned about a physical symptom and believe it is harmful to you, you can use this framework to come up with alternative explanations. This may look something like this:

Negative thought: I'm sweating so much I think I am having a heart attack

Evidence for: My heart is beating really fast I am sweating a lot	**Evidence against**: My heart is beating fast as I am in a fearful situation and my fight/flight response is activated to prepare my body I am sweating because my heart is beating fast

New thought: My increased heart rate and sweating is because my body is having a normal and natural response to the situation

Using these techniques, you can help to avoid feeling more fearful and anxious; this can also help to reduce the anxiety you are experiencing. If this does not seem to work, another mindfulness technique you could implement is called mindfulness with shifting awareness. This helps redirect your attention to what is going on around you which can give your sense of control back, as you choose what to focus on, whilst also removing your focus on the physical sensations you are experiencing.

How to Do This

Firstly, find a place to sit with your eyes closed in a comfortable position, begin to notice your five senses. Then focus on yourself: how does your breathing feel as you take deep, slow breaths into your nose and out through your mouth? After a few minutes, refocus your attention to the external environment once more, has anything changed in those few minutes? Are you noticing anything new with your five senses, or is everything the same? Finally, once you feel ready, gradually open your eyes and bring your attention back to your next task.

If you are experiencing anxiety, for instance social anxiety, there are a few ways that you can alter mindfulness to be more targeted.

For more information on this, or any of the techniques mentioned above take a look at Margaret Wehrenberg's 'The 10 Best-Ever Anxiety Management Techniques Workbook' [40] to help reduce burnout and anxiety further.

Stress Management Techniques

Another set of techniques that can prove useful to practitioners to help reduce burnout and anxiety is around stress management. Similar to mindfulness, there are a variety of different sub-set techniques that can be used such as: progressive muscle relaxation and autogenic training, breathing and stretching exercises, sense imagery and meditation, mini-relaxation, problem-solving, exposure and desensitisation [53].

For this section, the focus will be on autogenic training, sense imagery and problem solving.

If you would like to learn more about the stress management techniques mentioned in this section or those not included, Smith [53] provides a detailed description of these techniques and more.

Autogenic training aims to lower blood pressure and decrease breathing to promote the natural relaxation response your body has, which in turn helps to reduce burnout and anxiety. Each step is repeated six times before moving onto the next one and will take just a few minutes overall:

1. Take a few, even, slow breaths to calm yourself whilst quietly repeating to yourself 'I am completely calm'
2. Whilst focusing your attention on your arms, maintaining your level breathing, repeat 'My arms are heavy' before finishing with 'I am completely calm'

3. Maintaining focus on your arms, repeat to yourself slowly 'My arms are very warm' before finishing with 'I am completely calm'
4. Turning your attention to your legs, slowly repeat 'My legs are heavy', before finishing with 'I am completely calm'
5. Again, focusing on your legs, slowly and quietly repeat to yourself 'My legs are very warm, before finishing with 'I am completely calm'
6. Turn your attention to your heartbeat and repeat six times 'My heartbeat is calm and regular' before finishing with 'I am completely calm'
7. Next, turn to your breathing and say 'My breathing is calm and regular' quietly and slowly, before saying 'I am completely calm'
8. Following this, focus next on your abdomen and slowly say six times 'My abdomen is warm' before finishing with 'I am completely calm'
9. Focusing your attention on your forehead, say 'My forehead is pleasantly cool' before saying 'I am completely calm'
10. Finally, once you have spent some time enjoying the leftover feeling of warmth and relaxation, quietly and calmly say 'Arms firm, breathe deeply, eyes open', before opening your eyes and continuing with your day

Sense imagery is another stress management technique which can be used to reduce both stress, burnout, and anxiety. It works by having the individual create a daydream of a situation that is relaxing, involving no goal-directed activity. It uses all five senses to help the individual fully immerse themselves into their chosen relaxing situation. For example, the calming place may be a forest and you may note hearing a soft stream flow by and see squirrels chasing each other through the trees. You may feel the softness of the mossy-green forest floor and smell the sweetness of nature around you. You may even imagine you are eating some chocolates and tasting the smooth richness of the food. If you choose to undertake this technique, ensure you are in a comfortable place first and away from interruption, taking some deep breaths before you close your eyes and start picturing the scene. Some individuals may prefer to go directly to their calming place, whereas others may prefer to imagine themselves travelling

to that place first: picturing themselves going further away from the stressful situation and closer to their safe and relaxing place. It can help to use your five senses again to ground yourself back to your day and the room around you.

Problem solving is another stress management technique that can be used to help practitioners reduce burnout and anxiety. This technique can be used for a variety of different situations and settings and is a practical approach to help individuals consider solutions to issues that are stress inducing:

Step 1	Identify the problem	Firstly, identify a problem that you would like to address: one example could be that you are quite stressed because you feel you are being overworked and are struggling to keep up with the high intensity workload
Step 2	Consider all solutions	At this stage, you can think of all solutions regardless of how irrational they may seem. With the situation above, a few may be to: talk to your manager about reducing your caseload, cry, talk to a colleague about seeing if they can pick up a few cases, change your job role
Step 3	Analysing the solutions	Whenever you feel all possible solutions have been noted, you can then progress to analysing the solutions. With this, you take each solution and draw up the strengths and weaknesses of carrying them out. For example, if looking at the 'change your job role' solution, some advantages may be that it would stop the stress and anxiety immediately and that you had the possibility to work in a less demanding role. Some disadvantages could be that you would have reduced income, finding a new job may be challenging and cause you anxiety in itself
Step 4	Choose an outcome	After weighing up the advantages and disadvantages of each solution, you can then choose an outcome which you feel is most appropriate and positive. Once a solution has been chosen, you can then plan out how you will go about carrying out this solution, which can be broken down into smaller steps if the solution is quite large
Step 5	Carry it out	Finally, once the solution has been planned, the next step is to plan and carry it out

By encouraging informal debrief talks between colleagues, providing individuals with knowledge of mindfulness and stress management techniques, and having monthly-check ins with managers who can help to provide solutions to decrease mammographer stress, the chance of burnout, and anxiety, occurring in practitioners should reduce.

Errors

There are two aspects of errors to consider when thinking about how to reduce practitioner anxiety: pre-mistake and post-mistake. Considering ways to prevent errors from occurring in the first place is beneficial. Three steps can be undertaken to help reduce the likelihood of a mistake occurring: (1) Education, (2) Observation and (3) Obtaining a second opinion.

Education	The more educated you are in a particular subject, the less likely you are to make a mistake. Whilst all practitioners are educated for qualification, it is beneficial to undertake continued professional development. By doing this, practitioners will have increased clinical self-efficacy and clinical skills, reducing the likelihood of errors being made along with reduced anxiety [54]
Observation	This second step is through observation of the practitioner and observation by the practitioner. Following an educational refresher course for example, it is beneficial for the practitioner to be observed to ensure they are confident in their abilities. This would also allow for any errors to be highlighted and corrected. Practitioners can also observe colleagues performing that task, allowing them to visualise the correct way for that task to be undertaken
Second opinions	Encouraging practitioners to ask for a second opinion if they are uncertain of their techniques or decisions is beneficial. By doing so, the practitioner can be assured that their way of thinking is correct, or be provided with an alternative, so that the chance of a mistake being made is reduced

There will still be occasions where errors occur, and this is often anxiety provoking. By encouraging openness and transparency in the workplace around errors and discussing any

thoughts around those errors with peers and managers, this will help reduce any anxiety felt and allow for a safe space to problem-solve solutions. The practitioner can also utilise some anxiety reducing techniques (as listed in previous sections) to further help reduce any anxiety.

Challenging Situations

As mentioned previously, difficult patients can often provoke anxiety in practitioners, therefore providing support and techniques to reduce this anxiety is beneficial. One of the ways this can be achieved is by providing general support for practitioners. As talking has been found to reduce anxiety [55], having managers schedule specific times for practitioners to come and see them could be advantageous. This can allow practitioners time to voice their concerns and discuss anxiety related issues, also providing a chance for any problems to be resolved, or for a plan of action to be put into place. Additionally, providing practitioners with easy access to protocols would further be beneficial. These protocols could be presented as flowcharts in staff rooms, for example, listing the first point of contact and subsequent processes to follow after an abusive patient.

Another way to reduce practitioner anxiety is to provide them with a serenity room with a variety of items to appeal to all five senses. This helps by refocusing their attention away from the previous situation to the calming environment around them [30]. A study by Salmela et al. [56] investigated the benefits of the inclusion of a serenity room in an emergency department for staff. The room included items such as vinyl artwork, a reclining chair and a three-way light bulb to provide dimmer lighting, all of which contributed to reduced stress in professionals using the room. The average member rated the room to be effective for reducing stress, refocusing attention and relaxing (74%). Furthermore 94% of respondents believed that having a serenity room within other departments would be beneficial, as such, including a similar room within mammography settings would be advantageous for reducing practitioner anxiety.

Result Disclosure

Many clinicians will have knowledge of client results but will be unable to disclose that result. This can induce anxiety and stress in practitioners who have to maintain a normal and positive attitude with clients. Some of this anxiety may come from clinicians being unsure on how to act towards the client, for others the anxiety may come about due to the information they have found. For those who have to disclose results, they may also find this stressful and anxiety provoking, as they have to remain calm and professional in an emotional situation.

For both situations similar solutions to decrease anxiety can be put in place. To begin with, implementing education techniques to help inform practitioners who are unable to disclose results how to appropriately act upon seeing a bad result/where clients ask questions around their results is useful in reducing the likelihood of the practitioner panicking 'in the moment', whilst also helping to decrease anxiety around the situation. For practitioners who do disclose results, the education provided can discuss how best to disclose difficult results and deal with responses in a professional and sensitive manner. By having additional knowledge on what to do in these situations, anxiety can decrease.

In both situations a few things can be put in place to reduce the amount of anxiety practitioners experience post client contact. For example; ensuring practitioners are aware that they can discuss any stressful or anxiety provoking situations with their manager, and ensuring practitioners are educated on anxiety reducing techniques such as mindfulness and deep breathing exercises. Furthermore, a serenity room [56] can provide practitioners with a safe space to let out their emotions and help them decrease their anxiety; they can then return to their working day with minimal disruption.

Gallagher et al. [57] discovered that a variety of radiologists were reluctant to disclose their errors to clients due to the discomfort of the situation, stress, anxiety and the challenges that can occur because of this. Having interventional strategies such as education and providing support to practitioners via their managers, peers or leads, may help to reduce this reluctance to disclose errors.

> Practitioner anxiety: a summary
>
> Anxiety can occur because of burnout, errors, difficult situations and result disclosure. To help reduce this anxiety, practitioners can implement regular check-ins with managers, educate themselves on mindfulness and stress management techniques, undertake observation roles, be encouraged to ask for a second opinion, and have access to a serenity room. In using all these elements practitioner anxiety will reduce, supporting a reduction to sick leave and errors, improved wellbeing and allowing for a smoother procedure for both client and practitioner.

Future Considerations

Aspects which future researchers may find beneficial to investigate are:

- Determining if environmental changes can positively influence anxiety levels such as: conducting mammograms in a cool room and/ or a blue room to reduce patient anxiety and promote practitioner productiveness
- Investigating if the introduction of informational leaflets in waiting rooms which explain the procedure, answer common questions and/ or include psychoeducation on the fight or flight system, to determine if this aids in patient anxiety reduction
- Encouraging patients to carry out relaxation exercises pre and during procedure to conclude if this benefits patient anxiety reduction
- Investigating if the inclusion of regular check-in sessions with practitioner managers, which provides a space for open discussion on any anxiety inducing aspects of practitioner life, will help to reduce anxiety
- Observing if the inclusion of continued professional development on various mammography topics/procedures will help reduce error rates and decrease practitioner anxiety. This can additionally include practitioners observing procedures carried out by those more experienced than them, and further being observed by managers/more qualified practitioners to ensure no errors are being made
- Determining if the inclusion of a serenity room for practitioners will help improve overall mental health and decrease anxiety

- Encouraging practitioners to educate themselves on, and utilise, mindfulness and stress management techniques, to determine if this will have a positive impact on anxiety reduction

Clinical Pearls

- Incorporating relaxation techniques and procedural knowledge into leaflets which clients can use can help to reduce anxiety and increase attendance rates
- As a clinician, using mindfulness and stress management techniques regularly, whilst communicating with your team and manager about any work-related problems, will help reduce anxiety

Chapter Review Questions
Review Questions

1. What are some common causes of anxiety in clients?
2. What are some common causes of anxiety in practitioners?

Answers

1. Staff interactions, pain and discomfort, waiting, fear, physical environment.
2. Burnout, errors, challenging situations, result disclosure.

Appendix

Test your learning and check your understanding of this book's contents: use the "Springer Nature Flashcards" app to access questions using https://sn.pub/dcAnWL.

To use the app, please follow the instructions in Chap. 1.

Flashcard code: 48341-69945-ABCB1-2A8C7-CE9D2.

Short URL: https://sn.pub/dcAnWL.

References

1. Public Health England. Guidance for breast screening mammographers. https://www.gov.uk/government/publications/breast-screening-quality-assurance-for-mammography-and-radiography/guidance-for-breast-screening-mammographers. Accessed 15 Aug 2021.
2. Aro AR, De Koning HJ, Absetz P, Schreck M. Two distinct groups of non-attenders in an organized mammography screening program. Breast Cancer Res Treatment. 2001;70(2):145–53.
3. Consedine NS, Magai C, Krivoshekova YS, Ryzewicz L, Neugut AI. Fear, anxiety, worry, and breast cancer screening behavior: a critical review. Cancer Epidemiol Prevent Biomarkers. 2004;13(4):501–10.
4. Lagerlund M. Factors affecting attendance at population-based mammography screening. Department of Medical Epidemiology and Biostatistics; 2002.
5. Brunton M, Jordan C, Campbell I. Anxiety before, during, and after participation in a population-based screening mammography programme in Waikato Province, New Zealand. N Z Med J. 2005;118(1209):1–10.
6. Jackson V. Pain psychology: an overview of concepts and methods. In: Hogans BB, Barreveld AM, editors. Pain care essentials. New York, NY: Oxford University Press; 2019. p. 75–89.
7. Maimone S, Morozov AP, Wilhelm A, Robrahn I, Whitcomb TD, Lin KY, Maxwell RW. Understanding patient anxiety and pain during initial image-guided breast biopsy. J Breast Imaging. 2020;2(6):583–9.
8. Montgomery M, McCrone SH. Psychological distress associated with the diagnostic phase for suspected breast cancer: systematic review. J Adv Nurs. 2010;66(11):2372–90.
9. Hu W, Wang G, Huang D, Sui M, Xu Y. Cancer immunotherapy based on natural killer cells: current progress and new opportunities. Front Immunol. 2019;10(1):1205.
10. Andersen BL, Farrar WB, Golden-Kreutz D, Kutz LA, MacCallum R, Courtney ME, Glaser R. Stress and immune responses after surgical treatment for regional breast cancer. J Natl Cancer Inst. 1998;90(1):30–6.
11. Witek-Janusek L, Gabram S, Mathews HL. Psychologic stress, reduced NK cell activity, and cytokine dysregulation in women experiencing diagnostic breast biopsy. Psychoneuroendocrinology. 2007;32(1):22–35.
12. Howell RT, Kern ML, Lyubomirsky S. Health benefits: meta-analytically determining the impact of well-being on objective health outcomes. Health Psychol Rev. 2007;1(1):83–136.
13. Hall LH, Johnson J, Watt I, Tsipa A, O'Connor DB. Healthcare staff wellbeing, burnout, and patient safety: a systematic review. PLoS One. 2016;11(7):e0159015.
14. Department of Health. The relationship between wellbeing and health. https://assets.publishing.service.gov.uk/government/uploads/system/uploads/attach-

ment_data/file/295474/The_relationship_between_
wellbeing_and_health.pdf. Accessed 10 Aug 2021.

15. Clark S, Reeves PJ. Women's experiences of mammography: a thematic evaluation of the literature. Radiography. 2015;21(1):84–8.

16. Drossaert CH, Boer H, Seydel ER. Monitoring women's experiences during three rounds of breast cancer screening: results from a longitudinal study. J Med Screen. 2002;9(4):168–75.

17. Office for National Statistics. Cancer survival in England: national estimates for patients followed up to 2017. https://www.ons.gov.uk/releases/cancersurvivalinenglandadultstageatdiagnosisandchildhoodpatientsfollowedupto2017. Accessed 10 Aug 2021.

18. American Psychiatric Association. Diagnostic and statistical manual of mental disorders. 5th ed. Washington, DC: American Psychiatric Association; 2013.

19. Carvalho AF, Stubbs B, Maes M, Solmi M, Vancampfort D, Kurdyak PA, Brunoni AR, Husain MI, Koyanagi A. Different patterns of alcohol consumption and the incidence and persistence of depressive and anxiety symptoms among older adults in Ireland: a prospective community-based study. J Affect Disord. 2018;238(1):651–65.

20. McLellan TM, Caldwell JA, Lieberman HR. A review of caffeine's effects on cognitive, physical and occupational performance. Neurosci Biobehav Rev. 2016;71(1):294–312.

21. Moylan S, Jacka FN, Pasco JA, Berk M. How cigarette smoking may increase the risk of anxiety symptoms and anxiety disorders: a critical review of biological pathways. Brain and Behavior. 2013;3(3):302–26.

22. Pasche S. Exploring the comorbidity of anxiety and substance use disorders. Curr Psychiatry Rep. 2012;14(3):176–81.

23. Meguerditchian AN, Dauphinee D, Girard N, Eguale T, Riedel K, Jacques A, Meterissian S, Buckeridge DL, Abrahamowicz M, Tamblyn R. Do physician communication skills influence screening mammography utilization? BMC Health Serv Res. 2012;12(1):1–8.

24. Louw A, Lawrence H, Motto J. Mammographer personality traits–elements of the optimal mammogram experience. Health SA Gesondheid. 2014;19(1):1–7.

25. Smalls TE. An evidence-based process change to improve mammography adherence [doctoral dissertation]. University of South Carolina; 2017.

26. Wanzer MB, Booth-Butterfield M, Gruber K. Perceptions of health care providers' communication: relationships between patient-centered communication and satisfaction. Health Commun. 2004;16(3):363–84.

27. Agius EC, Naylor S. Breast compression techniques in screening mammography–a Maltese evaluation project. Radiography. 2018;24(4):309–14.

28. Borkovec TD, Alcaine O, Behar E, Heimberg RG, Turk CL, Mennin DS. Avoidance theory of worry and generalized anxiety disorder. In: Heimberg RG, Turk CL, Mennin DS, editors. Generalised anxiety disor-

der: advances in research and practice. New York: Guilford Press; 2004. p. 77–108.

29. Newman MG, Llera SJ, Erickson TM, Przeworski A, Castonguay LG. Worry and generalized anxiety disorder: a review and theoretical synthesis of evidence on nature, etiology, mechanisms, and treatment. Annu Rev Clin Psychol. 2013;9(1):275–97.

30. Milosevic I, McCabe RE. Phobias: the psychology of irrational fear. Greenwood; 2015.

31. Simmons DR. Colour and emotion. In: Biggam CP, Hough CA, Kay CJ, Simmons DR, editors. New directions in colour studies. Amsterdam: John Benjamins Publishing Company; 2011. p. 395–414.

32. Xu AJ, Labroo AA. Incandescent affect: Turning on the hot emotional system with bright light. J Consum Psychol. 2014;24(2):207–16.

33. Scheer FA, Buijs RM. Light affects morning salivary cortisol in humans. J Clin Endocrinol Metab. 1999;84(1):3395–8.

34. Noelke C, McGovern M, Corsi DJ, Jimenez MP, Stern A, Wing IS, Berkman L. Increasing ambient temperature reduces emotional well-being. Environ Res. 2016;151(1):124–9.

35. Fogarty LA, Curbow BA, Wingard JR, McDonnell K, Somerfield MR. Can 40 seconds of compassion reduce patient anxiety? J Clin Oncol. 1999;17(1):371–7.

36. Richards D, Whyte M. Reach out: national programme student materials to support the delivery of training for psychological wellbeing practitioners delivering low intensity interventions. 3rd ed. Rethink Mental Illness; 2009.

37. Fernández-Feito A, Lana A, Baldonedo-Cernuda R, Mosteiro-Díaz MP. A brief nursing intervention reduces anxiety before breast cancer screening mammography. Psicothema. 2015;27(2):128–33.

38. Fernández-Feito A, Lana A, Cabello-Gutiérrez L, Franco-Correia S, Baldonedo-Cernuda R, Mosteiro-Díaz P. Face-to-face information and emotional support from trained nurses reduce pain during screening mammography: results from a randomized controlled trial. Pain Manag Nurs. 2015;16(6):862–70.

39. Sharaf AY, Hafeez NA. Effect of nursing interventions on pain and anxiety among women undergoing screening mammography. Int J Novel Res Healthc Nurs. 2019;6(3):454–69.

40. Wehrenberg M. The 10 best-ever anxiety management techniques: understanding how your brain makes you anxious and what you can do to change it. 2nd ed. WW Norton & Company; 2018.

41. Sambrook J. Relaxation exercises. https://patient.info/news-and-features/relaxation-exercises. Accessed 23 Aug 2021.

42. Jerath R, Crawford MW, Barnes VA, Harden K. Self-regulation of breathing as a primary treatment for anxiety. Appl Psychophysiol Biofeedback. 2015;40(2):107–15.

43. Al-Ayash A, Kane RT, Smith D, Green-Armytage P. The influence of color on student emotion, heart rate, and performance in learning environments. Color Res Appl. 2016;41(2):196–05.

44. O'Connor Z. Colour psychology and colour therapy: Caveat emptor. Color Res Appl. 2011;36(3):229–34.
45. IJzerman HR. Heartwarming: how our inner thermostat made us human. WW Norton & Company; 2021.
46. Miguel P. The effects of anxiety on cognitive performance [doctoral dissertation]. London: Royal Holloway, University of London; 2012.
47. Roy-Byrne PP, Davidson KW, Kessler RC, Asmundson GJ, Goodwin RD, Kubzansky L, Lydiard RB, Massie MJ, Katon W, Laden SK, Stein MB. Anxiety disorders and comorbid medical illness. Gen Hosp Psychiatry. 2008;30(3):208–25.
48. Layard R. Why we should spend more on mental health. Am J Med Res. 2016;3(1):188–206.
49. Mainiero MB, Parikh JR. Recognizing and overcoming burnout in breast imaging. J Breast Imag. 2019;1(1):60–3.
50. Ekpo EU, Alakhras M, Brennan P. Errors in mammography cannot be solved through technology alone. Asian Pac J Cancer Prev. 2018;19(2):291–301.
51. Thomas S, O'Loughlin K, Clarke J. The 21st century sonographer: role ambiguity in communicating an adverse outcome in obstetric ultrasound. Cogent Med. 2017;4(1):e1373903.
52. Fischer J, Alpert A, Rao P. Promoting intern resilience: individual chief wellness check-ins. MedEdPORTAL. 2019;15(1):1–7.
53. Smith JC. Stress management: a comprehensive handbook of techniques and strategies. New York, NY: Springer; 2002.
54. Shahsavari H, Ghiyasvandian S, Houser ML, Zakerimoghadam M, Kermanshahi SS, Torabi S. Effect of a clinical skills refresher course on the clinical performance, anxiety and self-efficacy of the final year undergraduate nursing students. Nurse Educ Pract. 2017;27(1):151–6.
55. Bourne EJ. The anxiety and phobia workbook. 5th ed. Oakland, CA: New Harbinger Publications; 2011.
56. Salmela L, Woehrle T, Marleau E, Kitch L. Implementation of a "Serenity Room": promoting resiliency in the ED. Nursing. 2020;50(10):58–63.
57. Gallagher TH, Cook AJ, Brenner RJ, Carney PA, Miglioretti DL, Geller BM, Kerlikowske K, Onega TL, Rosenberg RD, Yankaskas BC, Lehman CD, Elmore JG. Disclosing harmful mammography errors to patients. Radiology. 2009;253(2):443–52.

Client-Practitioner Interactions Within Breast Care Services

14

Rita M. Borgen and Joleen K. Eden

Learning Objectives
- Identify the commonly reported themes that influence client/patient experience
- Discuss how client/patient anxiety can potentially be reduced
- State practitioner strategies which could improve re-attendance for breast screening
- Outline the benefits of advanced communication skills training

Introduction

Although there are a variety of models internationally, within the United Kingdom (UK) breast care services are delivered within one of two models. Clients presenting with breast symptoms (*symptomatic*) are assessed within a 'one stop' (within one hospital attendance) out-patient setting whilst asymptomatic clients in the UK aged 50–70 (*screening*) are invited for 3 yearly breast screening by the National Health Service Breast Screening Programme (BSP). A proportion of the latter are recalled for further assessment should a mammographic abnormality be suspected (*assessment clients*). Many other health care systems around the world also offer these three breast care approaches (symptomatic, screening and assessment services), though the timeframe between screening invitations and the age range of clients varies within the screening services [1] (Chap. 2).

These services are delivered by a multidisciplinary group of health professionals supported by other vital staff such as receptionists and support workers, and all require a high level of communication skills. It is important to remember that for an individual client each interaction is a unique experience which should leave them with a sense of value and recognition of their individuality.

The importance of the health care professional to recognise and acknowledge individual client needs to provide a satisfactory client experience is recognised internationally and has been highlighted in UK guidelines [1]. Within screening environments, the health care professional is likely to be a qualified radiographer with postgraduate mammography education and training (mammographer) or a mammography associate or assistant. However, clients attending either symptomatic or assessment clinics will meet a range of different health professionals within a

R. M. Borgen (✉) · J. K. Eden
Breast Screening Service, East Lancashire Hospitals
NHS Trust, Burnley General Hospital, Burnley, UK
e-mail: rita.borgen@elht.nhs.uk;
joleen.eden@elht.nhs.uk

single clinic attendance including mammography associate or assistants, practitioners, breast care nurses, clinicians (radiologists or breast surgeons), health care assistants and receptionists. It is important that all of these staff groups are able to communicate effectively and compassionately, and in the UK the completion of advanced communication skills training is a requirement for those core members of the team who have direct contact with those clients on the breast cancer pathway [2]. However, concerns have been raised in several annual UK peer review exercises regarding poor compliance with this national requirement [3, 4], so it is important not to be complacent. This chapter will now explore the nature and challenges of practitioner-client interactions within the routine screening setting and the assessment/symptomatic clinic.

The Breast Screening Experience

Research has demonstrated that clients who participate in breast screening are generally positive about their experience [5]. Clark and Reeves identified in a recent literature review that clients experienced diagnostic breast procedures in unique and diverse ways, and they identified five commonly reported themes that influenced the experience: fear, pain and discomfort, waiting, the physical environment and staff interactions [5]; this was explored in detail within Chap. 13. In particular, Clark and Reeves argued that poor communication or interaction by the practitioner can have a negative influence on patient experience, a finding also supported by Davey [6]. It is important that the nature of any negative experiences are understood, including the impact they may have on the client and their wider social network. A poor experience may be communicated to friends and family, heightening anxiety in those who may subsequently be invited for screening. Indeed, Sharp et al. [7] found that clients were influenced by accounts from others, often via social media (Chap. 15). Some may have been embellished, but they were nevertheless very 'real' to them at the time, possibly causing increased anxiety.

The client experience may be influenced by the beliefs and values of the practitioner performing the examination [8], who is engaged in a complex decision-making process that involves a range of human and technological facets (Fig. 14.1) [9].

Clients may experience a range of emotions during the procedure and some degree of discomfort related to the application of compression force. Although the number of women experiencing pain has been reported to be as low as 6% [10], moderate pain may be experienced in up to 50% of women [11]. While Poulos identified that discomfort, rather than pain, is a more appropriate descriptor of the mammography experience [12], one recent qualitative study noted that almost without exception mammography was described by women as painful [13]. Dibble et al. [14] estimate that up to 8% of women consider delaying or missing screening appointments due to the pain experienced at previous examinations. Most interventions to reduce mammography pain or discomfort (for example pre-examination pain relief) have not been successful, however the provision of written and verbal information were identified within a systematic review to be the most helpful intervention in counteracting the

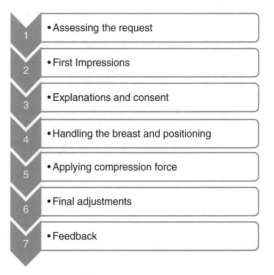

Fig. 14.1 Complex decision making and problem solving in mammography—the seven stages of the mammography examination. (Taken from Nightingale et al. [8] reprinted with permission from Elsevier)

'experienced' discomfort [15]. However negative experiences are also associated with factors other than pain, such as a perceived lack of information, especially about benign breast conditions, and the demeanor and attitude of the practitioner [16].

Socio-demographic variables such as age, family history and breast size do not seem to be consistently associated with the amount of pain experienced during a mammogram [6]. Conversely, nervousness and anxiety have been found to be associated with painful mammograms [6], suggesting that there is an emotional component to the experience and/or tolerance of pain. This link offers practitioners a brief window of opportunity to potentially influence the degree of perceived discomfort, by initiating strategies to reduce nervousness and anxiety. Chapter 13 discusses this in wider detail.

Practitioner Strategies

Nightingale et al. [9] identified rapid practitioner decision-making on first meeting the client that enabled a range of anxiety-reducing strategies to be implemented (Fig. 14.2). Practitioners employ various strategies to produce quality diagnostic images whilst demonstrating empathy and professionalism. These include facilitating a degree of client empowerment by encouraging the clients to comment on the level of compression force themselves, or at least advising when the level is uncomfortable [8, 9].

Clarke and Iphofen [17] offered an individual patient perspective which identified that being encouraged to say 'stop' during a procedure was very empowering. Bruyninckx et al. also stressed that this very act of speaking out could reduce perceived pain levels [18]. However, some clients

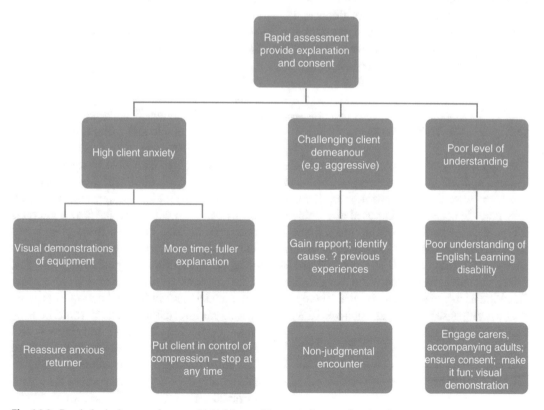

Fig. 14.2 Psychological approaches—rapid decision making upon first meeting the client. (Adapted from Nightingale et al. [8] reprinted with permission from Elsevier)

may insist on ceasing the application of compression force when it is insufficient for acceptable image quality, thus giving the practitioner a dilemma. How the practitioner addresses this dilemma will have implications for either image quality, client experience, or both, and these difficult practitioner-client interactions are found to be influenced to some extent by the values and behaviours of the individual practitioner, and indeed the culture of the wider screening unit.

Murphy et al. [8] identified within some mammography screening units what they described as 'tribal' cultural influences upon mammography practitioners, where (compression) practice was not necessarily supported by an evidence base but more associated with local social factors. They recognised that the mammography practitioner-client interaction was a paradox of humanistic caring against the demands of imaging technologies, presenting difficult challenges and decisions for individual practitioners [8]. Therefore, from the study of Murphy et al. it is reasonable to suggest that the client experience may differ from one practitioner to another, and between different screening units [8].

Compression Techniques

The application of compression force varies between and within practitioners [19]. Since the numerical scale for compression force is rarely referred to in some units, but used as a guide in others, the look and feel of the breast tissue is often considered to be a better indicator of optimum compression force [8, 9], Chaps. 27 and 28 will expand upon compression force application. Practitioners included in Murphy et al.'s study [8] refer to a response to verbal and non-verbal feedback from the client.

Client Anxieties

Although the application of compression force appears to provoke anxiety in lots of women, several studies have identified other causes of anxieties as being very significant in the overall client experience. This includes issues associated with privacy, dignity, the process itself and understandably the implications of finding breast cancer [5, 6]. Murphy et al. [8] found that practitioners identified overt differences in behaviours and anxiety levels between clients attending screening for the first time (*prevalent screen*) and those attending for follow up screening (*incident screen*), and this prompted different practitioner responses. First attenders were often extremely anxious and a more detailed explanation was required, often including a demonstration of the equipment. Repeat attenders were often influenced by a prior 'poor' experience, requiring a degree of gentle persuasion by the practitioners [8, 9]. In some cases 'white lies' (harmless mistruths told in the belief it will benefit the client) about new and improved equipment were told to reassure clients that the discomfort they previously experienced will be reduced [8].

Client Engagement

Various client groups may have additional concerns that result in poor engagement with the screening programme. Such groups might arise from different ethnic and cultural backgrounds [20], those who may be unable to communicate in the language spoken in that country, those with learning difficulties [21], or those with lack of mobility [22]. Engagement with such groups can be challenging [23], and interpersonal relationships between these clients and their social networks (family and close friends) influences breast screening behaviour [24, 25]. A requirement for close working with local group leaders and individual carers to provide clear client information leaflets would be beneficial (including language translations and visual guides for learning disability), but there is no substitute on these occasions for an open and friendly approach to welcoming the client. However, for some of these 'hard to reach' client groups, there may be a growing role for positive local, regional and national social media to encourage attendance for breast screening (Chap. 15).

The Breast Clinic Experience

Following breast screening a client may be recalled for a repeat mammography examination (*technical recall*) because the images are deemed to be non-diagnostic. Within the UK, practitioners should record no more than 3% technical recalls with a target of 2% [1]. Technical recalls use additional resources, result in additional radiation dose and are inconvenient for the client, increasing their anxiety about the potential diagnosis.

Some clients, however, are referred to a breast clinic for additional investigations because an abnormality is suspected, and these include both symptomatic clients and screening assessment clients. There is inevitably a high degree of anxiety about potential findings for both client groups. Symptomatic clients will have identified a physical sign of breast disease (for example: breast lump, nipple discharge) which their doctor considers requires urgent referral. While this will clearly be worrying for the symptomatic client, breast screening clients subsequently recalled to a breast assessment clinic are likely to experience an additional feeling of 'shock' [26].

Assessment clinic appointment letters which arrive unexpectedly have been criticised by low-income ethnic minority women in one American study as being difficult to understand [27]. In the UK, there may be a delay of several days between informing the client of the need for their breast clinic appointment and the date of the actual appointment. In other countries the delay can be longer. These few days of delay may be filled with worry for the client, their friends and relatives; while some studies report that support from significant others is comforting, it does not diminish the women's anxiety [28]. The quality of the invitation letter and information leaflet are very significant in this pre-attendance period; personal contact by telephone from a health professional has also been found to be very beneficial in this early 'waiting' stage [28].

It is understandable that clients referred to a breast clinic will have anxiety related to the potential diagnosis of breast cancer. As this is the most common female cancer in Western civilisations, with a one in seven lifetime risk of women developing the disease [29], it is highly likely that many clients will have been in some way 'affected' by the disease, either through friends or relatives with the condition. Clients with a strong family history of the disease across several generations may experience heightened anxiety that is disproportionate to the actual risk factors [30] because they may be unaware of significant improvements in early diagnosis, treatment options and survival in recent years. Severe worry has been identified as a barrier to mammography use in higher risk women, but this is also found in normal risk populations [31]. There is once again a vital role for accurate verbal and written communication of appropriate information with clients. Nevertheless, the degree of anxiety experienced by clients could be extremely high on entering the clinic, since they have had several days to consider the potential outcomes.

Client Interventions

Clients attending a screening assessment or symptomatic clinic are likely to have a combination of additional tests in a single visit, including clinical consultations and breast assessment such as standard mammography, additional mammographic projections, ultrasound scan, and interventional procedures such as aspirations and biopsies. While the 'one-stop' visit may be resource efficient and give a more rapid diagnosis, inevitably the clients may feel they are on a diagnostic 'conveyor-belt', being passed from one room to another with little continuity. Similarly, there is potential for the client to receive information very quickly which may not give them sufficient time to process and come to terms with the diagnosis, although in a survey by Hodgson et al. [32] ($n = 46$) all participants either agreed or strongly agreed that they had received sufficient information and enough time for discussion within their breast assessment clinic visit.

The assessment client journey could involve several individual staff-client interactions with a range of health care professions. While individual staff-client encounters are expected to be highly professional and empathetic, there is the potential for information overload and in some cases insufficient information being provided to the client. While staff are likely to make significant efforts to gauge the understanding and information needs of their clients, O'Connell et al. identified that many of the medical terms used in consultation with breast surgeons was not understood and this adversely affected the patient experience [33]. For this reason, the appointment of a named individual to act as a guide to escort the client through the clinic experience, where resources allow, may be beneficial. Alternatively having the same person to 'open' the patient journey (initial greetings and explanations of the procedure) and to 'close' the journey at the end (summary of findings and next step), preferably in a pleasant and private environment, would facilitate personalised care.

Interventional Procedures

Clients where suspicion of cancer is high may require a biopsy, and these procedures may be associated with discomfort or even pain, although in one study the discomfort was categorised as only 'minimal' [34]. In most cases the biopsy results may take several days to be processed, requiring the client to return several days later. This additional wait can add to the client's anxiety, although in many centres the client will be placed under the care of a breast care nurse who will 'escort' them through the process and be a point of contact within the intervening period. They may also be their point of contact throughout their treatment should this be required.

Difficult Client Conversations

Following on from Chap. 13, difficult conversations with clients such as communicating bad news, is a necessary task within a breast clinic. The most senior staff will often be expected to engage in these conversations, which may leave a

lasting impression on the client and any accompanying relatives. Sasson et al. [35] found that radiology staff experienced stress explaining results to patients and responding to their emotions. Collins analysed 100 consultations and found a distinction between doctors using technical language and nurses who disclosed results with a more patient-centred approach [36]. Kalber suggests that healthcare professionals working predominantly within an oncology setting may be better equipped in delivering results [37]. This coincides with the theory that mammographers demonstrate increased emotional intelligence compared with general radiographers [38].

While accredited communication skills training exists to better prepare staff to engage in these difficult conversations, peer support and debriefing is likely to be required to ensure the continuing well-being of the staff working regularly in this challenging environment. Burnout and fatigue is often reported within obstetric sonography; however informal debriefing sessions have shown to alleviate emotional burden [39]. Warnock et al. reports an array of emotional challenges from various healthcare professionals which may lead to anxiety [40].

The application of a communication model during difficult client conversation has been found to ensure understanding whilst reducing distress [41]. Various communication models exist including BREAKS [42] and COMFORT [43], however these often focus on pre-planned consultations; the SPIKES communication model is often taught and applied to the UK NHS 'Connected' communication skills training [44].

Improving Re-attendance

While attendance at a screening assessment clinic is not the only factor to influence a clients' decision to participate in subsequent screening, the assessment clinic experience is intensely stressful, with increases in anxiety, worry and intrusive thoughts occurring in the short and medium term [45]. One study also identified negative effects

6 months after a false positive result, but noted surprisingly that these were experienced at a similar level to women who had received a diagnosis of cancer [46]. Even after 3 years these clients still reported greater negative psychosocial consequences compared to those with normal screening findings [46]. This 3 year timeframe coincides with an invitation for the next UK routine screen—just receiving such an invitation has been shown to increase negative thoughts [26].

Screening units should be proactive in encouraging re-attendance for clients with previous false positive results, as well as those from client groups which are often under-represented in screening, using a variety of methods such as reminder letters and follow up phone calls [47]. However, the most important predictor for encouraging re-attendance for breast screening is an effective client experience, which, albeit constrained by time and resources, is within the gift of the practitioners working within the screening service.

Delivering Results

Core members of the breast team, particularly those directly involved with assessment clinics, should undergo accredited advanced communication skills training. Within the UK, although traditionally, radiographers are not involved in the disclosure of results, the possibility of role extension requires consideration. The NHSBSP assessment guidelines [48] states that 'all women with a diagnosis of breast cancer should receive their results in the presence of a clinician and a clinical nurse specialist in breast care'. This may be interpreted to include an advanced practitioner radiographer delivering results, in conjunction with a clinical breast care nurse for those patients with a malignant outcome.

A recent study explored the perceptions of advanced practitioner radiographers in delivering breast biopsy results within a single UK screening centre [49]. The findings suggested that role extension is within the radiographer scope of practice, and although further training is required

with radiology support, this has been successful. Radiographers have repeated interaction with clients throughout their care journey, from screening to biopsy during assessment, and whilst that continuity of care may be unique within the context of mammography, there is a familiarity of the role. Additionally, advanced practitioners have experience and advanced knowledge in imaging and biopsy procedures.

It is considered essential for those working within results clinics to have interventional experience, advanced communication skills training and a supportive radiological environment. Participation in the multi-disciplinary team meetings is crucial to understand appropriate patient management, whilst increasing clinician confidence in the delivery of the result. Given the increasing pressures on the radiology workforce, skill-mix with the development of advanced practitioners is essential [50]. Field and Snaith report clinical resistance to advanced practice, with radiologists often the main impediment [51]. However, supportive radiology units have shown to blur the professional boundaries to improve patient outcomes with radiographers performing many of the tasks traditionally undertaken by radiologists. Radiographers who report images have shown to positively impact on the workload with practitioners reporting to a comparable standard to radiologists [52–54].

Inclusion of advanced practitioners delivering results may increase efficiency, enabling radiologists to concentrate on other tasks. Increased role development and team cohesion is also likely with experience. Although patient satisfaction remains unexplored, the paternalistic hierarchy of medicine may be unjustified given the continuity of care provided by other healthcare workers. Within the UK, radiographer led practice without the need for medical (doctor) input is becoming more commonplace with autonomous radiographer decision making in interventional procedures and client/patient discharge. The collaboration of various professional roles highlights the patient centred approach which is significant in breast imaging.

Clinical Pearls

- Advanced communication skills training can be considered an essential requirement for all core members of the breast care team
- Application of a communication model such as SPIKES can assist during difficult conversations whilst ensuring understanding and reducing overall distress
- Good client experience can impact positively on re-attendance for breast screening

Chapter Review Questions
Review Questions

1. Discuss the main challenges of client-practitioner interactions in the breast care service setting.
2. What reasons may clients be recalled from screening?
3. Consider the benefits of advanced practitioner radiographers in delivering breast biopsy results within the breast screening service.

Answers

1. Client experience is influenced by fear, discomfort, waiting, physical environment and staff interactions. Practitioner engagement using communication strategies, compression techniques. Relevant, comprehensible information to alleviate anxiety. Misinformation, cultural beliefs, communication difficulties and social media behaviours may all induce fear. The waiting following a recall letter for further assessment and the physical environment of an unfamiliar clinical setting.
2. Technical issue with the images for example non diagnostic. Additional imaging required such as digital breast tomosynthesis or ultrasound. Triple assessment approach (further imaging including ultrasound, clinical breast examination and/or biopsy). Clinical symptom as indi-

cated at the time of screening. Asymptomatic abnormality which requires follow up.
3. Radiologist workforce pressures and increasing workload to breast imaging services.

    Role development, within the scope of the advanced practitioner. Impact on increasing continuing professional development with development of advanced communication skills through an accredited training programme. Team cohesiveness within the breast imaging unit with potential for enhanced patient satisfaction due to reduced waiting times and improved patient experience.

Appendix

Test your learning and check your understanding of this book's contents: use the "Springer Nature Flashcards" app to access questions using https://sn.pub/dcAnWL.

To use the app, please follow the instructions in Chap. 1.

Flashcard code: 48341-69945-ABCB1-2A8C7-CE9D2.

Short URL: https://sn.pub/dcAnWL.

References

1. Public Heath England. Breast screening: guidance for breast screening mammographers. https://www.gov.uk/government/publications/breast-screening-quality-assurance-for-mammography-and-radiography. Accessed 12 Feb 2022.
2. National Cancer Peer Review Programme. Manual for cancer services: breast cancer measures version 1.1. https://assets.publishing.service.gov.uk/government/uploads/system/uploads/attachment_data/file/216117/dh_125890.pdf. Accessed 12 Feb 2022.
3. National Cancer Peer Review Programme. Report 2009/2010: breast MDTs. https://www.gov.uk/government/publications/national-cancer-peer-review-programme-report-2010-11. Accessed 12 Feb 2022.
4. National Cancer Peer Review Programme. Report 2011/2012: breast MDTs. https://assets.publishing.service.gov.uk/government/uploads/system/uploads/attachment_data/file/216205/dh_131669.pdf. Accessed 12 Feb 2022.
5. Clark S, Reeves PJ. Women's experiences of mammography: a thematic evaluation of the literature. Radiography. 2015;21(1):84–8.

6. Davey B. Pain during mammography: possible risk factors and ways to alleviate pain. Radiography. 2007;13(3):229–34.

7. Sharp PC, Michielutte R, Freimanis R, Cunningham L, Spangler J, Burnette V. Reported pain following mammography screening. Arch Intern Med. 2003;163(7):833–6.

8. Murphy F, Nightingale J, Hogg P, Robinson L, Seddon D, Mackay S. Compression force behaviours: an exploration of the beliefs and values influencing the application of breast compression during screening mammography. Radiography. 2015;21(1):30–5.

9. Nightingale JM, Murphy FJ, Robinson L, Newton-Hughes A, Hogg P. Breast compression—an exploration of problem solving and decision-making in mammography. Radiography. 2015;21(4):364–9.

10. Poulos A, McLean D, Rickard M, Heard R. Breast compression in mammography; how much is enough? J Med Imaging Radiat Oncol. 2003;47(2):121–6.

11. Bai JY, He ZY, Dong JN, Yao GH, Chen HX, Li KA. Correlation of pain experience during mammography with factors of breast density and breast compressed thickness. J Shanghai Jiaotong Univ. 2010;30(9):1062–6.

12. Poulos A. Having a mammogram: how does it feel? Radiographer. 2004;51(3):129–31.

13. Mathers SA, McKenzie GA, Robertson EM. 'It was daunting': experience of women with a diagnosis of breast cancer attending for breast imaging. Radiography. 2013;19(2):156–63.

14. Dibble SL, Israel J, Nussey B, Sayre JW, Brenner RJ, Sickles EA. Mammography with breast cushions. Womens Health Issues. 2005;15(2):55–63.

15. Miller D, Livingstone V, Herbison GP, Vermeulen H. Interventions for relieving the pain and discomfort of screening mammography 1. Nederlands Tijdschrift Voor Evid Based Pract. 2013;11(1):15–6.

16. Robinson L, Hogg P, Newton-Hughes A. The power and the pain: mammographic compression research from the service-users' perspective. Radiography. 2013;19(3):190–5.

17. Clarke KA, Iphofen R. Breast cancer: a personal reflective account. Synergy. 2006;27:12–6.

18. Bruyninckx E, Mortelmans D, Van Goethem M, Van Hove E. Risk factors of pain in mammographic screening. Soc Sci Med. 1999;49(7):933–41.

19. Mercer CE, Hogg P, Szczepura K, Denton ERE. Practitioner compression force variation in mammography: a 6-year study. Radiography. 2013;19(3):200–6.

20. Jafri NF, Ayyala RS, Ozonoff A, Jordan-Gray J, Slanetz PJ. Screening mammography: does ethnicity influence patient preferences for higher recall rates given the potential for earlier detection of breast cancer? Radiology. 2008;249(3):785–91.

21. Wilkinson JE, Deis CE, Bowen DJ, Bokhour BG. 'It's easier said than done': perspectives on mammography from women with intellectual disabilities. Ann Family Med. 2011;9(2):142–7.

22. Liu SY, Clark MA. Breast and cervical cancer screening practices among disabled women aged 40-75: does quality of the experience matter? J Women's Health. 2008;17(8):1321–9.

23. Watson-Johnson LC, DeGroff A, Steele CB, Revels M, Smith JL, Justen E, Barron-Simpson R, Sanders L, Richardson LC. Mammography adherence: a qualitative study. J Women's Health. 2011;20(12):1887–94.

24. Kaltsa A, Holloway A, Cox K. Factors that influence mammography screening behaviour: a qualitative study of Greek women's experiences. Eur J Oncol Nurs. 2013;17(3):292–301.

25. Browne JL, Chan AYC. Using the Theory of Planned Behaviour and implementation intentions to predict and facilitate upward family communication about mammography. Psychol Health. 2012;27(6):655–73.

26. Brett J, Bankhead C, Henderson B, Watson E, Austoker J. The psychological impact of mammographic screening. A systematic review. Psychooncology. 2005;14(11):917–38.

27. Marcus EN, Drummond D, Dietz N. Urban women's preferences for learning of their mammogram result: a qualitative study. J Cancer Educ. 2012;27(1):156–64.

28. Pineault P. Breast cancer screening: women's experiences of waiting for further testing. Oncol Nurs Forum. 2007;34(4):847–53.

29. Cancer Research UK. Cancer statistics. https://www.cancerresearchuk.org/about-cancer/breast-cancer/about. Accessed 2 Dec 2020.

30. Sauven P. Guidelines for the management of women at increased familial risk of breast cancer. Eur J Cancer. 2004;40(5):653–65.

31. Andersen MR, Smith R, Meischke H, Bowen D, Urban N. Breast cancer worry and mammography use by women with and without a family history in a population-based sample. Cancer Epidemiol Biomark Prev. 2003;12:314–20.

32. Hodgson L, Dixon AM, Turley L, Sharma N. Vote of confidence. Imag Ther Pract. 2013;101:5–10.

33. O'Connell RL, Hartridge-Lambert SK, Din N, St John ER, Hitchins C, Johnson T. Patients' understanding of medical terminology used in the breast clinic. Breast. 2013;22(5):836–8.

34. Brandon CJ, Mullan PB. Patients' perception of care during image-guided breast biopsy in a rural community breast center: communication matters. J Cancer Educ. 2011;26(1):156–60.

35. Sasson JP, Zand T, Lown BA. Communication in the diagnostic mammography suite: implications for practice and training. Acad Radiol. 2008;15(4):417–24.

36. Collins S. Explanations in consultations: the combined effectiveness of doctors' and nurses' communication with patients. Med Educ. 2005;39(8):785–96.

37. Kalber B. Breaking bad news—whose responsibility is it? Eur J Cancer Care. 2009;18(4):330.

38. Mackay SJ, Hogg P, Cooke G, Baker RD, Dawkes T. A UK-wide analysis of trait emotional intelligence within the radiography profession. Radiography. 2012;18(3):166–71.

39. Thomas S, O'Loughlin K, Clarke J. The 21st century sonographer: role ambiguity in communicating an adverse outcome in obstetric ultrasound. Cogent Medicine. 2017;4(1):1373903.

40. Warnock C, Buchanan J, Tod AM. The difficulties experienced by nurses and healthcare staff involved in the process of breaking bad news. J Adv Nurs. 2017;73(7):1632–45.

41. Maguire P, Pitceathly C. Key communication skills and how to acquire them. BMJ. 2002;325(7366):697–700.

42. Narayanan V, Bista B, Koshy C. 'BREAKS' protocol for breaking bad news. Indian J Palliat Care. 2010;16(2):61.

43. Villagran M, Goldsmith J, Wittenberg-Lyles E, Baldwin P. Creating COMFORT: a communication-based model for breaking bad news. Commun Educ. 2010;59(3):220–34.

44. Baile WF, Buckman R, Lenzi R, Glober G, Beale EA, Kudelka AP. SPIKES—a six-step protocol for delivering bad news: application to the patient with cancer. Oncologist. 2000;5(4):302–11.

45. Rimer BK, Bluman LG. The psychosocial consequences of mammography. J Nat Cancer Inst Monogr. 1997;22:131–8.

46. Brodersen J, Siersma VD. Long-term psychosocial consequences of false-positive screening mammography. Ann Fam Med. 2013;11(2):106–15.

47. Costanza ME, Luckmann R, White MJ, Rosal MC, Cranos C, Reed G, Clark R, Sama S, Yood R. Design and methods for a randomized clinical trial comparing three outreach efforts to improve screening mammography adherence. BMC Health Serv Res. 2011;11(1):1–11.

48. Wallis M, Borrelli C, Cohen S, Duncan A, Given-Wilson R, Jenkins J, Kearins O, Pinder S, Sharma N, Sibbering M, Steel J. Clinical guidance for breast cancer screening assessment. 4th ed. London: Public Health England; 2016.

49. Eden JK, Borgen R. Exploring the perceptions of advanced practitioner radiographers at a single breast screening unit in extending their role from delivering benign to malignant biopsy results; a preliminary study. Br J Radiol. 2020;93:20200423.

50. The Royal College of Radiologists. Clinical radiology UK workforce census 2016 report BFCR(17)6. London: The Royal College of Radiologists; 2017.

51. Field LJ, Snaith BA. Developing radiographer roles in the context of advanced and consultant practice. J Med Radiat Sci. 2013;60(1):11–5.

52. Thom SE. Does advanced practice in radiography benefit the healthcare system? A literature review. Radiography. 2018;24(1):84–9.

53. Torres-Mejía G, Smith RA, de la Luz C-FM, Bogart A, Martínez-Matsushita L, Miglioretti DL, Kerlikowske K, Ortega-Olvera C, Montemayor-Varela E, Angeles-Llerenas A, Bautista-Arredondo S. Radiographers supporting radiologists in the interpretation of screening mammography: a viable strategy to meet the shortage in the number of radiologists. BMC Cancer. 2015;15(1):1–2.

54. Wivell G, Denton ER, Eve CB, Inglis JC, Harvey I. Can radiographers read screening mammograms? Clin Radiol. 2003;58(1):63–7.

Digital Health Technologies

15

Marie Griffiths, Beverley Scragg, Julie R. Stein-Hodgins, and Cathy Ure

Learning Objectives

- Recognise and understand the digital health and social media landscape for practitioners
- Recognise the appropriateness of the different platforms/social media for health promotion in breast screening
- Understand how social media can enhance and support communication around breast screening attendance
- Develop a critical awareness of the current practitioner practices when using social media

- Recognise the benefits of becoming involved in health promotion via digital health
- Participate in professional social media use to enhance Continuing Professional Development (CDP) portfolio

M. Griffiths (✉)
Salford Business School, University of Salford, Manchester, UK
e-mail: m.griffiths@salford.ac.uk

B. Scragg · C. Ure
School of Health and Society, University of Salford, Manchester, UK
e-mail: b.c.scragg1@salford.ac.uk;
c.m.ure1@salford.ac.uk

J. R. Stein-Hodgins
Pennine Breast Unit, Bradford, UK

The Concept of Digital Health for Promoting Health

Defining the concept of digital health is problematic given that its current scope encompasses broad areas of health, fitness and well-being. How digital health is consumed, and by who, adds different layers of complexity when attempting to agree common terminology and theorise 'digital health'. For instance, the lexicon of digital health encompasses eHealth, health apps, telehealth and 'the quantified self'—the cultural phenomenon of self-tracking [1]. The digital transformation of health draws on emerging concepts such as Health 4.0, connected health, healthcare big data, the Internet of Medical Things (IoMT), cloud computing, augmented reality and block chain [2]. In an attempt, to clarify such complexities in this burgeoning area, the World Health Organisation (WHO) formulated a detailed taxonomy of digital health [3]. However, whilst we have demonstrated the difficulty in arriving at a definition, for the purposes of this chapter, we will consider digital health as an umbrella term for the use of digital technologies that have transformed or are transforming the way healthcare services are conceived and delivered. We suggest it does this through three basic features providing: information, personal support, and improved access.

- Firstly, digital health offers individuals easily accessible information in a range of formats that empowers them to track, self-manage and control their own and their family's health. Smartphone penetration in the United Kingdom (UK) has continued to grow year on year and in 2021 has now reached 92% [4]. The digital health app space is already crowded. In 2020, 90,000 new apps were brought to the global market, amounting to more than 350,000 apps currently available to consumers. More specifically, 47% of digital health apps are now focused upon managing health conditions [5].
- Secondly, digital health refers to the technological developments that underpin its ability to provide personal support including, but not limited to: the world wide web (www), cloud computing, social media, mobile devices and global positioning systems (GPS), as well as bio-sensing technologies and wearables that are cost-effective, portable, and non-evasive. The size of this market is demonstrated by spending on wearable devices forecast globally to be in the region of $81.5 billion in 2021 [6].
- Thirdly, digital health provision seeks to improve and increase access to healthcare whilst improving the quality of service, reducing costs and delivering an increasingly personalised service. Other improvements include remote monitoring and the use of digital messaging to remind and alert individuals to their treatments, prescriptions or appointments [7]. For instance, these include text messaging reminder services to reduce the number of missed breast screening appointments in England, UK [8]. In all areas, digital

healthcare is growing exponentially providing enormous potential for future improvements.

Using Social Media for Health Promotion

The umbrella of digital healthcare provision includes social media—a set of tools that can be used for health promotion [9, 10]. For the purpose of this chapter, we consider that social media refers to a group of internet-based applications that allow the creation and exchange of user-generated content [11]. It is an umbrella term for a range of user-generated platforms including Facebook, YouTube and Twitter (Fig. 15.1). By utilising a range of these applications, patients or clients can generate and access content related to health education, information, networking, research, support, goal-setting and tracking personal progress [12]. In the UK, 82% of users use at least one social networking site (an 18% increase since our original chapter published in 2015 [13]), with Facebook (86%), Instagram (47%), YouTube (39%), and Twitter (31%) being the most popular [14].

In the first edition of Digital Mammography, Robinson et al. argued that extending patient/client participation beyond the physical space of the doctor's surgery or healthcare unit was achievable if clinicians, academics, and the public could harness social media effectively [13]. No-one could have foreseen the impact of the COVID-19 pandemic and the swift mobilization of clinicians and patients to engage virtually [15, 16]. While some argue that social media has fundamentally altered health promotion and how health care professionals (HCPs) interact with patients [9], others argue the use of social media platforms by healthcare professionals for professional purposes are still very much at the embryonic stage [17]. In a study of Australian healthcare professionals ($n = 219$) working in hospitals, clinics, and other clinical environments, only 19% used Facebook, 12% used Twitter, 25% used YouTube,

Types of social media	Examples	Why are they used?
Social networks	Facebook, LinkedIn, TikTok	To connect with people (or brands e.g., UK National Health Service Breast Screening Programme, NHSBSP) online
Media sharing networks	Instagram, Snapchat, YouTube	To find and share media online including photos, video, live video
Blogging and publishing networks	WordPress, Tumblr	To publish, find or comment on, content online

Fig. 15.1   Types of social media

21% used LinkedIn, 7% utilised blog sites, and 11% used other platforms professionally [17]. Later in this chapter, we will explore how some UK breast units have developed a social media presence since the first edition of this chapter.

Using Social Media in Breast Screening and Symptomatic Contexts

In the previous edition of this book [13], it was argued that there was sparse evidence that social media has been employed to its full potential within medical imaging and, more specifically, the asymptomatic breast imaging service in the UK. Globally, it is the case that the amount of research exploring online discourse around breast screening has increased significantly in recent years. This research, however, is dominated by secondary analysis. In other words, naturally occurring conversation on a range of social media platforms has been analysed, including Facebook [18, 19], YouTube [20, 21] and Twitter [22–27]. In a systematic review of online breast cancer screening discourse (n = 17 studies), Döbrössy et al. reported most online discussion is driven by non-healthcare professional lay people [28]. Indeed, the absence of professional input and the need for more active involvement from practitioners in online breast screening online was reported in many of the studies. It remains the case therefore, that evidence remains limited regarding online interaction with asymptomatic breast imaging practitioners and clients. In the

next section, we discuss how the UK focused WoMMeN (Word of Mouth Mammography e-Network) project explored how to support online conversations between practitioners and clients.

Using Social Media to Communicate with Clients

Within the UK, the WoMMeN project started in 2013, with the aim of creating an online space to inform clients about breast screening. The central premise of WoMMeN was to explore the concept of enabling supportive conversations between breast screening professionals and clients. A feasibility study, comprising 94 survey questionnaires and two focus groups, found that women users of the UK's National Health Service Breast Screening Programme (NHSBSP) broadly felt an online breast screening digital social network would be useful in helping them prepare for a mammogram [29]. Consequently, the WoMMeN project explored how interaction in a 'digital space' would work from two different perspectives. Firstly a 'digital space' was designed using participatory methods in a closed 'user design' Facebook group (n = 71 members). Here, discussion between clients, and the project team (consisting of a patient involvement researcher, mammographers, radiographers, business/social media experts and media psychologists) led to the design of a prototype 'digital space' in which breast screening professionals and clients could 'talk'.

Research analysis showed subtle differences in the emphasis placed on requirements from a 'digital space'. While practitioners emphasised concern over the provision of accurate information, clients focused on experiential (subjective) information and control over the amount of information they wanted [30]. A moderated space, with access to a variety of information sources ranging in complexity was identified as key. Interestingly, further conversation analysis work explored contributions in the User Design Group between clients and our subject experts [31]. In terms of interacting on social media, this has provided some useful insights. We found that when engaging on social media with breast screening clients, practitioners need to be careful not to diminish or downplay lay experiences and inadvertently close down conversation/communication. At the same time, it was recognised that there was a need to understand how practitioners might feel about 'talking' to clients online and using social media as part of their role. NHSBSP practitioners ($n = 78$) were specifically asked about any perceived challenges [32]. These were framed as the requirement to:

- Work within boundaries (including professional/legal; time; and in relation to the provision of accurate information).
- Have support from the employer to use social media as part of their role (including access to technology; skills development; and supportive practices) and having managerial support.

The WoMMeN project team found that practitioners' reluctance to engage with clients through social media was fueled by the thought of an error being amplified by a rogue social media post 'going viral' [32]. Their feelings were possibly reinforced by perceptions relating to social media use aligned to their working environment. In a sample of UK National Health Service (NHS) employers' social media policies, HCP's use of social media was viewed negatively on the whole [33]. To support practitioner social media use to engage with clients online, work by the WoMMeN project team has led to The Society of Radiographers developing a new guidance document for practitioners in the UK [34]. Detailed

below are eight tips for staying safe on social media from that guidance [34]:

- Choose the appropriate platform for the audience/community you want to engage with.
- Represent your profession with integrity and pride.
- Know the boundaries of your expertise and be willing to signpost to other sources of information.
- Speak out when you witness inappropriate online behaviour.
- Respect confidentiality and dignity of colleagues, employers, and service-users.
- Be professional in your communication at all times.
- Only say what you would be willing to say face-to-face and in any public arena.
- Check your employer's policy on Social Media use

Despite the trepidation surrounding the use of social media for direct communication between practitioner and client, it should be recognised that the reach of digital communication far outweighs face to face or telephonic means. It is this increased reach that can be exploited to support mass screening programmes. The potential reach of social media can be measured, although there is no way to tell whether this 'reach' will translate into action. An early United States pilot study found that a targeted information campaign for public health on Google Search, Facebook and Twitter reached 17 million people, translating into 51,397 active engagements (users clicking onto the advertisements), and that in 2014 this could be achieved for less than $1 for each active engagement [35]. This does demonstrate that although the most popular social media platforms are free to use, for organisational use they are not cost neutral, and thus in the resource stretched environment of the UK's NHS this may be a substantial barrier to use without proven benefits. Overall evidence of the effectiveness of social media in relation to public health (health promotion) is lacking [36]. That said, qualitative benefits have been identified in relation to psychosocial support and psychological functioning [36]. The authors recommend that future studies need careful design, taking into account cost-effectiveness and patient outcomes.

As we have seen, contrary to a national strategy in the UK of 'digital by default' [37], evidence that online discourse between practitioners and clients is still not plentiful. Anecdotally, however, Facebook pages seem to be the most utilised method by which two-way communication happens for this group of clients. Traditionally, health promotion campaigns in the field of cancer screening are difficult to evaluate in terms of patient outcomes, as the time lag required for a benefit to become apparent makes it difficult to then link to the campaign which provoked the necessary action [38]. However, the NHS Digital's Widening Digital Participation Programme used social media to improve breast screening rates by 13% over 4 years in Stoke-On-Trent (UK) [39], a North Midlands local authority with higher than average deprivation, in the prevalent round attenders over one screening round. This was achieved by linking with other health providers, such as primary care practices and community groups via their Facebook pages to promote the service and by also being open to accepting direct messages from potential clients [40]. The Kings Fund—a UK independent think tank—recently championed this activity by practitioners, in their framework document on tackling inequalities. They stated:

> Radiographers in the North Midlands used social media to help improve breast screening rates across the region. They used Facebook and other methods to communicate screening-specific information to service users to increase the reach of this information despite limited funds. [41].

It is well recognised that significant challenges relate to using social media both personally and in a professional context including, but not limited to: the volume of data, misinformation, fake news, patient data privacy, poor quality information; the practitioner/client boundary management and social media management [9, 28, 32, 42, 43]. The absence of practitioner engagement on social media, potentially because of concerns relating to these issues, means that lay persons create the majority of content, with lay misunderstandings of the harms and benefits of mammography still prevalent [28]. Significantly,

scientifically reliable information attracts the same amount of engagement as lay misunderstandings and misinformation, potentially leading to the distrust of social media as a source of valid information about mammography [28], with the new phenomena of 'fake news' in this context revealing itself to be more akin to the old adage "Falsehood flies, and the Truth comes limping after it". The study authors argue this will only be counteracted with more direct interaction between healthcare providers and clients, which in turn may improve the efficacy of health promotion. With continuing calls for practitioners to engage with clients through social media, we now turn to exploring use in a professional context for ongoing development.

Using Social Media for Continuing Professional Development

Continuing Professional Development (CPD) is expected by professional bodies within the UK; indeed, it is a regulatory requirement [44]. CPD should also be recorded as evidence, not only that the activity was completed, but that learning occurred and that it had impact upon professional practice and patient outcomes, if possible.

Social Media has the capacity to inform, debate and discuss within a media-rich environment and thus should be able to provide an arena in which CPD can occur. Social media is used for professional development in other healthcare professions including the successful #We Communities Tweet Chats on Twitter which were started by a nurse. In response, the medical radiation community in the UK set up a monthly online journal club using Twitter. This blends the traditional CPD method of journal clubs with the online use of social media, thereby increasing reach from individual hospitals to global participation. Open Access journal articles are used for the basis of a discussion lasting 1 h and accessed by filtering Twitter content using the hashtag #MedRadJClub. One such tweet chat, about how people used the journal club, was analysed by Bolderston et al. in 2018 [45]. They found evidence that the discourse was influencing practice and that professionals used the tweet chats as evidence for CPD, with one person commenting that they would use the available Twitter transcript as evidence. However, it must be noted that this does not present evidence that learning has occurred.

While studies of social media use for continuous development are available [45, 46], the evidence that social media is used for CPD activities by practitioners remains scant [46]. CPD for UK practitioners has been mandatory for longer than Irish practitioners, which was introduced in 2015. A 2018 study sought to identify barriers and motivators around CPD participation, mechanisms of CPD delivery and confidence of practitioners in using e-learning [46]. At this time, 48% of the cohort ($n = 453$) considered that social media was acceptable for delivering CPD, however those in the 50–59 age group were more resistant to its use in this way. The study authors concluded that there was a broad willingness, regardless of age, to engage in CPD using hand-held technologies and social media to facilitate what they called "on the go" CPD engagement. The erosion of the private-professional boundary was identified as a cause for concern by half of the cohort when identifying barriers to using social media, although the barriers to CPD itself were mainly funding, time and location. Social media can overcome many of these traditional barriers, but the erosion of the boundaries between work and home life is a different matter and is a legitimate concern. Some may argue that CPD time has never been given adequately by employers, and that much of this work has been undertaken in the practitioner's own time. To date, a complete picture of this has not been captured by research. We conclude this chapter by exploring how other digital technologies may change the screening environment.

What's Next? Blue Sky Thinking

While there has been some moderate use of digital health in the sector, these trail far behind digital health technologies exponential growth. In the UK, the NHSBSP has national targets. One of the key performance indicators (KPIs) is to increase the numbers of women attending for first and subsequent appointments. The innovative use of digital health technology by the NHSBSP could

enhance the client experience and therefore positively influence these KPIs. The following suggestions take the reader through the client's NHSBSP journey, identifying potential points throughout this journey where the three benefits of digital health discussed in the first part of this chapter—information, personal support and improved access—might be realised.

Pre-examination

First, it is imperative that practitioners identify their role in health promotion and take an active involvement in breast cancer awareness campaigns. Successful examples of social media used for this purpose include the practitioners previously discussed, who use a dedicated Facebook page to communicate with clients and raise awareness [39–41]. We acknowledge that this Breast Screening Unit (BSU) is, sadly, currently in the minority in the UK.

Usually, the first contact with the client is via the invitation letter and an information leaflet, which is in likely to be in the country's native language. Information about digital resources could be included in the letter as QR codes which could open up communication opportunities. Information provided at this initial contact point means all clients, attenders and non-attenders, would be made aware of sources of support. For example, many clients will have a similar set of Frequently Asked Questions (FAQs), which have been answered by the screening programme and presented in the information leaflet. Others are using DVDs to help promote awareness [47] and in the UK's Bedfordshire and Hertfordshire BSU, this includes DVDs with sign language. However, there may be instances where a client requires other questions to be answered, or requires information in another language and here, digital technology could provide more options, alternative channels and flexibility for communication.

Appointment

Currently in the UK, screening appointments are block booked, with no gaps or clear spaces between clients. The 'smart clinic' probability booking system is also popular; whereby appointment slots are 'overbooked' with several clients allocated the same time slot. The system does this based upon the probability that only one client will turn up at that time, and for the most part this system does work as intended, with the consequence that the BSU maximises efficiency and evens out the peaks and troughs of demand for the service [48]. However, if we look at this from the point of view of the client, their appointment is allocated at the service providers' convenience, with no chance of change unless someone else cancels their appointment, leaving a space. Appointments cannot be changed or altered without contacting the screening office within office hours, or by email giving suggested dates and times, with the resultant effect of making the service less accessible to working women.

It is suggested that the simple action of leaving spaces and allowing women to alter their appointments digitally would improve accessibility to the service. In the NHS Long Term Plan, this 'digital first' option is proffered as a goal for the whole of the NHS, and it follows that this should include screening programmes [49]. Some NHS services already use SMS appointment reminders; these are linked to options to cancel appointments via text, lessening the chance of did not attends (DNAs), but could also, with smartphone technology offer links to forums and information—again coupling the client to useful sources of support. Discussion boards and forums could be used to respond through a wider audience thus dealing with the anxieties of several clients simultaneously.

During the Examination

The physical environment has been criticised by clients as being clinical and unwelcoming [50]. Equipment manufacturers are addressing this, with a common feature now being 'mood lighting' as an addition to new mammography equipment. Furthermore, some BSU's have incorporated biophilic design into their mobile trailers by including whole wall murals of natural vistas in their examination rooms. If this is not available, digital screens displaying relaxing imagery in the waiting room

and X-ray room may be effectively employed to address such criticisms. These have been found to have a positive impact on patient pain thresholds and to reduce anxiety in breast imaging contexts [51]. Music has also been found to have a calming effect [52] and the possibility should be explored of enabling the client to choose a song from a playlist via a tablet, as they are getting changed, so that their preferred music is playing throughout the examination (refer to Chap. 13).

Post examination

It is common to see feedback mechanisms in the retail industry, designed to capture customers perceptions of their services at the point of contact simply and quickly via 'smiley face' terminals. It is suggested that these could be employed in BSU's to capture quantitative data, or to capture important client feedback so that the screening programme can address any issues raised.

The UK NHS Long Term Plan champions the person taking control of their own health record to reduce the amount of time spent repeating medical history to various health practitioners [53]. Results of tests should be made available digitally, although here a note of caution is to be raised about allowing a client to receive cancer results potentially without any other emotional support available. The timing of release of definitive results should be carefully managed. The initial screening result, whether routine recall or recall to assessment, could certainly be transmitted digitally to the client's health record.

The UK NHS App

Recently, the UK NHS App has been developed and has allowed General Practitioners/primary care physicians to offer patients various services including ordering prescriptions, booking appointments, and secure messaging. It is suggested that the screening service could also utilise this app to improve accessibility without losing efficiency in the ways suggested above—appointment bookings, providing results and information, in different languages. As the App is in its infancy, services are limited, but the question remains whether there is scope for support forums or networking to be included within the app at a later date. Not only clients, but also practitioners, would benefit from being digitally connected across a dedicated social and professional network, such as the one the WoMMeN (Word of Mouth e-Network) project initiated. Such networks promote the sharing of best practice, learning, research and innovation, enabling practitioners to ensure the service they deliver is current and evidence based. In short, the potential for the NHS App is limitless, but requires a leap of faith from the breast imaging community in the UK to realise the potential [54].

Summary

Globally, the exponential growth of digital healthcare signals continuing change in the workplace to support the achievement of KPIs. Increasing screening attendance rates, through gaining wider reach, improving knowledge, reducing fear and building supportive relationships, are strategies that can all be supported through positive adoption of digital communication including social media. Further research is needed in this field as practitioners integrate its use into their professional practice.

Clinical Pearls

- Practitioners can successfully use social media for lifelong learning and CPD purposes.
- Digital health innovations have the potential for use by clients to improve access and communication with the breast screening programme. This also allows people to 'watch or follow', thus learning from others.
- The use of digital platforms supports the drive to be inclusive. Information can be visual and easily translated. It must allow invites and results to be online for the diverse communities.

Chapter Review Questions
Review Questions

1. Explain how digital health can empower the client to improve the breast screen experience?
2. Describe how you can use social media to enhance your practice and life-long learning?

Answers

1. The chapter first provides a backdrop of the different characteristics that make up digital health and this is complimented with statistics of this growing sector. Digital health has huge potential for clients having increased access to health care, to have a personalised service and to join online communities. This chapter includes a useful structure of the different digital health activities that a client can access at the various stages of the breast screening journey. Useful examples have been given with associated research; Facebook communities being linked with other screening services; text reminders and being able to direct message practitioners. There is a good balance given of the challenges and opportunities that may impact the breast screening experience.
2. The process of using social media to enhance practice and life-long-learning must be first understood and decided if that is a suitable route for the practitioner. Research indicates that some practitioners are hesitant. For those who engage in social media, there is a wealth of opportunities, such as joining journal papers discussions, contributing to tweet chats and being part of a global community. There are also exemplars across social media of how other medical professions have grown their digital presence. It is important to ensure how evidence can be captured for the CPD process, but others have used tweet exchanges and transcripts from on-line discussions.

Appendix

Test your learning and check your understanding of this book's contents: use the "Springer Nature Flashcards" app to access questions using https://sn.pub/dcAnWL.

To use the app, please follow the instructions in Chap. 1.

Flashcard   code: 48341-69945-ABCB1-2A8C7-CE9D2.

Short URL: https://sn.pub/dcAnWL.

References

1. Lupton D. The quantified self. Malden, MA: Polity; 2016.
2. Müschenich M, Wamprecht L. Health 4.0—how are we doing tomorrow? Bundesgesundheitsbl Gesundheitsforsch Gesundheitsschutz. 2018;61(3):334–9.
3. World Health Organization. Classification of digital health interventions v1.0 : a shared language to describe the uses of digital technology for health. 2018. https://www.who.int/reproductivehealth/publications/mhealth/classification-digital-healthinterventions/en/. Accessed 11 Aug 2021.
4. Statista. UK: smartphone ownership by age from 2012-2021. 2021. https://www-statista-co.salford.idm.oclc.org/statistics/271851/smartphone-owners-in-the-united-kingdom-uk-by-age/. Accessed 9 Aug 2021.
5. Olsen E. Digital health apps balloon to more than 350,000 available on the market, according to IQVIA report. 2021. https://www.mobihealthnews.com/news/digital-health-apps-balloon-more-350000-available-market-according-iqvia-report. Accessed 10 Aug 2021.
6. Gartner. Gartner forecasts global spending on wearable devices to total $81.5 billion in 2021. https://www.gartner.com/en/newsroom/press-releases/2021-01-11-gartner-forecasts-global-spending-on-wearable-devices-to-total-81-5-billion-in-2021. Accessed 9 Aug 2021.
7. Robotham D, Satkunanathan S, Reynolds J, Stahl D, Wykes T. Using digital notifications to improve attendance in clinic: systematic review and meta-analysis. BMJ Open. 2016;6(10):e012116.
8. Public Health England Screening. Setting up reminder text messaging services in the NHS Breast Screening Programme. 2020. https://phescreening.blog.gov.uk/2020/11/19/reminder-texts-breast-screening-programme/. Accessed 27 Aug 2021.
9. Khan MI, Loh J. Benefits, challenges, and social impact of health care providers' adoption of social media. Soc Sci Comput Rev. 2021. https://doi.org/10.1177/08944393211025758. Accessed 27 Aug 2021.
10. Wallace C, McCosker A, Farmer J, White C. Spanning communication boundaries to address health inequalities: the role of community connectors and social media. J Appl Commun Res. 2021;49(6):1–9.
11. Kaplan AM, Haenlein M. Users of the world, unite! The challenges and opportunities of social media. Business Horizons. 2010;53(1):59–68.
12. Househ M, Borycki E, Kushniruk A. Empowering patients though social media: the benefits and challenges. Health Inform J. 2014;20(1):50–8.
13. Robinson L, Griffiths M, Ure CM, Wray J, Hodgins JS, Shires G. The use of digital health technology and social media to support breast screening. In: Hogg P, Kelly J, Mercer C, editors. Digital mammography: a holistic approach. New York: Springer; 2015. p. 105–11.
14. Ofcom. Adults' media use and attitudes 2021: interactive report. https://www.ofcom.org.uk/research-and-data/media-literacy-research/adults/adults-media-use-and-attitudes/interactive-tool-2021. Accessed 15 Aug 2021.
15. Bestsenny O, Gilbert G, Harris A, Rost J. Telehealth: a quarter-trillion-dollar post-COVID-19 reality? 2021. https://www.mckinsey.com/industries/healthcare-systems-and-services/our-insights/telehealth-a-quarter-trillion-dollar-post-covid-19-reality. Accessed 15 Aug 2021.
16. Monaghesh E, Hajizadeh A. The role of telehealth during COVID-19 outbreak: a systematic review based on current evidence. BMC Public Health. 2020;20(1):1–9.
17. Khan MI, Saleh MA, Quazi A. Social media adoption by health professionals: a TAM-based study. Informatics. 2021;8(1):6.
18. Huesch M, Chetlen A, Segel J, Schetter S. Frequencies of private mentions and sharing of mammography and breast cancer terms on Facebook: a pilot study. J Med Internet Res. 2017;19(6):201.
19. Klippert H, Schaper A. Using Facebook to communicate mammography messages to rural audiences. Public Health Nurs. 2019;36(2):164–71.
20. Basch CH, Hillyer GC, MacDonald ZL, Reeves R, Basch CE. Characteristics of YouTube™ videos related to mammography. J Cancer Educ. 2015;30(4):699–703.
21. Rosenkrantz AB, Won E, Doshi AM. Assessing the content of YouTube videos in educating patients regarding common imaging examinations. J Am Coll Radiol. 2016;13(12):1509–13.
22. Lyles CR, López A, Pasick R, Sarkar U. "5 mins of uncomfyness is better than dealing with cancer 4 a lifetime": an exploratory qualitative analysis of cervical and breast cancer screening dialogue on Twitter. J Cancer Educ. 2013;28(1):127–33.
23. Nastasi A, Bryant T, Canner JK, Dredze M, Camp MS, Nagarajan N. Breast cancer screening and social media: a content analysis of evidence use and guideline opinions on Twitter. J Cancer Educ. 2018;33(3):695–702.

24. Rosenkrantz AB, Labib A, Pysarenko K, Prabhu V. What do patients tweet about their mammography experience? Acad Radiol. 2016;23(11):1367–71.

25. Seimenis I, Chouchos K, Prassopoulos P. Radiation risk associated with X-ray mammography screening: communication and exchange of information via Tweets. J Am Coll Radiol. 2018;15(7):1033–9.

26. Thackeray R, Burton SH, Giraud-Carrier C, Rollins S, Draper CR. Using Twitter for breast cancer prevention: an analysis of breast cancer awareness month. BMC Cancer. 2013;13(1):508.

27. Wong KO, Davis FG, Zaïane OR, Yasui Y, Dietz J, Aveiro D, Bernardino J. Sentiment analysis of breast cancer screening in the United States using Twitter. KDIR. 2016:265–74.

28. Döbrössy B, Girasek E, Susánszky A, Koncz Z, Győrffy Z, Bognár VK. "Clicks, likes, shares and comments": a systematic review of breast cancer screening discourse in social media. PLoS One. 2020;15(4):e0231422.

29. Robinson L, Griffiths M, Wray J, Ure CM, Shires G, Hodgins JS, Hill C, Hilton B. Preparing women for breast screening mammography: a feasibility study to determine the potential value of an on-line social network and information hub. Radiography. 2015;21(4):308–14.

30. Galpin A, Meredith J, Ure C, Robinson L. "Thanks for letting us all share your mammogram experience virtually": developing a web-based hub for breast cancer screening. JMIR Cancer. 2017;3(2):17.

31. Meredith J, Galpin AJ, Robinson L. Examining the management of stake and interest in a participatory design Facebook group. Qualitative Research Psychology. 2020;19(3):658–77. https://doi.org/10.1 080/14780887.2020.1780354.

32. Scragg B, Shaikh S, Shires G, Hodgins JS, Mercer C, Robinson L. An exploration of mammographers' attitudes towards the use of social media for providing breast screening information to clients. Radiography. 2017;23(3):249–55.

33. Scragg B, Shaikh S, Robinson L, Mercer C. Mixed messages: an evaluation of NHS Trust social media policies in the North West of England. Radiography. 2017;23(3):235–41.

34. Society & College of Radiographers (SCor). SoMeRAD: guidance for the radiography workforce on the professional use of social media. 2015. https://www.sor.org/learning-advice/professional-body-guidance-and-publications/documents-and-publications/policy-guidance-document-library/somerad-guidance-for-the-radiography-workforce-on. Accessed 1 Aug 2021.

35. Huesch M, Galstyan A, Ong MK, Doctor JN. Using social media, online social networks, and internet search as platforms for public health interventions: a pilot study. Health Serv Res. 2016;51(S2):1273–90.

36. Giustini D, Ali SM, Fraser M, Boulos MN. Effective uses of social media in public health and medicine: a systematic review of systematic reviews. Online J Public Health Inform. 2018;10(2):15.

37. Visram S, Hussain W, Goddard A. Towards future healthcare that is digital by default. Future Healthcare J. 2020;7(3):180.

38. Plackett R, Kaushal A, Kassianos AP, Cross A, Lewins D, Sheringham J, Waller J, von Wagner C. Use of social media to promote cancer screening and early diagnosis: scoping review. J Med Internet Res. 2020;22(11):e21582.

39. NHS Digital. More women attend for breast screening thanks to success of digital inclusion project. 2018. https://digital.nhs.uk/news/2018/more-women-attend-for-breast-screening-thanks-to-success-of-digital-inclusion-project. Accessed 21 June 2021.

40. Public Health England Screening. How the North Midlands breast screening team uses Facebook to increase breast screening uptake. 2019. https://phescreening.blog.gov.uk/2019/04/09/how-the-north-midlands-breast-screening-team-uses-facebook-to-increase-breast-screening-uptake/. Accessed 27 Aug 2021.

41. Dougall D, Buck D. My role in tackling health inequalities: a framework for allied health professionals. 2021. https://www.kingsfund.org.uk/publications/tackling-health-inequalities-framework-allied-health-professionals. Accessed 12 Aug 2021.

42. Chou WS, Oh A, Klein WMP. Addressing health-related misinformation on social media. JAMA. 2018;320(23):2417–8.

43. George DR, Rovniak LS, Kraschnewski JL. Dangers and opportunities for social media in medicine. Clin Obstet Gynecol. 2013;56(3):453–62.

44. Society & College of Radiographers (ScoR). Continuing professional development: professional and regulatory requirements. https://www.sor.org/getmedia/81bc25a9-1b84-4f21-aaa2-887ff64456a0/Continuing%20Professional%20Development_%20Professional%20and%20Regulatory%20Requirements_1. Accessed 2 Aug 2021.

45. Bolderston A, Watson J, Woznitza N, Westerink A, Di Prospero L, Currie G, Beardmore C, Hewis J. Twitter journal clubs and continuing professional development: an analysis of a #MedRadJClub tweet chat. Radiography. 2018;24:3–8.

46. Grehan J. The introduction of mandatory CPD for newly state registered diagnostic radiographers: an Irish perspective. Radiography. 2018;24(2):115–21.

47. Greenhough B, Dembinsky M, Dyck I, Brown T, Robson J, Homer K, Sajani C, Carter L, Duffy SW, Ornstein M. Evaluating a DVD promoting breast cancer awareness among black women aged 25–50 years in East London. J Epidemiol Community Health. 2016;70(7):678–82.

48. Public Health England. Achieving and maintaining the 36 month round length. 2019. https://www.gov.uk/government/publications/breast-screening-set-and-maintain-round-length/achieving-and-maintaining-the-36-month-round-length-aug19. Accessed 6 Aug 2021.

49. NHS England. NHS long term plan chapter 5: digitally enabled care will go mainstream across the NHS. https://www.longtermplan.nhs.uk/online-version/chapter-5-digitally-enabled-care-will-go-mainstream-across-the-nhs/. Accessed 6 Aug 2021.

50. Robinson L, Hogg P, Newton-Hughes A. The power and the pain: mammographic compression research from the service-users' perspective. Radiography. 2013;19(3):190–5.

51. Minard M. Moving essence nature art therapy installations (MENAT). http://www.movingessence.net/ArtisticOverview.pdf. Accessed 30 July 2021.

52. Zain NM, Mut NA, Ruslizan NF, Norsuddin NM, Suhaimi SA, Dahari MA, Hasan NA. Mammogram: does music therapy helps? Eur J Med Health Sci. 2020;2(3):1–4.

53. NHS England. NHS long term plan. 2020. https://www.longtermplan.nhs.uk/. Accessed 15 June 2021.

54. NHS Digital. NHS app. 2022. https://digital.nhs.uk/services/nhs-app. Accessed 16 August 2022.

Pain and Discomfort in Mammography

16

Patsy Whelehan, Deborah Nelson, and Rebecca Berry

Learning Objectives

- Understand the concepts, extent and importance of discomfort and pain and how they may be measured
- Describe what steps may be taken to minimise the amount of discomfort and pain and its impact on mammography clients

---

Introduction

Pain in mammography has long been recognised by clinicians and researchers as a problem worthy of attention. Furthermore, a quick internet search or glance at social media confirms the public consciousness of mammography as a potentially painful examination. There are two main aspects of the standpoint that painful mammography is a problem needing to be addressed.

P. Whelehan (✉)
Breast Screening and Imaging Department,
NHS Tayside, Ninewells Hospital and Medical
School, Dundee, UK
e-mail: p.j.whelehan@dundee.ac.uk

D. Nelson · R. Berry
Breast Radiology Department, Tameside and Glossop
Integrated Care NHS Foundation Trust,
Ashton-under-Lyne, UK
e-mail: debbie.nelson@tgh.nhs.uk;
Rebecca.Conlon@tgh.nhs.uk

The first is simply the humane aspect—the ethos of minimising harm in the course of healthcare. The second aspect is the potential deterrent effect of pain expectations on mammography participation, particularly in the context of breast screening. It is a key principle of screening that the test should be acceptable to the population [1].

Although studies concentrating on breast screening participation have addressed experiences of the actual examination to some degree, qualitative research focusing in detail on patient experience in mammography has been surprisingly sparse. However, the following quote from a qualitative study back in 2005 [2] exemplifies both the painfulness of the examination and the potential adverse effect of pain on future mammography participation:

> Well, when I went the first time … it hurt quite a bit, and then when … she said, ok, we're going to give you an appointment for your [next] mammogram, and I said OK. And so I walked out and pretended I didn't know it was going to be there, so I left. And so I never got my second one [2, p. 27].

Despite the length of time that the problem of pain in mammography has been discussed in the literature, it was asserted as recently as 2015 that 'concerns about pain may have been underestimated and deserve more systematic attention in the future' [3, p. 489]. A 2017 qualitative study has confirmed that, despite mammography being a mature technique with the technology having improved over time, pain continues to be a problem for some patients:

I got to the point where I just thought, "I can't, you know I really can't take this anymore" because I know they have to compress the breast but I just thought, when is she going to stop this? It was really, really painful [4, p. 8].

This quote also reminds us of the mammography practitioner's integral and crucial role in the patient experience, adding to the weight of responsibility involved in performing mammography. This chapter will address understanding and measuring pain, and how its importance as a problem in mammography is quantified. It will also explore the factors that can affect how painful the examination is, and review interventions that may be capable of alleviating the pain.

Defining, Describing, and Measuring Pain

Physical pain is defined by the International Association for the Study of Pain (IASP) as 'an unpleasant sensory and emotional experience associated with, or resembling that associated with, actual or potential tissue damage' [5]. Thus, even in the context of specifically physical pain, it is acknowledged that there are affective (emotional) dimensions alongside or arising from the sensory perceptions [6]. Furthermore, it is emphasised that pain is always a personal experience, influenced by biological, psychological, and social factors [7]. It has been argued that, rather like hunger or thirst, pain is a motivational state whose primary function is to guide behaviour [8]. Whereas in some circumstances, pain may motivate people in positive ways such as taking rest and recovery, in the context of mammography screening, pain—once experienced—may delay or prevent future participation.

In the mammography literature, discomfort—either as well as or instead of pain—is often considered. It is therefore important to understand

distinctions in meaning between pain and discomfort. Discomfort can describe both physical and psychological states while physical discomfort can be caused by physical perceptions other than pain [9]. It is clear that some mammography researchers have considered physical discomfort to be the same phenomenon as physical pain but simply less severe, and indeed the Oxford English Dictionary suggests that discomfort can mean 'slight physical pain' [10]. However, discomfort is often considered as distinct from pain, as evidenced within qualitative mammography research: 'It doesn't really hurt, it's just uncomfortable.' [11, p. 413].

For measuring pain, self-report is generally the preferred method because of the personal, subjective nature of pain. Unfortunately, rather than using existing validated pain measures, published mammography studies have often used unvalidated pain measures developed by the authors themselves [12, 13], thus limiting the reliability of the findings. Furthermore, pain and discomfort terms have on occasions been combined within single scales, despite evidence that pain and discomfort are distinct.

The three simplest and best known pain intensity scales are the 100 mm visual analogue scale (VAS), the 0–10 numerical rating scale (NRS), and the four point verbal rating scale (VRS)—no pain, mild pain, moderate pain, severe pain [14]. In the case of the VAS and NRS, "anchors" are terms used at each end to denote the extremes of the scale, for example as shown in the NRS in Fig. 16.1. A valuable review of the advantages and disadvantages of these scales, plus one other, was published in 2018 [15]. Whereas pain scale responses were traditionally captured orally or on paper, electronic means are now available, for example capturing VAS data using a sliding cursor on a mobile app or computer screen [16], or using hand pressure exerted on a sensor to capture pain intensity electronically in real time.

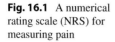

Fig. 16.1 A numerical rating scale (NRS) for measuring pain

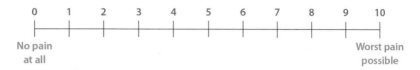

The Extent and Importance of the Problem of Pain in Mammography

The extent of the problem of pain in mammography can be considered according to the proportions of patients affected, the levels of experienced pain, or the proportions experiencing a particular level of pain. Reported percentages of those experiencing any level of pain during mammography, in studies published between 2000 and 2021, range from 7% to 96% [17–26]. The wide variation is largely a reflection of the variety of pain measurement methods used and the thresholds assigned to no pain versus any pain. More recent and interventional studies are more likely than older, observational studies to use validated pain scales, with the 0–10 NRS and the 0–100 VAS being the most common.

Twelve studies published between 2000 and 2021 [27–38] that used a standard NRS pain scale have reported mean or median values in a sample of patients who were not selected by any particular characteristic, or who were the control group in an interventional study. The mean NRS score ranged from 1.5 to 6.1 [27–38]. The median pain score on a 0–10 NRS was reported in one study as 2 [37] and in another as 6 [38]. Using a standard VAS, the mean pain score in five studies ranged from 14.3 to 61.5 [17, 34, 39–41]. Thus, the evidence suggests that—on average—women experience mild to moderate pain during mammography. However, studies using validated pain scales to assess the proportions of patients experiencing specific levels of pain have shown that around 10% of patients feel severe pain during mammography [17, 21, 22]. In one of these studies, the rate of severe pain was greater in women who had been treated for breast cancer, at 19% [22].

A few studies have investigated pain persisting for some time after the mammogram. For example, a large breast screening study found that approximately 6% of participants reported pain persisting up to two weeks after mammography [42].

Another way to consider the importance of the problem of pain in mammography is according to its ability to affect screening participation. A systematic review published in 2013 explored that question, in terms of assessing the numbers of women who either gave pain as a reason for not reattending for mammography screening, or who did not reattend following a measured painful experience at an index examination [43]. As of 2021, no new primary studies meeting the inclusion criteria for that systematic review had been published. The review found that among non-reattenders asked for their reasons, 11–46% cited pain. In the best-quality primary studies that had investigated statistical associations between painful mammography and subsequent non-reattendance [44–46], the combined relative risk of not returning was 1.34 (95% confidence interval 0.94–1.91).

The problem of pain in mammography has proven difficult to quantify, even using a range of approaches. However, taken together, the qualitative and quantitative evidence suggests that it remains a significant problem meriting continued attempts at amelioration.

Factors Associated with Pain in Mammography

Many factors hypothesised to be related to mammography pain have been studied but the results are often inconclusive. Here we consider some of the best-quality and clearest evidence for relationships between mammography pain and a range of potential influencing factors.

Regarding potential psychological influences on pain in mammography, anxiety is reasonably well-evidenced as a risk factor [22, 30, 41, 47]. This is covered in depth within Chap. 13. Positive associations between expected pain and experienced pain have also been convincingly demonstrated [21, 22, 24, 34, 40, 47, 48]. Qualitative research reveals that the expectation that mammography will be painful may result either from prior personal experience or word-of-mouth accounts from other women [49, 50].

Concerning physical factors, there is reasonably good evidence for a positive association between greater mammography pain and pre-existing breast pain or tenderness [22, 33, 47], as well as an association with previous breast conserving surgery [40, 51]. Evidence regarding breast size and mammography pain is mixed and overall inconclusive, while evidence linking breast density to mammography pain is extremely weak. A single, albeit large, study has found a 33% (95%CI 1.07–1.65) higher relative risk of severe versus no mammography pain in patients with pre-existing shoulder or neck pain [38]. It is possible that the shoulder or neck pain was a marker of more general co-morbidities that may predispose to mammography pain, rather than there being a direct relationship between pain in the neck or shoulder and pain in mammography.

Among demographic factors covered in the literature, only higher educational levels among clients have been reliably shown to correlate with greater mammography pain [20, 21, 52].

The importance of the practitioner's role in patient experience in mammography is prominent in the qualitative literature, including indications that a lack of compassionate care may exacerbate perceived pain:

> She didn't talk, she just shoved and pushed, didn't even say now turn around and do this … her attitude was bad and it made my time miserable and it was more painful [2, p. 27].

Surprisingly, however, there is little strong quantitative evidence concerning the influence of the practitioner on pain in mammography. There is some evidence that lower satisfaction with care or attention, and perceiving the practitioner's handling to be rough, are predictive of discomfort [21, 52], while politeness, gentleness and competence have been linked to less pain [26]. Only one published study has directly investigated possible links between variations in mammographic positioning and pain and it is a small and preliminary study that found no association [53].

Interventions to Minimise Pain in Mammography

There is only one published systematic review of interventions to reduce pain in mammography. It was published in 2008 and, as of 2021, has not been updated [54]. The review was restricted to randomised controlled trials. One of the review's key findings, based on a single primary study, was that provision of procedural information before the mammogram could reduce pain [55]. A further finding of the review was that giving patients more control over the compression had the potential to reduce pain but with concerns over effects on image quality [56]. Finally, cushioning pads for the equipment were found to have an effect but again with some image-quality concerns [34]. The review authors gave the following assessment of the body of evidence:

> Differences in interventions, and inconsistency in measures, validation of pain scales, and in assessment of mammogram quality, mean that results of these studies cannot be combined. All results are based on single studies. Further research is required [54, p. 2].

In later primary studies, interventions that are designed to reduce pain by reducing the amount of compression force applied have shown little evidence of success. One reason may be that practitioners probably already tend to tailor the compression force to what women find tolerable, to some degree at least. Conversely, when patients are given a degree of actual physical control over the application of compression, pain is reduced without any significant compromise on the tissue thickness reduction that the compression is designed to achieve [57]. However, this intervention was found to be time-consuming. Meanwhile, there is modest evidence for the effectiveness of cushioning pads [28, 54, 58] but premedication with oral analgesics has not been shown to be effective [36, 47].

There is little evidence for the effect of relaxation techniques and music interventions in reducing mammography pain but physical exercise prior to mammography has been found to be effective, albeit potentially difficult to implement in high-volume population-based screening programmes [39]. Intervention studies involving mammographic practice are rare and have shown little evidence of effectiveness. There is some evidence that optimising provision of information to patients can reduce mammography pain but at least one of the two such reported interventions was not delivered by the mammography practitioner [35].

Summary

Pain is a challenging topic to investigate, and it is important that researchers and services use only validated measures when attempting to quantify levels or rates of pain. The main factors that have been robustly shown to affect pain experienced during mammography are patient anxiety, expectation or prior experience of pain, and breast tenderness. The standard of care by mammographers has been shown in qualitative research to be very important to patients and there is a small amount of quantitative evidence linking poor care to greater mammography pain. Effective interventions for reducing mammography pain remain scarce. Researchers should therefore continue to seek new and better ways to minimise pain in mammography. Meanwhile, practitioners should recognise the importance of their role in minimising pain, optimising patient experience, and influencing the willingness of patients to continue to participate in mammography.

Clinical Pearls
- Pain is a problem for many clients during mammography and risks reducing future mammography participation.
- Politeness, gentleness and competence on the part of practitioners have been shown to be associated with lower perceptions of pain.
- Higher client anxiety, expectation of pain or previous painful mammography, previous breast conserving surgery, and breast tenderness are associated with greater pain from mammography. Prior to performing the examination, practitioners should try to ascertain whether any of these factors are present and should tailor their care accordingly.

Chapter Review Questions
Review Questions

1. Name three validated pain measures that can be used to study pain in mammography.
2. Roughly what percentage of women experience severe pain during mammography?
3. Which aspects of care by mammographers have been shown to be linked to less pain?

Answers

1. Visual analogue scale (VAS), Numerical Rating Scale (NRS), Verbal Rating Scale (VRS). (Other answers are possible, eg Wong-Baker Faces Scale, McGill Pain Questionnaire, but those are not directly mentioned within the chapter.)
2. Roughly 10%.
3. Politeness, gentleness, competence.

Appendix

Test your learning and check your understanding of this book's contents: use the "Springer Nature Flashcards" app to access questions using https://sn.pub/dcAnWL.

To use the app, please follow the instructions in Chap. 1.

Flashcard   code: 48341-69945-ABCB1-2A8C7-CE9D2.

Short URL: https://sn.pub/dcAnWL.

References

1. Andermann A, Blancquaert I, Beauchamp S, Déry V. Revisiting Wilson and Jungner in the genomic age: a review of screening criteria over the past 40 years. Bull World Health Organ. 2008;86:317–9.
2. Engelman KK, Cizik AM, Ellerbeck EF. Women's satisfaction with their mammography experience: results of a qualitative study. Women Health. 2006;42(4):17–35.
3. Morris N. When health means suffering: mammograms, pain and compassionate care. Eur J Cancer Care. 2015;24(4):483–92.
4. Whelehan P, Evans A, Ozakinci G. Client and practitioner perspectives on the screening mammography experience. Eur J Cancer Care. 2017;26(3):e12580.

5. International Association for the Study of Pain. IASP terminology. Available from: https://www.iasp-pain.org/resources/terminology/#pain. Accessed 6 Feb 2022.

6. Bueno-Gómez N. Conceptualizing suffering and pain. Philos Ethics Humanit Med. 2017;12(1):1–11.

7. Raja SN, Carr DB, Cohen M, Finnerup NB, Flor H, Gibson S, Keefe FJ, Mogil JS, Ringkamp M, Sluka KA, Song XJ, Stevens B, Sullivan MD, Tutelman PR, Ushida T, Vader K. The revised International Association for the Study of Pain definition of pain: concepts, challenges, and compromises. Pain. 2020;161(9):1976–82.

8. Wall PD. On the relation of injury to pain the John J. Bonica lecture. Pain. 1979;6(3):253–64.

9. Ashkenazy S, Ganz FD. The differentiation between pain and discomfort: a concept analysis of discomfort. Pain Manag Nurs. 2019;20(6):556–62.

10. Oxford University Press. Discomfort. Available from: https://www.oed.com/view/Entry/53820?rskey=T95QCz&result=1#eid. Accessed 13 Feb 2022.

11. Bobo JK, Dean D, Stovall C, Mendez M, Caplan L. Factors that may discourage annual mammography among low-income women with access to free mammograms: a study using multi-ethnic, multiracial focus groups. Psychol Rep. 1999;85(2):405–16.

12. Andrews FJ. Pain during mammography: implications for breast screening programmes. Australas Radiol. 2001;45(2):113–7.

13. Pagliarin F, Pylkkanen L, Salakari M, Deandrea S. Are women satisfied with their experience with breast cancer screening? Systematic review of the literature. Eur J Pub Health. 2021;31(1):206–14.

14. Jensen MP, Karoly P. Self-report scales and procedures for assessing pain in adults. In: Turk DC, Melzack R, editors. Hand pain assess. 3rd ed. New York: The Guildford Press; 2011. p. 19–44.

15. Karcioglu O, Topacoglu H, Dikme O, Dikme O. A systematic review of the pain scales in adults: which to use? Am J Emerg Med. 2018;36(4):707–14.

16. Escalona-Marfil C, Coda A, Ruiz-Moreno J, Riu-Gispert LM, Gironès X. Validation of an electronic visual analog scale mHealth tool for acute pain assessment: prospective cross-sectional study. J Med Internet Res. 2020;22(2):e13468.

17. Asghari A, Nicholas MK. Pain during mammography: the role of coping strategies. Pain. 2004;108(1–2):170–9.

18. Drossaert CH, Boer H, Seydel ER. Does mammographic screening and a negative result affect attitudes towards future breast screening? J Med Screen. 2001;8(4):204–12.

19. Gosein MA, Pereira SM, Narinesingh D, Ameeral A. Breast cancer and mammography: knowledge, attitudes, practices and patient satisfaction post-mammography at the San Fernando General Hospital, Trinidad. J Health Care Poor Underserved. 2014;25(1):142–60.

20. Gupta R, Nayak M, Khoursheed M, Roy S, Behbehani AI. Pain during mammography: impact of breast pathologies and demographic factors. Med Princ Pract. 2003;12(3):180–3.

21. Keemers-Gels ME, Groenendijk RP, Van Den Heuvel JH, Boetes C, Peer PG, Wobbes TH. Pain experienced by women attending breast cancer screening. Breast Cancer Res Treat. 2000;60(3):235–40.

22. Nelson DJ, England A, Cheptoo M, Mercer CE. A comparative study of pain experienced during successive mammography examinations in patients with a family history of breast cancer and those who have had breast cancer surgery. Radiography. 2020;26(1):76–81.

23. Papas MA, Klassen AC. Pain and discomfort associated with mammography among urban low-income African–American women. J Community Health. 2005;30(4):253–67.

24. Sapir R, Patlas M, Strano SD, Hadas-Halpern I, Cherny NI. Does mammography hurt? J Pain Symptom Manag. 2003;25(1):53–63.

25. Goethem MV, Mortelmans D, Bruyninckx E, Verslegers I, Biltjes I, Hove EV, Schepper AD. Influence of the radiographer on the pain felt during mammography. Eur Radiol. 2003;13(10):2384–9.

26. Wiratkapun C, Lertsithichai P, Wibulpolprasert B, Leelaswattanakul M, Detakarat J, Jungjai P. Breast pain and service satisfaction during digital mammography. J Med Assoc Thai. 2006;89(11):1864.

27. Agasthya GA, D'Orsi E, Kim YJ, Handa P, Ho CP, D'Orsi CJ, Sechopoulos I. Can breast compression be reduced in digital mammography and breast tomosynthesis? AJR. 2017;209(5):W322.

28. Chan HH, Lo G, Cheung PS. Is pain from mammography reduced by the use of a radiolucent MammoPad? Local experience in Hong Kong. Hong Kong Med J. 2016;22(3):210–5.

29. Sharp PC, Michielutte R, Freimanis R, Cunningham L, Spangler J, Burnette V. Reported pain following mammography screening. Arch Intern Med. 2003;163(7):833–6.

30. Zavotsky KE, Adrienne Banavage MS, Patricia James RN, Kathy Easter MS, Pontieri-Lewis V, Lynn Lutwin MS. The effects of music on pain and anxiety during screening mammography. Clin J Oncol Nurs. 2014;18(3):E45.

31. de Groot JE, Broeders MJ, Grimbergen CA, den Heeten GJ. Pain-preventing strategies in mammography: an observational study of simultaneously recorded pain and breast mechanics throughout the entire breast compression cycle. BMC Womens Health. 2015;15(1):1–9.

32. De Groot JE, Broeders MJ, Branderhorst W, Den Heeten GJ, Grimbergen CA. A novel approach to mammographic breast compression: improved standardization and reduced discomfort by controlling pressure instead of force. Med Phys. 2013;40(8):081901.

33. de Groot JE, Branderhorst W, Grimbergen CA, den Heeten GJ, Broeders MJ. Towards personalized compression in mammography: a comparison study between pressure-and force-standardization. Eur J Radiol. 2015;84(3):384–91.

34. Dibble SL, Israel J, Nussey B, Sayre JW, Brenner RJ, Sickles EA. Mammography with breast cushions. Womens Health Issues. 2005;15(2):55–63.

35. Fernández-Feito A, Lana A, Cabello-Gutiérrez L, Franco-Correia S, Baldonedo-Cernuda R, Mosteiro-Díaz P. Face-to-face information and emotional support from trained nurses reduce pain during screening mammography: results from a randomized controlled trial. Pain Manag Nurs. 2015;16(6):862–70.

36. Freitas-Junior R, Martins E, Metran-Nascente C, Carvalho AA, da Silva MF, Soares LR, Ximenes CA. Double-blind placebo-controlled randomized clinical trial on the use of paracetamol for performing mammography. Medicine. 2018;97(13):e0261.

37. Jeukens CR, Van Dijk T, Berben C, Wildberger JE, Lobbes MB. Evaluation of pressure-controlled mammography compression paddles with respect to force-controlled compression paddles in clinical practice. Eur Radiol. 2019;29(5):2545–52.

38. Moshina N, Sagstad S, Sebuødegård S, Waade GG, Gran E, Music J, Hofvind S. Breast compression and reported pain during mammographic screening. Radiography. 2020;26(2):133–9.

39. Cardoso de Almeida T, Marques de Mello L, Saraiva de Castro Mattos J, Soares da Silva A, Aparecido Nunes A. Evaluation of the impact of physical exercise in reducing pain in women undergoing mammography: a randomized clinical trial. Pain Med. 2018;19(1):9–15.

40. Kornguth PJ, Keefe FJ, Wright KR, Delong DM. Mammography pain in women treated conservatively for breast cancer. J Pain. 2000;1(4):268–74.

41. Mattsson P. Mammography-related breast pain is associated with migraine. Cephalalgia. 2009;29(6):616–23.

42. Brotherton J, Taylor R, Ivanov O, Tewson R, Page A. "It's much easier than going to the dentist": high levels of satisfaction in a mammography screening program. Aust N Z J Public Health. 2007;31(4):353–9.

43. Whelehan P, Evans A, Wells M, MacGillivray S. The effect of mammography pain on repeat participation in breast cancer screening: a systematic review. Breast. 2013;22(4):389–94.

44. Orton M, Fitzpatrick R, Fuller A, Mant D, Mlynek C, Thorogood M. Factors affecting women's response to an invitation to attend for a second breast cancer screening examination. Br J Gen Pract. 1991;41(349):320–2.

45. Marshall G. A comparative study of re-attenders and non-re-attenders for second triennial National Breast Screening Programme appointments. J Public Health. 1994;16(1):79–86.

46. Edwards SA, Chiarelli AM, Ritvo P, Stewart L, Majpruz V, Mai V. Satisfaction with initial screen and compliance with biennial breast screening at centers with and without nurses. Cancer Nurs. 2011;34(4):293–301.

47. Lambertz CK, Johnson CJ, Montgomery PG, Maxwell JR. Premedication to reduce discomfort during screening mammography. Radiology. 2008;248(3):765–72.

48. Shrestha S, Poulos A. The effect of verbal information on the experience of discomfort in mammography. Radiography. 2001;7(4):271–7.

49. Tejeda S, Thompson B, Coronado GD, Martin DP. Barriers and facilitators related to mammography use among lower educated Mexican women in the USA. Soc Sci Med. 2009;68(5):832–9.

50. Peek ME, Sayad JV, Markwardt R. Fear, fatalism and breast cancer screening in low-income African-American women: the role of clinicians and the health care system. J Gen Intern Med. 2008;23(11):1847–53.

51. De Groot JE, Broeders MJ, Branderhorst W, Den Heeten GJ, Grimbergen CA. Mammographic compression after breast conserving therapy: controlling pressure instead of force. Med Phys. 2014;41(2):023501.

52. Dullum JR, Lewis EC, Mayer JA. Rates and correlates of discomfort associated with mammography. Radiology. 2000;214(2):547–52.

53. Whelehan P, Pampaka M, Boyd J, Armstrong S, Evans A, Ozakinci G. Development and validation of a novel measure of adverse patient positioning in mammography. Eur J Radiol. 2021;140:109747.

54. Miller D, Livingstone V, Herbison GP, Vermeulen H. Interventions for relieving the pain and discomfort of screening mammography 1. Nederlands Tijdschrift voor Evid Based Pract. 2013;11(1):15–6.

55. Alimoğlu E, Alimoğlu MK, Kabaalioğlu A, Çeken K, Apaydin A, Lüleci E. Mammography-related pain and anxiety. Tani Girisim Radyol. 2004;10(3):213–7.

56. Rimer BK, Conaway MR, Kornguth PJ, Stout AL, Catoe KE, Brackett JS. Effects of force, race, and coping style on pain during patient-controlled mammography. J Women's Heal. 1993;2(3):249–55.

57. Henrot P, Boisserie-Lacroix M, Boute V, Troufléau P, Boyer B, Lesanne G, Gillon V, Desandes E, Netter E, Saadate M, Tardivon A. Self-compression technique vs standard compression in mammography: a randomized clinical trial. JAMA Intern Med. 2019;179(3):407–14.

58. Markle L, Roux S, Sayre JW. Reduction of discomfort during mammography utilizing a radiolucent cushioning pad. Breast J. 2004;10(4):345–9.

Tissue Viability and Skin Tearing in Mammography

17

Melanie Stephens, Sheba Pradeep, and Fiona Dobson

Learning Objectives
- Understand the risks of mammography on skin and tissues of the breast of men and women
- Review the anatomy and physiology of the skin
- Describe the risk factors that makes a client's skin more vulnerable to skin damage
- Classify the types of skin damage that can occur
- Identify prevention and management strategies for the care of clients undergoing mammography

Introduction

It has been acknowledged that some women are more sensitive to the handling and pressure exerted on their breasts during a mammogram than others [1]. This sensitivity can include heightened feelings of pain, skin reddening, tin-

gling and bruising [2]; these are considered to be acceptable risks. A small proportion of women after mammography, however, can go on to experience breast pain for days. Also, they may develop pressure ulcers or skin tears. Internationally, healthcare associated harm is recognised as a risk to public health and wellbeing [3]. Estimates of the number of healthcare associated harms that occur in hospitals in high income countries equates to one in every ten patients [4]. The causes are multifaceted however, nearly 50% of them are preventable [5]. Pressure ulcers or skin tears from women who have undergone mammography are very rarely reported. With the advent of safer care for patients and the reporting of avoidable harm through reporting systems [6], the area of tissue viability needs to be addressed.

Recording Information

Recording clients and family's experiences can assist in the identification of everyday actions in clinical practice, reducing future risk and influencing the delivery of safer healthcare. Documenting experiences of harm enriches client safety incident reporting and analysis and is consider the foundation for future learning [7]. A search of the data and literature within the specialty of breast screening and mammography proffers one case study of a client who developed a haematoma after mammography, which pro-

M. Stephens (✉) · S. Pradeep
School of Health and Society, University of Salford, Manchester, UK
e-mail: m.stephens@salford.ac.uk; s.pradeep@salford.ac.uk

F. Dobson
Medicines Support Team, Burnley General Teaching Hospital, Burnley, UK

© The Author(s), under exclusive license to Springer Nature Switzerland AG 2022
C. Mercer et al. (eds.), *Digital Mammography*, https://doi.org/10.1007/978-3-031-10898-3_17

gressed to an aggressive inflammatory carcinoma three months later [8]. Whereas a general search of the internet using the search terms 'skin tears' and 'mammography' leads to multiple stories found on medical companies' websites, blogs, and message boards [8–11]. It is within these pages that the extent of the issue is reported, and the term traumatic mammography injury (TMI) is used.

Case Studies

The next three client stories provide practitioners with insight into this area of tissue viability, all names have been changed in accordance with confidentiality and data protection [12, 13].

Case Study 1 (Fig. 17.1)

Kennedy attended her appointment for a mammography at her local hospital. Whilst having the left breast compressed the technologists pulled and tugged at her breast which hurt. When the examination was completed, she found a skin tear under her breast which was 15 cm long. She initially found the mammography practitioners rude, aggressive, and not attending to personal and protective hygiene controls. Whilst having the left breast compressed, the practitioners pulled and tugged at her breast which hurt and Kennedy's comment regarding the pain was quickly dismissed. Kennedy reported once more

that she felt like her skin was ripping and she was informed that this was normal. When the examination was completed, she found a skin tear under her breast which was 15 cm long. When showing the tear to the practitioner, Kennedy's injury was dismissed as a common injury during mammography. Kennedy rebutted this claim from her previous experience of mammography and discussion with her friends after theirs. She asked for an incident form but became upset as the practitioners did not know the procedure to file such an injury and asked them to call their supervisor. Kennedy spoke via telephone to the supervisor about the incident and was asked to send a picture of the skin tear, the supervisor would then complete an incident report. After, she was provided with some simple dressings and offered some cream (of which she was allergic to). Kennedy did receive a reply to the incident form that was completed where it was explained that skin tears were a possible complication of mammography.

Case Study 2 (Fig. 17.2)

Leslie had a mammogram to rule out a lump in her breast. During and immediately after the mammogram, Leslie was in a lot of pain and whilst getting dressed she realised that she had developed a 10-cm skin tear underneath her breast which had begun to bleed.

When Leslie had a mammogram to rule out a lump in her breast the mammography practitioner

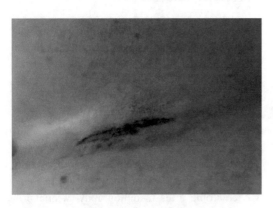

Fig. 17.1 Breast skin tear of client

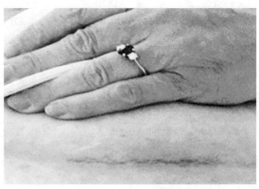

Fig. 17.2 Skin tear from a mammogram

began with taking some images. She then switched to using some small paddles and this is when the procedure began to really hurt. Leslie was informed that smaller paddles compress the breast 'thinner' and that is why it increases the discomfort she felt. Leslie was in a lot of pain and whilst getting dressed she realised that she had developed a skin tear underneath their breast which had begun to bleed. Once dressed, Leslie spoke to the practitioners about the skin tear and bleeding and was informed that this does happen sometimes. She felt their response was uncaring and dismissive. Leslie was left with a 10-cm skin tear. She returned to work that day but had to leave as her bra was rubbing on the open wound. She went to buy dressings and returned home to dress the skin tear. This episode of care has left Leslie wondering whether all mammograms are like this.

Case Study 3

Alex wanted to share her experiences of compression variability in breast screening as she has attended four breast screening examinations at the same unit. The process of attending the appointments caused Alex some degree of anxiety, stating that she felt both embarrassed and vulnerable. She is reported to find any medical appointment where she must remove clothing uncomfortable. The practitioners who use the machines are pleasant and attentive and do their best to make Alex feel comfortable, but she does not find mammography to be a comfortable or pleasant experience.

One aspect that really concerns Alex is variability in the amount of compression that is used, and she reflects on a routine mammography appointment in 2016/2017.

> At that screening there was a massive difference in compression for the 'up-down' mammogram between my left and right breasts. The practitioner applied considerably more compression to my left breast. At the time I wanted to pull away from the machine. As well as being extremely painful at the time it had lasting effects. It was traumatic. The skin above my breast was torn and there was a graze and because of this I felt some pain for a

while after my mammogram. I wondered at the time if the operator was inexperienced. I went back to work after the appointment and showed one of my colleagues the torn skin. She commented that it might be a good idea to report the incident to the head of the mammography unit. I did this, not because I wanted to complain, but because I thought the compression might be excessive and they needed to know. The longer lasting implication relates to how I now feel about mammography as that episode really does make me anxious about attending further screening events, not just about what might be found but also about the procedure itself. I've since had another mammography and the experience was better. I've spoken to friends and colleagues who have said they too have anxieties about attending screening appointments because of the feeling of vulnerability and the worry about what might be discovered. The operators do their best to make their patients feel comfortable and some are more successful than others at this but to them it's a job that they do many times a week. The patient sees it differently, it's a big deal for the patient. They are taking time out of their day to attend the appointment and they are the ones standing there half naked feeling vulnerable. I suppose people react to situations differently. Some people prefer the approach to be clinical and quite "matter of fact" and over with quickly. Whereas other people (me) like a more friendly approach. I don't want to feel like I'm an inconvenience or that I'm just one of many people that day, I want to feel appreciated.

Client stories that refer to undergoing a mammogram found on websites and information leaflets are ones that promote the importance of breast cancer screening. Complications such as skin tears and pressure damage are not referred to despite the plethora of stories. To understand the extent and impact of skin damage from mammography in the United States, two surveys were sent out to clients who attended one of 222 breast imaging centres and their staff [14]. The results from the anonymised responses found that 4.7% of the 778 women who replied had experienced a skin tear during a mammogram. 35.1% of these women noticed their skin tear only after leaving the breast imaging centre, and only 40.5% contacted the centre to report the issue. Within this survey the breast imaging centre staff reported an annual skin tear rate of 0.49%, whilst others reported 10% or more skin tear incidents post mammography.

The researcher also found that the impact of developing a skin tear on the client and their lives included quite significant reactions such as not returning for their next mammogram, delaying the next mammogram or switching to a different breast imaging centre. The participants also reported increased fear and anxiety when attending for routine mammograms.

The investigator also explored the impact of skin tears on the imaging unit's workload. Analysis of the surveys found reports of added workload on staff, as after a skin tear had occurred, charts and incident reports had to be completed. They were required to assess and manage the skin damage or wound. There was also extra work managing follow-up calls and managing fearful clients who were more difficult to position when they returned for subsequent screening or were delaying future mammograms.

A limitation of the survey is that it was conducted by the president of a company who produces mammography protective plate covers and the findings could potentially increase sales of their product. This could be considered as sponsorship bias and creates a conflict of interest in the conclusions made. However, the findings do make for interesting reading about the extent of tissue damage that occurs during breast screening and its apparent under reporting by both staff and clients. Moving forward, change is required, and use of the stories of women can assist in informing future practice, developing healthcare professions education on assessment and management of tissue viability in mammography, accurate incident reporting and development of the information provided to women on other risks of mammograms.

Risks of Mammography to the Skin

To ensure a high-quality mammogram image, that separates tissue components and reduces the dosage of radiation, compression of the breast is essential [15]. However, applying compression force to the breast also increases the risk of tissue damage from pressure, shear, and friction forces, resulting in iatrogenic injuries [16]. The National Pressure Ulcer Advisory Panel (NPUAP) and the European Pressure Ulcer Advisory Panel (EPUAP) [17, 18] definitions of shear stress and friction clearly explain the risk mammography can cause from either applying forces to the breast, which causes two adjacent parts (the skin and underlying structures) to distort in the transverse plane or the rubbing of two surfaces together. The resultant damage can appear as a blister (friction), ulceration or tear of the epidermis or even skin breakdown that occurs days after the mammogram (pressure and shear). The risks of skin breakdown are heightened when clients undergoing mammography are considered to be more at risk due to predisposing risk factors such as age, gender, dry and fragile skin or if the client already has intertrigo, skin abrasions or lesions.

Anatomy and Physiology of the Skin

The skin consists of two layers: the superficial layer called the epidermis and a deep layer known as the dermis. The dermis lies over the subcutaneous tissue, which contains fat cells also known as lipocytes [19]. The skin is the largest weighing organ of the body and constitutes to about 15% of the total body weight [19]. The thickness of the epidermis varies from region to region, with the thinnest layer found on the eyelid and the thickest layer noted on the palm of the hand and soles of the feet. The epidermis is made up mostly of Keratinocytes (about 90%) but there are also other cells such as the Melanocytes (which produce pigment melanin responsible for skin colour); Merkel cells (which help with the sensation of touch); and Langerhans cells (which are part of the immune response) found in this layer [20]. The Keratinocytes are arranged in layers, with the deepest layer of Stratum Basale cells followed by Stratum spinosum, Stratum granulosum, Stratum lucidum and Stratum corneum, (which is the top layer of cells) [20]. As the cells mature, they migrate to the top, acquiring a protein known as keratin through a process of keratinisation, and eventually shed off. As the cells migrate away from the Stratum basale layer, they receive less nutrition and eventually undergo apoptosis (a self-programmed cell death) [21].

The dermis is made up of two layers, the outer papillary dermis and deeper reticular dermis, and is responsible for providing nutrition and support to the epidermis [20]. The collagen and elastic fibers produced by the fibroblast cells of the reticular dermis increases the tensile strength of the skin [21]. Ageing decreases the collagen content and elasticity of the dermis and increases the susceptibility for skin breakdown due to stretching because of mammography.

The epidermis forms undulating ridges with the dermis known as rete ridges. These not only help to anchor the epidermis onto the dermis, providing a structural integrity, but also allow for exchange of nutrients [21]. Shearing and external frictional forces may cause the two layers to become separated. Loss of rete ridges due to ageing risks skin breakdown due to these shearing forces [22]. Compression forces applied during mammography may exert an additional force by stretching of the skin.

Defining Skin Tears and Pressure Ulcers

A pressure ulcer, according to the European Pressure Ulcer Advisory Panel, National Pressure Injury Advisory Panel and Pan Pacific Pressure Injury Alliance [23], is defined as

> …localised damage to the skin and/or underlying tissue as a result of pressure in combination with shear, pressure injuries usually occur over a bony prominence but may be related to a medical device or other object.

Device related pressure ulcers result from devices, equipment, furniture, and everyday objects that have applied pressure to the skin and unintentionally created skin damage. In mammography, when pressure damage has occurred from carrying out a diagnostic procedure, the practitioner should record this as medical device related pressure injury (MDRPI). The injury should also be staged using a recognised classification system [23].

Skin tears are considered to be traumatic injuries, varying from minor to complex wounds, which can result in the development of partial or full thickness injuries, where the epidermis has separated from the dermis or both layers of skin have separated from the underlying structures [24]. The problem arises when the damage has been caused through shear or friction forces, as the type of wound that subsequently occurs can be categorised as both a pressure ulcer or skin tear. More research is needed to improve diagnosis of these types of wounds.

Where Do They Occur?

Pressure ulcers most commonly develop over bony prominences; however, Fletcher [25] notes that device-related pressure ulcers can occur on other parts of the body, such as the breast. Skin tears can occur on any anatomical location, however in relation to mammography, common places can be the inframammary fold or upper (inner or outer) aspects of the breast.

Predisposing Risk Factors

There are many predisposing risk factors that can contribute to the development of pressure ulcers and skin tears; they can either be intrinsically or extrinsically related. Extrinsic factors can be linked to direct pressure, shear, and friction forces. Intrinsic factors are those that affect the physical, social, and mental wellbeing of clients. For mammography these factors can include:

- *Age:* As aging occurs the skin thins and flattens. In conjunction, there is a loss in the number of blood vessels, nerve endings and collagen. This leads to a reduction in sensation, moisture balance, elasticity, and temperature control. Atrophy and contraction of the dermis causes wrinkles and folds, whilst sebaceous glands reduce their level of activity causing the skin to dry out. The consequences of all these changes include skin fragility, furrowing and wrinkling of the skin [26–28].

- *History of previous skin damage, bruising, abrasions and intertrigo:* Some clients may present with current bruising, skin abrasions, sores, or tears and this increases the risk of further skin breakdown or worsening of their current skin condition [29]. For these cases, breast imaging units should consider having local protocols in relation to informing the client of the risks of continuing with screening. According to Wingfield [30] dry, fragile skin is frequently related to other skin diseases (eczema), illnesses (hypothyroidism) or environmental factors (central heating) and once the skin dries out it is more susceptible to cracks and splits. These may develop into infected wounds and sores.
- *Medication:* Can affect skin structure and function and increase the risk of skin breakdown. For example, steroids can cause thinning of the skin; non-steroidal anti-inflammatories can cause irritant dermatitis [31].
- *Diet and weight:* A lack of adequate fats, carbohydrates, proteins, minerals, vitamins, fibre and water may predispose a client to increased risk of skin damage and delayed wound healing. Therefore, clients who are either obese or emaciated are associated with a higher risk due to a lack of essential nutrition and hydration which promotes skin cell turgidity, elasticity and function [32].
- *Sensory impairment:* Clients with altered cognitive or sensory impairment are at an increased risk of skin breakdown as they may not be able to perceive pain from pressure, shear and friction forces.
- *Co-morbidity:* Many clients present with comorbidities that affect skin status. These can include conditions such as cardiovascular, renal, endocrinology and respiratory diseases, which can alter the blood flow, oxygenation and nutrient levels and the removal of toxic waste from the skin.

Prevention of Tearing and Ulceration from Mammography

Preventing pressure ulcers and skin tears is complex in mammography as the device which potentially causes the damage forms the essential part of the diagnostic investigation. Nevertheless, assessment of the client's skin and risk factors when attending for mammography is vital. The mammography practitioner should note relevant factors which are reported by the client or observed through skin inspection before and after the mammogram. Findings should be documented in the client's notes. If required, if skin abrasions, tears or lesions are present, discussions of the risks of further skin damage should be carried out with the client. As there is a lack of research in the prevention and management of pressure ulcers and skin tears, current best practice includes consideration of:

- Reduction or elimination of pressure, shear, and friction forces
- Correct positioning and alignment of breasts during the mammogram
- Obtaining pre-mammogram information in regards of skin tone, skin care, nutrition and hydration, treatment of current lesions, intertrigo, and skin tears
- Protection of susceptible skin areas during the mammography maybe be necessary

If a client develops a pressure ulcer or skin tear during or after the mammogram, it is important to document accurately the wound and refer to the appropriate healthcare professional for advice and further management.

Healthcare professionals should also be culturally aware of the differences in skin tone when they assess clients. Two classification systems for objectively assessing human skin colour include the Munsell skin tone chart [33], which can assist with predicting pressure ulcer risk, and the 6 Fitzpatrick [34] skin types for assessing risk of damage from ultraviolet light.

Pressure Ulcer and Skin Tear Classification Systems

In order to provide consensus across Europe in the care and management of pressure ulcers, EPUAP [23] developed a common classification system in 2014 which is still used today.

When assessing the skin post mammogram for potential pressure damage the healthcare practitioner would examine the breasts and look for the following [23]:

- *Category/Stage I: Non blanchable Erythema Intact skin with non-blanchable redness of a localized area usually over a bony prominence. Darkly pigmented skin may not have visible blanching; its colour may differ from the surrounding area. The area may be painful, firm, soft, warmer or cooler as compared to adjacent tissue. Category/Stage I may be difficult to detect in individuals with dark skin tones. May indicate "at risk" individuals (a heralding sign of risk).*
- *Category/Stage II: Partial Thickness Skin Loss Partial thickness loss of dermis presenting as a shallow open ulcer with a red/pink wound bed, without slough. May also present as an intact or open/ruptured serum filled blister. Presents as a shiny or dry shallow ulcer without slough or bruising.* This Category/Stage should not be used to describe skin tears, tape burns, perineal dermatitis, maceration or excoriation. *Bruising indicates suspected deep tissue injury.*
- *Category/Stage III: Full Thickness Skin Loss Full thickness tissue loss. Subcutaneous fat may be visible but bone, tendon or muscle are not exposed. Slough may be present but does not obscure the depth of tissue loss. May include undermining and tunneling. The depth of a Category/Stage III pressure ulcer varies by anatomical location. The bridge of the nose, ear, occiput and malleolus do not have subcutaneous tissue and Category/Stage III ulcers can be shallow. In contrast, areas of significant adiposity can develop extremely deep Category/Stage I I pressure ulcers. Bone/tendon is not visible or directly palpable.*

- *Category/Stage IV: Full Thickness Tissue Loss Full thickness tissue loss with exposed bone, tendon or muscle. Slough or eschar may be present on some parts of the wound bed. Often include undermining and tunneling. The depth of a Category/Stage IV pressure ulcer varies by anatomical location. The bridge of the nose, ear, occiput and malleolus do not have subcutaneous tissue and these ulcers can be shallow. Category/Stage IV ulcers can extend into muscle and/or supporting structures (e.g., fascia, tendon or joint capsule) making osteomyelitis possible. Exposed bone/tendon is visible or directly palpable.*
- *Unstageable: Depth Unknown Full thickness tissue loss in which the base of the ulcer is covered by slough (yellow, tan, grey, green or brown) and/or eschar (tan, brown or black) in the wound bed. Until enough slough and/or eschar is removed to expose the base of the wound, the true depth, and therefore Category/Stage, cannot be determined. Stable (dry, adherent, intact without erythema or fluctuance) eschar on the heels serves as 'the body's natural (biological) cover' and should not be removed.*
- *Suspected Deep Tissue Injury: Depth Unknown Purple or maroon localized area of discoloured intact skin or blood-filled blister due to damage of underlying soft tissue from pressure and/or shear. The area may be preceded by tissue that is painful, firm, mushy, boggy, warmer or cooler as compared to adjacent tissue. Deep tissue injury may be difficult to detect in individuals with dark skin tones. Evolution may include a thin blister over a dark wound bed. The wound may further evolve and become covered by thin eschar. Evolution may be rapid exposing additional layers of tissue even with optimal treatment.*

Skin Tears

Payne and Martin [35] were the first practitioners to develop a classification system for skin tears and this is divided into categories and subcategories depending on the severity of the tear.

- Category 1: Skin tears without loss of tissue
- Category 2: Skin tears with partial tissue loss
- Category 3: Skin tears with complete tissue loss

Since 1993, subsequent studies have explored the inter-rater reliability of the classification system and general use in clinical practice, which has led to the development of a more universally acceptable classification Skin Tear Audit Research (STAR) Classification System [35, 36]. This system comprises three categories and two subcategories of skin tears. The STAR Classification System is generally used in Australia, with early indications of implementation reported across the UK. When assessing the skin post mammogram for potential skin tears the healthcare practitioner would examine the breasts and look for the following:

- Category 1a: A skin tear where the edges can be realigned to the normal anatomical position (without undue stretching) and the skin or flap colour is not pale, dusky or darkened.
- Category 1b: A skin tear where the edges can be realigned to the normal anatomical position (without undue stretching) and the skin or flap colour is pale, dusky or darkened.
- Category 2a: A skin tear where the edges cannot be realigned to the normal anatomical position and the skin or flap colour is not pale, dusky or darkened.
- Category 2b: A skin tear where the edges cannot be realigned to the normal anatomical position and the skin or flap colour is pale dusky or darkened.
- Category 3: A skin tear where the skin flap is completely absent.

Intertrigo

Intertriginous dermatitis has been defined as *'an inflammatory dermatosis [dermatitis] involving the body folds, notably those of the sub-mammary [under the breasts] and genitocrural regions'* [37]. It is caused by perspiration trapped in skin folds plus the effect of friction of the skin layers rubbing together. Intertrigo usually starts with erythema and inflammation and can lead to lesions or ulceration of the skin due to maceration and wet oedema. Factors that increase the risk of developing intertrigo include increased stratum corneum ph (predisposing the risk to yeast infections), obesity (increased moisture and heat in the skin folds), atophy (genetic predisposition to develop allergic reactions), and age (the moisture barrier decreasing with age) [38].

Intertrigo in the inframammary area is directly linked to women (and men) with large or pendulous breasts. This creates a warm and moist environment which can lead to intertrigo. Common symptoms include itching, burning, or stinging. However, some experience no symptoms at all. Candidiasis can occur and presents as satellite papules or pustules with a bright red colour or merging erythema [39].

Management and Other Considerations

If the mammography practitioner finds a pressure ulcer, skin tear, intertrigo or abrasion on the breast pre or post mammography procedure, it is imperative to discuss with the client subsequent management. This may include the practitioner carrying out some simple wound management and/or a referral to other services.

Simple steps to consider include:

1. Control of any bleeding and cleaning of the wound according to local policy.
2. If the wound is a skin tear and it is feasible and viable, to realign any skin flap or tear.

3. Assessment of the client, their wound and the peri wound area adhering to local policy documents, to assess the degree of tissue damage or loss. This may include the use of either a pressure ulcer or skin tear classification tool, depending on the diagnosis.
4. Apply appropriate dressings according to local policy dressing formulary.
5. Referral to appropriate healthcare practitioner for follow up dressings or treatment of intertrigo and candidiasis.
6. Discussion with the client regards to findings and health education and promotion.
7. Completion of any clinical incident or safety report forms.

Clinical Pearls

- Prior to carrying out the mammography, gain consent from the client to examine the skin of the breast. Check for intertrigo, any splits, sores or cracks, and dry skin. Record this examination in the notes.
- If a client is informing you that they are in pain from the procedure and their skin feels as though it is ripping or tearing, stop the procedure and check the client and their skin where it hurts or feels damaged. A mammogram should not hurt so much that it deters future tests.
- After the mammogram, gain consent to examine the skin once more, checking for tears, bruising, signs of pressure damage and recording this examination in the notes.
- Advise clients to contact the department and their local healthcare provider if during the next 24–48 h they develop skin damage for follow up and complete any clinical incident or safety report forms.

Chapter Review Questions
Review Questions

1. Which of the following are not acceptable risks of mammography?
   (a) Bruising
   (b) Reddening or warmth of the skin that dissipates after 15 min once the mammogram has finished.
   (c) Pressure Ulcers and skin tears.
   (d) Tingling
2. What are clients calling damage to their skin after mammography?
3. Why is it important to document a client's skin assessment pre and post mammography?

Answers

1. Pressure Ulcers and skin tears.
2. Traumatic Mammography Injury
3. It is good practice and aids diagnosis and management if skin damage was to occur.

Acknowledgments The authors would like to thank Beekley Medical for the kind permissions to use the images of skin tears from mammography.

Appendix

Test your learning and check your understanding of this book's contents: use the "Springer Nature Flashcards" app to access questions using https://sn.pub/dcAnWL.

To use the app, please follow the instructions in Chap. 1.

Flashcard code:
48341-69945-ABCB1-2A8C7-CE9D2.

Short URL: https://sn.pub/dcAnWL.

References

1. NHS Breast Screening Programme. Information and advice for health professionals in breast screening. Sheffield: NHS Cancer Screening Programme; 2002.
2. Cancerbackup. NHS breast screening: helping you decide. Available from: http://www.cancerscreening.nhs.uk/breastscreen/publications/nhsbsp.pdf. Accessed 17 Jan 2022.
3. Avery AJ, Sheehan C, Bell B, Armstrong S, Ashcroft DM, Boyd MJ, Chuter A, Cooper A, Donnelly A, Edwards A, Evans HP. Incidence, nature and causes of avoidable significant harm in primary care in England: retrospective case note review. BMJ Qual Saf. 2021;30(12):961–76.
4. Slawomirski L, Auraaen A, Klazinga N. The economics of patient safety: strengthening a value-based approach to reducing patient harm at national level. Paris: OECD; 2017.
5. de Vries EN, Ramrattan MA, Smorenburg SM, Gouma DJ, Boermeester MA. The incidence and nature of in-hospital adverse events: a systematic review. Qual Saf Health Care. 2008;17(3):216–23.
6. World Health Organisation. Patient safety- Global action on patient safety. Report by the Director-General. Geneva: World Health Organization; 2019.
7. Donaldson LJ. The wisdom of patients and families: ignore it at our peril. BMJ Qual Saf. 2015;24:603–4.
8. Vibberts M. Skin-tears-in-mammography-happen… but-do-they-have-to. Available from: https://blog.beekley.com/skin-tears-in-mammography-happen%E2%80%A6but-do-they-have-to. Accessed 17 Jan 2022.
9. Vibberts M. When a breast skin tear becomes more important than diagnosis. Available from: https://blog.beekley.com/when-a-breast-skin-tear-becomes-more-important-than-diagnosis. Accessed 17 Jan 2022.
10. Steady Health. Excessive breast pain after mammogram. Available from: https://www.steadyhealth.com/topics/excessive-breast-pain-after-mammogram?page=1. Accessed 17 Jan 2022.
11. 2PeasRefugees. Tear/micro-tears under breast after mammogram? Available from: https://2peasrefugees.boards.net/thread/39692/micro-tears-breast-after-mammogram. Accessed 17 Jan 2022.
12. Nursing and Midwifery Council. The code. Available from: https://www.nmc.org.uk/standards/code/. Accessed 17 Jan 2022.
13. UK Public General Acts. Data protection act 2018. Available from: https://www.legislation.gov.uk/ukpga/2018/12/contents/enacted. Accessed 17 Jan 2022.
14. Shonyo M. The impact of skin tears on patients and breast imaging centers: viewpoints from two different perspectives. Available from: https://beekley.com/Portals/0/Resource%20Library/Case%20Studies%20&%20White%20Papers/Mammography/Impact%20of%20Skin%20Tears%20on%20Patients%20and%20Breast%20Imaging%20Centers.pdf?utm_source=blog&utm_medium=blog-skin-tears&utm_campaign=blog-patient-fears-skin-tears. Accessed 17 Jan 2022.
15. Dustler M, Andersson I, Brorson H, Fröjd P, Mattsson S, Tingberg A, Zackrisson S, Förnvik D. Breast compression in mammography: pressure distribution patterns. Acta Radiol. 2012;53(9):973–80.
16. Stekelenburg A, Oomens CW, Strijkers GJ, Nicolay K, Bader DL. Compression-induced deep tissue injury examined with magnetic resonance imaging and histology. J Appl Physiol. 2006 Jun;100(6):1946–54.
17. National Pressure Ulcer Advisory Panel. Friction induced skin injuries – are they pressure ulcers? Available from: https://www.npuap.org/wp-content/uploads/2012/01/NPUAP-Friction-White-Paper.pdf. Accessed 17 Jan 2022.
18. National Pressure Ulcer Advisory Panel. Shear force initiative presentation. Available from: http://www.npuap.org/wp-content/uploads/2012/03/Shear_slides.pdf. Accessed 17 Jan 2022.
19. Kolarsick PAJ, Kolarsick MA, Goodwin C. Anatomy and physiology of the skin. J Dermatol Nurses Assoc. 2011;3(4):203–13.
20. Tortora GJ, Derrickson BH. Principles of anatomy and physiology: organisation, support and movement and control systems of the human body, vol. 1. 12th ed. Hoboken NJ: Wiley; 2009.
21. McLafferty E, Hendry C, Farley A. The integumentary system: anatomy, physiology and function of skin. Nurs Stand. 2012;27(3):35–42.
22. Langton AK, Halai P, Griffiths CEM, Sherratt MJ, Watson REB. The impact of intrinsic ageing on the protein composition of the dermal-epidermal junction. Mechan Age Develop. 2016;156:14–6. https://doi.org/10.1016/j.mad.2016.03.006.
23. European Pressure Ulcer Advisory Panel and Pan Pacific Pressure Injury Alliance. Prevention and treatment of pressure ulcers/injuries: clinical practice guideline: the international guideline. EPUAP/NPIAP/PPPIA; 2019.
24. LeBlanc K, Baranoski S. Skin tears: state of the science: consensus statements for the prevention, prediction, assessment, and treatment of skin tears©. Adv Skin Wound Care. 2011;24(9):2–15.
25. Fletcher J. Device related pressure ulcers made easy. Available from: http://www.woundsinternational.com/pdf/content_10472.pdf. Accessed 17 Jan 2022.
26. Voegeli D. Factors that exacerbate skin breakdown and ulceration, Skin breakdown, the silent epidemic. Hull: Smith and Nephew Foundation; 2007.
27. Baranoski S, Ayello EA. Wound care essentials, practice principles. Springhouse: Lippincott, Williams and Wilkins; 2004.
28. Mistiaen P, van Halm-Walters M. Prevention and treatment of intertrigo in large skin folds of adults: a systematic review. BMC Nurs. 2010;9(12):1–9.
29. Stephen-Haynes J, Carville K. Skin tears made easy. Wounds Int. 2011;2(4):1–6.

30. Wingfeld C. Managing dry skin conditions. Wound Essent. 2011;6:50–9.
31. British National Formulary. British National Formulary online. Available from: http://www.bnf.org/bnf/index.htm. Accessed 17 Jan 2022.
32. Johnston E. The role of nutrition in Tissue Viability. Available from: http://www.woundsinternational.com/pdf/content_182.pdf. Accessed 17 Jan 2022.
33. Fitzpatrick TB. The validity and practicality of sunreactive skin types I through VI. Arch Dermatol. 1988;124(6):869–71.
34. Konishi N, Kawada A, Morimoto Y, Watake A, Matsuda H, Oiso N, Kawara S. New approach to the evaluation of skin color of pigmentary lesions using Skin Tone Color Scale. J Dermatol. 2007;34(7):441–6.
35. Payne RL, Martin ML. Defining and classifying skin tears: need for a common language. Ostomy Wound Manag. 1993;39(5):16–20.
36. Carville K, Lewin G, Newall N, Haslehurst P, Michael R, Santamaria N, Roberts P. STAR: a consensus for skin tear classification. Prim Intent. 2007;15(1):18–28.
37. McMahon R, Buckeldee J. Skin problems beneath the breasts of in-patients: the knowledge, opinions and practice of nurses. J Adv Nurs. 1992;17(10):1243–50.
38. White W. Skin tears: a descriptive study of the opinions, clinical practice and knowledge base of RNs caring for the aged in high care residential facilities. Prim Intent. 2001;9(4):138–49.
39. Sibbald RG, Kelley J, Kennedy-Evans KL, Labrecque C, Waters N. A practical approach to the prevention and management of intertrigo, or moisture-associated skin damage, due to perspiration: expert consensus on best practice. Wound Care Canada. 2013;11(2):1–21.

Part III

Mammography Equipment

18

Ioannis Sechopoulos and Cláudia Sá dos Reis

Learning Objectives
- Understand the basic function of the different components of a mammography system.
- Describe the similarities and differences between the equipment used for the different x-ray-based breast imaging modalities.
- Describe the basic concepts of image processing and display after image acquisition.

Introduction

Being one of the most technically demanding examinations in radiography, mammography requires X-ray technology designed specifically

I. Sechopoulos (✉)
Department of Medical Imaging, Radboud University Medical Center, Nijmegen, The Netherlands

Technical Medical Centre, University of Twente, Enschede, The Netherlands

Dutch Expert Centre for Screening (LRCB), Nijmegen, The Netherlands
e-mail: ioannis.sechopoulos@radboudumc.nl

C. S. dos Reis
Escola Superior de Tecnologia da Saúde de Lisboa, Lisbon School of Health Technology, Lisbon, Portugal
e-mail: claudia.reis@estesl.ipl.pt

for the task. The pathology to be imaged ranges from small, 20–100 μm, high density calcifications to ill-defined low contrast masses. These must be imaged against a background of mixed densities. This makes demonstrating pathology challenging. Because of its use in asymptomatic screening, mammography must also employ as low a radiation dose as possible while still yielding an adequate image for the task at hand [1, 2].

In the past three decades, revolutionary technological developments in breast imaging have taken place [1, 2]. The main goal pursued by the mammography equipment industry has been to develop practical, inexpensive, and harmless equipment which is both appealing and effective in identifying, localising, and characterising abnormal tissues and signs of pathology within the breast [3–5]. Currently available technologies for breast imaging are used to identify structural or morphological differences in tumours, such as calcifications, soft tissue masses, asymmetry and architectural distortion. Some of the more recently developed techniques, especially with the use of intravenous contrast agents, can provide information about the biological or functional differences between tumours and normal tissues.

Mammography is based on the differential attenuation of X-ray photons in the breast tissues and this process is optimised when low-energy photons are used [6, 7]. The varying composition and densities of the adipose and fibroglandular tissues produce singular contrasts represented as dark and bright areas in the mammography image. However, the composition and density of fibroglandular tissue and carcinoma are similar and therefore, for the most part, non-calcified lesions are distinguished by their morphology, not their contrast.

The need for lower energy X-ray spectra to enhance contrast, for high spatial resolution to aid in the visibility and characterisation of calcifications, and for breast compression to reduce tissue overlap (among many other reasons), promotes the refinement of dedicated X-ray equipment for mammography. These systems count with specialised X-ray tubes, detectors, and overall acquisition geometries [6].

Technological advances over the last several decades have greatly improved the diagnostic performance of mammography. However, probably the most important milestone was the introduction of digital mammography systems in the 1990s. The possibility of advanced acquisitions and post-processing of the images opened the door to new imaging techniques that have great expanded the possibilities of X-ray breast imaging. Over the last two decades, three new X-ray modalities have been developed aimed at addressing the two most important limitations of standard mammography, its two-dimensional nature and its anatomical-imaging only nature.

Digital breast tomosynthesis (DBT) [8–10] and dedicated breast computed tomography (BCT) [11–13] have finally introduced tomography, to varying degrees, to X-ray breast imaging. The former, although only a pseudo-three-dimensional modality, shares the same platform as standard mammography, and therefore results in equivalent installation requirements and very similar workflow and interpretation. This has established DBT as the new standard in X-ray breast imaging, in many countries practically replacing standard mammography completely [14]. BCT involves a completely new system geometry and acquisition setup. However, BCT imaging requires no breast compression, making it attractive for the patients, and is fully three-dimensional, promising to further enhance clinical performance. Therefore, interest in BCT is

high, and its best placement in the clinical realm remains to be ascertained.

While still two-dimensional, contrast-enhanced spectral mammography (CESM) results in functional images in which the blood flow and uptake in (malignant) lesions are depicted [15–17]. This capability has made CESM be of great interest, being a potential alternative to breast MRI while being considerably more affordable and with fewer contraindications.

The Mammographic X-Ray Unit

Mammography is performed using dedicated equipment usually with a "C" shaped arm aimed at facilitating breast positioning. The C arm can be adjusted in height and angular orientation to adjust the compression paddle and the breast support to the client standing or sitting position. The X-ray tube and digital receptor table assembly are mounted in opposition: the X-ray tube for the generation of the photon beam along with a face protector on the top head, and a compression paddle, the image receptor system on the lower arm (Fig. 18.1).

The stages for production of mammography images are acquisition, processing, display, and post processing for interpretation and storage. In digital mammography, each step is performed by an individual system that can be independently assessed and optimised. The image acquisition system is composed of an X-ray tube, breast compression paddle, and image receptor system [7]. The distance from the X-ray focus to the breast support platform is commonly around 60 cm. A moving anti-scatter grid is normally used, which is situated just behind the low-attenuation (often carbon-fibre) tabletop and in front of the image receptor. Some designs work without an anti-scatter grid and make a software correction for the large-scale effects of scattered radiation in the image [18, 19].

Due to the requirements for very high spatial resolution, X-ray focal spot sizes must be small. Focal spots of approximately 0.3×0.3 mm are used for conventional mammography, with a size

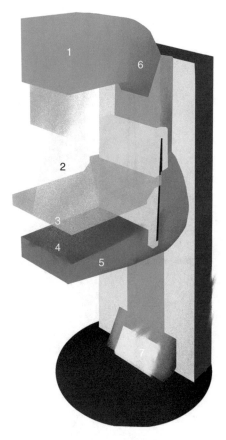

Fig. 18.1 Integrated direct digital mammography system. 1 X-ray tube, 2 X-ray beam, 3 compression paddle, 4 breast support, 5 detector, 6 C-arm, 7 monitor for angle, breast thickness, and compression force

The Mammographic X-Ray Spectrum

The X-ray spectrum from a conventional tungsten target, glass encapsulated, aluminium filtered X-ray tube is not necessarily optimal for mammography. The optimal photon energy considering subject contrast between the different breast tissues and dose is around 20 keV, which is much lower than that used in normal radiography [7]. Increasing photon energy will reduce contrast and reducing photon energy will lead to inadequate penetration of the breast and a large increase in patient dose, so the X-ray spectrum is critical. A range of mammographic spectra are used for digital mammography.

The X-ray tube target may well be switchable (depending on the design) between molybdenum and rhodium, or consist only of tungsten, which has now become the most common X-ray tube target in mammography systems. Due to the low-energy spectra, to maximize tube output, the tube has a low attenuation beryllium output window. The beam is then filtered with either molybdenum, rhodium, silver, or aluminium filters, with other filter materials, like copper, titanium, or tin, being used or investigated for use in CESM [8, 9]. The X-ray tube is operated, in general, at a voltage in the range of 25–35 kV, although somewhat higher voltages may be used for DBT, while, of course, CESM requires the use of voltages in the range of 45–49 kV for the acquisition of the second, high-energy projection.

Figure 18.2 shows the spectrum of a rhodium target, rhodium filtered beam at a tube voltage of 30 kV. Rhodium has characteristic X-ray peaks at 20.2 and 22.7 keV, which contribute strongly to the limited range spectrum. Rhodium is again used as the filter because, due to the K-edge absorption, it strongly attenuates energies just above its own K-characteristic peaks as well as attenuating lower energies. The end result is a spectrum with most photons lying in a narrow band of energies.

Although molybdenum and rhodium targets are no longer the most common X-ray sources used in mammography, these are still in use and Fig. 18.2 is a good example of how the right com-

of 0.15 × 0.15 mm selectable for magnified views, where the breast is raised away from the image receptor on a special magnification table to produce a geometrically magnified view [7].

The X-ray tube is positioned within the unit so that the anode heel effect is employed to reduce X-ray intensity towards the nipple side of the field where the breast will be thinner. Heavy reliance is placed on the automatic exposure control system of modern mammography units. These systems can sense the thickness and composition of the compressed breast and then automatically select the tube potential, target and filter combination, and tube current-exposure time product required to give the optimal imaging exposure within the constraints of patient dose limitations [7].

Fig. 18.2 X-ray spectrum for a typical rhodium target, rhodium filtered mammographic X-ray beam at 30 kV. The spectrum peaks around 20 keV due to the characteristic X-ray emissions of the rhodium target. This spectrum is suitable for imaging moderate-sized breasts

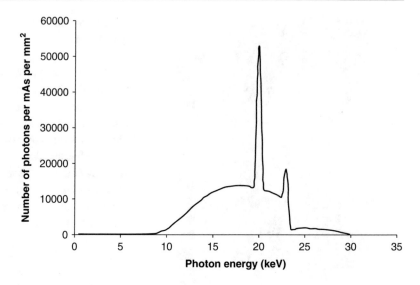

Fig. 18.3 X-ray spectrum for a typical tungsten target, aluminium-filtered mammographic X-ray beam at 30 kV

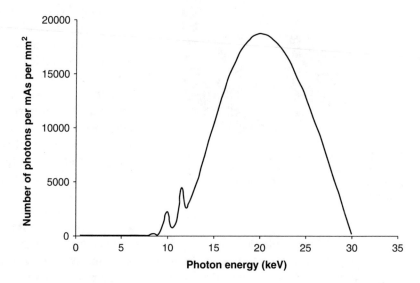

bination of target and filter material are used to maximize the number of X-ray photons in the beam that are close to the optimal energy. Since the introduction of digital mammography, sources with tungsten targets have become more common, and they have been paired with a variety of different filters. Fig. 18.3 shows the spectrum of a tungsten target, aluminium-filtered beam again at a tube voltage of 30 kV, with the X-ray tube again having a beryllium output window.

The shape of the spectrum is quite different from Fig. 18.2 even though the tube voltage is the same. The tungsten target has no K-characteristic X-ray peaks in this energy range, and the aluminium filter, which similarly does not have a K-absorption edge in this energy range, does not preferentially attenuate the higher energy end of the spectrum.

Compression Paddle Design

In mammography the breast is compressed using a rigid transparent plastic compression paddle that is motor driven. The use of compression force reduces the thickness of the breast and holds it in place, which gives several advantages [7]:

- Reduced tissue superposition. Compressing the breast makes the tissues spread out over a larger area, reducing the possibilities for normal fibroglandular tissue masking pathology (reducing sensitivity) and of separate normal tissues projecting onto the image in a way that mimics a suspicious lesion (reducing specificity).
- Better spatial resolution. The breast is brought closer to the imaging receptor so that magnification and focal spot blurring is reduced.
- Reduced movement blur, even at the relatively long exposure times (1 s typical) common in mammography.
- Less scattered radiation in the image. The beam path length through the breast is shorter, so there is less material to do the scattering. Reducing the proportion of scattered radiation in the image improves image contrast.
- Lower radiation dose to the breast. Due to the same reduction of the beam path length through the breast, there is overall less absorption of X rays in the breast, so lower exposure levels are needed.
- Improved image uniformity. Compression spreads the breast tissue out more evenly across the image and makes pathology easier to detect.
- Diminished exposure time given the need for lower total exposure for an adequate acquisition [20, 21].
- The reduced path length makes practicable the use of lower energy (less penetrating) X-ray spectra. This gives greater subject contrast.

Compression in mammography is one of the few occasions in radiography where a technical advantage is gained without detriment to other aspects of the image, although there is a disadvantage in patient discomfort. Mammography systems measure the increasing amount of force resulting from a given small increase in compression to stop the motorised movement at a given compression. The compression force maximum limit set on mammography systems is 200 Newtons. A range of compression paddles are normally supplied with a digital mammography system to cover different types of projections [7]. Some typical types are:

- Flat rigid paddle - The basic flat paddle that covers the whole of the area of the digital image receptor and is used for full-field mediolateral oblique (MLO) and cranio-caudal (CC) views. The paddle maintains its shape parallel to the plane of the receptor and deforms only slightly when the compression force is applied.
- Tilting flat paddle - A flat paddle used for full-field MLO and CC views that allows rotation against a spring resistance so that during compression the chest-wall side of the breast will be thicker than the nipple side. The advantages are claimed to be that the design holds the breast in place more firmly.
- Sliding compression paddle - Suitable for imaging smaller breasts where the full area of the image receptor is not required. By sliding the paddle to one side or the other, the MLO view can be achieved using the edge of the breast support table to improve positioning.
- Spot compression paddle - This paddle has a raised cylindrical area that applies extra compression force over a small area. The advantages to spot compression are that better compression over the small area of interest is obtained, with all of the advantages above, but also that the spreading of surrounding parenchyma allows the outline of masses to be better visualised. Whereas features in superimposed tissue will spread out, mechanically harder malignant tissues will tend to retain their shape. Spot views are an additional examination often performed at assessment.

Magnification Compression Paddle

For magnification views, an add-on breast support table is used that raises the breast away from the plane of the image receptor by some 30 cm (depending on the magnification factor and focus-to-receptor distance), so that the image is geometrically magnified. The compression paddle for this is smaller, as the X-ray field is smaller closer to the focus, and often has a step in the support arm to allow it to fix to the compression system at a point lower than the magnification support table. Please refer to Chap. 30.

Biopsy Compression Paddle

Various specialist compression paddles may be required for biopsy systems where the paddle has an aperture to accommodate the biopsy needle or device (Chap. 30).

Multiple advances have been proposed to lessen the uncomfortable aspect of breast compression, although the tolerance to it is variable (Chap. 16) while maintaining its advantages. Some such paddles have different levels of tilt, allowing for superior compression of the mid and anterior breast with less client discomfort. Another paddle has a curve in the center, more closely following the expected anatomy of the breast, especially in the CC view, allowing for superior compression towards the periphery of the breast compared to the central portion.

Another advance that does not involve only the re-design of the paddle is the use of a compression system that measures compression pressure (pressure = force/area) instead of force. Chapter 28 provides more details on this approach to breast compression. No recommendation is provided regarding the suitable compression force to consider the characteristics of the breast, namely compressibility, composition, and thickness. Several studies [22–27] investigated the best compression force in terms of dose, image quality, and client tolerance. One of these studies concluded that the amount of compression force has noticeable effects on image quality. Moreover, better image quality rates were consistently associated with higher compression forces [22], although the tolerance to compression is variable (Chap. 27). However, a study has also reported lower sensitivity at screening at the highest levels of compression force [28]. So, it is possible that the application of too high a compression level is not only detrimental to client comfort, but also to the clinical performance of the exam. Furthermore, another study evaluated the increase in compressed breast thickness, possibility for motion artifacts, and loss of tissue coverage if the compression force used was reduced by half, and no detrimental effects were found, while the level of comfort for the client was significantly increased [29]. Clearly, there is still room for further research in the area of breast compression.

Digital Mammographic Image Receptors

Digital image capture was first introduced into mammography as 'small-field digital mammography' for needle and core biopsy guidance, using detectors typically approximately 15 cm in size. Full-field digital mammography, with detector sizes up to the equivalent of the 24 × 30 cm was developed later.

The imaging advantages of digital mammography include a wide and linear dynamic range and the separation of the image capture and image display functions, so that the image display can be varied to optimally show the full range of recorded X-ray intensities [7]. This provides good visualisation of the skin line and nipple and has advantages when imaging dense breasts and younger clients [30]. Although a wide range of competing image capture technologies for digital mammography have been introduced since the introduction of digital detectors to this imaging modality, only two technologies, both consisting of full-field detectors, remain widely in use: the amorphous selenium-based direct and the scintillator-based indirect detectors [31].

General Features of Digital Mammographic Images

A digital image is not a continuous distribution of bright and dark but is composed of a finite number of points (or 'pixels'), where each pixel has a value of brightness dictated by a stored numerical value. Digital images have the advantage that they can be enhanced and manipulated by computer to extract the maximum amount of diagnostic information. Digital images can be stored, transferred, copied without detriment, and retrieved in a very efficient manner using computer mass data storage techniques [32]. They have the disadvantage of a limit to spatial resolution caused by the finite pixel size. Digital mammography receptors have a very linear response between pixel value and the radiation dose incident on the pixel over a very wide dynamic range, typically a factor of some 10,000:1. The choice of what dose is required for digital mammography is therefore driven by the signal-to-noise ratio required for a diagnostic image rather than a specific radiation dose to the receptor [7].

The Direct Digital Detector: Amorphous Selenium

In direct conversion detectors the X-ray interaction is converted directly to an electrical signal using an amorphous selenium (a-Se) layer, behind which lies an amorphous silicon microcircuit layer, which in turn is supported by a rigid substrate (Fig. 18.4) [7]. Selenium is a photoconductor, so is an electrical insulator in the dark, and a conductor when exposed to light or X-rays. The amorphous selenium is employed as a mammographic image receptor in the form of a thin layer (~0.5 mm) with a voltage applied between a large area electrode across the front surface, and an array of charge collection electrodes, one per pixel, on the back surface. These are linked to capacitors to accumulate the charge released during the exposure. These are linked, in turn, to

thin-film-transistor switches to provide a line-by-line read out arrangement in which the charge stored for an individual pixel is passed pixel-by-pixel along the line until it can be measured by electronics external to the imaging sensor. Incoming X-ray photons interact photoelectrically in the a-Se layer producing electrons and 'holes' (the vacancy where an electron should be). Because of the high voltage gradient across the thin a-Se layer, the electrons move towards the positive surface electrode and the holes towards the negative charge collection electrodes. The electrons and holes do not move sideways as they must follow the direction of the electric field gradient, so image blurring from this source is minimal and the spatial resolution of the detector is good. At the end of the exposure, the charge signals (proportional to the radiation detected) from each pixel are read out via the thin-film-transistor switches and data lines. The charge signals are converted to digital values via charge amplifiers and with a digital-to-analogue converter and sent to the computer for assembly into an image.

The photoconductor is a layer of amorphous selenium that allows electrons to flow across it when exposed to X-ray photons [7]. The capacitor builds up a charge, proportional to the X-ray exposure for that pixel. The charge is transferred out of the device via the switch at the end of the exposure and converted to a numerical pixel value.

The a-Se layer has good photon capture characteristics in the mammographic energy range, and the lack of sideways spread of the electrons and holes carrying the image information allow the a-Se layer to be made relatively thick, resulting in an efficient detector. As the receptor is

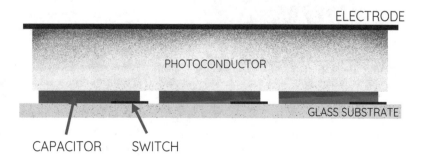

Fig. 18.4 Cross-section through a direct digital mammography image receptor

mounted rigidly in the breast support table of the mammography unit, it is always in the same position with respect to the X-ray beam, allowing the use of 'flat-fielding'. This is an important image calibration in which the receptor is exposed to the unattenuated X-ray beam under test conditions, so that variation in the X-ray intensity across the field and variations in pixel-to-pixel sensitivity can be removed from subsequent images. The removal of these fixed noise sources further improves the efficiency of the receptor.

The Indirect Digital Detector: Scintillator and Amorphous Silicon

Indirect digital mammography detectors use a two-step process for X-ray detection [6, 7, 18]. This type of receptor is similar to that commonly employed in digital radiography and consists of a thin crystalline scintillator layer closely coupled to an amorphous silicon microcircuit layer which is supported by a rigid substrate. Indirect conversion detectors work by first converting the incident X-ray distribution into a light image, then converting the light distribution into electrical signals addressable to a pixel location on the detector [6, 33, 34] (Fig. 18.5).

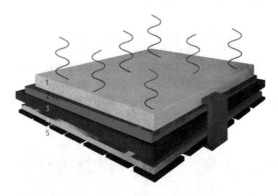

Fig. 18.5 Basic structure of detectors for digital mammography in integrated systems. *Layer 1*—detector material: CsI scintillator + transparent electrode or a-Se (amorphous selenium), *Layer 2*—a-Si array (amorphous silicon), *Layer 3*—base plate, *Layer 4*—driver board— readout board—driver board and *Layer 5*—glass substrate (Reproduced courtesy of Mário Oliveira)

The most successful scintillator is thallium-activated caesium iodide [7]. This has excellent X-ray absorption characteristics and can be grown in a channeled crystal structure that acts like a fibre optic guide to prevent light spreading sideways, giving to the detector improved spatial resolution. It is similar to the input phosphor material of X-ray image intensifiers. The scintillator layer is deposited onto an amorphous silicon micro-circuit array of light sensitive photodiodes and associated electronics to measure the signal from each photodiode. After the X-ray exposure is completed, a switching array of thin-film transistors and associated data lines allow the signals from the photodiodes to be fed out of the receptor array in sequence. These signals are then digitised and transferred to the computer to be assembled into an image.

This type of receptor is also mounted rigidly in the breast support table of the mammography unit, so the important flat-fielding correction described above can also be used, with the same removal of fixed pattern noise and resulting efficiency improvement [7].

The introduction of DBT and CESM resulted, for some systems, in some advances or modifications in these digital detectors. In the case of DBT, detector readout needed to be fast enough to allow for the acquisition of all the DBT projections within a short period. Although acquisition protocols vary substantially across DBT systems, some systems acquire 15 projections in ~2–4 s. Such acquisition protocol requires a detector readout rate that is much faster than what was needed for standard mammography. This rapid projection acquisition also required electronic advances to reduce detector lag, the latent signal from a previous acquisition that remains as a faint shadow in subsequent acquisitions [35]. For CESM, due to the use of a considerably higher-energy X-ray spectrum than that in standard mammography and DBT, the X-ray stopping layer, be it the a-Se layer or CsI scintillator, has to be thick enough to achieve a reasonable detection efficiency for these higher-energy photons [36].

Legacy Devices

Multiple detector technologies were used with different success in digital mammography [7]. Some of these, although not widely commercialised anymore, still have an important installed footprint, especially in countries where medical imaging equipment is not replaced at a relatively rapid pace. Probably the most common of these is computed radiography (CR) [7]. CR systems have been especially popular due to their being an affordable entry point to digital imaging. CR is used with traditional screen-film mammography systems, replacing only the screen-film cassette for the CR-based detector, which is then read out by a special scanner. As such, to introduce some level of digitisation to the mammography clinic, with CR it is not necessary to completely replace the imaging systems. As a result, CR systems continue to be prevalent in many countries with limited resources to allow for installation of full-digital systems. CR is based on the phenomenon of photo-stimulable luminescence.

When X-rays are incident on a material such as europium-doped barium fluorohalide, they produce high-energy photoelectrons that in turn produce ionisation that results in many lower energy electron–hole pairs. In conventional screen-film mammography, this happens in a screen in close contact with the film where the electron–hole pairs recombine to emit light that then exposes the film [7]. In photo-stimulable luminescence, however, less than 50% of the electron–hole pairs recombine, the others are trapped apart due to the presence of the doped sites in the phosphor. These electron traps are crystal lattice defects where halogen ion vacancies occur in the otherwise regular ionic lattice. These so-called 'F' or 'Colour' centres are created during manufacture by prolonged irradiation of the imaging plate with high intensity X-rays and ultra-violet light.

Following exposure, electrons can remain trapped at these defects for many hours or days, although the stored image gradually fades with time. The concentration of trapped electrons is proportional to the locally incident X-ray exposure. The electrons are trapped in this state until they are stimulated by light of a suitable wavelength in a CR plate reader, whereupon they are free to travel to the holes, recombine and emit light. The emitted light, which is linearly proportional to the locally incident X-ray intensity is then detected by a photomultiplier and digitised to form an image. The plate reader works by scanning an intense laser beam across the image plate on a line-by-line basis while the plate is slowly drawn through. A red laser is used to add enough energy to the trapped electrons to get them out of their traps and into the conduction band of the material. They can then move and recombine with a positive ion, dropping back to the ground energy state, and in doing so emit their excess energy as a photon of blue light. This weak light signal is picked up by a light guide and sent via a blue filter (to keep out the red light of the stimulating laser) to a photo-multiplier tube that measures the amount of light. This signal is then digitised to produce the raw 'pixel value' associated with that particular location on the image plate.

The scanning laser is focused to a diameter of approximately 0.1 mm to define the pixel of the image (although note that the imaging plate is continuous and not divided into physical pixels). Following read-out, the image plate is exposed to high-intensity light to completely erase any traces of the previous image, then reloaded into the cassette and ejected from the reader ready for reuse.

Because the CR cassette is not mounted rigidly in position, and several cassettes will normally be used in rotation, it is not possible to apply flat-fielding corrections in CR mammography, and the efficiency of the detector is reduced by the fixed pattern noise in the image arising from non-uniformity of the crystalline photo-stimulable phosphor. There is also an element of light spread in the phosphor from the read-out laser that leads to some blurring. Although, as mentioned, CR is a stepping stone to digital imaging, it has been found that CR is too inefficient, resulting in considerably higher doses and lower clinical performance than even screen-film mammography [37, 38].

A quite different type of digital mammography system that is no longer marketed is that employing a scanning fan beam of X-rays coupled to a moving one-dimensional photon-counting detector. This geometry is attractive in terms of its ability to reject scattered photons using a slit collimator at the detector, so no anti-scatter grid is required. The photon-counting detector, based on those used in high-energy experimental physics, counts each individual photon detected, and the pixel brightness is dictated by the total photons counted during the time the X-ray beam was swept over the pixel position. This has the advantage that low-level fluctuations caused by thermal excitation in the amplifiers and electronics can be rejected, leaving only the higher energy photon counts, so one source of image noise can be negated. In addition, later generations of these detectors included more advanced electronics allowing for the energy of the detected photon to be determined, and therefore photons of different energy levels could be discriminated.

Although this energy resolution is limited, it does allow for the simultaneous acquisition of at least two images, one consisting of the detected low-energy X rays and the other only including the high-energy X-rays. This is ideal for CESM acquisitions. However, the motorised movements of the scanning beam are complex, the X-ray tube loading tends to be high, and the scan time is generally longer than the exposure time for a two-dimensional receptor. These issues, among others, resulted in this technology, for now, not being pursued further for mammography.

The Automatic Exposure Control System

In the 1980s the automatic exposure control (AEC) system was implemented in mammography equipment with the aim to provide the most optimal optical density on the film. For the most part, current mammography AEC systems adjust the exposure time, while the tube current is often fixed or varied only across very few settings. Mammographic AECs can be very sophisticated, making allowance for the attenuation of the breast,

the energy of the beam, and able to automatically select not only the exposure time, but in some implementations also the target/filter combination and tube voltage for the breast being imaged. For this, most current digital mammography systems use part of the digital detector itself as the AEC sensor. The image acquisition starts with a short low-dose exposure, called pre-exposure or scout image, of the breast and the resulting signal is sampled automatically to identify the area with the lowest signal level, which usually corresponds to the densest areas of the breast. This information, in combination with the compressed breast thickness obtained from an electronic readout of the position of the arm of the compression paddle, is used to select the optimal image acquisition settings.

In some systems, the breast thickness alone determines the target/filter (for systems that have more than one of either) and the tube voltage to be used, while the pre-exposure is only used to set the tube current-exposure time product. In other systems, all these image acquisition settings are determined based on the pre-exposure [7]. The most sophisticated AEC systems can detect non-breast tissue on the pre-exposure image, so the AEC can be used when imaging breasts with implants or some medical device.

The AEC system is usually programmed to provide a constant contrast-to-noise ratio with increasing compressed breast thickness, although at the largest thicknesses the signal-to-noise ratio is allowed to decrease slowly, to avoid the largest increase in doses for the largest breasts.

Optimisation of Digital Mammography

The linear response and wide dynamic range of digital mammographic receptors means that images can be successfully acquired over a large range of doses [7]. This provides several possibilities for image optimisation and dose reduction, but equally also allows systems with sub-optimal setups to acquire images at higher patient doses than are necessary. The phenomenon of 'exposure creep' has been identified in general digital radiography, where average patient doses can rise due to the natural human inclination to make the images look better, and the fact that images are not rejected for being 'too good'. Modern automatic exposure control software may offer alternative combinations of automatic exposure factors that either optimise for contrast (at the expense of higher dose) or dose (at the expense of poorer contrast-to-noise ratio).

Given the sophisticated AEC systems now available, after adequate installation and commissioning, there are few instances, if any, for which it is justified to perform mammographic acquisitions with manual settings. As mentioned, some systems do not have AECs sophisticated enough to perform correctly in the presence of breast implants or implanted medical devices, and therefore the use of manual settings in this case is justified and necessary.

Display Devices

With a pixel size of 0.05–0.1 mm, and a typical field size for full-field digital mammography of 24 × 30 cm, a digital mammography image may well be composed of over ten million pixels [7]. Specialist medical-grade display monitors are required to provide an adequate display for primary reporting. Lower specification displays may be used as 'review' monitors in the mammography room for the practitioner to confirm the quality of image acquisition, but these should not be used for primary reporting. By now, it is exceedingly rare to see cathode-ray-tube-based digital mammography monitors, all of them having been replaced by LCD flat-panel displays.

Although there can be some flexibility in the format of simultaneous image display for reporting, in general two high-resolution (approximately 2000 × 2500 pixels = 5 megapixels) monitors in portrait orientation will be required for a reporting workstation as usually two images need to be compared. Over the last few years, 10 to 12 MP monitors have been introduced, so one monitor, in landscape mode, is used instead of two 5 MP portrait monitors. An additional low-resolution monitor may be required to display patient information, worklists, and other textual diagnostic reports.

It is not generally expected that the display monitor will be capable of displaying the full resolution of the recorded image as a complete frame, but that magnification, pan, and zoom within the image will be used to display all pixels when this is needed. With current 5-megapixel monitors, only a proportion of the breast image can be displayed at full resolution.

An important distinguishing feature of medical-grade displays is their maximum luminance. Ideally this should be 450 cd/m² or higher (much brighter than standard computer displays) so that a large ratio between maximum and minimum can be maintained, and susceptibility to the effects of ambient lighting is reduced. Careful consideration to the design of the viewing room is still required, however, as the brightness of the monitor itself will light up the room (as well as more obvious light sources such as open doors and windows) and structured reflections of room surroundings and indeed the observer superimposed on the viewed image will reduce its contrast and may introduce distracting features. Since the introduction of DBT, tomosynthesis-ready mammographic monitors have been developed, which support a rapid enough refresh rate to allow for the quick scanning through the different reconstruction planes without any motion blur.

The DICOM Greyscale Standard Display Function

DICOM is the medical image interchange standard that allows varied imaging-related systems to communicate images and image-related information, such as radiation dose structured reports. One element to DICOM that is particularly important from the radiological reporting standpoint is the Greyscale Standard Display Function (GSDF). This is based on a psychophysical model of the human visual system and is designed to maximise the number of 'just noticeable differences' that a given display can reproduce, and to give a perceptually linear greyscale, with the same small change in contrast visible in a dark part of the image as in a light part. Usually, the GSDF boosts the signal in the lighter side of the greyscale range. If the GSDF is correctly implemented for a given monitor, it should give the best display that monitor is capable of in the viewing conditions where it is used. The GSDF attempts to make the best of the display's capabilities but cannot make a sub-par display in poor viewing conditions as good as an expensive megapixel grey-scale monitor in good viewing conditions.

Display Tools

Display workstations would be expected to provide a user interface providing an efficient throughput of images and a range of display tools, typically including:

- Magnification, zoom, and pan (roam)
- Contrast and brightness adjustment (windowing)
- Image flip and rotation
- Black/white inversion
- Spatial measurement
- Edge enhancement and noise reduction (spatial frequency filtering)
- For DBT: manual scanning as well as automatic cine mode through the DBT slices

Some of these features are further explained below.

Windowing

Post-processing of digital images by windowing is a very powerful feature of digital imaging that also applies to CT, MR, and radioisotope imaging [32]. As the brightness of a pixel is dictated by an integer number (the 'pixel number') in a digital image, there are a finite number of values that the brightness level can take. Digital mammography systems might typically digitise to 12 bits (4096 grey levels), whereas the display monitor will probably only have a capability of displaying 1024 levels of luminance (10 bits). In addition, the human visual system is only capable of distinguishing about 100 grey levels at one time in an image, even under ideal viewing conditions, so it follows that if all the information present in a digital image was displayed on the monitor at once, small differences in contrast, although recorded successfully, would not be distinguishable.

The solution to this problem is to display only a selected range of pixel values, thus increasing the displayed contrast for that subset of levels. This 'window' of pixel number values is defined by a window 'width' and window 'level' (Fig. 18.6). By altering the display window width and level settings, the observer can optimise the display of the range of grey levels for the diagnostic task being undertaken, and any contrast

Fig. 18.6
Diagrammatic representation of image display windowing. The display width and level define a subset of the stored image grey levels which is expanded to fit the full luminance range of the display device

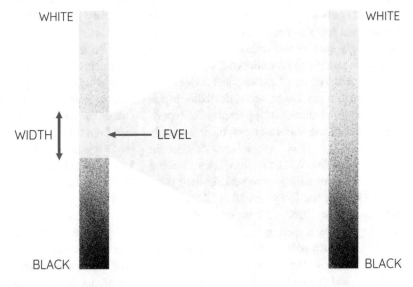

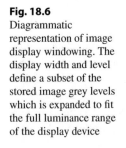

WHITE

WHITE

WIDTH

LEVEL

BLACK

BLACK

STORED IMAGE DATA

DISPLAYED IMAGE

recorded in the image can be displayed, but the time taken to make many such adjustments can become a factor in reporting high volumes of images. Therefore, preset window levels are usually set and used when a mammographic image is displayed, while the user interface for window width and level adjustment is usually quite intuitive, using a dedicated keypad, in addition to the computer mouse or trackball.

Spatial Frequency Filtering

Images can be thought of and analysed as sets of spatial frequencies. In general, low spatial frequencies are associated with uniform greyness or slowly changing gradients, whilst high spatial frequencies are associated with sudden changes in brightness such as at sharp edges or patterns of dots or lines [32]. By applying a spatial frequency filter, ranges of spatial frequencies can be enhanced or attenuated. Enhancing high spatial frequencies enhances the contrast of sharp edges, e.g., calcifications and linear structures, and generally 'sharpens' the image. Unfortunately, high frequency enhancement comes at the price of also boosting the noise that lies in this frequency band, so subtle enhancement is the most effective.

Attenuating high frequencies effectively blurs the image, and this can be used to reduce the appearance of quantum noise in some situations. Various layers of image processing, including spatial frequency filtering, are routinely used in digital mammography. Whilst this processing can make improvements to clinical images, it can also cause problems with quality control phantom images, for which the image processing often must be deselected.

Quality Control of Display Devices

Monitor performance reduces with age, and regular quality control checks are required. Regular user checks should include the system-

atic visual checking of a test pattern, such as the SMPTE pattern, the AAPM TG18 pattern (Fig. 18.7), and/or the more recent AAPM TG270 patterns.

Images of a suitable pattern should be accessible from the reporting workstation and for review monitors. Quantitative tests of the monitor performance, which include measurements of luminance over a range of grey levels, and assessment of the number of 'just noticeable differences' that the monitor can deliver in the lighting conditions where it is used. It is common for medical-grade monitors to support self-calibration, where the monitor makes measurements of its own luminance output and adjusts its calibration accordingly. The calibration takes account of room lighting conditions, so problems can arise if the lighting in the room at the time of self-calibration is not the same as when it is used for reporting.

A systematic review of viewing conditions and monitor specifications in mammography was performed in 2020 by Papathanasiou and colleagues [39]. This review provides an overview and further information which would be useful for the reader.

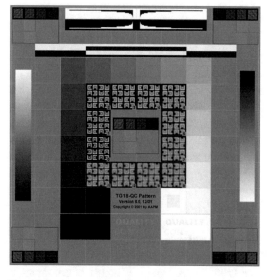

Fig. 18.7 A common quality control test object for display monitor testing. This is the AAPM Topic Group 18 (TG18) test pattern. The pattern features grey scale, image alignment, high spatial resolution and low contrast tests

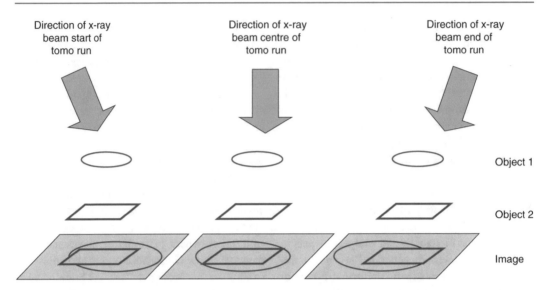

Fig. 18.8 Tomosynthesis image acquisition - The breast is held compressed against the stationary support table, and a sequence of small exposures is made as the tube gantry moves through an angle

Digital Breast Tomosynthesis

The use of MLO and CC views in standard mammography ameliorates, to some degree, the impact of tissue superposition on sensitivity and specificity. However, acquiring two planar images of the breast cannot replace obtaining the more ideal image, which would be a 3-D array of X-ray attenuation, from which it would be possible to display any desired image plane. DBT falls some way short of that ideal but does provide some useful depth information. This benefit, combined with the ease of introduction of DBT due to it sharing the same imaging platform as mammography, has resulted in it being quickly taking up for X-ray breast imaging in the clinic. Further information on tomosynthesis is available in Chap. 37, some aspects are summarised below.

Image Acquisition

For DBT acquisition, the breast is compressed against the image receptor as normal, but instead of one exposure with the X-ray central ray orthogonal to the image plane, a sequence of shorter exposures is made as the tube gantry

moves through an arc. The result is a series of images, taken with the source of X-rays stepping through the swing angle that can range from ±7.5° to ±25° of the normal vertical position. The projections will be subtly different, as the X-ray shadow of objects close to the top of the breast will appear to move relative to the image frame as the X-ray focus moves, but objects close to the support table will be imaged in the same place (Fig. 18.8).

Reconstruction

To produce the tomographic image, the series of projections must be reconstructed into a single image that emphasises features at a particular depth within the breast. In the simplest form of tomosynthesis, this could be done by shifting the projection images with respect to the image frame, so that the features at a selected depth all appear in the same place within the frame. These shifted images are then added together. The addition reinforces the contrast of features in the selected plane, where they are in the same position, but tends to blur out objects in other planes.

The degree of blurring (or technically streaking, as the blur occurs in the direction of X-ray tube movement) increases with distance from the selected plane. The result of image reconstruction is therefore an image reminiscent of film-screen tomography, where the observer can focus on objects in the intended image plane but tends to 'see through' the blurred features in other planes. This is distinct from true tomography (e.g., CT), where each image is a true cross-sectional cut through the object with no overlying or underlying structure. More sophisticated DBT image reconstruction methods based on filtered back projection (a variant of CT reconstruction) or iterative techniques are used in commercial DBT designs, but because of the very limited range of angles at which the projections in DBT are recorded, these still cannot recover enough information to produce pure tomographic slices.

Image Interpretation

To create an image stack suitable for mammographic reporting, the tomosynthesis reconstruction process is repeated with the calculated in-focus plane shifted, typically, one millimetre down from the previous one [9]. This cycle is repeated to eventually produce an image stack of perhaps 50 or 60 tomosynthesis images, for a typical compressed breast thickness. The entire stack of tomosynthesis images can be reconstructed from just the one set of projections. It should be noted that the information contained within one of these in-focus planes pertains to a lot more than 1 mm of tissue, but rather ~5 to 10 mm of breast tissue content, or more, depending on the contrast of the features, can appear in the plane being depicted.

To report the images, the viewer controls the selected in-focus plane shown on the display screen, and this can be rapidly swept up and down through the image stack [40]. The act of stepping through the images on the display allows the observer to build up a 3-D impression of the relative positions of features within the volume of the breast. For example, a small detail feature, such as a cluster of calcifications, will gradually come into sharp focus as the displayed

in-focus plane approaches its true depth, then will fade out of focus as displayed image moves beyond it.

Radiation Dose for Tomosynthesis

The radiation dose to the patient from DBT would be expected to be marginally higher than for conventional 2-D views, because the X-rays forming the projection views at the extremes of the angular swing have to traverse a greater thickness within the compressed breast. Most commercial implementations aim to keep the dose for DBT comparable with conventional 2-D views.

Synthetic Mammograms

Acquiring a standard mammogram in addition to a DBT would result in, at least, doubling the dose of an exam. To avoid this, the information acquired in the DBT projections can be used to reconstruct not only the DBT pseudo-3D image, but also a single planar image, the synthetic mammogram. This planar image is useful to both compare the current exam to priors, and to provide the interpreting radiologist with an overview of the breast, so that they can determine if there is an area they want to focus on, in addition to the review of the entire image stack.

There are two approaches to creating this synthetic mammogram. In the first place, the aim could be to create an image that is as close to what the real mammogram of that imaged breast would be [41]. Another approach is to create a planar image that includes all the interesting features found in the DBT image, and nothing more [42]. Of course, this latter approach is much more challenging, and requires some level of automated interpretation of the DBT image to identify the features of interest. With the advent of artificial intelligence-based image interpretation methods, we can expect that this latter approach to synthetic images will become more common.

Dedicated Breast CT

Dedicated breast CT (BCT) is a newer technology that delivers fully tomographic images of the breast [11–13, 43]. To achieve this, BCT uses the same principles as conventional (body) CT, but it is optimised, in terms of acquisition geometry, X-ray source, and detector, to imaging the breast. In addition to its true tomographic capabilities, BCT has the advantage that it does not involve any breast compression, increasing client comfort.

From the equipment point of view, BCT involves a horizontal gantry involving an X-ray source and a digital X-ray detector, both rotating around a vertical axis. This gantry is placed under the client table, on which the client lies prone, with the breast to be imaged pending through a hole on the table. The vertical axis of rotation of the gantry is located at the center of the hole for the breast.

To date, there are two implementations of BCT: cone-beam BCT and spiral BCT [11–13, 43]. In the former, the whole breast is included in each projection, and the detector is an energy-integrating flat-panel detector, similar to the indirect detectors described above for mammography. A single cone-beam BCT image consists of the acquisition of 300–500 projections during an entire 360° revolution around the breast, in 10–16 s. In the current implementation of spiral BCT, a fan-beam of x-rays and a narrow photon-counting detector strip are used, and these two revolve around the breast while also translating downwards. In this implementation, the detector behaves similarly to the photon-counting detectors that are described above as previously having been used in some mammography systems.

BCT has many advantages over mammography and DBT. It does not involve breast compression and results in a fully tomographic image. In some implementations, the dose for a BCT acquisition is equivalent to that of the acquisition of two views of mammography, resulting in the same dose for a complete exam of one breast. In addition, presenting a calcification cluster in its true three-dimensional distribution should make characterising it easier for an interpreting image reader. In addition, for low-contrast soft-tissue masses, the tomo-graphic nature of BCT should make them easier to detect and characterise. Finally, since BCT is performed with higher X-ray energies than mammography and DBT, it is ideal for contrast-enhanced imaging, with the spectra being very well tuned for iodine imaging [13].

However, the installed clinical, and research, base of BCT is, for now, much smaller than that for DBT and CESM, so the clinical evidence of its performance and its most suitable clinical use is still lacking. Since, as opposed to DBT and CESM, BCT requires a completely new system, its acceptance has not yet been as widespread as that of these other two modalities. Therefore, it remains to be seen what, if any, will be the clinical impact of BCT.

Contrast-Enhanced Spectral Mammography

As mentioned, CESM has been introduced over the last few years to breast clinics with the aim of providing functional information in addition to the anatomical information obtained with standard mammography. Just like DBT, CESM shares the same platform with standard mammography with only relatively minor modifications, and now the typical mammography system can perform the three types of imaging [17]. In fact, the modifications to a mammography system needed for CESM are fewer than those needed for DBT [44]. Usually, mammography systems already were able to use tube voltages of up to 45 or 49 kV. Therefore, only specific additional filters, such as copper or titanium, were needed to allow for adequate high-energy image acquisition. As discussed previously, the use of higher-energy x-rays could also necessitate a thickening of the X-ray absorption layer of the digital detector, to ensure an adequate stopping power, avoiding a substantial increase in dose.

To obtain the recombined, iodine-only, image, in CESM two images are acquired of the breast during one compression event: a low and a high energy image. The low energy image is the equivalent of a standard mammogram. The high energy image is acquired immediately thereafter, with the higher tube voltage, ~45–49 kV, and an additional filter. The aim of this higher energy spectrum is for it to include all or most of the photons above the k-absorption edge of iodine, which is 33.2 keV.

At this energy, the rate of absorption of x-rays of iodine increases substantially, while breast tissue does not have any k-edge present within the mammographic spectrum range. Therefore, in the presence of iodine, a specific mathematical combination of the low and high energy images results in an image that depicts only the iodine. Since the iodinated contrast agent is mixed in the blood, the recombined CESM image depicts the distribution of blood in the breast and in any pathology present. Due to the chaotic nature of blood vessels in the tumor growing rapidly through angiogenesis, blood leaks out from the tumor vasculature, resulting in tumors appearing enhancing in these images. More information on CESM can be found in Chap. 38.

Acknowledgments The authors would like to acknowledge one of the two previous authors of this chapter from the first edition: John Kotre. In addition, the authors would like to pay particular thanks to Penelope Booth art.penelope.booth@gmail.com for the illustrations contained within this chapter.

Appendix

Test your learning and check your understanding of this book's contents: use the "Springer Nature Flashcards" app to access questions using https://sn.pub/dcAnWL.

To use the app, please follow the instructions in Chap. 1.

Flashcard   code: 48341-69945-ABCB1-2A8C7-CE9D2.

Short URL: https://sn.pub/dcAnWL.

References

1. Thierry-Chef I, Simon SL, Weinstock RM, Kwon D, Linet MS. Reconstruction of absorbed doses to fibroglandular tissue of the breast of women undergoing mammography (1960 to the present). Radiat Res. 2012;177(1):92–108.

2. Gold RH, Bassett LW, Widoff BE. Highlights from the history of mammography. Radiographics. 1990;10(6):1111–31.

3. Nass SJ, Henderson IC, Lashof J. Mammography and beyond: developing technologies for the early detection of breast cancer. 1st ed. Washington, DC: National Cancer Policy Board – Institute of Medicine; 2001.

4. Joy JE, Penhoet EE, Petitti DB. Saving women's lives – strategies for improving breast cancer detection and diagnosis. Washington DC: The National Academies Press; 2005.

5. Fass L. Imaging and cancer: a review. Mol Oncol. 2008;2(2):115–52.

6. Public Health England. Commissioning and routine testing of full field digital mammography systems. NHSBSP Equipment Report 0604, version 3. NHS Cancer Screening Programmes; 2009.

7. Bushberg J, Seibert JA, Leidholdt E Jr, Boone J. The essential physics of medical imaging. 2nd ed. Philadelphia: Lippincott Williams & Wilkins; 2002.

8. Sechopoulos I. A review of breast tomosynthesis. Part I. The image acquisition process. Med Phys. 2013;40(1):014301.

9. Sechopoulos I. A review of breast tomosynthesis. Part II. Image reconstruction, processing and analysis, and advanced applications. Med Phys. 2013;40(1):014302.

10. Dobbins JT III. Tomosynthesis imaging: at a translational crossroads. Med Phys. 2009;36(6 Pt 1):1956–67.

11. Boone JM, Nelson TR, Lindfors KK, Seibert JA. Dedicated breast CT: radiation dose and image quality evaluation. Radiology. 2001;221(3):657–67.

12. Lindfors KK, Boone JM, Nelson TR, Yang K, Kwan AL, Miller DF. Dedicated breast CT: initial clinical experience. Radiology. 2008;246(3):725–33.

13. Sechopoulos I, Feng SS, D'Orsi CJ. Dosimetric characterization of a dedicated breast computed tomography clinical prototype. Med Phys. 2010;37(8):4110–20.

14. Conant EF, Zuckerman SP, McDonald ES, Weinstein SP, Korhonen KE, Birnbaum JA, Tobey JD, Schnall MD, Hubbard RA. Five consecutive years of screening with digital breast tomosynthesis: outcomes by screening year and round. Radiology. 2020;295(2):285–93.

15. Diekmann F, Freyer M, Diekmann S, Fallenberg EM, Fischer T, Bick U, Pöllinger A. Evaluation of contrast-enhanced digital mammography. Eur J Radiol. 2011;78(1):112–21.

16. Fallenberg EM, Dromain C, Diekmann F, Engelken F, Krohn M, Singh JM, Ingold-Heppner B, Winzer KJ, Bick U, Renz AD. Contrast-enhanced spectral mammography versus MRI: initial results in the detection of breast cancer and assessment of tumour size. Eur Radiol. 2014;24(1):256–64.

17. Fallenberg EM, Schmitzberger FF, Amer H, Ingold-Heppner B, Balleyguier C, Diekmann F, Engelken F, Mann RM, Renz DM, Bick U, Hamm B. Contrast-

enhanced spectral mammography vs. mammography and MRI–clinical performance in a multi-reader evaluation. Eur Radiol. 2017;27(7):2752–64.

18. Van Peteghem N, Bemelmans F, Adversalo XB, Salvagnini E, Marshall N, Bosmans H, Van Ongeval C. Grid-less imaging with antiscatter correction software in 2D mammography: the effects on image quality and MGD under a partial virtual clinical validation study. In: Medical Imaging 2016, editor. Physics of medical imaging. International Society for Optics and Photonics; 2016. p. 97832K.

19. Monserrat T, Prieto E, Barbés B, Pina L, Elizalde A, Fernández B. Impact on dose and image quality of a software-based scatter correction in mammography. Acta Radiol. 2018;59(6):649–56.

20. Andolina V, Lyllé S. Mammographic imaging – a practical guide. 3rd ed. Baltimore: Wolters Kluwer Health-Lippincott Williams & Wilkins; 2011.

21. Bassett LW, Hoyt AC, Oshiro T. Digital mammography: clinical image evaluation. Radiol Clin. 2010;48(5):903–15.

22. O'Leary D, Teape A, Hammond J, Rainford L, Grant T. Compression force recommendations in mammography must be linked to image quality. Vienna: ECR; 2011.

23. Poulos A, McLean D. The application of breast compression in mammography: a new perspective. Radiography. 2004;10(2):131–7.

24. Poulos A, Llewellyn G. Mammography discomfort: a holistic perspective derived from women's experiences. Radiography. 2005;11(1):17–25.

25. Spuur K, Poulos A, Currie G, Rickard M. Mammography: correlation of pectoral muscle width and the length in the mediolateral oblique view of the breast. Radiography. 2010;16(4):286–91.

26. Bentley K, Poulos A, Rickard M. Mammography image quality: analysis of evaluation criteria using pectoral muscle presentation. Radiography. 2008;14(3):189–94.

27. Spuur K, Hung WT, Poulos A, Rickard M. Mammography image quality: model for predicting compliance with posterior nipple line criterion. Eur J Radiol. 2011;80(3):713–8.

28. Holland K, Sechopoulos I, Mann RM, Den Heeten GJ, van Gils CH, Karssemeijer N. Influence of breast compression pressure on the performance of population-based mammography screening. Breast Cancer Res. 2017;19(1):1–8.

29. Agasthya GA, D'Orsi E, Kim YJ, Handa P, Ho CP, D'Orsi CJ, Sechopoulos I. Can breast compression be reduced in digital mammography and breast tomosynthesis? AJR. 2017;209(5):W322.

30. Pisano ED. DMIST Investigators Group. Diagnostic accuracy of digital versus film mammography: exploratory analysis of selected population subgroups in DMIST. Radiology. 2008;246:376–83.

31. Pisano ED, Yaffe MJ. Digital mammography. Radiology. 2005;234(2):353–62.

32. Gonzalez RC, Woods RE. Digital Image Processing. 2nd ed. Tennessee: Pearson Education; 2008.

33. Smith A. Fundamentals of digital mammography: physics, technology and practical considerations. Radiol Manage. 2003;25(5):18–24.

34. Yaffe MJ, Rowlands JA. X-ray detectors for digital radiography. Phys Med Niol. 1997;42(1):1.

35. Ren B, Ruth C, Wu T, Zhang Y, Smith A, Niklason L, Williams C, Ingal E, Polischuk B, Jing Z. A new generation FFDM/tomosynthesis fusion system with selenium detector. In: Medical Imaging 2010, editor. Physics of medical imaging. International Society for Optics and Photonics; 2010. p. 76220B.

36. Ren B, Ruth C, Zhang Y, Smith A, Kennedy D, O'Keefe B, Shaw I, Williams C, Ye Z, Ingal E, Polischuk B. Dual energy iodine contrast imaging with mammography and tomosynthesis. In: Medical Imaging 2013, editor. Physics of medical imaging. International Society for Optics and Photonics; 2013. p. 86680U.

37. Séradour B, Heid P, Estève J. Comparison of direct digital mammography, computed radiography, and film-screen in the French national breast cancer screening program. AJR. 2014;202(1):229–36.

38. Mackenzie A, Warren LM, Wallis MG, Cooke J, Given-Wilson RM, Dance DR, Chakraborty DP, Halling-Brown MD, Looney PT, Young KC. Breast cancer detection rates using four different types of mammography detectors. Eur Radiol. 2016;26(3):874–83.

39. Papathanasiou S, Walton LA, Thompson JD. A systematic review of viewing conditions and monitor specifications in mammography. Radiography. 2020;26(4):325–31.

40. Reiser I, Glick S. Tomosynthesis imagine (imaging in medical diagnosis therapy). CRC Press; 2014.

41. Gur D, Zuley ML, Anello MI, Rathfon GY, Chough DM, Ganott MA, Hakim CM, Wallace L, Lu A, Bandos AI. Dose reduction in digital breast tomosynthesis (DBT) screening using synthetically reconstructed projection images: an observer performance study. Acad Radiol. 2012;19(2):166–71.

42. Lång K. Mounting evidence for synthetic mammography in breast cancer screening. Radiology. 2020;297(3):554–5.

43. Glick SJ, Breast CT. Annu Rev Biomed Eng. 2007;9:501–26.

44. Huang H, Scaduto DA, Liu C, Yang J, Zhu C, Rinaldi K, Eisenberg J, Liu J, Hoernig M, Wicklein J, Vogt S. Comparison of contrast-enhanced digital mammography and contrast-enhanced digital breast tomosynthesis for lesion assessment. J Med Imag. 2019;6(3):031407.

Artificial intelligence (AI) in Mammography

19

Richard Sidebottom, Iain Lyburn, and Sarah Vinnicombe

Introduction

Artificial intelligence (AI) systems can be described as machines that perceive and act and hopefully choose actions that will achieve their objectives [1] and that 'improve their achievement of objectives through experience'. Over the last decade or so there have been significant improvements in computing power and advancements in machine learning techniques, leading to the development of AI systems for image classification that appear powerful enough to be clinically valuable. Mammographic breast screening provides an ideal scenario for developing such systems given the large volumes of imaging data coupled with outcome measures. In addition, the accuracy of breast screening is not perfect, and delivery of this service is becoming increasingly challenging because of a workforce shortage. This provides an opportunity where AI systems could play a role in improving screening accuracy and performance and, more mundanely, mitigate some of the workload problems experienced by population screening services worldwide.

However, it is important to be cognisant of the fact that the implementation of AI systems could be detrimental without careful evaluation, prospective clinical trials and ongoing quality assurance. There are a number of potential pitfalls. Problems could arise when integration of the AI tool into the clinical workflow results in inferior accuracy than was anticipated from studies done using retrospective data. The introduction of AI systems could exacerbate the harms from screening which currently occur, such as the problem of 'overdiagnosis' of a cancer which would never have caused harm in the individuals lifetime. A change to the characteristics of the cases identified could alter the balance of risks and benefits for the worse. For these, and other reasons, it is important to have an understanding of these emerging technologies, including methods of development and assessment.

Background

Researchers have been experimenting with using computers to analyse mammograms since the 1970s. Initial approaches used basic image processing techniques and involved expert radiologists and computer scientists working to create mathematical descriptions of the features that we look for in mammograms such as shape, size, and density. The next step was using artificial intelligence techniques based on advanced statistics

R. Sidebottom (✉)
Thirlestaine Breast Centre, Gloucester Hospitals NHS Foundation Trust, Cheltenham, UK

AI Imaging Hub, The Royal Marsden NHS Foundation Trust, London, UK
e-mail: richard.sidebottom@nhs.net

I. Lyburn · S. Vinnicombe
Thirlestaine Breast Centre, Gloucester Hospitals NHS Foundation Trust, Cheltenham, UK
e-mail: iain.lyburn@nhs.net;
sarah.vinnicombe@nhs.net

and machine learning to classify these hand-crafted features. This is the basis of 'traditional' CAD systems that have been in clinical use over the last two decades [2].

However, these CAD systems came nowhere close to human levels of specificity. They were shown to increase recall rates [3] and therefore have never gained traction in Europe, though they have been widely used in the USA. Use of such systems is now questioned and in 2015 a large US study analysing over 1/2 million cases concluded that 'CAD does not improve diagnostic accuracy of mammography' [4].

The recent renewed commercial and scientific interest in medical image classification have resulted from the development of machine learning techniques known as 'deep learning' which use a multi-layered architecture, loosely inspired by biological neural networks. These networks are iteratively trained by exposure to patient data. Internal network factors that lead to successful categorisation of data become strengthened and these complex networks become 'trained'. The term 'deep' signifies a large number of layers or steps over which incremental information processing occurs. This method aims to uncover internal relationships within the data and is a more successful approach to medical image analysis than previous methods of computer analysis requiring explicitly programmed feature extraction. These networks 'learn' features within training sets of images which allow successful image classification. These features are not determined by the people designing the system, but rather, are learned by the algorithm. The abstract intermediate features that the system determines are contained within the vastly complex trained network and are not explicit, making the process by which classification is performed obscure to the user, thus presenting some difficulties with interpreting the output of these systems.

Computing Architecture and Patient Data Are Both Vital for AI Development

Training deep learning systems requires large volumes of reliable data and vast computing power. Advancements in data science and computing power have made these systems feasible for use in medical imaging in the last decade. The large volume of imaging data held within hospital PACS systems, together with pathology and follow up data make breast screening an obvious suitable application for this approach.

The quality of the data on which the training is performed is crucial. 'Ground truth' is a term used for the values on which AI systems are trained. Underlying truth (for example the presence or absence of cancer at a point in time) may be obscure, but a pathologically confirmed cancer can be considered truth and, whilst it is more difficult to establish that a mammogram is 'normal', long term follow up data allows characterisation of an earlier study as normal if no cancer has developed in the interim period. This allows the objectives for the AI to be defined in terms of classification of screening mammograms as cancer or no cancer, and the possibility exists within large enough datasets to set objectives in terms of classifying different types of cancer, aiming to prioritise the identification of the most biologically significant subtypes.

A deployed AI system may use a combination of methods for analysis, however the predominant architectures currently used for medical image classification are called deep convolutional neural networks (CNN). Data science is currently a very fast-moving area and recently alternative architectures known as transformer networks are beginning to outperform CNN's in image classification and undoubtedly further advancements will also be applied to medical image classification.

Process of Training a Model

Convolutional neural networks are usually trained using a process known as supervised learning, where every example case has a 'ground truth' value. This may be simply 'cancer' or 'no cancer' and in the case of breast screening can be determined from pathology data and follow up data that is typically collected during routine clinical care. The untrained network will typically produce a classification on a continuous scale eg. 0 (no cancer) to 1 (cancer). The error of this result will then inform the learning through a process called back propagation, where multiple internal parameters throughout the network are altered. This happens iteratively, and incrementally the performance of the output is improved towards the 'ground truth'. Pixel level data for annotations of cancers may also be used as an input. Architectures of AI systems are varied and evolving and can combine various strategies in an ultimate output for image classification.

Datasets used in AI Development

Three sets of data are required to develop an AI system. These are a training set, a tuning/validation set, and an independent test set. A training dataset is used to incrementally alter the internal network parameters and will be accessed in the process of learning repeatedly. This data must contain examples from the breadth of variety required for use, for example if a single manufacturer is used for training, then performance on an alternative may be unreliable. However, it need not be representative of the use case – for example training sets may contain a much higher percentage of cancers than are seen in a typical screening population. When training these systems, a problem known as 'overfitting' may occur whereby the model in some way memorises the cases in the training set, or learns spurious correlations which will not allow generalisation to other similar data. A separate dataset known as a 'validation set' or 'tune set' is used by the developers to optimise the design of the algorithm to avoid overfitting and aims to ensure generalisability. This tuning set is often a subset of the same data used for training that has been withheld from model training. Confusingly the term 'validation set' is often used in the computer science community for this dataset, whereas the clinical community may use the same term to refer to the dataset used to demonstrate final performance.

Finally, an independent test set is required to demonstrate the performance of the system. This should closely match the use case and should ideally be representative in terms of population including ethnicities, and local screening methods including the mammography manufacturers and screening strategies. If a reliable measure of performance is to be demonstrated then this dataset must be large enough for statistical measures to be used, likely to require tens of thousands of cases.

Analysis of System Performance

Performance of AI systems is often reported in terms of AUC, the 'area under the (ROC) curve'. A Receiver Operator Characteristic (ROC) curve is a graph where the true positive rate (TPR) is plotted against the false positive rate (FPR) across the range of possible threshold values [5]. The closer the AUC is to 1, the better the performance, and 0.5 is equal to chance [6]. Because the operating point of an AI system can be varied continuously, this graph can be plotted. This AUC can be useful for assessing or comparing AI algorithms (providing the same dataset is used) but is not such a meaningful comparison to the clinical reality of human readers. Only a single point may be plotted for a clinical reader's performance, determined from the sensitivity and specificity over multiple reads.

Rather than using AUC measures, more familiar ways of understanding performance are by fixing the positive/negative threshold of the AI system, then documenting true positive, false positive, true negative and false negative rates with resultant sensitivity and specificity. Thankfully this approach is increasingly used in reports of AI performance, which may report sensitivity when matching the clinically acceptable specificity rate or vice versa. It is also important to note whether an assessment of performance has been made at the 'lesion' level, the 'breast' level or for the woman overall. If not at the lesion level, then a positive classification could be spuriously based on a different lesion (not on the true cancer) and will give misleading results 6].

Definitions of Cancer Cases

When assessing the performance of an AI system against current screening performance it is important to consider how to determine what constitutes a positive case. If only the screen detected cancers are used, then this 'gatekeeper effect' would of course bias the results. This can be overcome by also defining prior screens as positive cases for women who go on to develop interval cancers or even screen detected cancers diagnosed at the next screening round. This longer follow up is an advantage of using retrospective data for these studies.

Current Performance

Current standalone performance of these AI systems on retrospective datasets appears to be around the level of a single human reader in several different publications [7–9]. A recent publication by the UK national screening committee reviewed the current evidence and concluded that there is currently insufficient evidence to support implementation of AI in UK breast screening [10]. Several prospective studies are underway at the time of writing and the volume and quality of evidence should improve. Interestingly the use of hybrid human/AI has been shown to outperform either in several studies [8, 11].

Possible Use Cases

Reader Assist

Until very recently, AI applications for image classification have mainly focused on reader assist, effectively working as a much more accurate version of traditional CAD systems. Some systems taking this approach allow users to interrogate the image with the system providing an AI classification of user defined areas [12].

Independent Reader

In the European double read screening workflow, an obvious application is to replace one of the readers with AI. In addition to workflow efficiency, a potential advantage of this approach is that if the cases recalled by humans and those

recalled by AI are less similar than those recalled by two human readers, then the sensitivity of a human/AI double read has the potential to improve over a two human double read, provided that arbitration is successfully performed. This would be at the cost of an increased burden of arbitration cases [13].

Stratified Screening

Risk adapted screening offers the potential to enhance the overall benefits of screening [14]. AI solutions may facilitate effective personalisation of screening protocols, such as to modify the screening interval or the screening test, for example adding DBT, ultrasound, contrast-enhanced mammography or abbreviated MRI. Analysing personal risk factors, current and prior images, pathology data and genomics could all contribute to this approach. This would require the development of richer datasets containing the information required to optimise for this wider and more ambitious objective.

Triage and Workflow

It has been suggested in simulation studies that low risk mammograms could be triaged for AI read only [15], and higher risk cases prioritised for early reading. An alternative approach would be to use immediate AI output at the time of imaging, which could allow for further imaging such as tomosynthesis or referral for assessment to happen at the time of the initial screening and could radically change screening workflows.

Problem of Interpretability

Although it is conceivable that ultimately the best reading performance will be reached by an AI system without human intervention, such a scenario is probably distant. It will be important to understand how use of an AI tool might influence behaviour of human readers. With currently used deep learning systems, it is not possible to explicitly determine how a classification decision has been made [16]. A system can however be designed to describe features of interest in an interpretable manner, most importantly lesion location. This interpretable output will be essential to inform the clinician when making difficult decisions such as will be encountered if arbitrating a human/AI discrepancy.

Some method of developing a good understanding of the strengths and weaknesses of a particular AI system will be crucial. This may be achieved by clinical experience, specific research endeavour, or perhaps informed by output from the AI model itself. As a crude example, it would be important to know that an AI system was usually superior to human performance for subtle distortions and consistently inferior to human performance when evaluating calcifications.

Quality Assurance and Monitoring

Breast screening performance is highly monitored in the UK and Europe and the quality assurance of screening programmes must be maintained and updated to allow monitoring of AI performance. This is important because it is possible that these complex systems could behave unpredictably, for example, it is possible that a change to a different mammography unit could result in an unexpected change in performance. Because it is conceivable that such a scenario could be difficult to detect, deteriorating performance of an AI should be detected by quality monitoring so that it can be rectified quickly. Some degree of integration into national screening infrastructure will be beneficial to optimise workflow and allow for large scale monitoring [17].

Conclusion

The development of powerful AI systems has the potential to improve our performance in breast screening and positively impact population health. These advancements bring exciting possibilities but also potential problems, as we have discussed. Whilst the computing methods are currently quickly advancing and will change and improve over time, the power of these systems will depend on the data on which they are trained and tested. The overall effectiveness of this adjunct to screening will be determined by the objectives which we define.

Ultimately the objective of breast screening is to reduce the chances of breast cancer specific mortality and morbidity. We use mammography to achieve this aim, coupled with some risk stratification for women judged to be at moderate or higher risk. Most current AI approaches aim to improve screening using the objective of improving mammography screening accuracy. By using more diverse datasets containing long term outcome data, it may be possible to address these more general objectives of breast screening. Whatever the proposed use, prospective studies are required to ensure that these innovations can deliver real world benefits in the near future.

Appendix

Test your learning and check your understanding of this book's contents: use the "Springer Nature Flashcards" app to access questions using https://sn.pub/dcAnWL.

To use the app, please follow the instructions in Chap. 1.

Flashcard code:
48341-69945-ABCB1-2A8C7-CE9D2.

Short URL: https://sn.pub/dcAnWL.

References

1. Russell S. BBC Reith Lecture 2021. Living with artificial intelligence. https://www.bbc.co.uk/news/technology-59326684; http://downloads.bbc.co.uk/radio4/reith2021/BBC_2021_Reith_Lecture_2021_1.pdf. Accessed 5/12/2021
2. Bitencourt A, Naranjo ID, Gullo RL, Saccarelli CR, Pinker K. AI-enhanced breast imaging: where are we and where are we heading? Eur J Radiol. 2021;142:109882.
3. Gilbert FJ, Astley SM, Gillan MG, Agbaje OF, Wallis MG, James J, Boggis CR, Duffy

SW. Single reading with computer-aided detection for screening mammography. N Engl J Med. 2008;359(16):1675–84.

4. Lehman CD, Wellman RD, Buist DS, Kerlikowske K, Tosteson AN, Miglioretti DL. Breast Cancer Surveillance Consortium. Diagnostic accuracy of digital screening mammography with and without computer-aided detection. JAMA Intern Med. 2015;175(11):1828–37.

5. Park SH, Goo JM, Jo CH. Receiver operating characteristic (ROC) curve: practical review for radiologists. Korean J Radiol. 2004;5(1):11–8. https://doi.org/10.3348/kjr.2004.5.1.11.

6. Wallis MG. Artificial intelligence for the real world of breast screening. Eur J Radiol. 2021;144:109661. https://doi.org/10.1016/j.ejrad.2021.109661.

7. Rodríguez-Ruiz A, Krupinski E, Mordang JJ, Schilling K, Heywang-Köbrunner SH, Sechopoulos I, Mann RM. Detection of breast cancer with mammography: effect of an artificial intelligence support system. Radiology. 2019;290(2):305–14.

8. Wu N, Phang J, Park J, Shen Y, Huang Z, Zorin M, Jastrzębski S, Févry T, Katsnelson J, Kim E, Wolfson S. Deep neural networks improve radiologists' performance in breast cancer screening. IEEE Trans Med Imaging. 2019;39(4):1184–94.

9. McKinney SM, Sieniek M, Godbole V, Godwin J, Antropova N, Ashrafian H, Back T, Chesus M, Corrado GS, Darzi A, Etemadi M. International evaluation of an AI system for breast cancer screening. Nature. 2020;577(7788):89–94.

10. Freeman K, Geppert J, Stinton C, Todkill D, Johnson S, Clarke A, Taylor-Phillips S. Use of artificial intelligence for image analysis in breast cancer screening programmes: systematic review of test accuracy. BMJ. 2021;374:n1872.

11. Schaffter T, Buist DS, Lee CI, Nikulin Y, Ribli D, Guan Y, Lotter W, Jie Z, Du H, Wang S, Feng J. Evaluation of combined artificial intelligence and radiologist assessment to interpret screening mammograms. JAMA Netw Open. 2020;3(3):e200265.

12. FDA. ScreenPoint medical FDA clearance. 2020. https://www.accessdata.fda.gov/cdrh_docs/pdf19/K193229.pdf

13. Sharma N, Ng AY, James JJ, Khara G, Ambrozay E, Austin CC, Forrai G, Glocker B, Heindl A, Karpati E, Rijken TM. Large-scale evaluation of an AI system as an independent reader for double reading in breast cancer screening. MedRxiv. 2021.

14. Gilbert FJ, Hickman SE, Baxter GC, Allajbeu I, James J, Carraco C, Vinnicombe S. Opportunities in cancer imaging: risk-adapted breast imaging in screening. Clin Radiol. 2021;76(10):763–73.

15. Dembrower K, Wåhlin E, Liu Y, Salim M, Smith K, Lindholm P, Eklund M, Strand F. Effect of artificial intelligence-based triaging of breast cancer screening mammograms on cancer detection and radiologist workload: a retrospective simulation study. The Lancet Digital Health. 2020;2(9):e468–74.

16. Kelly CJ, Karthikesalingam A, Suleyman M, Corrado G, King D. Key challenges for delivering clinical impact with artificial intelligence. BMC Med. 2019;17(1):1–9. https://doi.org/10.1186/s12916-019-1426-2.

17. Sidebottom R, Dunbar K, Wilkinson L. Harnessing the benefits of AI in the breast imaging pathway. RAD Mag 48. 2022;560:19–20. Master-article (rad-magazine.com).

Radiation Dose in Mammography

Raed Mohammed Kadhim M. Ali

Learning Objectives
- Assess the radiation risk from mammographic examination
- Understand and explain the radiation dose received by body tissues and organs other than examined breast

Introduction

Medical imaging represents the major source of man-made ionising radiation for people [1, 2]. In the United Kingdom (UK), radiographic examinations constitute 90% of artificial radiation sources and have resulted in a 23% increase of the UK per caput dose between 1998 and 2008 [3]. In the United States (US), a sixfold increase in medical radiation exposure was reported between 1980 and 2012, making medical radiation to be the cause of 50% of the US per caput dose [4]. Therefore, for all radiographic procedures, an acceptable image quality should be produced with the least possible radiation dose; doses should be kept as low as reasonably practicable (ALARP). ALARP is a radiation protection approach to deal with and control the radiation dose to patients to as low as reasonable limits.

ALARP does not mean the reduction of radiation dose to zero, but it means the reduction of radiation dose to an acceptable level eliminating the deterministic effects and minimising the stochastic effects of radiation [5].

Biological Effects of Radiation

The radiation risk refers to the damage produced by ionising radiation due to energy deposition in tissues. This energy may result in ionisation within the tissues if the photons pass near an orbital electron and provide sufficient energy for an electron to be liberated from the atom [6]. The amount of damage is related to radiation dose, type of radiation, whether it is internal or external, time of exposure, radiation distribution (type of exposed tissue), and the individual's sensitivity which is influenced by gender and age [7]. Females are at higher risk of radiation-induced cancer than males [8]. Younger people are at a higher risk because they have a longer remaining life span. For example, the risk of radiation damage for a 20-year-old is twice that of a 40-year-old. The latter has double the risk when compared to a 60-year-old. The radio-sensitivity of young children is 3–4 times more than that of adults [9].

In general, the radiation interactions with tissue are either direct, wherein the radiation energy is directly transferred to the DNA causing structural changes in its molecules, or indirect interaction, where the radiation energy is absorbed by

R. M. K. M. Ali (✉)
Faculty of Medicine, University of Kufa, Najaf, Iraq
e-mail: Raedm.kadhim@uokufa.edu.iq

water molecules forming free radicals which in turn cause damage to DNA molecules. It has been found that for X-rays with 100 mGy, 30–40% of the DNA damage is due to direct interaction and the remaining 60–70% of the damage results from indirect interactions [10]. The adverse health effects of radiation can be classified into two groups:

- Deterministic effects: follow high radiation doses and result in relatively immediate and predictable tissue reactions and damage. This damage can occur within minutes, hours, days and even weeks.
- Stochastic effects: follow low radiation doses and may result in cancer development [11]. Development is based on probability. The lag period between irradiation and cancer development for stochastic effects is at least 5 years and may reach to 10 or 20 years [9].

Stochastic effects usually occur due to mutations in DNA which occur randomly. In general, the probability of stochastic effects' occurrence increases as the radiation dose increases. However, the severity of the resultant disease is not related to radiation dose because the cancer produced by a 2 Sv radiation dose is not more severe than cancer produced by 0.2 Sv radiation dose. Stochastic effects are classified into radiation-induced cancer and reproductive cell damage, which affects sperm and ova and causes defects in offspring [6].

For radiological doses ranging from 5 to 100 mSv, no strong evidence is available to describe the relationship between the risk of radiation-induced cancer and these low doses [12].

Persistent controversy exists in literature regarding the risk of radiation-induced cancer from low dose ionising radiation. This creates a big challenge for epidemiological studies. In this context, the controversy arises in questions about the dose threshold of cancer production, linearity and gradient of dose-response curves [13]. Overall, there are two opposing risk models to estimate the risk of low radiation doses. The first adopts the linear no-threshold principle. According to this model, any dose, however

small, can result in cancer incidence. However, the second model proposes that there is a specific threshold for radiation-induced cancer and below this threshold the radiation dose can be considered as safe [14]. Although, the International Commission on Radiation Protection (ICRP) [11] and the National Academy of Sciences (NAS) [15] have adopted the linear no-threshold (LNT) model, United Nations Scientific Committee on the Effects of Atomic Radiation (UNSCEAR) [16] considered the LNT to be uncertain at radiation doses less than 100 mSv and it is no longer recommended for radiation-induced cancer assessment from such doses. This motivates many researchers to investigate the reliability of this model using different data sources.

The risk of radiation-induced cancer within the mammographic dose range was experimentally estimated by Brenner et al. [17]. In this work, cells were irradiated in vitro using a 15–25 keV mono-energetic X-ray beam. The analysis of oncogenic transformation indicated that mammography increases the risk of breast cancer development by approximately twofold; this effect is age dependent, making screening mammography commencing at the age of 50 more beneficial than that which commences at 40 [17].

In conclusion, the accurate determination of radiation-induced cancer from low radiation dose is not easy. The limited data available about the risk from low radiation dose (used in mammography) has resulted in controversy and uncertainty [12, 18]. According to the available data, the risk of radiation-induced cancer from low dose radiation is very small but unlikely to be zero [19]. Therefore, the linear no-threshold model may be the best reasonable risk model for describing the relationship between the exposure to low energy radiation and solid cancer incidence [11, 15, 20]. To overcome uncertainty about the LNT model [21, 19] recommended the classification of low dose radiation cancer risk into four categories as follow:

- Negligible risk (<1 case per million)
- Minimal risk (1–10 case per million)
- Very low risk (>10–100 case per million)
- Low risk (>100–1000 case per million)

Radiation Protection in Mammography

For mammographic radiation protection four aspects must be considered [22]:

- Benefit to risk ratio: mammographic procedures should not be achieved unless the benefit from the examination outweighs the risk associated with the procedure
- Client/Patient protection: when the mammographic procedure is required, the client/patient should be protected from undesirable radiation
- Staff protection: mammography staff should be adequately protected from excessive radiation
- General public in mammographic vicinity should be well protected from radiation exposure

Mammography Dosimetry

With more than 50 years of mammography development, large changes have been made in mammographic dosimetry. It has been reported that breast radiation dose is reduced from about 150 mGy when using industrial film to less than 2 mGy for full field digital mammography (FFDM) [23].

Incident radiation exposure (R) at breast surface and the entrance surface dose (ESD), which is measured by thermo-luminance dosimeter (TLD) at the breast surface, were the early quantities used to determine the radiation risk of mammography [24]. However, since mammography uses low energy X-ray photons, the dose inside the breast rapidly reduces as the depth increases [25]. Accordingly, different quantities were suggested as measures for mammographic radiation risk, such as midline breast dose and total breast energy [24].

In 1976, the use of breast glandular tissue radiation dose as a measure for mammographic radiation risk was firstly proposed. It was utilised to study dose distribution within a mixture of alcohol and water breast phantom to compare the radiation

dose of different image receptors which resulted in equivalent mammographic image qualities [26]. Later, in 1987, a mean glandular dose (MGD) for breast dosimetry was recommended by the ICRP [27]. Mammography is a common screening practice and it is considered to be one of the most highly optimised techniques [23].

Mean Glandular Dose (MGD)

The risk of radiation-induced cancer from breast X-ray examination is small and is generally related to mean glandular dose (MGD) [28]. MGD is the amount of energy imparted from ionising radiation per unit mass of breast glandular tissue; glandular tissue has the highest radiation sensitivity among breast tissues [29]. MGD is utilised as a standard quantity in breast dosimetry, which is an essential part in quality control protocols of mammography, and is recommended by several international committees such as ICRP, National Council on Radiation Protection and Measurements (NCRP), and Institute of Physics and Engineering in Medicine (IPEM).

MGD is considered to be an important element of mammographic quality assurance programmes. This is because it can be used as a parameter to evaluate the mammographic system performance, patient risk assessment, and different mammographic imaging techniques with regards to dosimetry [30]. Accordingly, MGD has been of great interest to a large number of researchers [25, 31–35]. MGD is fundamentally related to [25, 36, 37]:

1. Target/filter combination (radiation spectrum)
2. X-ray tube output (kV, mA, and time)
3. Breast density (glandularity)
4. Breast size (compressed breast thickness)

Target/Filter Combination

The first commercial mammography system was with molybdenum/molybdenum (Mo/Mo) target/filter combination [38]. For mammographic

Table 20.1 Lists s factor for different target/filter combinations [41, 42]

Target/filter combination	s factor
Mo/Mo	1.000
Mo/Rh	1.017
Rh/Rh	1.061
W/Rh	1.042
W/Ag	1.042
W/Al	1.069–1.212[a]

[a]Depending on compressed breast thickness

imaging, the useful part of the molybdenum X-ray beam is the characteristic radiation of molybdenum, because the energy of its K-edge characteristic radiation is approximately 20 keV, wherein the majority of its other characteristic radiations have energies around 19 keV [39]. The use of molybdenum target tubes resulted in the production of lower energy radiation, with a more limited energy range than that produced by conventional radiography tubes. This resulted in optimum image contrast [38].

Since the Mo/Mo target/filter combination was suitable for average breasts only, other target/filter combinations were introduced such as molybdenum/rhodium (Mo/Rh), rhodium/rhodium (Rh/Rh), tungsten/rhodium (W/Rh), tungsten/aluminum (W/Al) and tungsten/silver (W/Ag). The target/filter combination is determined by compressed breast thickness and breast composition (density) [39]. Also, tubes with dual track anodes have been produced. One of these tracks was Mo and the other was either Rh or W. Filters are automatically selected depending on the track material [40]. Overall, target/filter combination may result in up to 20% difference in calculated MGD. Table 20.1 demonstrates the spectral correction factor which is used to correct for different target/filter combinations [41, 42].

X-ray Tube Output

X-ray tube output is directly related to the product of tube current and time (mAs) and to the square of the tube potential (kVp) [43].

Breast Density (Glandularity)

Breast density is a measure of breast composition. It reflects the percentage of glandular tissue in the breast. Since it is basically assessed by mammography, it is expressed as mammographic density [44]. The validity of breast dose estimation could be improved by accurate measurement of breast density because the breast composition is an essential factor in breast dosimetry [45].

Breast Size (Compressed Breast Thickness)

Breast size and shape differ in relation to many factors: race, diet, age, status of female parity, and menopausal status [46]. Breast thickness is non-uniform. It is thicker closer to the chest wall than when compared to the nipple side. In order to compensate for this, the compression paddle is usually tilted during breast compression. Paddle tilting results in variations in the breast thickness readout accuracy for fixed and flexible paddles [47]. The breast thickness readout variation may result in up to 20% difference in calculated MGD. More variations in MGD may be introduced if the thickness readout variation leads to a different target/filter combination selection [48].

Both breast density and size change with age and consequently affecting the mammographic MGD. A lower MGD in older women is reported because both breast density and compressed breast thickness decrease with age [49, 50]. It has been found that there is a linear inverse relationship between woman age and the reduction percentage of required mAs [49].

MGD Estimation

MGD has to be calculated from multiplying the incident air kerma (kinetic energy released per unit mass) by conversion factors, obtained by Monte Carlo simulation, as published by Dance et al. [42]. This method is recommended in IPEM report 89 [37], International Atomic Energy Agency

Fig. 20.1 g-factor as a function of compressed breast thickness (cm) for different beam HVL

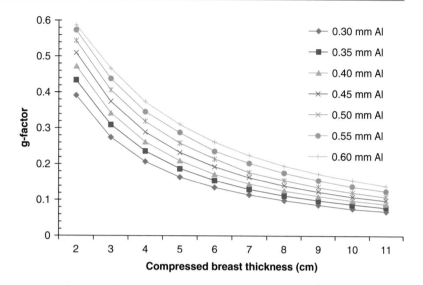

(IAEA) [29], and the European Commission [51]. However, conversion factors published by Wu et al. [52] have been recommended by the American College of Radiology [32].

Thus, the MGD can be calculated using the equation defined by Dance et al. [42] as follows:

$$MGD = K\, g_t\, c_t\, s$$

- K is the incident air kerma measured at the top surface of PMMA breast phantom without backscatter.
- g_t is a factor to convert the incident air kerma to MGD for a simulated breast of thickness t (Fig. 20.1) [36, 41].
- c_t is a conversion factor which allows for the density of a standard breast (50% glandularity) of thickness t. Since the c_t factor is related to breast density, it has been tabulated for 5 different breast densities (0.1%, 25%, 50%, 75%, 100%) at different breast thicknesses and different HVL (Fig. 20.2) [41].
- Both g_t and c_t factors are dependent on beam quality which represented by beam half-value layer (HVL). Accordingly, for MGD calculation, the HVL which is related to target-filter combination and kV have to be determined.
- s is the spectral correction factor which is used to correct for different target/filter combinations (Table 20.1) [41, 42].

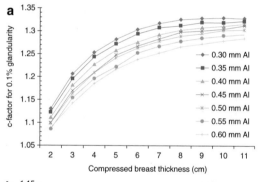

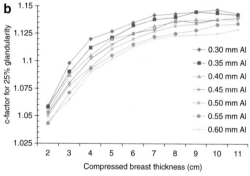

Fig. 20.2 c-factor as a function of compressed breast thickness (cm) for different beam HVL (**a**) for 0.1% breast glandularity, (**b**) for 25% breast glandularity, (**c**) for 75% breast glandularity, and (**d**) for 100% breast glandularity

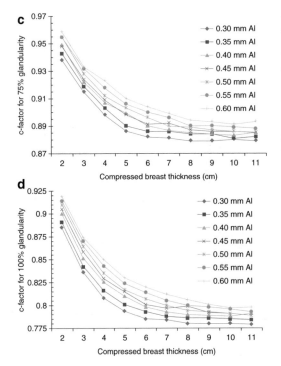

Fig. 20.2 (continued)

The main limitation of MGD calculations using conversion factors is that, during Monte Carlo simulation, a homogenous breast phantom of different breast densities was used. The use of this homogenous phantom results in significant MGD overestimation. The greatest value of MGD overestimation has been recorded at low photon energies. This overestimation decreases as the photon energy increases [53]. It has been reported that the use of conversion factors may result in up to a 43% difference in calculated MGD due to glandular tissue spatial distribution [54]. Accordingly, total energy imparted in glandular tissue (GIE) is recently suggested to be used instead of MGD [55].

MGD Estimation for Digital Breast Tomosynthesis (DBT)

DBT produces several cross-sectional high spatial resolution and low dose breast images to minimise breast tissue overlapping resulting in more clearly defined lesions, especially within high-density breast where mammographic sensi-

tivity and specificity reduce [56]. It is achieved by taking multiple exposures of the breast from different angles. The image acquisition geometry of DBT is comparable to that of FFDM [57]. Similar to FFDM, MGD has been recommended for use as a radiation risk indicator in DBT [58].

In the early stage of DBT development, it was reported that DBT caused comparable MGD to that from single view screen-film mammography [59]. However, MGD from single view DBT is currently stated to be one to two times more than that from FFDM [60]. In general, MGD resulted from DBT is higher than MGD from FFDM and this difference increases as the breast thickness increase [61].

For the estimation of MGD from DBT, two-dimensional FFDM equation described by Dance et al. [58] is formalised to be:

$$D(\theta) = K\,gcs\,t(\theta)$$

where $D(\theta)$ is the radiation dose results from the exposure of a single projection at angle θ, t is the 'tomo' factor at angle θ and K is the incident air kerma measured at the $0°$ projection using the exposure factors and the X-ray spectrum of θ angle projection. Therefore, radiation dose at $0°$ angle is equal to that from the two-dimensional FFDM and t = 1 [58].

The MGD for single view DBT is the total MGDs of all projections in the tomographic scan. The estimation of MGD for complete tomographic scan is related to the tomographic geometry. For fixed image receptor geometry,

Table 20.2 T-factors for different DBT systems of different geometries (Hologic Selenia Dimensions, Siemens Inspiration and Sectra) [58]

Breast thickness (mm)	T-factor Hologic	T-factor Siemens	T_s-factor Sectra
20	0.997	0.980	0.983
30	0.996	0.974	0.958
40	0.996	0.971	0.935
50	0.995	0.968	0.907
60	0.994	0.966	0.883
70	0.994	0.965	0.859
80	0.993	0.964	0.833
90	0.992	0.962	0.806
100	0.993	0.961	0.783
110	0.992	0.960	0.759

such as Hologic Selenia Dimensions system and Siemens Inspiration, the total MGD is calculated as follow [58]:

$$D_T = K_T \, gcs \, T$$

The T-factor is determined by definition the ratio between the dose for conventional projection mammography and the dose for tomosynthesis when the same exposure factors and X-ray spectrum are used. T-factor values are listed in Table 20.2 as published by Dance et al. [58].

For the other DBT geometry, with moving image receptor as in Sectra system, the incident air kerma is determined for a complete scan at the same exposure factors. The 3D dose is found from the following equation:

$$D_S = K_S \, gcs \, T_S$$

K_S is the incident air kerma calculated for a single scan of the Sectra system and the factor T_S is listed in Table 20.2 as published by Dance et al. [58].

Mammography: Dose to Organs Other than the Examined Breast

A limited number of studies have estimated the radiation dose received by organs and tissues, other than the exposed breast, from mammography. Most of these studies utilised mathematical models to simulate mammography. Sechopoulos et al. [62] utilised the Geant 4 Monte Carlo toolkit to estimate the radiation dose to all body tissues other than the breast [62]. The same procedure has more recently been used by Sechopoulos and Hendrick [63] to estimate the radiation dose received by the thyroid gland during mammography. The thyroid dose is considered to be negligible in regard to radiation-induced cancer - four-view mammography would result in 1 cancer case per 166 million women. Leidens et al. [64] used the Monte Carlo PENELOPE toolkit to estimate lung, heart and red bone marrow radiation dose during standard craniocaudal (CC) mammography with film-screen systems. They reported that only the lung received a considerable radiation dose, while doses to the others were negligible [64].

A study by Whelan et al. [65] used TLDs for the direct measurement of radiation dose received by women's skin overlying the thyroid during standard screening mammography (CC and MLO views for each breast) and diagnostic mammography. This study concluded that the average measured thyroid dose was insignificant compared to that received by the breast tissue. Hatziioannou et al. [66] also utilised TLDs accommodated inside an upper body anthropomorphic Lucite phantom to simulate female body contour. This was done to investigate the in vivo measurement of dose to the breast, sternum red bone marrow (SRBM), thyroid, liver, lung, stomach, and oesophagus during screening mammography. They found that the breast dose contributes over 98% of the overall effective dose. SRBM and thyroid receive a considerable radiation, and the other organ doses were negligible [66].

Other organs radiation dose from FFDM and DBT were investigated by Baptista et al. [60]. They utilised Monte Carlo MCNPX toolkit with mathematical "Laura" voxel phantom to estimate the organ dose from the CC position. For both digital mammography and DBT, the estimated organs dose data showed that the radiation dose received by the contralateral lung and thyroid ranked as second and third highest dose in relation to the examined breast.

An extended study was conducted by M.Ali et al. [67] to estimate organs radiation dose for 16 FFDM screening machines within the UK. They used ATOM dosimetry phantom to simulate screening clients' bodies with PMMA-Polyethylene breast phantom. They found that the highest radiation dose, after exposed breast, was received by contralateral breast tissue and sternum red bone marrow, respectively. The same procedure was used by M.Ali et al. [57] to compare the organs radiation dose from DBT with those from FFDM. They found that the use of DBT for breast cancer screening increases the radiation dose received by body tissues and organs and the highest other tissue doses were received by contralateral breast tissue, thyroid and lung tissue, respectively [57].

In summary, there is evidence to suggest that the radiation dose received by organs other than the breast requires further consideration, as the radiation dose and the risk associated with it is not captured by MGD. For a more thorough and accurate estimation of the radiation risk from mammography, the dose to all organs should be taken into account.

> **Clinical Pearls**
> - An unnecessary radiation dose, however small, should be avoided
> - It is necessary for any medical screening procedure involving ionising radiation to be justified in term of its benefits and risk

Chapter Review Questions
Review Questions

1. What is the standard method of MGD estimation?
2. What is the main limitation associated with the use of MGD as a predator for radiation risk assessment from mammography?

Answers

1. MGD is estimated by indirect method using incident air kerma and conversion factors as described by Dance's equation.
2. The main limitation of MGD is that it cannot capture the radiation risk to body tissues and organs other than exposed breast.

Appendix

Test your learning and check your understanding of this book's contents: use the "Springer Nature Flashcards" app to access questions using https://sn.pub/dcAnWL.

To use the app, please follow the instructions in Chap. 1.

Flashcard   code: 48341-69945-ABCB1-2A8C7-CE9D2.

Short URL: https://sn.pub/dcAnWL.

References

1. Zenone F, Aimonetto S, Catuzzo P, Peruzzo Cornetto A, Marchisio P, Natrella M, Rosano AM, Meloni T, Pasquino M, Tofani S. Effective dose delivered by conventional radiology to Aosta Valley population between 2002 and 2009. Br J Radiol. 2012;85(1015):e330–8.
2. Olarinoye IO, Sharifat I. A protocol for setting dose reference level for medical radiography in Nigeria: a review. Bayero J Pure Appl Sci. 2010;3(1):138–41.
3. Hart D, Wall BF, Hillier MC, Shrimpton PC. Frequency and collective dose for medical and dental x-ray examinations in the UK, 2008. Oxfordshire: Health Protection Agency; 2010.
4. Linet MS, Slovis TL, Miller DL, Kleinerman R, Lee C, Rajaraman P, Berrington de Gonzalez A. Cancer risks associated with external radiation from diagnostic imaging procedures. CA Cancer J Clin. 2012;62(2):75–100.
5. Sezdi M. Dose optimization for the quality control tests of X-ray equipment. Available from: https://www.intechopen.com/chapters/22140. Accessed 24 Jan 2021.
6. Statkiewicz-Sherer MA, Visconti PJ, Ritenour ER. Radiation protection in medical radiography. 6th ed. London: Mosby; 2010.
7. Health Protection Agency (HPA). Risk of solid cancers following radiation Exposure: estimates for the UK population. Oxfordshire: Health Protection Agency; 2011.
8. Balonov MI, Shrimpton PC. Effective dose and risks from medical X-ray procedures. Ann ICRP. 2012;41(3–4):129–41.
9. Lin EC. Radiation risk from medical imaging. Mayo Clin Proc. 2010;85(12):1142–6.
10. Suzuki K, Yamashita S. Low-dose radiation exposure and carcinogenesis. Jpn J Clin Oncol. 2012;42(7):563–8.
11. ICRP. The 2007 Recommendations of the International Commission on Radiological Protection. ICRP publication 103. Ann ICRP. 2007;37(2–4):1–332.
12. Brenner DJ. What we know and what we don't know about cancer risks associated with radiation doses from radiological imaging. Br J Radiol. 2014;87(1035):20130629.
13. Griffey RT, Sodickson A. Cumulative radiation exposure and cancer risk estimates in emergency department patients undergoing repeat or multiple CT. AJR Am J Roentgenol. 2009;192(4):887–92.
14. Prasad KN, Cole WC, Hasse GM. Health risks of low dose ionizing radiation in humans: a review. Exp Biol Med. 2004;229(5):378–82.
15. National Academy of Sciences (NAS). Health risks from exposure to low levels of ionizing radiation: BEIR VII – phase 2. Washington: National Academies Press; 2006.
16. United Nations Scientific Committee on the Effects of Atomic Radiation (UNSCEAR). UNSCEAR 2006

report vol. I. Annex A: Epidemiological studies of radiation and cancer. 2008.

17. Brenner DJ, Sawant SG, Hande MP, Miller RC, Elliston CD, Fu Z, Randers-Pehrson G, Marino SA. Routine screening mammography: how important is the radiation-risk side of the benefit-risk equation? Int J Radiat Biol. 2002;78(12):1065–7.

18. de González AB, Darby S. Risk of cancer from diagnostic X-rays: estimates for the UK and 14 other countries. Lancet. 2004;363(9406):345–51.

19. Wall BF, Kendall GM, Edwards AA, Bouffler S, Muirhead CR, Meara JR. What are the risks from medical X-rays and other low dose radiation? Br J Radiol. 2006;79(940):285–94.

20. Little MP, Wakeford R, Tawn EJ, Bouffler SD, Gonzalez AB. Risks associated with low doses and low dose rates of ionizing radiation: why linearity may be (Almost) the best we can do. Radiology. 2009;251(1):6–12.

21. Dobrzynski L, Fornalski KW, Feinendegen LE. Cancer mortality among people living in areas with various levels of natural background radiation. Dose-Response. 2015;13(3):1559325815592391.

22. Health Canada. Radiation protection and quality standards in mammography: safety procedures for the installation, use and control of mammographic X-ray equipment - Safety Code 36 In: Canada. CH, editor. Ottawa, ON: Health Canada; 2013.

23. Huda W, Nickoloff EL, Boone JM. Overview of patient dosimetry in diagnostic radiology in the USA for the past 50 years. Med Phys. 2008;35(12):5713.

24. Dance DR, Skinner CL, Carlsson GA. Breast dosimetry. Appl Radiat Isot. 1999;50(1):185–203.

25. Di Maria S, Barros S, Bento J, Teles P, Figueira C, Pereira M, Vaz P, Paulo G. TLD measurements and Monte Carlo simulations for glandular dose and scatter fraction assessment in mammography: A comparative study. Radiat Meas. 2011;46(10):1103–8.

26. Karlsson M, Nygren K, Wickman G, Hettinger G. Absorbed dose in mammary radiography. Acta Radiol Ther Phys Biol. 1976;15(3):252–8.

27. ICRP. Statement from the 1987 Como meeting of the International Commission on Radiological Protection. Ann ICRP. 1987;17(4):i–v.

28. Myronakis ME, Zvelebil M, Darambara DG. Normalized mean glandular dose computation from mammography using GATE: a validation study. Phys Med Biol. 2013;58(7):2247–65.

29. IAEA. Quality assurance programme for digital mammography. Austria: IAEA in Austria; 2011.

30. Säbel M, Aichinger H. Recent development in breast imaging. Pysics Med Biol. 1996;41(3):315–68.

31. Tyler NJ, Strudley C, Hollaway P, Peet DJ. Patient dose measurements in full field digital mammography and comparison with dose to the standard breast. Munich: World Congress on Medical Physics and Biomedical Engineering; 2009.

32. Tsai HY, Chong NS, Ho YJ, Tyan YS. Evaluation of depth dose and glandular dose for digital mammography. Radiat Meas. 2010;45(3–6):726–8.

33. Dong SL, Chu TC, Lan GY, Lin YC, Yeh YH, Chuang KS. Development of an adjustable model breast for mammographic dosimetry assessment in Taiwanese women. Am J Roentgenol. 2011;196(4):W476–81.

34. Nsiah-Akoto I, Andam AB, Adisson EK, Forson AJ. Preliminary studies into the determination of mean glandular dose during diagnostic mammography procedure in Ghana. Res J Appl Sci Eng Technol. 2011;3(8):720–4.

35. Geeraert N, Klausz R, Muller S, Bloch I, Bosmans H. Breast characteristics anddisimetric data in X ray mammography - a large sample worldwide survey. Germany: International Conference on Radiation Protection in Medicine; 2012.

36. Dance DR. Monte Carlo calculation of conversion factors for the estimation of mean glandular breast dose. Pysics Med Biol. 1990;35(9):1211–9.

37. IPEM. The commissioning and routine testing of mammographic X-ray systems. York: IPEM; 2005.

38. Vyborny CJ, Schmidt RA. Mammography as a radiographic examination: An overview. Radiographics. 1989;9(4):723–64.

39. Law J. The development of mammography. Phys Med Biol. 2006;51(13):R155–67.

40. Säbel M, Aichinger H. Recent development in breast imaging. Phys Med Biol. 1996;41(3):315–68.

41. Dance DR, Skinner CL, Young KC, Beckett JR, Kotre CJ. Additional factors for the estimation of mean glandular breast dose using the UK mammography dosimetry protocol. Phys Med Biol. 2000;45(11):3225–40.

42. Dance DR, Young KC, van Engen RE. Further factors for the estimation of mean glandular dose using the United Kingdom, European and IAEA breast dosimetry protocols. Phys Med Biol. 2009;54(14):4361–72.

43. Bushong SC. Radiologic science for technologists: physics, biology, and protection. 12th ed. Elsevier; 2020.

44. Boyd NF, Martin LJ, Yaffe MJ, Minkin S. Mammographic density and breast cancer risk: current understanding and future prospects. Breast Cancer Res. 2011;13(6):223.

45. Alonzo-Proulx O, Packard N, Boone JM, Al-Mayah A, Brock KK, Shen SZ, Yaffe MJ. Validation of a method for measuring the volumetric breast density from digital mammograms. Phys Med Biol. 2010;55(11):3027–44.

46. Standring S, Gray H. Gray's anatomy: The anatomical basis of clinical practice. 40th, anniversary ed. Edinburgh: Churchill Livingstone/Elsevier; 2008.

47. Diffey J, Hufton A, Beeston C, Smith J, Marchant T, Astley S. Quantifying breast thickness for density measurement. In: Krupinski EA, editor. Digital mammography: 9th International Workshop, IWDM 2008 Tucson, AZ, USA, July 20–23, 2008 Proceedings. Berlin, Heidelberg: Springer; 2008. p. 651–8.

48. Hauge IH, Hogg P, Szczepura K, Connolly P, McGill G, Mercer C. The readout thickness versus the measured thickness for a range of screen film mammography and full-field digital mammography units. Med Phys. 2012;39(1):263–71.

49. Beckett JR, Kotre CJ. Dosimetric implications of age related glandular changes in screening mammography. Phys Med Biol. 2000;45(3):801–13.
50. Suad K, Suada K, Samek D, Amila H, Samir K. Analysis of application of mean glandular dose and factors on which it depends to patients aged 65 to 80. J Phys Sci Appl. 2013;3(6):387–91.
51. European Commission. European guidline for quality assurance in breast cancer screening and diagnosis: fourth edition supplements. Belgium; 2013.
52. Wu X, Gingold EL, Barnes GT, Tucker DM. Normalized average glandular dose in molybdenum target-rhodium filter and rhodium target-rhodium filter mammography. Radiology. 1994;193(1): 83–9.
53. Sechopoulos I, Bliznakova K, Qin X, Fei B, Feng SS. Characterization of the homogeneous tissue mixture approximation in breast imaging dosimetry. Med Phys. 2012;39(8):5050–9.
54. Dance DR, Hunt RA, Bakic PR, Maidment AD, Sandborg M, Ullman G, Alm Carlsson G. Breast dosimetry using high-resolution voxel phantoms. Radiat Prot Dosim. 2005;114(1–3):359–63.
55. Geeraert N, Klausz R, Muller S, Bloch I, Bosmans H. Evaluation of exposure in mammography: limitations of average glandular dose and proposal of a new quantity. Radiat Prot Dosim. 2015;165(1–4): 342–5.
56. Destounis S, Gruttadauria JL. An overview of digital breast tomosynthesis. J Radiol Nurs. 2015;34(3):131–6.
57. M.Ali RMK, England A, Tootell AK, Hogg P. Radiation dose from digital breast tomosynthesis screening: a comparison with full field digital mammography. J Med Imag Radiat Sci. 2020;51(4):599–603.
58. Dance DR, Young KC, van Engen RE. Estimation of mean glandular dose for breast tomosynthesis: factors for use with the UK, European and IAEA breast dosimetry protocols. Phys Med Biol. 2011;56(2):453–71.
59. Niklason LT, Christian BT, Niklason LE, Kopans DB, Castleberry DE, Opsahl-Ong BH, Landberg CE, Slanetz PJ, Giardino AA, Moore R, Albagli D. Digital tomosynthesis in breast imaging. Radiology. 1997;205(2):399–406.
60. Baptista M, Di Maria S, Barros S, Figueira C, Sarmento M, Orvalho L, Vaz P. Dosimetric characterization and organ dose assessment in digital breast tomosynthesis: measurements and Monte Carlo simulations using voxel phantoms. Med Phys. 2015;42(7):3788–800.
61. Feng SSJ, Sechopoulos I. Clinical digital breast tomosynthesis system: dosimetric characterization. Radiology. 2012;263(1):35–42.
62. Sechopoulos I, Suryanarayanan S, Vedantham S, D'Orsi CJ, Karellas A. Radiation dose to organs and tissues from mammography: Monte Carlo and phantom study. Radiology. 2008;246(2):434–43.
63. Sechopoulos I, Hendrick RE. Mammography and the risk of thyroid cancer. AJR Am J Roentgenol. 2012;198(3):705–7.
64. Leidens M, Goes E, Nicolluci P. Use of Monte Carlo method to determine radiation dose to organs and tissues from mammography. Med Phys. 2013;40(6):139.
65. Whelan C, McLean D, Poulos A. Investigation of thyroid dose due to mammography. Australas Radiol. 1999;43(3):307–10.
66. Hatziioannou KA, Psarrakos K, Molyvda-Athanasopoulou E, Kitis G, Papanastassiou E, Sofroniadis I, Kimoundri O. Dosimetric considerations in mammography. Eur Radiol. 2000;10(7):1193–6.
67. M.Ali RMK, England A, Mercer C, Tootell A, Walton L, Schaake W, Hogg P. Mathematical modelling of radiation-induced cancer risk from breast screening by mammography. Eur Radiol. 2017;96(Suppl C):98–103.

Image Quality, System Optimisation and Quality Control

21

Katy Szczepura and Cláudia Sá dos Reis

Learning Objectives
- Understand the parameters that are assessed during quality control
- Recognise the role of quality control and its implications for justification and optimisation
- Identify the main quality control tests for mammography CR and DR systems, required equipment, frequency and expected results

Introduction

Mammography is the only medical imaging technology that is designed to image only one organ. Mammography machines are required to deliver the highest quality medical images of all the imaging modalities, the reason for this is twofold. Firstly, cancer produces very small physical changes, and the masses can look similar to the background glandular tissue, leading to poor inherent contrast [1, 2]. This means that very high levels of contrast resolution are required to be able to distinguish cancer from background structures [3]. Secondly, calcifications may be present and an indicator of disease, and although they are high electron density, and so have high inherent contrast, they are very small, meaning very good spatial resolution is required [3, 4].

Image Quality Parameters

All QC tests will test the system's capacity in terms of image quality and dose [5]. Although tests may vary, there are fundamental parameters that are linked to clinical image quality, that ascertain the baseline system capability. These are discussed below.

Contrast Resolution

Contrast resolution in any medical imaging modality is defined as the ability of the system to distinguish between differences in image intensity [1, 2]. Contrast resolution is essential for the conspicuity of pathology in mammography [6]. If an object blends in with its background, the object cannot be seen, therefore low contrast means the image is less optimal for detection and diagnosis [6].

K. Szczepura (✉)
School of Health and Society, University of Salford, Manchester, UK
e-mail: K.Szczepura@salford.ac.uk

C. S. dos Reis
School of Health Sciences (HESAV), University of Applied Sciences and Arts Western Switzerland (HES-SO), Lausanne, Switzerland
e-mail: claudia.sadosreis@hesav.ch

© The Author(s), under exclusive license to Springer Nature Switzerland AG 2022
C. Mercer et al. (eds.), *Digital Mammography*, https://doi.org/10.1007/978-3-031-10898-3_21

Contrast is an essential measure of the diagnostic capability of a system. Contrast to noise ration and signal to noise are standard measures used to represent this in quality control [1, 2, 7]. They are both size independent if they are used in isolation as quantitative measures of image quality [6]. They represent the difference in signal amplitude between the object and the noise within the background [1, 2]. In digital mammography, it is important to distinguish between inherent (or subject) and image contrast.

Inherent Contrast

Inherent, or subject contrast, is a result of the differences in attenuation between the tissues within the path of the X-rays [6]. This is affected by the exposure parameters, as well as the electron densities and thicknesses of the different tissues. Exposure parameters have a strong impact on inherent contrast, next we will consider kVp, as well as target and filter materials.

kVp As kVp increases, inherent contrast reduces, this is due to the increased transmission through the tissues, making them less distinct from one another [1, 2]. Although increasing kVp increases radiation dose if done in isolation, the increased transmission allows for a lower mAs to be used, reducing radiation dose overall. Low kVp can be used in mammography as only soft tissues are being imaged, and compression helps to reduce the thickness of tissue [8].

Target and Filter Combination The target material defines the line spectrum, and materials are chosen to give appropriate line spectrum energies for the thickness and density of a breast [8]. Filter material is used to remove the continuous spectrum, whilst still allowing transmission of the line spectrum. This improves inherent contrast resolution and reduces radiation dose. In mammography, low kVp and high levels of filtration are used to ensure the highest level of contrast resolution possible whilst keeping doses ALARA [8].

Image Contrast

One huge advantage of digital imaging over film is the ability to adjust and optimise image contrast after the image has been acquired. Image contrast is not fixed and, alongside brightness, can be adapted to enhance areas or tissues of interest to suit the observer. As long as the exposure factors are within a range that ensures there is suitable inherent contrast, image contrast is not a fixed, measurable parameter within clinical imaging [9, 10]. The acceptable range of exposures is very wide within digital imaging, the biggest risk is overpenetration, and losing inherent contrast due to too high kVp [10].

Spatial Resolution

Spatial resolution refers to the ability of the imaging system to differentiate between two objects adjacent to each other and display them as distinct objects in the image [1, 2]. Limiting spatial resolution is defined as the smallest object that can be resolved by the system [11]. Spatial resolution is an important criterion in mammography, as calcifications can be very small, and so the limiting spatial resolution needs to be of high enough quality to resolve these features. Often spatial resolution is described as the *sharpness* of an image, and is impacted by the *unsharpness*, which is often referred to as image blur [10].

Unsharpness

Many things can affect the unsharpness of an image, the main parameters are focal spot size, motion, receptor performance, and geometry [1, 2]. Focal spot size will impact on the penumbra of an image, and therefore contributes to the unsharpness of an image. Using a smaller focal spot size can reduce the penumbra, improving spatial resolution, however the use of a smaller focal spot can impact on the tube performance and longevity. Commonly there are two focal spot size options in mammography, with nominal sizes of 0.1 and 0.3 mm [12], with the smaller focal spot sized being used when unsharpness may be more of an issue, such as during magnification imaging. The amount of motion unsharpness in an image is directly related to the speed of the motion in comparison to the speed of the system. Client/patient motion is the biggest cause of motion unsharpness in mammography [4], compression is utilised to immobilise the breast to reduce motion unsharpness [3].

Noise

There are different types of noise in mammography, it is easiest to separate them into system noise and structural or anatomical noise.

System noise is a random fluctuation of image intensity and appears as speckles in an image. In digital systems noise can occur due to electrical and quantum noise [5]. In screen-film systems images are very susceptible to noise, and mAs needs to be high enough to ensure noise is not seen on the image, additionally, too high a mAs can cause over exposure in film.

With digital imaging, there is less impact from noise, and mottle only typically appears if the exposure is approximately half of the ideal level [11]. Due to the wide latitude of digital imaging, over exposure is almost impossible to see on the image, however it can cause an increase in scatter, which will deteriorate image quality [13]. In digital mammography, it is often beneficial to move to a higher energy spectrum than with film-screen mammography, since image noise is lower and the resulting loss in image contrast can be compensated for by adjusting the window setting [11].

Structural noise constitutes normal tissue structures in an image, and can prevent the image reader from seeing the pathology they are looking for [14]. It can mask or imitate pathology and lead to reduced conspicuity within the image. Compression is used to attempt to reduce the impact of overlying structure to reduce structural noise.

In QC, homogeneous test tools are used to ensure that there is no structural noise present to ensure the noise of the system is only being measured [14].

Quality Control and Implications for Justification and Optimisation

Justification and optimisation are part of the fundamental basis of radiation protection [15] and although they can be complex clinical tasks, quality control is an essential tool to ensure consistency and enable the processes to be as accurate as possible.

The *principle of optimisation* requires that the likelihood of potential exposure, the number of people exposed and the magnitude of their individual exposure, should all be kept as low as reasonably achievable, taking into account economic and societal factors [16]. Although optimisation of an individual exposure is patient/client dependent, QC ensures that the equipment is functioning optimally, and is not deviating from is baseline parameters. This enables the operator to ensure they are using equipment that is in appropriate condition for them to be able to apply the individual optimisation process.

For screening programmes, the optimisation process is more complex, as the exposure is to an asymptomatic population. This is often why AECs are implemented in mammography, to ensure exposure is optimised for each individual, and why QC is performed more regularly than in other imaging modalities [17].

The *principle of justification* requires that any decision that impacts on an exposure to ionising radiation should do more good than harm; to either the individual or societal benefit [18]. This is an intellectual process of weighing up the potential benefit of a medical exposure against the detriment for that individual. It must include consideration of techniques which involve less or no ionising radiation [19]. Although quality control is not directly linked to the justification process, knowledge of the potential detriment of the exposure is important to enable the decision-making task to be completed.

QC ensures doses are consistent over time and can identify any changes in dose delivery by the system early on so that any problems can be rectified. As well as regular QC tests, an appropriate QA programme, dose audits are an essential part of this process [17]. Additionally, when mammography is used as a screening tool, the exposure is to an asymptomatic population, and justification is often performed at a national level where clients have to meet set criteria to be included in the screening programme [18]. QC is an essential tool to ensure the maintenance of the justification of the screening programme on a national level.

Processes for Quality Assurance and Quality Control

Processes and individual tests can vary from country to country, and even from manufacturer to manufacturer, however, there are fundamental principles that can be undertaken to ensure equipment is functioning optimally. These will now be discussed further.

Acceptance Testing and Commissioning

Acceptance and commissioning of imaging equipment is a part of the purchasing of new equipment. Acceptance assures that the facility is getting the equipment and performance that was specified in the purchase agreement. Once the integrity and performance of the equipment has been assured, commissioning provides information necessary for clinical use and establishes base line measurements for future quality control checks [20, 21].

Acceptance testing should occur at two time points. Firstly, it should happen immediately after the equipment is installed (before commissioning); and best practice is that it should happen again approximately 1 month before the end of the warranty period. The second acceptance test assures that the equipment still meets the specifications before the warranty expires. This provides sufficient time to notify the manufacturer and have the issues resolved within the warranty period.

During commissioning baseline scanning protocols are established such as AEC settings. If manufacturer provided protocols are to be used, image quality and dose need to be optimised within those protocols. Acceptance tests and commissioning needs to be undertaken by qualified medical physicists working in conjunction with the service engineers [22–25].

Baseline Measurements and Acceptable Ranges

For some QC tests, baseline measurements need to be established to ensure that the equipment is not deviating from the acceptable performance established during commissioning. Baseline measurements are set to enable comparison of performance in the future as part of the ongoing quality control program. For some tests there are acceptable ranges of deviation from the baseline measurements and provides and indicator for when action is required.

Regular Quality Control

Regular QC testing may be performed by the practitioner, or by medical physicists. Practice varies from country to country, but most countries have different levels of tests that are performed by medical physicists or local practitioners.

Although several tests, as described next in this chapter, can be performed by local practitioners, there are more elaborate measurements that should be undertaken by medical physicists who are trained and experienced in diagnostic radiology and specifically trained in mammography QC [22–25]. Comparability and consistency of the results from different centres is best achieved if data from all measurements, including those performed by local practitioners are collected and analysed centrally [22–25].

Quality Control Tests

Quality Assurance (QA) programmes and Quality Control (QC) tests provide a framework for continuous assessment to ensure that issues are identified and resolved before problems arise. QC tests can provide early identification of when equipment starts to deviate from optimum performance and can implement appropriate interventions. The first stage of optimisation within the mammography imaging chain is to ensure the machines are performing optimally at all times. Quality Assurance (QA) aims to provide systematic and constant improvement through a feedback mechanism to address the technical, clinical and training aspects [5, 26]. Quality Control (QC), in relation to mammography equipment, comprises a series of tests to determine equipment performance characteristics. The introduction of digital technologies promoted changes in QC tests and protocols and there are some tests that are specific for each manufacturer [26].

Within each country, specific QC tests should be compliant with regulatory requirements and guidance [5]. Ideally, one mammography practitioner should take overarching responsibility for QC within a service, with all practitioners having responsibility for actual QC testing. All QC results must be documented to facilitate troubleshooting, internal audit and external assessment [22, 23].

Generally speaking, the practitioner's role includes performing, interpreting and recording the QC tests as well as reporting any out of action limits to their service lead. They must undertake additional continuous professional development to maintain their QC competencies [22]. They are usually supported by technicians and medical physicists; in some countries the latter are mandatory. Technicians and/or medical physicists often perform many of the tests indicated within this chapter. In Europe it is a legal requirement that some tests are performed by a certified Medical Physics Expert (MPE) or representative [27].

It is important to recognise that this chapter is an attempt to encompass the main tests performed within European countries. Specific tests related to the service that you work within must be familiarised with and adhered too.

The QC tests in this chapter are based on recommendations from various organisations and documents, specifically: Institute of Physics and Engineering in Medicine (IPEM); National Health Service Breast Screening Programme (NHSBSP) [25, 28]; European Protocol (EP) (EUREF [23, 29, 30]); European Federation of Organisations in Medical Physics (EFOMP) [31]; and International Atomic Energy Agency (IAEA).

EP and EFOMP guidelines have been included because they aim to promote harmonisation of mammography practices within EU countries. EP guidance is disseminated within Europe and to date is adopted in more than 15 countries [32–39]. The NHSBSP guidance (United Kingdom) is used by various countries worldwide [5, 40].

IAEA and EFOMP guidelines are the most up-to-date documents for digital mammography QC [22]. For general QC tests, all the above documents provide guidance on periodic testing, to address image acquisition, detection systems, image processing, image display, and others tests (e.g. electrical and mechanical tests) [22, 25, 28, 30, 41–43].

The tests that are commonly recommended in all the guidance documents are now presented in this chapter.

Tests for Acquisition Systems

X-Ray Tube and Generator

Various tests (reproducibility and accuracy, focal spot size, tube output, HVL, etc.) can be performed to assess this part of the equipment. However, with the introduction of digital technologies the majority are no longer done by mammography practitioners due to the stability of the X-ray generators that are currently in use. The QC tests that are in use are those related to dosimetry—tube output and Half Value Layer (HVL) [31].

Procedure and Materials	The performance of the X-ray system is assessed through measurements of the X-ray tube output (in air). Measurements should be undertaken with a calibrated dosimeter [31].
	The dosimeter should be positioned at 4 cm from the chest wall edge laterally centred on the image receptor (the Perspex it is not positioned on the image receptor but on top of breast support platform) and irradiated using a collimated radiation beam. The compression paddle should be removed for the measurements [23]. Tube output should be measured for all target-filter combinations used in clinical practice (e.g. Mo/Mo, Mo/Rh, Rh/Rh, W/Rh, W/Ag). Repeating this test with the paddle on can be done if you want to ascertain the attenuation of the paddle for dosimetry purposes.
	Output measurements need to be repeated using 2 mm aluminium filtration (or 4.5 cm PMMA) attached to the tube port using a broad X-ray beam geometry to mimic the attenuation and scatter of the breast. The output should be measured across a range of mAs values (10, 20, 40, 80, 120 and 180). This data is required to characterise the detector response function (signal transfer function—STP).
Frequency	At equipment acceptance and annual checks.
	Within the UK this is every 6 months.
Expected Results	Output at 28 kVp for target filter Mo/Mo—the reference acceptable and achievable X-ray tube output values recommended by EUREF are >30 μGy/mAs and >40 μGy/mAs, respectively.

Tests for Detection Systems

Alignment of X-Ray Field to Optical Field

The aim of this test is to evaluate coincidence of X-ray and light fields. The chest wall edge is most important. Misalignment may result in breast tissue being missed or non-breast tissue being imaged: the latter increases dose for no benefit; the former could mean pathology is missed.

Procedure and Materials	The light field edges must be identified using radio-opaque markers, an X-ray image is then produced and evaluated. Difference between X-ray and light fields is assessed.
Frequency	At equipment acceptance and annual checks.
	Within the UK this is every 6 months.
Expected Results	Misalignment should be less than 5 mm along any edge [23, 28].

Compression Force and Thickness Accuracy

Some systems use compressed breast thickness to auto-select kVp and T/F, consequently it is important to assess the thickness indicator accuracy; thickness reduction is achieved by the application of compression force [22].

Procedure and Materials	Prior to testing compression force, the compression paddle should be inspected to identify physical damage (e.g. cracks). Compression force can be evaluated by placing weighing scales on the breast platform and centred under the compression paddle. The compression paddle should be moved up to the maximum compression force supported by the system (generally 180 or 200 N). Care must be exercised so as not to damage the mammography equipment. Results from the mammography machine and weighing scales should be compared. The next test considers compression force maintenance over 30 s or 1 min—to identify if there is any compression force drop over time [22, 23].
	To verify breast thickness readout accuracy display, a rectangular poly-methyl methacrylate (PMMA) phantom with three different thickness (20, 45 and 70 mm) is used. This is aligned with the chest wall and centred on breast platform. Typically, 80 N is applied and the machine given thickness readout is recorded. Phantom and machine given readout thickness are then compared.
Frequency	Monthly, or more frequently as required by guidance.
Expected Results	The display value for compression force readout on the mammography machine should be within ±20 N of the display on the weighing scales
	If the display on the weighing scales is higher than 200 N the machine should be taken out of action and reported immediately. For breast thickness indicator should be ±5 mm [22, 23].

Signal Transfer Function

Procedure and Materials	The signal transfer property (STP) establishes the relationship between the entrance air kerma at the detector and the pixel value in pre-processed images. It is useful to understand how the detector transforms the input into an output signal.
	Measurement of STP can be performed using images produced with an attenuated beam by having 2 mm thick aluminium plate attached to the tube port to mimic the attenuation of a standard breast. The compression paddle (optional) and the grid are removed for the image acquisition. Non-processed (raw) images can be acquired either (a) a standard tube voltage (28 kVp) across a wide range of entrance air kerma values (nominal 12.5, 25, 50, 100, 200 and 400 µGy) or (b) in the UK factors selected by the AEC when exposing a standard breast. The mAs values required to produce the aimed receptor air kerma values are determined from the output measurements previously performed [44].
	For each image, measurements of the mean pixel value and standard deviation must be undertaken in the Region of Interest (ROI) of 1 cm^2 at 6 cm from the image chest wall edge [23].
	For mammography systems with a linear STP response (DR systems) the mean pixel value should be plotted against the entrance air kerma; linearity is assessed using software [44].
Frequency	For equipment acceptance and six monthly checks.
Expected Results	Correlation coefficient should be R^2 > 0.99 [23, 44]

Automatic Exposure Control System (AEC)

The AEC controls the exposure to the detector; its performance testing is crucial as it has a direct impact on image quality and patient dose. This test is recommended because it provides information regarding the global performance of mammography equipment [5].

Various methods have been proposed and metrics have been developed, e.g. detector air kerma, detector dose index, pixel value, Signal to noise Ratio (SNR) and Signal difference to Noise Ratio (SdNR) equivalent to Contrast to Noise Ratio (CNR). Here the SdNR method is explained. SdNR is measured from images produced with a PMMA phantom and a low contrast object (aluminium 0.2 mm thick, >99.9% purity). Figure 21.1 demonstrates this [44].

SdNR and dose should be measured in at least three different thicknesses (20, 45 and 70 mm) which are considered to mimic attenuation and scatter provided by a thin, average and large breast. The PMMA breast phantom is composed of various 0.5 or 1 cm slabs piled up on top of each other to produce the necessary thickness. A small aluminium square (1 cm × 1 cm and 0.2 mm thickness) must be positioned below the top slab at 6 cm from the chest wall edge. In the UK it is placed on top of the bottom slab and then built up with additional PMMA on top.

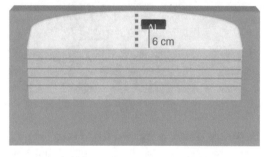

Fig. 21.1 PMMA phantom used to perform the AEC testing

The PMMA phantom is placed on the Perspex, it is not positioned on the image receptor but on top of breast support platform, with an overhang of 5 mm out from the chest wall edge and laterally centred in the image field. The radiation field size should be collimated to cover the complete phantom.

The compression paddle must be positioned in contact with the PMMA slabs and a consistent compression force is recommended e.g. 60 N. For AEC systems with options for positioning the AEC (X-ray sets associated with CR systems and some DR e.g. Hologic Dimensions) the midline position is selected and a region that would not be affected by the Aluminium square.

Images should be acquired using AEC and associated exposure settings typically used in clinical practice. Images are acquired for the three PMMA thicknesses. For the standard thickness (45 mm PMMA) the procedure should be repeated three times.

For thicknesses ≥40 mm, low attenuation material spacers can be positioned at the edges of the phantom to achieve the intended equivalent [breast] thickness. This is important because some mammography systems adjust the X-ray settings according to the detected breast thickness or compression force.

Only raw images with the processing algorithm turned off are used, acquired in a "raw", "unprocessed" or DICOM "for processing" format depending on the system used.

For each image, measurements of the mean pixel value and its standard deviation are performed in ROIs (1 cm²) in aluminium and the surrounding background. Pixel values are corrected using STP data and SdNR is calculated as (refer to Fig. 21.1) (Table 21.1):

$$SdNR = \frac{\text{mean pixel value}(\text{signal}) - \text{mean pixel value}(\text{background})}{\text{background standard deviation}}$$

| Frequency | Every 6 months, or more frequently as required within the UK: Daily for Radiographers at 4 cm and monthly for 2 and 6/7 cm. |
| Expected Results | Using the SdNR method, the IAEA reference values can be used (Table 21.1). |

Detector Uniformity and Artefacts

Image receptor uniformity is essential and uniformity testing should be performed regularly. Uniformity problems in digital systems can be caused by inappropriate calibrations of the image field or due to artefacts caused by defects on the detector [31, 45]. There are also noted problems with the target, filters, grid, and paddle if looking at the system rather than just detector.

Procedures and Materials

Uniformity can be assessed using flat field uniform images produced with an attenuated

X-ray beam with a 2 mm Al foil attached to the tube port. Most manufacturers supply a large area block of PMMA which can sit over the breast support platform as an alternative to Al over the tube. The image receptor can be imaged using clinical exposure parameters to achieve an air kerma of approximately 100 μGy at the image detector. The images can be acquired either (a) without grid and without compression paddle and also without processing (raw images) or (b) with the grid to assess the system clinically. A large radiation field should be used (broad beam), typical for clinical use.

Pixel values should be corrected using STP data before making ROI measurements. The mean pixel value should be measured for five ROI (1 cm² each), distributed as shown in Fig. 21.2: one at the centre of the image and the other four at the centre of each quadrant [44].

Table 21.1 Acceptable (Accep.) and Achievable (Achiev.) reference levels for SdNR in mammography proposed by IAEA for thicknesses of 20, 45 and 70 mm [22]

| Mammography system | Compressed breast thickness [mm] | | | | | |
| | 20 | | 45 | | 70 | |
	Accep.	Achiev.	Accep.	Achiev.	Accep.	Achiev.
GE 2000D—DR	8.9	12.9	7.9	11.5	6.9	10.0
GE DS—DR	8.9	12.9	7.9	11.5	6.9	10.0
GE Essential—DR	12.7	18.4	11.3	16.5	9.9	14.4
Fuji Amulet—DR	6.1	8.7	5.5	7.8	4.8	6.8
Siemens Inspiration—DR	4.4	6.3	3.9	5.7	3.4	5.0

Frequency

Following equipment service to tube or detector and more frequently as required by protocol. Within the UK: Every 6 months by technicians/physicists and monthly by Radiographers.

Expected Results

The images should be artefact free. Importantly, dead pixels, missing lines or columns should not be visible in the area that is clinically relevant.

Mean SNR, calculated for all five ROIs should present a maximum deviation of ≤15% [23].

The images can be assessed for artefacts. Image artefacts can have different origins, including client, practitioner and equipment related.

The artefacts related to the client can be caused by motion or due to the anatomical characteristics (for instance the thin breast artefact (<20 mm) that is caused because it is possible

Fig. 21.2 Reference ROIs for uniformity measurements

that during compression, the paddle edges may be included at the corners of the image creating the artefact) [46].

The practitioner can introduce artefacts during the positioning of the breast, improper detector handling (CR systems) and inadequate screen cleaning procedures (CR systems) than can cause white dots due to dust and parts of the coating of the cassette [47].

The most common artefacts related to the equipment are those related to software processing errors and those that are caused by the specific architecture of the detector, namely geometric distortion due to incorrect stitching of sub-images and inhomogeneities towards the lateral sides of the image. Absence of detector calibration can also cause artefacts due to imperfections and differences in gain of each individual segments of the detector. The grid lines can also appear causing artefacts due to the stopping or slowing down of grid and also misplacement and vibration [45–47].

Test to Evaluate Image Retention (Ghosting)

In some digital imaging systems signal retention in the image receptor may be observed following radiation exposure, e.g. a ghost image superimposed on the subsequent image. This effect may cause artefacts and degrade image quality (Fig. 21.3).

Procedure and Materials	Image retention can be tested by irradiating a rectangular PMMA phantom with dimensions $18 \times 24 \times 45$ mm^3, using typical clinical exposure settings with grid in.
	The first image should be produced with the phantom positioned with the longest side perpendicular to the chest wall edge, covering half of the Perspex it is not positioned on the image receptor but on top of breast support platform. A second image is obtained with the phantom repositioned, centred in the breast platform covering it as much as possible with an 0.1 mm thick Al sheet placed (centred) on top to generate a low contrast signal. A time interval of 1 min should occur between both exposures and the two images need to be acquired in raw format (no processing).
	The mean pixel value is measured in three ROI (1 cm^2), within the area attenuated by the Al foil and in the surrounding background as illustrated in Fig. 21.3. The measured pixel values need to be corrected with STP data and then used to calculate an image retention factor:
	$$\text{Image retention factor} = \frac{\text{mean pixel value}\left(\text{ROI3}\right) - \text{mean pixel value}\left(\text{ROI2}\right)}{\text{mean pixel value}\left(\text{ROI1}\right) - \text{mean pixel value}\left(\text{ROI2}\right)}$$
Frequency	Yearly or after detector replacement. Within it is every 6 months.
Expected Results	The results can be compared with a reference value of 0.3 as proposed by EP [23].

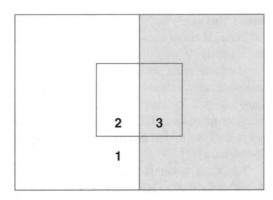

Fig. 21.3 Image retention—positioning of ROI measurements to determine image retention factor. *White area* represents the area with the PMMA attenuation during first exposure

Image Quality Assessment Using Phantoms

A common method to assess image quality (IQ) uses images produced with test objects and phantoms. This method has limitations due to the models in use. The models do not perfectly represent the breast characteristics and for that reason it is very difficult to establish an acceptable level of diagnostic IQ related to clinical images. However, it is accepted that when a technical image offers adequate quality, the clinical image should also be adequate [31]. It is also easier to implement a technical approach with test objects to monitor the quality due to the reproducibility.

There are several phantoms for IQ monitoring. For each, the details that are analysed vary; similarly, the methodologies and reference/tolerance values also vary [5]. IQ can be assessed by observers or software. A limiting factor of observer studies concerns variability; variability is eliminated in software-based approaches. The training of observers is very important to minimise intra- and inter-observer variability; training should also improve validity. Observer studies and software analysis both have a place in IQ analysis.

EFOMP guidelines outline seven different phantoms for mammography image quality (IQ) analysis: American College of Radiology (ACR) mammography accreditation phantom, CIRS Phantom (model 011A), TORMAS, TORMAX, TORMAM, CDMAM and MAM/DIGI. These guidelines are valuable when assisting with the selection phantom for services and also to identify the test methodologies [31]. There are other phantoms, including DMAM2 and QUART, and those dedicated to other breast modalities such as VOXMAX and CIRS (model 020 BR3D for tomosynthesis systems) [48, 49]. Regardless of phantom, it is necessary to define a baseline in order to identify changes over time [31].

Next we will consider a methodology to assess images produced with a phantom that is composed of two parts technical and clinical (TORMAM).

TORMAM (Assessment of Low Contrast Detail)

TORMAM is designed for quick and easy use on a routine basis to provide regular IQ assessment.

One part of the phantom contains a range of filaments, micro-particles and low-contrast detail that aim to mimic pathological features in the breast: six groups of multi-directional filaments, six groups of micro-calcification in the range 300–100 μm and six groups of three low-contrast detail subgroups. These details are sensitive to the dynamic range of mammography, noise and unsharpness and can be used to obtain an IQ score.

Another part of the phantom contains a structure that mimics the appearance of breast tissue; it contains micro-calcification clusters, fibrous material and nodules. This part provides a more realistic breast image (Figs. 21.4 and 21.5).

Procedure and Materials	Images should be produced using 3 cm rectangular or D shaped PMMA on breast support and then TORMAM on top of PMMA. A compression force of 60 N should be applied and the images are acquired using the AEC mode in clinical practice (Figs. 21.4 and 21.5).
	When TORMAM images are reviewed by observers' ambient light level should be low and the monitor should be free from reflections.

Frequency	Practitioners: Weekly.
	Physicists/technicians: 6 monthly.
Expected Results	No established acceptability criteria for this phantom yet the scores are established for the mammography system and compared for any degradation over time.
	The maximum possible score is 72 for the fibrous component, 18 for microcalcifications and 54 for nodules. The maximum score is 144.
	It is accepted that a higher score corresponds to better IQ. Using CDMAM phantom it is also possible to perform software analysis of IQ, thereby providing an objective and highly reproducible alternative to using observers.

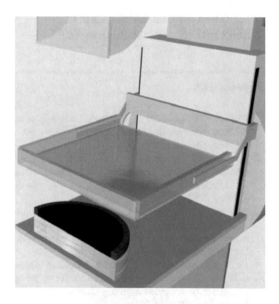

Fig. 21.4 TORMAM phantom on the top of D shaped PMMA for image acquisition (Courtesy of Mário Oliveira)

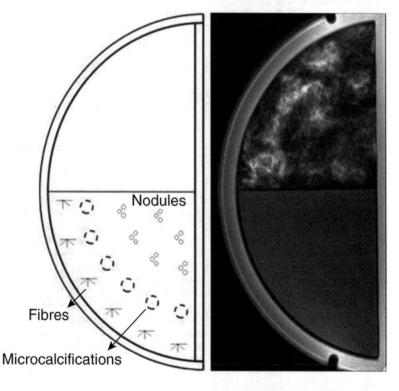

Fig. 21.5 TORMAM phantom: phantom: schematic and radiographic [48]

Nodules

Fibres

Microcalcifications

Appendix

Test your learning and check your understanding of this book's contents: use the "Springer Nature Flashcards" app to access questions using https://sn.pub/dcAnWL.

To use the app, please follow the instructions in Chap. 1.

Flashcard code:
48341-69945-ABCB1-2A8C7-CE9D2.

Short URL: https://sn.pub/dcAnWL.

References

1. Bushong SC. [Radiologic science for technologists: physics, biology, and protection] St. Louis, MO; London: Elsevier Mosby; 2008.
2. Bushberg JT, Seibert JA, Leidholdt EM, et al. [The essential physics of medical imaging]. Philadelphia, PA; London: Wolters Kluwer/Lippincott Williams & Wilkins; 2012.
3. Holland K, Sechopoulos I, Heeten G, et al. Performance of breast cancer screening depends on mammographic compression. Cham: Breast imaging, Springer; 2016. p. 183–9.
4. Holland K, Sechopoulos I, Mann RM, et al. Influence of breast compression pressure on the performance of population-based mammography screening. Breast Cancer Res. 2017;19(1):126.
5. Reis C, Pascoal A, Sakellaris T, et al. Quality assurance and quality control in mammography: a review of available guidance worldwide. Insights Imaging. 2013;4(5):539–53.
6. Szczepura KR, Manning DJ. Validated novel software to measure the conspicuity index of lesions in DICOM images. Proc SPIE. 2016;9787:978703-978703-15.
7. Waade GG, Sanderud A, Hofvind S. Compression force and radiation dose in the Norwegian Breast Cancer Screening Program. Eur J Radiol. 2017;88:41–6.
8. Markey M. [Physics of mammographic imaging]; 2014.
9. Kanal KM, Krupinski E, Berns EA, et al. ACR-AAPM-SIIM practice guideline for determinants of image quality in digital mammography. J Digit Imaging. 2013;26(1):10–25.
10. Carroll QB. Radiography in the digital age: physics, exposure, radiation biology. Springfield, IL: Charles C. Thomas; 2011.
11. Bick U, Diekmann F. Digital mammography: what do we and what don't we know? Eur Radiol. 2007;17(8):1931–42.
12. Tanaka N, Naka K, Kumazawa S, et al. Imaging properties of digital magnification mammography. In: World Congress on Medical Physics and Biomedical Engineering, September 7–12, 2009, Munich, Germany; 2009. p. 64–6.
13. Seeram E. [Digital radiography: physical principles and quality control].
14. Bochud F, Verdun F, Valley J-F, et al. [Importance of anatomical noise in mammography]. Proc SPIE. 3036 74 (1997).
15. ICRP. [The 2007 Recommendations of the International Commission on Radiological Protection]; 2007.
16. ICRP. P101 Representative person and optimisation - ANIB_36_3. Ottawa, ON: International Commission on Radiological Protection; 2006.
17. ICRP. [Managing patient dose in digital radiology. ICRP Publication 93]; 2004.
18. ICRP. [ICRP Publication 103]; 2007.
19. B. I. o. Radiology. IR(ME)R - Implications for clinical practice in diagnostic imaging, interventional radiology and diagnostic nuclear medicine. 2020. https://www.rcr.ac.uk/system/files/publication/field_publication_files/irmer-implications-for-clinical-practice-in-diagnostic-imaging-interventional-radiology-and-nuclear-medicine.pdf.
20. IAEA. Human health campus - acceptance and commissioning of imaging equipment. Vienna: IAEA; 2022.
21. E. Commission. [Criteria for acceptability of medical radiological equipment used in diagnostic radiology, nuclear medicine and radiotherapy]; 2012.
22. IAEA. [Quality assurance programme for digital mammography]; 2011.
23. Perry N, Broeders M, de Wolf C, et al. European guidelines for quality assurance in breast cancer screening and diagnosis. Fourth edition--summary document. Ann Oncol. 2008;19(4):614–22.
24. England PH. [Routine quality control tests for full-field digital mammography systems Equipment report 1303: fourth edition]; 2013.
25. Kulama E. [Commissioning and routine testing of full field digital mammography systems]; 2009.
26. Andolina V, Lillé S. [Mammographic imaging: a practical guide]. Philadelphia, PA: Wolters Kluwer/Lippincott Williams & Wilkins Health; 2011.
27. European Commission. European guidelines on medical physics expert. Brussels: EC; 2014. p. 174.
28. Moore AC; Institute of Physics and Engineering in Medicine (Great Britain). [The commissioning and routine testing of mammographic X-ray systems: a protocol produced by a Working Party of the National Breast Screening Quality Assurance Coordinating Group for Physics]. York: Institute of Physics and Engineering in Medicine; 2005.
29. Bosmans H, Engen RV, Heid P, et al. EUREF type testing protocol. Nijmegen: European Communities/EUREF; 2011.
30. Lelivelt H, Ongeval CV, Jacobs J, et al. EUREF type testing – clinical evaluation protocol. Nijmegen: European Communities/EUREF; 2010.
31. E. F. o. O. f. M. Physics; 2022.

32. Ciraj-Bjelac O, Faj D, Stimac D, et al. Good reasons to implement quality assurance in nationwide breast cancer screening programs in Croatia and Serbia: results from a pilot study. Eur J Radiol. 2011;78(1):122–8.
33. Thierens H, Bosmans H, Buls N, et al. Typetesting of physical characteristics of digital mammography systems for screening within the Flemish breast cancer screening programme. Eur J Radiol. 2009;70(3):539–48.
34. Ng KH, Jamal N, DeWerd L. Global quality control perspective for the physical and technical aspects of screen-film mammography--image quality and radiation dose. Radiat Prot Dosim. 2006;121(4):445–51.
35. Avramova-Cholakova S, Vassileva J. Pilot study of patient and phantom breast dose measurements in Bulgaria. Pol J Med Phys Eng. 2008;14(1):21–32.
36. Zdesar U. Reference levels for image quality in mammography. Radiat Prot Dosim. 2008;129(1–3):170–2.
37. Nikodemová D, Horváthová M, Salát D. Implementation of QA and QC standards in radiology in Slovakia. Radiat Prot Dosim. 2005;117(1–3): 274–6.
38. Shannoun F, Schanck JM, Scharpantgen A, et al. Organisational aspects of mammography screening in digital settings: first experiences of Luxembourg. Radiat Prot Dosim. 2008;129(1–3):195–8.
39. Hemdal B, Herrnsdorf L, Andersson I, et al. Average glandular dose in routine mammography screening using a Sectra MicroDose Mammography unit. Radiat Prot Dosim. 2005;114(1–3):436–43.
40. I. o. Medicine, and N. R. Council. Saving women's lives: strategies for improving breast cancer detection and diagnosis. Washington, DC: The National Academies Press; 2005.
41. Bosmans H, Engen RV, Heid P, et al. EUREF type testing protocol. Nijmegen: European Communities/EUREF; 2010.
42. N. H. S. B. S. Programme. [Guidance notes for equipment evaluation: protocol for user evaluation of imaging equipment for mammographic screening and assessment NHSBSP equipment report 0703]. Sheffield; 2007.
43. International Atomic Energy Agency. [Quality assurance programme for screen film mammography]. Vienna: IAEA; 2009.
44. Mackenzie A, Doylo P, Honey I, et al. [Measurements of the performance characteristics of diagnostic X-ray system: digital imaging system]. IPEM report 32 Part VII. York.
45. Bick U, Diekmann F. [Digital mammography]. Berlin: Springer Verlag; 2010.
46. Ayyala RS, Chorlton M, Behrman RH, et al. Digital mammographic artifacts on full-field systems: what are they and how do I fix them? Radiographics. 2008;28(7):1999–2008.
47. Van Ongeval C, Jacobs J, Bosmans H. Artifacts in digital mammography. JBR-BTR. 2008;91(6):262–3.
48. Medical Imaging Phantoms. Leeds test objects. @ leedstestobject; 2022.
49. Hill ML, Liu K, Mainprize JG, Levitin RB, Shojaii R. Breast imaging. In: Maidment ADA, Bakic PR, Gavenonis S, editors. 11th International Workshop, IWDM 2012, Philadelphia, PA, July 8–11, 2012; 2022.

Automated Assessment of Breast Positioning in Mammography Screening

Ariane Chan, Jaimee Howes, Catherine Hill, and Ralph Highnam

Learning Objectives
- Understand the importance of breast positioning for cancer detection in mammography screening
- Appreciate the variation, subjectivity, and limitations in how breast positioning is currently assessed clinically
- Learn about automated breast positioning tools that are being developed
- Understand how automated breast positioning can integrate into clinical practice and improve quality

Note: The term 'technologist' is used within this chapter instead of the term 'practitioner'.

A. Chan · J. Howes · R. Highnam (✉)
Volpara Health Technologies,
Wellington, New Zealand
e-mail: ariane.chan@volparahealth.com;
jaimee.howes@volparahealth.com;
ralph.highnam@volparahealth.com

C. Hill
DetectedX, The University of Sydney, Sydney, NSW, Australia
e-mail: catherine.hill@detectedx.com

Introduction

Several randomized controlled trials [1] have clearly demonstrated the effectiveness of organised breast cancer screening on reducing breast cancer mortality, especially for women who actually attend screening and who have cancers diagnosed at an earlier stage [2–4]. The acquisition of high-quality full-field digital mammographic (FFDM) and digital breast tomosynthesis (DBT) images is crucial for ensuring optimal sensitivity and detection of cancers at their earliest signs. Image quality reviews of FFDM and synthetic mammograms reconstructed from DBT include both technical (e.g. contrast, exposure, noise, sharpness, and artifacts) and clinical factors (e.g. breast positioning and adequate breast compression).

Optimal breast positioning is arguably the most critical aspect of image quality, ensuring as much breast tissue as possible is visualised for diagnostic interpretation. Manual, visual assessment of breast positioning is the predominant method used clinically, but has several limitations:

- It is time-consuming in nature, making it impractical to evaluate breast positioning on a large scale.
- There is considerable variability in evaluation criteria and subjectivity across readers [5–7].
- There is no global consensus standard as to how breast positioning should be assessed, leading to regional differences in the criteria used for evaluation [5, 8].

© The Author(s), under exclusive license to Springer Nature Switzerland AG 2022
C. Mercer et al. (eds.), *Digital Mammography*, https://doi.org/10.1007/978-3-031-10898-3_22

Several studies have found an association between sub-optimal breast positioning and screening outcomes, as summarised in Table 22.1. Poor positioning has also been reported as the primary reason for critical failures in clinical image quality reviews [15, 16].

Automated assessment of breast positioning, the focus of this chapter, has the potential to mitigate many of these issues. As we describe, automated analysis of breast positioning can support both retrospective analysis for training and ongoing monitoring of image quality, as well as providing on the job training. Furthermore, a better understanding of what is reasonably achievable in clinical practice, based on large-scale benchmarking of breast positioning, can inform standards.

Assessment of Breast Positioning in Current Clinical Practice

There is significant variability in the specific criteria, and interpretation of such criteria, used to evaluate clinical image quality, in part because of the lack of global consensus standards. Moreover, there have been few studies that have reviewed breast positioning in the context of informing and defining minimum positioning standards [17, 18]. While these studies included relatively small sample sizes (170–1000 patients), they were informative in terms of highlighting potential differences in positioning challenges between modalities. They were also useful for presenting baseline targets to inform what is reasonably achievable for certain metrics, albeit in the study

Table 22.1 Summary of studies showing associations between breast positioning and screening performance measures. DBT, digital breast tomosynthesis; FFDM, full-field digital mammography; UK, United Kingdom; US, United States

References	Key clinical findings relating to breast positioning
Taplin et al. [9]	
• N = 492 screen-detected; 164 interval cancers	• Sensitivity dropped from 84% to 66.3% for images meeting and failing breast positioning criteria respectively
• US setting	• Interval cancers 2.57 times more likely after images failed positioning
• Film screen mammography	
Bae et al. [10]	
• N = 335 cancers detected with ultrasound after a negative mammogram	• 3% (9/335) of cancers not detected at mammography were due to difficult anatomic position or poor positioning
• South Korean setting	
Mercieca et al. [11]	
• N = 2291 images (60 of which were rejected)	• Mammography reject rate was 2.67%
• Maltese setting	• The majority of rejected images (71.6%) were attributed to positioning
Yeom et al. [12]	
• N = 188 second breast cancers (in women with personal history of early-stage breast cancer)	• 12% (9/74) second breast cancers not detected at mammography due to difficult anatomic location/poor positioning
• South Korean setting	
Salkowski et al. [13]	
• N = 274 technical recalls (from >48,000 screening studies)	• Sub-optimal breast positioning the predominant reason for technical recalls, compared to technical/artifacts or motion blur.
• US setting (three sites)	• Of the recalls, 47% of FFDM and 81% of DBT images were attributed to inadequate positioning
• FFDM and DBT	
Gilroy et al. [14]	
• N = 2134 technical repeats; 1340 accepted images	• Images scored as inadequate were significantly more frequent amongst technical repeats attributed to breast positioning issues compared to accepted images (41% versus 2%, respectively)
• UK setting	• Insufficient evaluation of the pectoral muscle being the most common deficiency
• FFDM	

by Huppe et al. [18], these baselines were obtained after technologist training and after excluding studies with extenuating circumstances, so may not be representative of a typical screening setting. While attempts have been made to define more reproducible standards based on international expert opinions [5], these are yet to be implemented in any widespread manner.

To highlight the heterogeneity in the evaluation of image quality, Table 22.2 summarises various international guidelines and provides an overview of the breast positioning metrics considered for evaluation. The underlying intent across each of these guidelines is consistent, that is, to assess that all breast tissue has been included on the image; however, not only do the specific criteria differ, subjective and inconsistent lan-

Table 22.2 Breast positioning criteria considered by various image quality guidelines developed for different regions around the world. Although specific language varies, black circles indicate that the metric is mentioned in the guidelines. CC, craniocaudal; IMF, inframammary fold; MLO, mediolateral oblique; PNL, posterior nipple line

Country		United States	United Kingdom	Australia	Netherlands	Belgium
Guidelines maintained by		American College of Radiology [19]	National Health Service [20]	BreastScreen Australia [21]	LRCB, Dutch Expert Centre for Screening [22]	European Commission [23]
Criteria (CC/MLO views)	Skin folds	●	●	●	●	●
	Asymmetry left vs. right		●	●	●	●
	Nipple is not in profile		●	●	●	●
	PNL > 1 cm between CC and MLO views	●		●		
	Breast tissue cut-off	●		●		●
	Absence of artefacts/ other body parts	●	●	●	●	●
	Fibroglandular disc/ triangle				●	
Criteria (CC view only)	Medial tissue not visualised	●		●	●	●
	Lateral tissue/axillary tail not visualised		●		●	●
	Posterior tissue not visualised	●	●			●
	Pectoral muscle/shadow visualised		●		●	●
	Excessive exaggeration	●				
Criteria (MLO view only)	IMF not well demonstrated/visualised	●	●	●	●	●
	IMF skin folds or IMF obscured					●
	Pectoral length to level of nipple/PNL		●			●
	Pectoral angle		●			●
	Full width/sufficient amount of pectoral muscle			●	●	
	Breast too high on receptor	●				
	Breast sag/droop	●	●			●
	Posterior tissue not visualised	●	●	●		

guage is often used. Moreover, assignment of a clinically relevant score to provide some indication as to whether an image is of diagnostic quality or needs to be repeated is varied, with some evaluation criteria leading to, for example:

- A binary classification, e.g. Acceptable/Inadequate [20]
- A three-point classification, e.g. Excellent/Adequate/Repeat (EAR) [7]
- A 4-point classification, e.g. Perfect/Good/Moderate/Inadequate (PGMI) [21]

Screening programs that have quality review processes often rely on a manual, subjective review of only a small number of randomly sampled images. In the United States (US), for example, ongoing certification to provide mammography services is mandated by the Food and Drug Administration Mammographic Quality Act and Program (FDA MQSA) standards [24]. Sites are only required to submit two screening studies every 3 years, as part of the clinical image review for machine accreditation, to an FDA-approved accreditation body (e.g. the American College of Radiology). For the more recent FDA Enhancing Quality Using the Inspection Program (EQUIP), sites need to demonstrate that they complete periodic quality image reviews [25].

Automated Breast Positioning

Increased adoption of digital technologies has accelerated the pace at which quantitative and automated tools are being developed for mammography screening, including the evaluation of image quality criteria. Automated analysis allows for the evaluation of breast positioning on a much larger scale than has previously been possible and supports both a better understanding of baseline positioning metrics and the impact of targeted initiatives to improve image quality. At the time of writing, several vendors have commercially available automated image quality software (in certain regions) that include breast positioning:

1. Volpara Live™/Analytics™ (Volpara Health Technologies)
2. MiaIQ™ (Khieron Medical Technologies)
3. Densitas qualityai™ (Densitas)

We focus here on Volpara Live and Analytics software, both of which leverage Volpara's TruPGMI™ scoring system. The definitions of the TruPGMI scores are described in Fig. 22.1, and can give an indication of the breast positioning quality of the images and study. TruPGMI scores are derived from how well each image met, partially met, or didn't meet certain metrics for key breast positioning criteria, taking into account best practices from different regions around the world. Scores are provided at both an image and study level (see overview of key metrics and high-level workflow schematic in Figs. 22.2 and 22.3, respectively).

One advantage of automated evaluation of breast positioning is the power of benchmarking. Comprehensive analysis of image quality trends for individual technologists can be compared across the organization, or against aggregated global benchmark data. Based on data obtained from a cloud-based benchmarking dataset (over

Perfect Highest Diagnostic Quality	Good	Moderate	Inadequate*** Lowest Diagnostic Quality
This mammogram is an example of excellent work by the technologist.	This mammogram is high quality.	This mammogram is acceptable quality; technologist would be unlikely to repeat image(s).	This mammogram is poor quality; technologist might repeat image(s).
		* Extenuating circumstances, such as body habitus or mobility issues, may limit the technologist's ability to obtain an adequate study.	** Mosaic or tiled images may be categorized as Inadequate.

Fig. 22.1 Volpara's TruPGMI scoring system and definitions

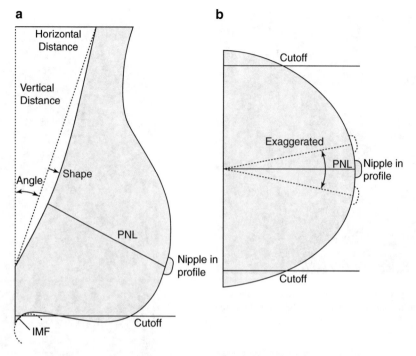

Fig. 22.2 Overview of breast positioning metrics assessed for TruPGMI on MLO views (**a**) and CC views (**b**)

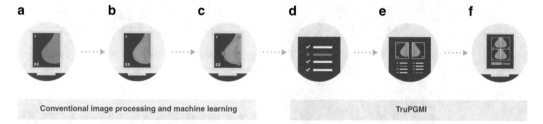

Fig. 22.3 Workflow overview of the generation of TruPGMI scores. Conventional image processing and machine learning are leveraged to first segment the breast tissue from the background (**a**), as well as the pectoral muscle on MLO views (**b**), so that key anatomical land-marks (e.g. the nipple) can be identified and localized (**c**). Automated TruPGMI scoring begins with the evaluation of key TruPGMI metrics as being met, partially met, or not met (**d**). TruPGMI scores are then derived for each image (**e**) and study (**f**) separately

three million studies), examples are provided for the four most common breast positioning issues identified:

1. Excessive exaggeration on craniocaudal (CC) view (Fig. 22.4)
2. Inframammary fold not visualised and open on mediolateral oblique (MLO) view (Fig. 22.5)
3. Pectoral muscle does not extend to within 1 cm of the level of the posterior nipple line (PNL) on MLO view (Fig. 22.6)

4. PNL lengths not within 1 cm for CC and MLO pairs (Fig. 22.7)

Several studies have found that interventional training or focused quality initiatives led to significant improvements in breast positioning quality, and even more so when individualised feedback was provided to technologists [6, 16, 26]. Pal et al. [6] estimated personnel costs of approximately US$1200 (i.e. 6 h) to audit 122 cases for breast positioning. Without an automated system, large scale review of breast positioning, for example to

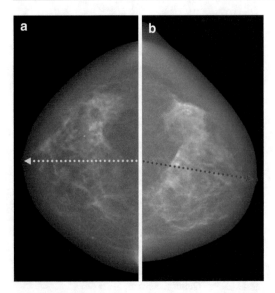

Fig. 22.4 Example of an optimal CC view with the nipple aligned to the midline (**a**) and an exaggerated CC (**b**) where the nipple is angled towards the medial aspect

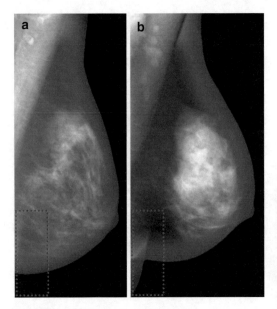

Fig. 22.5 Examples of MLO views where the inframammary fold is not visualised (**a**) or open (**b**)

assess the impact and success of quality initiatives, is not practical or cost-effective.

As described in the next section, automated evaluation of breast positioning can be integrated into the clinical workflow, to provide on the job training and as part of retrospective monitoring.

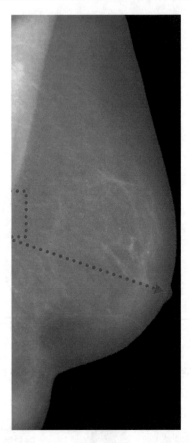

Fig. 22.6 Example of an MLO view where the inferior aspect of the pectoral muscle does not extend to within 1 cm of the level of the PNL

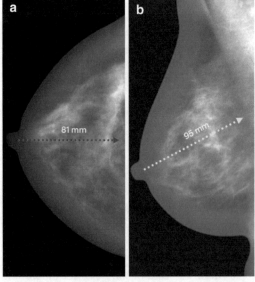

Fig. 22.7 Example where the PNL on the CC view (**a**) is not within 1 cm of the PNL on the MLO view (**b**). The difference in the PNL lengths in this example is 1.4 cm

Integration of Automated Breast Positioning into Clinical Practice

Using two product examples, we demonstrate how automated TruPGMI can integrate into clinical practice to improve image quality.

1. On the job training for breast positioning—Volpara Live™

    Images repeated or recalled for suboptimal quality are not only costly, but also add unnecessary dose and inconvenience for patients. The Live display (Fig. 22.8) appears on a dedicated tablet, soon after the first screening image is acquired. Live evaluates each image at the time of a screening study, to provide image- and study-level TruPGMI scoring, as well as alerts when there are images scored as "inadequate". Live can be configured to pro-

vide feedback on only images scored as inadequate, or on every image, for individualised training around key breast positioning metrics.

2. Continuous monitoring and feedback—Volpara Analytics™

    Analytics provides comprehensive analysis on a large scale, via web-based dashboards and automated reporting. Using examples from a particular customer who demonstrated excellent image quality, we illustrate the key benefits of Analytics software below:

    (a) Images from every study can be reviewed by technologists and centre managers in the web-based dashboards.

    - Positioning feedback provided at the metric, image, and study level, alongside vendor-neutral display images, to facilitate an understanding

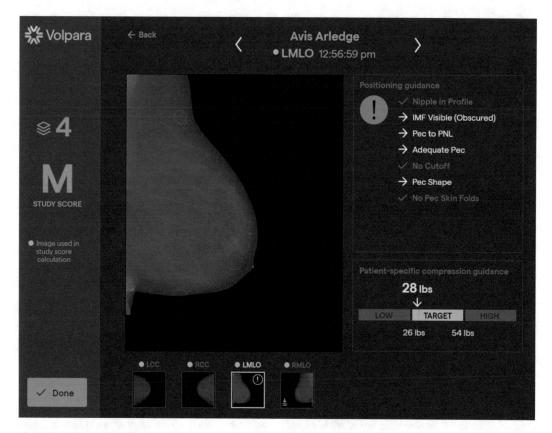

Fig. 22.8 Volpara Live display indicating a study scored as "M", i.e. Moderate, using the TruPGMI evaluation system. Feedback for key breast positioning metrics are provided for training purposes, for any individual images that are scored as "I", i.e. Inadequate

of the factors underlying the TruPGMI scores and areas for improvement.
- Feedback is paired with targeted positioning videos.

(b) Performance trends for individual technologist can be benchmarked against the whole organization and globally.
- Figure 22.9 highlights a technologist who has significantly improved over an 18-month period, with the percentage of Good and Perfect images exceeding organisation and global averages. This particular technologist also demonstrated good engagement with Analytics, with significantly more logins into the software compared to the average across the organisation.

(c) Lead technologists or centre managers may have access to a special role license that provides them with oversight across all technologists within their organisation.
- Figure 22.10 highlights the Team Quality overview, which shows where each individual technologist sits in relation to their breast positioning and compression quality scores, alongside global averages and excellence targets (i.e. 75th percentile globally).

(d) Automated Periodic Image Quality Review (PIQR) reporting.
- PIQR reports can be implemented by facilities to ensure a continuous focus on image quality compliance and ongoing review, in support of quality assurance programs around the world; e.g. FDA EQUIP [25], Royal

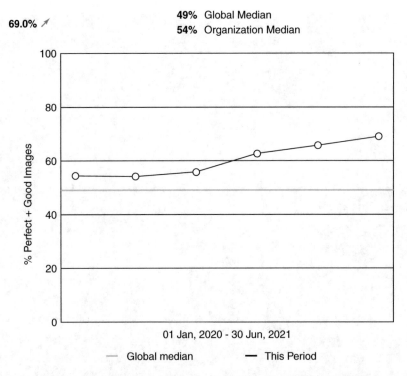

Fig. 22.9 Positioning trend analysis from Volpara Analytics, for an individual technologist over an 18-month period. The proportion of images scored as Perfect or Good using the TruPGMI evaluation system are presented for the individual technologist (black curve). For the April-June 2021 period, this technologist had 69% of studies scores as Perfect or Good, which was an increase (indicated by the upward green arrow) since the baseline January-March 2020 period. Their performance was also benchmarked against their organisation median for the same time period (49%), as well as against a global median (54%) for the January 2021–March 2021 time period (based on a benchmarking dataset of over three million studies)

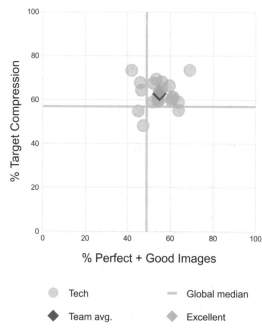

% Target Compression

% Perfect + Good Images

Tech — Global median

Team avg. ◆ Excellent

Fig. 22.10 Overview of team quality scores for the April-June 2021 period, based on the proportion of studies meeting compression pressure targets (7–15 kPa) and Perfect or Good TruPGMI scores. Blue circles indicate the quality scores for 20 individual technologists, alongside the team average across all technologists (blue diamond) for the same time period. Benchmarking is provided for global compression and breast positioning medians (green axis intersects) for the January 2021–March 2021 time period (based on a benchmarking dataset of over three million studies), with the "Excellent" performance target (green diamond) derived from the 75th percentile

Australian and New Zealand College of Radiologists' Mammography Quality Assurance Program (MQAP) [27], and the Canadian Association of Radiologists' Mammography Accreditation Program (MAP) [28].

(e) Identification of candidate studies of high breast positioning quality, to be submitted for accreditation.

Summary

Due to the subjectivity and time-consuming nature of visual inspection of image quality, it is challenging for technologists to receive consistent,

objective, and ongoing feedback about their breast positioning quality. Automated evaluation of breast positioning can help clinics by allowing:

- Individual technologists to review their own performance (overall and over time), as well as benchmarked results against the rest of their organisation and globally
- Managers to understand their team's performance, facilitate performance reviews and identify areas to target for team training
- Set realistic objectives and goals based on benchmarking and individualised trends
- Identify focus areas for improvement, by reviewing feedback down to the level of individual TruPGMI metrics, paired with the corresponding vendor-neutral display images

This automated approach to assessing positioning, based on best practices from around the world, enables breast imaging centers to train staff to:

- Achieve and maintain a high standard of mammographic image quality in breast screening
- Provide an objective training program to advance positioning performance
- More easily prepare for external inspections and quality assurance programs

Clinical Pearls
- Automated breast positioning software supports the evaluation and review of all mammographic images with comprehensive metric-, image- and study-level breast positioning feedback, supporting trend analyses, benchmarking, and targeted goal setting for positioning quality improvements
- Automated periodic image quality reporting can increase efficiencies for mammography screening providers, who are increasingly being expected to demonstrate that processes are in place that support a continuous focus on image quality compliance and ongoing review

Chapter Review Questions
Review Questions

1. What screening performance outcomes have been associated with sub-optimal breast positioning?
   Select all that apply:
   (a) Lowered sensitivity
   (b) Increased interval cancer rates
   (c) Increased false positive rates
   (d) Increased technical recalls and repeats
   (e) Increased recall rates

2. What are the top four breast positioning challenges identified as assessed using automated breast positioning software, on a large benchmarking dataset of over three million images?
   Select the correct four responses:
   (a) Nipple not in profile
   (b) Posterior nipple line lengths on craniocaudal and mediolateral oblique views not within 1 cm
   (c) Exaggerated craniocaudal view
   (d) Sagging breast tissue (mediolateral oblique view)
   (e) Inframammary fold not visualised or open (mediolateral oblique view)
   (f) Concave shape pectoral muscle on (mediolateral oblique view)
   (g) Pectoral muscle does not extend to within 1 cm of the posterior nipple line (mediolateral oblique view)

3. What is the main difference between Volpara Live and Volpara Analytics?
   Select the correct answer:
   (a) They use different positioning metrics to determine the TruPGMI score
   (b) They integrate at different points in the clinical workflow (i.e. at the time of image acquisition versus as part of retrospective review after the study)
   (c) Live only displays study-level analysis of breast positioning

4. What feature of Volpara Analytics best supports image quality compliance and ongoing review?
   Select the correct answer:
   (a) Integrated educational videos
   (b) Breast positioning quality benchmarking
   (c) Automated Periodic Image Quality Review Reporting
   (d) Managers' ability to have oversight across all technologists

Answers
Bold indicate correct answers

1. (a) **Lowered sensitivity**
   (b) **Increased interval cancer rates**
   (c) Increased false positive rates
   (d) **Increased technical recalls and repeats**
   (e) Increased recall rates
2. (a) Nipple not in profile
   (b) **Posterior nipple line lengths on craniocaudal and mediolateral oblique views not within 1 cm**
   (c) **Exaggerated craniocaudal view**
   (d) Sagging breast tissue (mediolateral oblique view)
   (e) **Inframammary fold not visualised or open (mediolateral oblique view)**
   (f) Concave shape pectoral muscle on (mediolateral oblique view)
   (g) **Pectoral muscle does not extend to within 1 cm of the posterior nipple line (mediolateral oblique view)**
3. (a) They use different positioning metrics to determine the TruPGMI score
   (b) **They integrate at different points in the clinical workflow (i.e. at the time of image acquisition versus as part of retrospective review after the study)**
   (c) Live only displays study-level analysis of breast positioning
4. (a) Integrated educational videos
   (b) Breast positioning quality benchmarking
   (c) **Automated Periodic Image Quality Review Reporting**
   (d) Managers' ability to have oversight across all technologists

Appendix

Test your learning and check your understanding of this book's contents: use the "Springer Nature Flashcards" app to access questions using https://sn.pub/dcAnWL.

To use the app, please follow the instructions in Chap. 1.

Flashcard code:

48341-69945-ABCB1-2A8C7-CE9D2.

Short URL: https://sn.pub/dcAnWL.

Acknowedgement The authors would like to thank Dr Jones & Partners Medical Imaging (Attunga Medical Centre, Toorak Gardens, SA, Australia) and their technologists for kindly allowing us to use screenshots from their Volpara Analytics dashboards.

References

1. Smith RA, Duffy SW, Tabár L. Breast cancer screening: the evolving evidence. Oncology. 2012;26(5):9–81, 85–86, 471–75.
2. Duffy SW, Tabár L, Yen AM-F, Dean PB, Smith RA, Jonsson H, Tornberg S, Chen SL, Chiu SY, Fann JC, Ku MM. Mammography screening reduces rates of advanced and fatal breast cancers: results in 549,091 women. Cancer. 2020;126(13):2971–9.
3. Tabár L, Chen TH-H, Yen AM-F, Chen SL-S, Fann JC-Y, Chiu SY-H, Ku MM, Wu WY, Hsu CY, Chen YY, Beckmann K. Effect of mammography screening on mortality by histological grade. Cancer Epidemiol Biomark Prev. 2018;27(2):154–7.
4. Tabár L, Yen AM-F, Wu WY-Y, Chen SL-S, Chiu SY-H, Fann JC-Y, Ku MM, Smith RA, Duffy SW, Chen TH. Insights from the breast cancer screening trials: how screening affects the natural history of breast cancer and implications for evaluating service screening programs. Breast J. 2015;21(1):13–20.
5. Taylor K, Parashar D, Bouverat G, Poulos A, Gullien R, Stewart E, Aarre R, Crystal P, Wallis M. Mammographic image quality in relation to positioning of the breast: a multicentre international evaluation of the assessment systems currently used, to provide an evidence base for establishing a standardised method of assessment. Radiography. 2017;23(4):343–9.
6. Pal S, Ikeda DM, Jesinger RA, Mickelsen LJ, Chen CA, Larson DB. Improving performance of mammographic breast positioning in an academic radiology practice. AJR Am J Roentgenol. 2018;210(4):807–15.
7. Moreira C, Svoboda K, Poulos A. Comparison of the validity and reliability of two image classification systems for the assessment of mammogram quality. J Med Screen. 2005;12(1):38–42.
8. Sweeney RI, Lewis SJ, Hogg P, McEntee MF. A review of mammographic positioning image quality criteria for the craniocaudal projection. Br J Radiol. 2017;91(1082):20170611.
9. Taplin SH, Rutter CM, Finder C, Mandelson MT, Houn F, White E. Screening mammography - clinical image quality and the risk of interval breast cancer. AJR Am J Roentgenol. 2002;178(4):797–803.
10. Bae MS, Moon WK, Chang JM, Koo HR, Kim WH, Cho N, Yi A, La Yun B, Lee SH, Kim MY, Ryu EB. Breast cancer detected with screening US: reasons for nondetection at mammography. Radiology. 2014;270(2):369–77.
11. Mercieca N, Portelli JL, Jadva-Patel H. Mammographic image reject rate analysis and cause – a national Maltese study. Radiography. 2017;23(1):25–31.
12. Yeom YK, Chae EY, Kim HH, Cha JH, Shin HJ, Choi WJ. Screening mammography for second breast cancers in women with history of early-stage breast cancer: factors and causes associated with non-detection. BMC Med Imaging. 2019;19(1):2.
13. Salkowski LR, Elezaby M, Fowler AM, Burnside E, Woods RW, Strigel RM. Comparison of screening full-field digital mammography and digital breast tomosynthesis technical recalls. J Med Imaging. 2019;6(3):031403.
14. Gilroy HM, Hill ML, Chan A, Halling-Brown M, Highnam RP. Automated breast positioning evaluation of screening mammograms in the UK. Poster presented at the European Congress of Radiology 2021. Vienna: ESR; 2021.
15. Guertin M, Theberge I, Dufresne M, Zomahoun HTV, Major D, Tremblay R, Ricard C, Shumak R, Wadden N, Pelletier E, Brisson J. Clinical image quality in daily practice of breast cancer mammography screening. Can Assoc Radiol J. 2014;65(3):199–206.
16. Rouette J, Elfassy N, Bouganim N, Yin H, Lasry N, Azoulay L. Evaluation of the quality of mammographic breast positioning: a quality improvement study. CMAJ Open. 2021;9(2):E607–E12.
17. Bassett LW, Hirbawi IA, DeBruhl N, Hayes MK. Mammographic positioning: evaluation from the view box. Radiology. 1993;188(3):803–6.
18. Huppe AI, Overman KL, Gatewood JB, Hill JD, Miller LC, Inciardi MF. Mammography positioning standards in the digital era: is the status quo acceptable? AJR Am J Roentgenol. 2017;209(6):1419–25.
19. American College of Radiology. Mammography accreditation clinical image review sheet. Reston, VA: ACR. https://www.acraccreditation.org/-/media/ACRAccreditation/Documents/Mammography/Clinical-Image-Review-Sheet%2D%2D-MAP.pdf?la=en. Accessed 31 Aug 2021.
20. National Health Services Breast Screening Program. Guidance for breast screening mammographers. 3rd ed. Sheffield: NHS Breast Screening Programme; 2017.
21. BreastScreen Australia Accreddation Review Commitee. National accreditation standards. Canberra, ACT: BreastScreen Australia National

Accreditation Standards (NAS). https://www.health.gov.au/. Accessed 31 Aug 2021.

22. LRCB. Dutch Expert Centre for Screening. Criteria regarding positioning techniques for mammography. Nijmegen: LRCB; 2009. https://www.lrcb.nl/en/download/criteria-regarding-positioning-techniques-for-mammography/. Accessed 31 Aug 2021.

23. Rijken H, Caseldine J, Laird O. Radiological guidelines. In: Perry N, Broeders M, de Wolf C, Tornberg S, Holland R, von Karsa L, editors. European guidelines for quality assurance in breast cancer screening and diagnosis. 4th ed. Luxembourg: Office for Official Publications of the Europeam Communities; 2006.

24. U.S. Food and Drug Adminstration. Mammography Quality Standards Act regulations. Silver Spring, MD: USFDA; 2002. https://www.fda.gov/radiation-emitting-products/regulations-mqsa/mammography-quality-standards-act-regulations#s90012. Accessed 31 Aug 2021.

25. U.S. Food and Drug Administration. EQUIP: enhancing quality using the inspection program. Silver Spring, MD: USFDA; 2017. https://www.fda.gov/radiation-emitting-products/mqsa-insights/equip-enhancing-quality-using-inspection-program. Accessed 31 Aug 2021.

26. Rauscher GH, Tossas-Milligan K, Macarol T, Grabler PM, Murphy AM. Trends in attaining mammography quality benchmarks with repeated participation in a quality measurement program: going beyond the mammography quality standards act to address breast cancer disparities. J Am Coll Radiol. 2020;17(11):1420–8.

27. Royal Australian and New Zealand College of Radiologists. Mammography quality assurance program. Wellington: RANZCR. https://www.ranzcr.com/fellows/clinical-radiology/quality-assurance-and-accreditation/mqap. Accessed 31 Aug 2021.

28. Canadian Association of Radiologists. Mammography accreditation program (MAP). Ottawa, ON: CAR. https://car.ca/patient-care/map/?__cf_chl_captcha_tk__=pmd_gkAOL-23GLnGIbPkvq.nu09KoPLPpkyV6diRec_bSouE-1629925597-0-gqNtZGzNA5CjcnBszQhl. Accessed 31 Aug 2021.

Radiographic Service Quality

23

Clare S. Alison and Caroline J. Dobson

Learning Objectives
- Demonstrate knowledge of the principles of visual image quality and the requirements for technical recalls and repeats.
- Apply principles and demonstrate how practitioners ensure they are working to the required standards.

Introduction

The success of breast cancer diagnosis requires consistent production of high-quality mammogram images to allow optimal visualisation of breast tissue. It is internationally recognised that the standards required in both screening programmes and symptomatic services need to be regularly monitored and audited. Individual practitioners are also required to regularly monitor and audit their work to maintain production of high-quality images and allow improved performance of the imaging service [1]. Within this chapter these will be defined by the Public Health England [2] guidelines for mammographers in the UK and Breast Screen Australia, National Accreditation Standards 2001 [3].

C. S. Alison (✉) · C. J. Dobson
Breast Imaging, Thirlestaine Breast Centre,
Cheltenham, UK
e-mail: clare.alison@nhs.net;
caroline.dobson3@nhs.net

Why Do Practitioners Require Service Quality Standards?

Standards are required to maintain a high-quality service and not allow individual interpretation of such standards to affect the overall service provision. They are also required to ensure maximum benefit and minimal harm to clients, whilst maximising cancer detection. Both physical and psychological needs of the client need to be observed to minimise discomfort, while still achieving the high standard required. The physical and psychological needs of the client are discussed more widely within Chaps. 11–14.

How Do Practitioners Ensure They Are Working to the Required Standards?

Practitioners should regularly measure, evaluate and audit their mammographic technique against the criteria for critically evaluating the mammogram detailed in The Quality Assurance Guidelines for Mammography, NHSBSP publication No. 63 [2]. The standard of mammography should be assessed using the PHE mammographic image assessment tool (Fig. 23.1). This is mandatory for use within the programme for image review at individual, peer and department levels. Peer review and formal appraisal are useful tools for ensuring the standard is maintained.

MAMMOGRAPHIC IMAGE ASSESSMENT

Dates of Assessment:																						Static/ Mobile		
Assessor(s):							Clinic Code						Date Taken				Mammographer							

Notes: No less than 20 exams should be reviewed, more if problems/trends are highlighted. No patient identifying numbers should be used. To view trends easily only place an X in boxes where criteria are NOT met

Column headings (left to right): Case No. | View | Correct patient ID & Markers (R/L) | Appropriate exposure (R/L) | Adequate compression to hold breast firmly - no movement (R/L) | Image sharp (R/L) | No artefacts obscuring image (R/L) | No obscuring skin folds (R/L) | Nipple in profile (R/L) | MLO's: Pectoral muscle to nipple level (R/L) | Pectoral muscle at appropriate angle (R/L) | IMF shown clearly (R/L) | CCs: Medial border demonstrated (R/L) | Back of breast clearly shown with some medial central & lateral (R/L) | Some axillary tail shown (R/L) | Symmetrical images | whole breast imaged | Comments

Case rows 1–10, each with MLO and CC view lines.

Fig. 23.1 Mammographic image assessment tool

These too should take place on a regular basis. These will be expanded upon later on in the chapter.

The 'perfect/good/moderate/inadequate' (PGMI) or 'excellent/acceptable/repeat' (EAR) methods to examine image quality are no longer acceptable [2]. An audit of a minimum of 20 mammograms every 2 months should be undertaken at service level.

Technical Repeats (TP) and Technical Recall (TC)

A qualified practitioner should be able to critically appraise their technique and the diagnostic quality of the mammographic images they have acquired and justify appropriate repeats. With the introduction of digital X-ray systems, the practitioner must utilise their expertise for instant decision making. Digital imaging has the advantage of generating an image instantly after exposure thus providing rapid feedback to the practitioner if the image is suboptimal [4]. Judgement on whether a repeat is required can be made while the client is present (TP), avoiding a recall for further imaging due to a technical error (TC) and unnecessary anxiety for the client.

A technical repeat (TP) is when a practitioner makes the decision to repeat the same projection after identifying an error when the client is still present [2]. If your service has Assistant/ Associate Practitioners working, it is important to follow protocols for any justification of repeat images [5].

Technical acceptability of an image may not always be adequately judged by the practitioner at time of acquisition. As an example, the acquisition stations utilised may not be of the same high specification as the reporting monitors. Often image blur is not identified until the point of image reading on the reporting workstation, thus subjecting the client to a possible technical recall (TC).

MAMMOGRAPHIC IMAGE ASSESSMENT

Case No.	View			Correct patient ID & Markers		Appropriate exposure		Adequate compression to hold breast firmly - no movement		Image sharp		No artefacts obscuring image		No obscuring skin folds		Nipple in profile		Pectoral muscle to nipple level		Pectoral muscle at appropriate angle		IMF shown clearly		Medial border demonstrated		Back of breast clearly shown with some medial central & lateral		Some axillary tail shown		Symmetrical Images	whole breast imaged	Comments
		R	L	R	L	R	L	R	L	R	L	R	L	R	L	R	L	R	L	R	L	R	L	R	L	R	L	R	L			

Dates of Assessment: / Static/ Mobile

Assessor(s): / Clinic Code / Date Taken / Mammographer / MLO's / CCs

1	MLO																							▨		▨		▨				
	CC																			▨		▨		▨		▨						
2	MLO																	▨		▨		▨		▨		▨						
	CC																							▨		▨		▨				
3	MLO																	▨						▨		▨		▨				
	CC																							▨				▨				
4	MLO																							▨								
	CC																	▨						▨		▨		▨				
5	MLO																	▨		▨		▨		▨		▨		▨				
	CC																							▨		▨		▨				
6	MLO																							▨		▨		▨				
	CC																	▨						▨		▨		▨				
7	MLO																							▨								
	CC																	▨						▨		▨		▨				
8	MLO																			▨				▨		▨						
	CC																	▨		▨		▨		▨		▨		▨				
9	MLO																							▨		▨		▨				
	CC																	▨		▨		▨		▨		▨		▨				
10	MLO																							▨		▨		▨				
	CC																	▨		▨		▨		▨		▨		▨				

Notes:No less than 20 exams should be reviewed, more if problems/trends are highlighted. No patient identifying numbers should be used. To view trends easily only place an X in boxes where criteria are NOT met

Fig. 23.2 Example of local protocol

Reasons for Repeat Images

Local protocols should be implemented, indicating to practitioners the reasons to repeat an image. The professional decision to repeat must remain with a suitably qualified practitioner. An example of a local protocol is that any image falling into the inadequate category be repeated, such protocols are subjective and thus open to individual interpretation (Fig. 23.2).

It is regarded as good practice for a department to audit and review TP and TC rates and the reasons for them, as they can provide evidence of both equipment and practitioner performance. This enables good management of underperformance in both areas.

Peer Review

The reliability of visual image quality grading, for example PGMI, can be further improved by peer review. Practitioners should be aware of their own proficiency but also how they compare to those of their peer group. Implementation of an organised peer review system with structured feedback and record keeping should aim to maintain high standards and disseminate good practice within the department [6]. If underperformance is identified an action plan should be agreed. This may include additional training and a review of working practice to ensure practitioners maintain the necessary expertise to reach the standard required.

QA Role and Visits

Peer review also takes place during a formal visit to the unit by the regional QA Radiographer during a QA visit within the U.K. screening service. During this visit the standard of mammography will be assessed using the Mammographic Image Assessment tool (Fig. 23.1). The aim of the QA visit is to confirm that the radiographic quality of the unit conforms to expected standards and to identify areas of underperformance.

Recommendations will be made where improvement is required.

Auditing Clinical Practice

Each practitioner should review and reflect on their clinical practice as part of regular personal performance monitoring and continuous professional development (CPD). Regular review of professional performance is essential as is formal annual appraisal. The annual appraisal needs to be a constructive process designed to assist staff in their jobs. By providing employees with constructive feedback and future objectives, this ensures they have the right knowledge and skills to undertake their role and supports them in their professional/personal development.

Breast Screening Programmes are responsible for recording, collating, and monitoring repeat examination data. All practitioners have a responsibility to regularly audit their number of repeat examinations against local protocols and national standards. The guidance on collecting, monitoring and reporting repeat examinations [7] gives clear detail on the collection of data; this guidance should be used when monitoring performance of the mammographic team and equipment.

Training needs can be identified from monitoring performance using the information from image quality assessment using visual grading together with TP, TC records. If underperformance is identified an action plan should be agreed. This may include additional training and a review of working practice to ensure practitioners maintain the necessary expertise to reach the standard required. To support the individual's audit of their clinical practice, the manager should regularly collect data from all repeat examinations (TR = TP + TC). The information collected should be [2]:

- The number and percentage of TRs
- Number and percentage of TCs by mammographer and by reason
- Number and percentage of TPs by mammographer and by reason
- TR rates which are <1% at service level (as repeat rates may not be recorded adequately on NBSS)

This data should be monitored locally, and the outcome of the audit should be available for feedback to the practitioners. If a problem is identified, a clear action plan with time scales should be agreed.

Continuous Professional Development (CPD)

All professional staff have a duty to continuously develop and improve themselves as a professional. CPD includes work-based learning, professional activities and formal educational learning. Evidence of CPD should be promoted and meet the learning requirements of the practitioner and should have, as its focus, the delivery of a high-quality mammography service. Examples of images, using the PGMI rating scale are now demonstrated.

Figures 23.3 and 23.4 demonstrate perfect CC and MLO images matching all image criteria.

Figures 23.5 and 23.6 highlight examples of Good CC images. In Fig. 23.5 there is a minor crease over the postero-lateral edge of the Right CC. It is not obscuring any breast tissue, therefore, this image does not need to be repeated. Within Fig. 23.6 the nipple on the Left CC is slightly laterally rotated, losing a little breast tissue at the back of the breast. However, the breast tissue is within 1 cm of that on the Left MLO, therefore, this image does not need to be repeated.

> **Learning Point**
> Check the lateral side of the breast under the paddle and the underside in contact with the detector for creases, smooth skin if necessary, before imaging.

> **Learning Point**
> Ensure the nipple is at 90° from the chest wall and optimal amount of breast tissue is pulled on to the detector before imaging.

Fig. 23.3 Perfect CC images matching all criteria

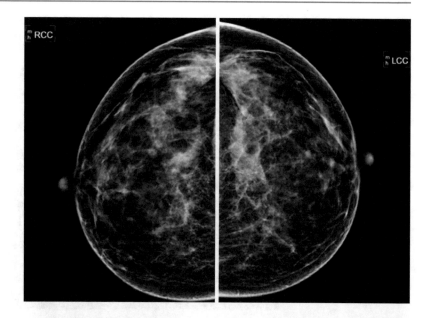

Fig. 23.4 Perfect MLO images matching all criteria

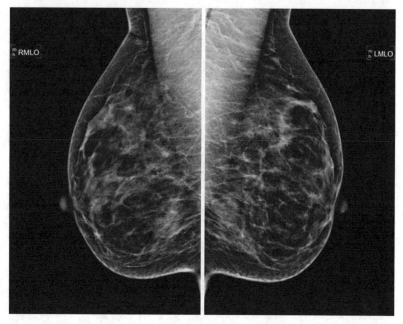

Figures 23.7 and 23.8 highlight examples of Good MLO images. On image 23.7 there is a minor crease in the Left axilla. This is not obscuring any breast tissue therefore is not a repeatable image. As demonstrated in Fig. 23.8 there is a minor crease in the Right infra-mammary fold (IMF). This is not obscuring any breast tissue therefore is not a repeatable image.

Learning Point
Lift the shoulder and smooth the axilla before applying compression.

Learning Point
Smooth the IMF downwards towards the feet before applying compression.

Fig. 23.5 Good CC images

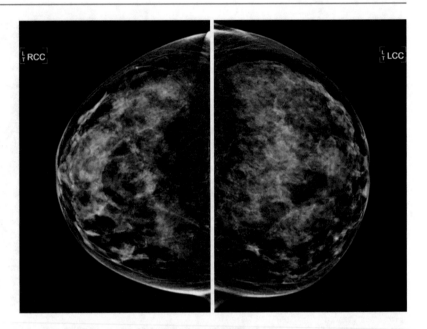

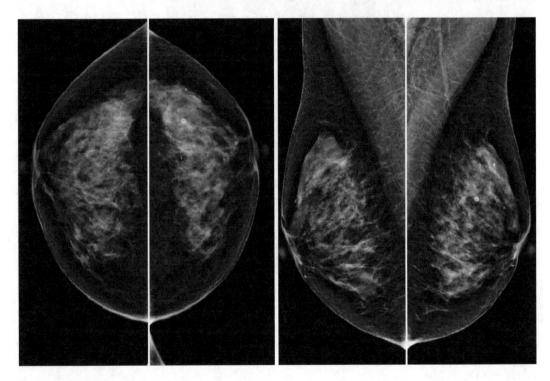

Fig. 23.6 Good CC images

Fig. 23.7 Good MLO images

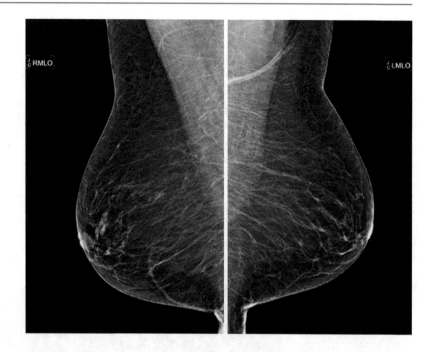

Fig. 23.8 Good MLO images

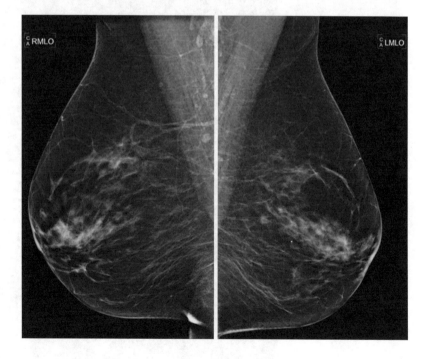

Figure 23.9 provides an example of Moderate images, the nipples are not in profile on the MLO views but are distinguishable from the retro-areolar tissue. There is slight asymmetry and the pectoral muscle is not at the correct angle, or down to nipple level, on the Right MLO. Most of the breast tissue is imaged, the IMFs are clearly demonstrated and, as the nipples are in profile on the CC images, these images do not need to be repeated.

Learning Point
Check that the nipples are in profile before compression, if they are not, re-position to bring more breast tissue onto the detector plate, either laterally or medially, depending on which way the nipples are turning. This will also ensure the pectoral muscle is down to nipple level. The uppermost corner of the detector plate must be placed at the back of the axilla to ensure the pectoral muscle is imaged at the correct angle.

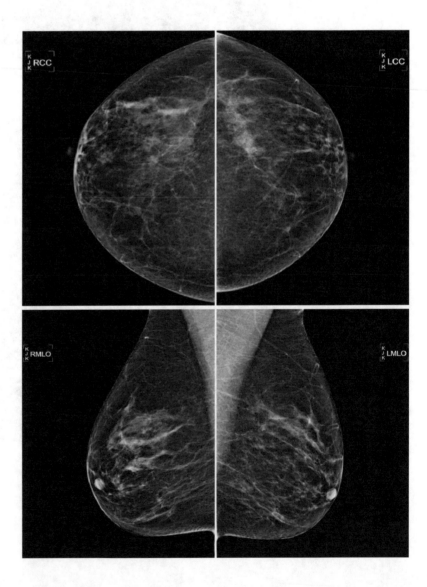

Fig. 23.9 Moderate images

Figure 23.10 further demonstrates moderate images. The nipples are not in profile on the MLO views but distinguishable from retro-areolar tissue and are in profile on the CC views. Nipples are not at 90° from chest wall on the CC views and the images are not asymmetric. The crease on the lateral aspect of the Right CC is obscuring a little breast tissue as is the artefact across the top of the Left MLO. The creases in both axilla are minor. The IMF on the Right is not clearly demonstrated. Most of the breast tissue is imaged therefore, these images do not need to be repeated.

Learning Point

Ensure the position of the breast for the CC's is central to the field of view to avoid asymmetry. Smooth crease. If nipples are not in profile and IMF's are not clearly demonstrated the client may be standing too close to the detector plate. A small side step away from the image receptor and moving slightly back will enable positioning for the MLO's easier. Ensure the clients chin is held up out of the field of view.

Fig. 23.10 Moderate images

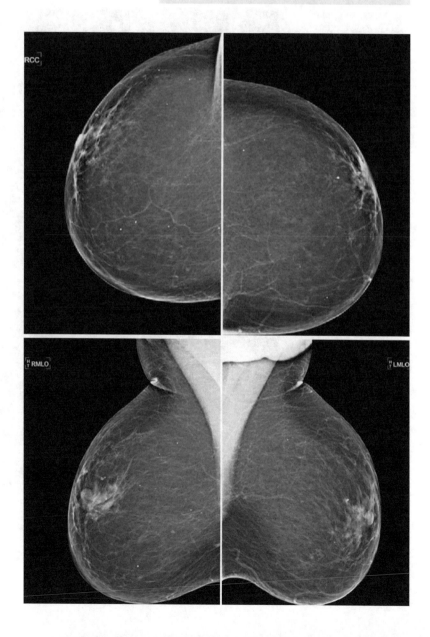

Figure 23.11 highlights moderate MLO images. The IMF on both MLO are not clearly demonstrated. The nipple is not in profile on the left and the pectoral muscles are not down to nipple level in both MLO, however, there is too much pectoral muscle imaged at the top. Most of the breast tissue is imaged, therefore, these images do not need to be repeated.

Learning Point

The image receptor is too high thus causing the client to be stretched up and standing too close. This has caused the loss of the IMF. The position of the client's feet is paramount for positioning the MLO views. A small side-step away from the image receptor, lowering of it will enable good positioning. The nipple must be in profile on the CC view in this case.

Fig. 23.11 Moderate MLO images

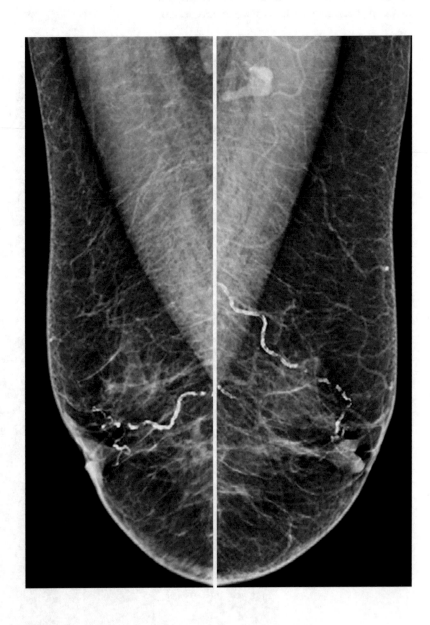

Figure 23.12 demonstrates a minor amount of breast tissue missing from the lateral edge of the Left CC. This part of the breast will be clearly demonstrated on a good MLO view and therefore does not need to be repeated.

Learning Point
Position the breast centrally within the field of view.

Within Fig. 23.13a–c, inadequate images are demonstrated. Both of the CC images have breast tissue missing off the back. The Right MLO is blurred. Some lesions can only be seen in one view and blurring could obscure small abnormalities, such as micro-calcifications, therefore these images are inadequate and need repeating. The repeat CC images above demonstrate how much breast tissue was missing from the initial ones. Further inadequate images are shown in Fig. 23.14; the pectoral muscles are not down to nipple level therefore breast is missing from the back on both views. The repeat images (b) dem-

onstrate how much tissue was missing from the initial images. The images shown in Fig. 23.14 are asymmetrical with breast missing from the bottom of the Left MLO thus not demonstrating the Left IMF. The images shown in Fig. 23.15 are asysymmetrical with breast missing from the bottom left MLO thus not demonstrating the left IMF.

Learning Point
Ensure the shoulder is pulled over adequately and the uppermost corner of the detector plate is positioned at the back of the axilla.

Learning Point
Ensure the feet are in the correct position for both views and that the detector plate is at the correct height. Check that the bottom of the breast is included in the field of view using the light beam. Lowering the lighting in the X-ray room may help.

Fig. 23.12 Moderate CC images

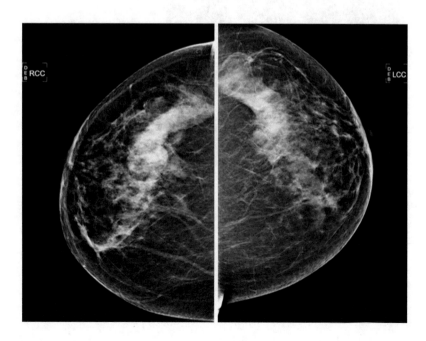

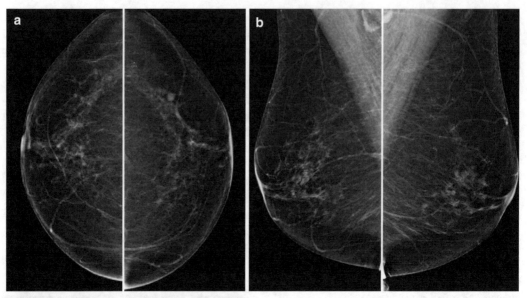

Repeat CC images

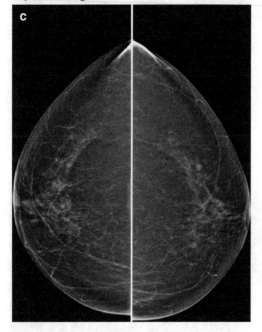

Fig. 23.13 (a–c) Inadequate images

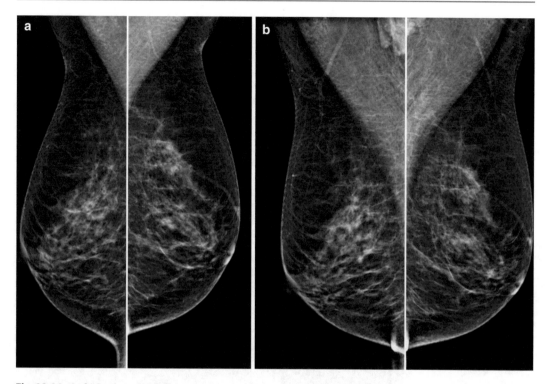

Fig. 23.14 (**a**, **b**) Inadequate MLO images

Fig. 23.15 Inadequate
MLO images

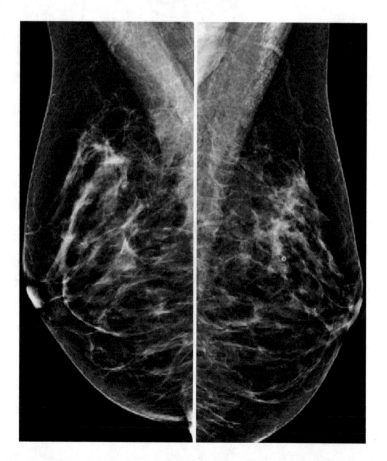

Further inadequate images are demonstrated in Fig. 23.16. There is breast missing from the top of both MLO's, particularly the Left. The IMF's are not demonstrated and the pectoral muscles are not down to nipple level. There is a significant amount of breast missing from these images therefore these should be repeated.

Learning Point

Ensure the detector plate is at the correct height, higher up in this case, and the client has taken a side step away from the plate. Lift the breast more onto the plate to bring the IMF's into the field of view.

Clinical Pearls

- Standards are required to maintain a high-quality service
- Practitioners should regularly measure and evaluate their technical imaging performance using a visual grading system
- An organised peer review system aims to maintain high standards and disseminate good practice within the department
- All practitioners have a responsibility to regularly audit their number of repeat examinations against local protocols and national standards
- CPD should be promoted and have at its focus the delivery of a high-quality mammography service

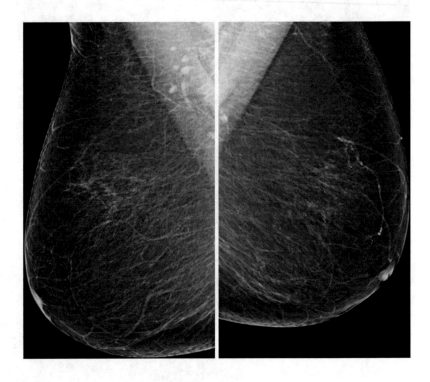

Fig. 23.16 Inadequate MLO images

Chapter Review Questions
Review Questions

1. How is a visual grading system (e.g. PGMI) useful for critically evaluating mammograms?
2. How is peer review a useful tool for critical evaluation?
3. Why is it important to audit clinical practice?

Answers

1. It is used to provide a standardisation of image reviewing and for setting guidance rules for use by both individual practitioners and reviewers assessing images.
2. Practitioners should be aware of how they compare to those of their peer group. It aims to maintain high standards and disseminate good practice within the department.
3. Training needs can be identified from monitoring performance. If underperformance is identified an action plan can be agreed. This may include additional training and a review of working practice to ensure practitioners maintain the necessary expertise to reach the standard required, thus providing a service acceptable to the general public.

Appendix

Test your learning and check your understanding of this book's contents: use the "Springer Nature Flashcards" app to access questions using https://sn.pub/dcAnWL.

To use the app, please follow the instructions in Chap. 1.

Flashcard code:
48341-69945-ABCB1-2A8C7-CE9D2.
Short URL: https://sn.pub/dcAnWL.

References

1. Moreira C, Svoboda K, Poulos A, Taylor R, Page A, Rickard M. Comparison of the validity and reliability of two image classification systems for the assessment of mammogram quality. J Med Screen. 2005;12(1):38–42.
2. Public Health England. Guidance for breast screening mammographers. London: PHE; 2020. https://www.gov.uk/government/publications/breast-screening-quality-assurance-for-mammography-and-radiography/guidance-for-breast-screening-mammographers.
3. The National Quality Management Committee of Breast Screen Australia. National Accreditation Standards: breast screen Australia quality improvement programme. Canberra, ACT: NAS; 2001.
4. Hashimoto BE. Practical digital mammography. New York, NY: Thieme; 2008.
5. The Society of Radiographers. The scope of practice for assistant practitioners in clinical imaging. London: The Society of Radiographers; 2012.
6. Starr L, Mercer C. Peer review – an essential part of learning and development. In: Symposium Mammographicum Conference, Bournemouth; 2014. https://sympmamm.org.uk/wp-content/uploads/2017/09/conf-symp.2014.pdf.
7. Public Health England. NHS Breast Screening Programme Guidance on collecting, monitoring and reporting technical recall and repeat examinations. London: PHE; 2017. https://assets.publishing.service.gov.uk/government/uploads/system/uploads/attachment_data/file/663899/Breast_screening_Guidance_on_collecting_recording_and_reporting_repeat_examinations.pdf.

Part IV

Recording Clinical and Client Information

Bernadette Bickley

Learning Objectives
- Demonstrate an understanding of the importance of accurate questioning and documentation
- Understand the implications of incomplete documentation
- Understand and demonstrate the importance of ascertaining history of breast augmentation or prior breast surgery

The mammography practitioner plays a vital role in ascertaining and documenting a relevant, accurate and complete clinical history prior to imaging, ensuring that the imaging workup is justified [1] and tailored to address the clinical needs of each individual [2].

The prevalent screen of a client refers to the first screening episode, where neither a history of any breast disease/treatment, nor any current breast symptoms, will be known. The incident screening episode refers to clients who have been screened previously, where a limited history may have been documented. However, any developing history since the previous screening episode, or any current breast symptoms that the client may

be experiencing, will not be known without appropriate questioning.

It may be necessary to recall a client for a clinical assessment given their current clinical symptoms, even if the mammographic assessment is normal [2]. It is therefore imperative that the mammography practitioner ensures a current and relevant clinical history is accurately documented at each screening attendance.

In the symptomatic setting, a request form (electronic or paper) completed by the requesting clinician will accompany the client. It is the responsibility of the requesting clinician to ensure that this is both legible and accurate. Furthermore, the practitioner must verify that both the client's demographics and the clinical history are relevant and accurate [1] prior to proceeding with the examination.

Initial Client Contact

It is essential that the practitioner firstly introduces themself and gives a relevant explanation of the mammographic procedure, establishing rapport with the client, thus facilitating full co-operation in both obtaining a relevant clinical history and the mammographic examination itself [3] (Chaps. 13 and 14). During this initial contact the individual needs of the client may be assessed. Clients who are anxious, have physical or learning difficulties, or indeed where English is not the functional language, may require

B. Bickley (✉)
Dudley, Wolverhampton and South West Staffordshire Breast Screening Service, Russells Hall Hospital, Dudley, West Midlands, UK
e-mail: bernadette.bickley@nhs.net

additional support and this can be sought prior to the commencement of the examination.

The practitioner must utilise excellent communication skills [4] and actively verify that the client's demographics (name, date of birth and address) are concordant with the request form/client sheet. Documentation to confirm concordance must be completed either by initialing the request form or by making an electronic record [1].

Previous Imaging

Once details have been verified and/or any changes have been made, it must then be established whether the client has undergone any previous breast imaging. If this is the case, it must be determined when the imaging occurred. Within the UK, a minimum interval period of 6 months is required for another screen in the screening service [5]. Within the symptomatic setting, a 6–12 months interval period between consecutive mammograms is required, dependent upon individual hospital protocol, with the exception of clinically suspicious findings [6]. This information is imperative to ensure that a mammogram is the appropriate imaging modality and conforms to both local imaging guidelines and ionising radiation regulations. It is also important to establish where the imaging was performed, thus enabling historical images to be obtained. Comparison with previous images may avoid unnecessary recall of unchanged longstanding breast lesions/calcifications and may also improve the appreciation of discrete mammographic changes, thus increasing sensitivity of breast cancer detection [7].

History Taking

There are several areas to focus upon when taking client history. These are expanded upon below:

- Any history of previous breast surgery must be ascertained, including when it was performed and the exact location within the breast (depicted with the aid of a breast diagram). A

post-operative scar may mimic an architectural distortion suspicious of malignancy [8]. If the previous surgical site is not clearly indicated this may result in avoidable additional imaging or an unnecessary recall, increasing client anxiety. Comparison with previous images is imperative when interpreting the post-operative breast. The density of scar tissue should either remain stable or reduce with time. Any increase in scar density or size would be considered suspicious of loco-regional recurrence and warrant further investigation [9].

- Information regarding any history of breast disease or previous breast interventional procedure (biopsy proven benign/malignant pathology or possible marker clip in situ) is also essential, as this will assist the reporting team in correlating pre-existing conditions with the corresponding imaging features, thus increasing specificity of diagnosis whilst also reducing unnecessary recall.

- Obtaining a history of breast augmentation will enable adaption of imaging technique and exposure parameters ensuring optimal imaging of the residual breast tissue [10]. If possible, the type of implant and site of implant (subglandular or submuscular) should be ascertained and documented. If the client reports any symptoms of breast change, whereby suspected implant rupture may be the cause, then screening should cease. The client should be provided with a letter to their G.P to seek further guidance as to whether the implant is ruptured, and if it is safe to proceed with screening. This should also be recorded on the electronic national database via notepad [11].

If implant rupture is not suspected, or where a stable longstanding rupture is reported, then the client may consent for screening, signing the consent form for special images with breast implant [11]. The Eklund technique must be offered to all those with breast augmentation attending for screening. It is essential that any previous history of injectable fillers be clearly documented, with the client being made fully aware of the consequential diagnostic limitations/reduced sensitivity and informed that additional imaging may be required [12].

- Documentation of any known skin lesions overlying the breast/axillary tissue (depicted with the aid of a breast diagram) reduces unnecessary recall, for example a sebaceous cyst may mimic a breast lesion whilst dermal calcifications within a skin lesion may result in a diagnostic dilemma [13].
- An accurate record of any family history of breast cancer is of importance; age of onset of disease and relationship to client will enable evaluation of the relevance and associated increased risk of breast cancer, identifying those that may be suitable for genetic counselling/testing and/or increased surveillance or additional use of MRI screening [14].
- Where appropriate, documentation of a pacemaker/heart-monitoring device or Hickman line will enable adaptation of mammographic technique, paying special attention not to compress the device or dislodge the line during the mammographic examination [2].
- Documentation of any current symptoms will alert the reporting team and may necessitate the need for a clinical recall in the absence of any abnormal mammographic findings.

> Any current breast symptoms that the client may be experiencing must be carefully documented, specifying the exact location and duration of symptoms [15], paying particular attention to the following:
> - A new lump or thickening in either breast
> - A lump or swelling in either axilla
> - Skin tethering, distortion or change in size or shape of the breast
> - Skin changes, for example *Peau d' orange*, rash or redness
> - Nipple discharge
> - Changes to the nipple such as recent nipple inversion/nipple eczema

- Duration of Hormone Replacement Therapy (HRT) or discontinuation of previous use must also be documented, as this information will aid the reporting team when considering any

associated change in breast density between imaging episodes.

- Any client limitations or mobility issues that may have a consequence on image quality also requires documentation. Whilst every effort should be made to obtain diagnostic quality images, consideration may be given to any pre-existing limitations. In exceptional circumstances it may be appropriate to record a partial examination, documenting the specific limitations of the examination and fully explaining the diagnostic consequences to the client, providing them with the NHS information leaflet on partial mammography.

> **Clinical Pearls**
> - Establish effective communication
> - Check for prior mammography
> - Ensure accurate and clear documentation

Chapter Review Questions
Review Questions

1. What additional views must be offered to those with breast augmentation attending for screening?
2. List six common breast symptoms that would necessitate the need for adding an alert at the time of screening.

Answers

1. Eklund views
2. (a) A new lump or thickening in either breast
   (b) A lump or swelling in either axilla
   (c) Skin tethering, distortion or change in size or shape of the breast
   (d) Skin changes, for example *Peau d' orange*, rash or redness
   (e) Nipple discharge
   (f) Changes to the nipple such as recent nipple inversion/nipple eczema

Appendix

Test your learning and check your understanding of this book's contents: use the "Springer Nature Flashcards" app to access questions using https://sn.pub/dcAnWL.

To use the app, please follow the instructions in Chap. 1.

Flashcard code:
48341-69945-ABCB1-2A8C7-CE9D2.

Short URL: https://sn.pub/dcAnWL.

References

1. IRMER. The ionising radiation (medical exposure) regulations 2017. London: Department of Health and Social Care; 2018. https://www.legislation.gov.uk/uksi/2017/1322/pdfs/uksi_20171322_en.pdf. Accessed 28 Oct 2021.
2. NHSBSP. Guidance for breast screening mammographers. Sheffield: Department of Health; 2020. https://www.gov.uk/government/publications/breast-screening-quality-assurance-for-mammography-and-radiography/guidance-for-breast-screening-mammographers. Accessed 28 Oct 2021.
3. SCOR. Code of professional conduct. London: The Society and College of Radiographers; 2013. https://www.sor.org/getmedia/dd242043-8c3a-449a-8f47-cc532e6d34f6/Code-of-Profressional-Conduct. Accessed 28 Oct 2021.
4. Donnelly E, Neville L. Communication, and interpersonal skills. Exeter: Reflect Press Ltd; 2008.
5. NHSBSP. Helping you decide. London: PHE; 2017. https://www.uhs.nhs.uk/Media/SUHTInternet/Services/BreastImagingUnit/NHS-Breast-Screening%2D%2D-helping-you-decide.pdf. Accessed 28 Oct 2021.
6. The Royal College of Radiologists. Guidance on screening and symptomatic breast imaging. 4th ed. London: The Royal College of Radiologists; 2019. https://www.rcr.ac.uk/system/files/publication/field_publication_files/bfcr199-guidance-on-screening-and-symptomatic-breast-imaging.pdf. Accessed 28 Oct 2021.
7. Hewang-Kobrunner SH, Dershaw DD, Schreer I. Diagnostic breast imaging. 2nd ed. New York, NY: Thieme; 2001.
8. Shaw de Paredes E. Atlas of mammography. 3rd ed. Philadelphia, PA: Lippincott Williams & Wilkins; 2007.
9. Cardenosa G. Breast imaging companion. 2nd ed. Philadelphia, PA: Lippincott Williams & Wilkins; 2001.
10. Andolina VF, Lillé SL. Mammographic imaging: a practical guide. 3rd ed. Philadelphia, PA: Lippincott Williams & Wilkins; 2011.
11. Public Health England. Screening women with breast implants. London: PHE; 2017. https://assets.publishing.service.gov.uk/government/uploads/system/uploads/attachment_data/file/624796/Screening_women_with_breast_implants_guidance.pdf. Accessed 28 Oct 2021.
12. MHRA. Medical device alert. London: Crown; 2014. http://www.mhra.gov.uk/Publications/Safetywarnings/MedicalDeviceAlerts/CON149825. Accessed 28 Oct 2021.
13. Barth V. Diagnosis of breast diseases: integrating the findings of clinical presentation, mammography, and ultrasound. New York, NY: Thieme; 2010.
14. NHSBSP. Protocols for surveillance of women at very high risk of developing breast cancer. London: Public Health England; 2021. https://www.gov.uk/government/publications/breast-screening-higher-risk-women-surveillance-protocols/protocols-for-surveillance-of-women-at-higher-risk-of-developing-breast-cancer. Accessed 28 Oct 2021.
15. Ikeda DM. Breast imaging; the requisites. 2nd ed. St. Louis, MO: Elsevier/Mosby; 2011.

Infection Control

Kathryn Taylor

Learning Objectives
- To understand the principles, preven-tion, monitoring and learning of infec-tion control
- To understand professional responsibili-ties in this area

Introduction

Infection is the establishment of one or more pathogenic agents, such as a bacteria, protozo-ans, or viruses, in or on the body of a suitable host. The close proximity and frequent physical contact in a shared working and living environ-ment all contribute to increased risk of trans-mission. Micro-organisms by their very nature are opportunistic, exploiting chances to colo-nise or enter the body, which may result in infection. Health care associated infections (HCAIs) may be caused by a large number of different microorganisms [1]. HCAIs, as described by the National Institute of Clinical Excellence (NICE):

cover any infection contracted as a direct result of treatment in, or contact with, a health or social care setting as a result of health care delivered outside a health care setting (e.g. mobile breast screening) and brought in by patients, staff or visi-tors and transmitted to others (for example, noro-virus) [1]

The majority of HCAIs, are caused by bacte-ria such as Staphylococcus aureus (SA) which are carried harmlessly by healthy people. SA is carried on the skin and in the nose causing no harm to the host and it is likely that many hospital staff may be passive carriers without showing any symptoms. However, they may transfer the bacteria from patient to patient usually via their hands. Similarly, patients themselves and visitors may harbour the bacteria. It has been indicated that SA frequently inhabits the nostrils in 30% of adults [2]. Other transmissible infections, such as influenza and norovirus, have the potential to spread from one patient to another causing infec-tion. Like SA, this is often on the hands of health-care workers via surfaces such as couches, equipment and floors. Some infections, such as Methicillin Resistant Staphylococcus Aureus (MRSA) pose the added complication of becom-ing resistant to treatment and all pose significant implications for health and social care facilities [1].

HCAIs are prevalent across the globe and in most developed countries 6–10% of patients who enter hospital are likely to acquire an infection of some sort [3]. This poses a significant financial burden. In the UK alone annual NHS cost of HCAIs is an estimated £2.6 billion/year with associated treatment, occupied bed days and

K. Taylor (✉)
Cambridge Breast Unit, Cambridge University Hospitals NHS Foundation Trust, Cambridge, UK
e-mail: Kathryn.taylor@addenbrookes.nhs.uk

C. Mercer et al. (eds.), *Digital Mammography*, https://doi.org/10.1007/978-3-031-10898-3_25

absenteeism among front-line healthcare professionals [4].

The occurrence of HCAIs is not new and is to some degree inevitable in any primary, community or secondary healthcare setting, however, a significant proportion of these are avoidable if sustainable and robust processes and systems are in place to manage risks associated with infection.

Principles of Prevention and Control

Infection prevention and control (IPC) is a scientific approach and practical solution designed to prevent harm caused by infection to patients/clients and health workers. It should not be viewed as a standalone element of professional practice, but rather as a set of principles fundamental to all activities which, when implemented, reduce the risks of a patient or person acquiring an infection. The focus should always be on the prevention of infection first, with control applied to outbreak or management scenarios. Effective IPC will:

1. Reduce the risk of antimicrobial resistance and support the preservation of effective antibiotics
2. Reduce morbidity (and in some cases mortality) from infection
3. Minimise healthcare costs in treating infection and any associated complications

As HCAIs are not confined to hospitals, health care workers who practice in the outpatient community settings (such as breast screening) have the same professional and clinical responsibilities as staff working in hospitals, to prevent opportunities for infection to occur, although the type and level of risk may vary.

Both prevention and control are underpinned by policies and procedures implemented locally and derived from both local and national guidance. In England, both NICE and Public Health England (PHE) have produced guidance pertaining to the prevention of HCAIs and every NHS hospital must have an infection prevention policy

in place [1, 5]. In addition, an NHS practice guide applies to staff in all disciplines in all care settings [6]. It covers responsibilities for organisations, staff and infection prevention and control teams.

Pandemic

Investigation of a cluster of cases of pneumonia of unknown cause identified the SARS-CoV-2 virus with an associated disease called COVID 19. Thus began a pandemic of global proportions and spanning several years. Hitherto accepted IC infection control measures rapidly became insufficient against the tidal wave of cases, many involving hospitalisation and even death particularly in those who were immuno suppressed for whatever reason. Although many IC principles formed the basis for measures against transmission rapidly applied research was able to inform precautionary measures specific to this disease. As such these have been applied and adjusted as the disease has evolved making it inappropriate to give current time specific advice here. Suffice to say there are many on line resources available to healthcare professional such as www.gov.uk, www.england.nhs.uk which track the history of the pandemic and provide current information. Guidance outlines the infection prevention and control principles required to prevent transmission of COVID-19 and other respiratory viruses and minimise disruption to health and care services. It should be used to inform operational implementation at country, regional and local levels to ensure appropriate application across different services/sectors.

Responsibilities

National policy

National policy aims to:

• Support a common understanding (making the right thing easy to do for every patient, every time)

- Reduce variation in practice and standardise care processes
- Improve how knowledge and skills are applied in infection prevention and control
- Help reduce the risk of healthcare-associated infection
- Help to align practice, education, monitoring, quality improvement and scrutiny

Within the UK, NHS England monitors the numbers of certain infections that occur in healthcare settings through routine surveillance programmes and advises on how to prevent and control infection in establishments such as hospitals, care homes and schools. NHS England also monitors the spread of antibiotic resistant infections and advises healthcare professionals about controlling antimicrobial resistance. Surveillance programmes are an important part of this as they provide essential information on what and where the problems are, along with how well control measures are working.

Organisation

The Health Act 2006 Code of Practice for the prevention and control of HCAIs puts a duty of care onto NHS bodies to ensure that healthcare workers are free of, and are protected from, exposure to communicable disease during the course of their work and are suitably educated in the prevention and control of HCAI between staff and patients [7]. In addition, there is a specific legal requirement on NHS bodies, as employers, to carry out risk assessments of biological agents that employees could be exposed to. Organisations must derive and follow local polices based on national policy, advice can be sought from the organisation infection control team, and service managers should recognise the need to develop and compile specific departmental policies which have a direct relevance to their staff.

Departments may wish to consider the development of the role of a link radiographer to the Trust (or equivalent) infection control team. That individual would act as a conduit for the provision of current and pertinent on-going advice and guidance, regarding the practical applications of infection control, within the clinical imaging department setting.

Healthcare Professional

It is the ethical responsibility of members of healthcare professions to:

- Report any communicable disease to obtain medical advice and, if found to be infected, to submit to regular medical supervision including counselling
- Act upon medical advice they have been given, which may include the necessity to cease practice either altogether or, in some areas of practice, to modify their practice
- Keep up to date with local and national policy and actively undertake the necessary precautions in relation to themselves and the healthcare environment in which they work

The UK Health Care Professions Council (HCPC) is clear about the requirements of health professionals in the matter of infection control and their duty of care towards patients, themselves and visitors in this respect [8].

You must take appropriate precautions to protect your patients, clients and users, their carers and families, your staff and yourself from infection. In particular, you should protect your patients, clients and users from infecting one another

Additional guidance can be sought from the Society of Radiographers [9].

Practicalities of Prevention and Control

To be able to minimise spread of infection we need to know the potential sources. These include:

- Blood and other body fluids secretions or excretions (excluding sweat)
- Non-intact skin or mucous membranes
- Any equipment or items in the care environment that could have become contaminated

Preventative Tasks

Standard infection control precautions (SICPs) should be used by all staff, in all care settings, at all times, for all patients, whether infection is known to be present or not, to ensure the safety of those being cared for, staff and visitors in the care environment [10]. SICPs are the basic infection prevention and control measures necessary to reduce the risk of transmission of infectious agent from both recognised and unrecognised sources of infection. The application of SICPs during care delivery is determined by a risk assessment—an assessment of risk to and from individuals—and includes [10]:

- The task
- Level of interaction and/or
- The anticipated level of exposure to blood and/or other body fluids

When all activities undergo this same assessment of risk, the correct level of SICPs will be applied to and transmission of infection minimised. Within breast imaging this will range from screening mammography in the community to complex percutaneous tissue sampling in the hospital setting. To be effective in protecting against infection risks, SICPs must be used continuously by all staff.

Hand Hygiene

Hand hygiene is considered an important practice in reducing the transmission of infectious agents which cause HAIs. The term hand hygiene includes handwashing, surgical scrub and the use of alcohol gel. The type of hand hygiene performed is dependent on the type of care that will, or has been, carried out and local protocol will guide on this and how to perform effective handwashing. Typically, hand hygiene will be performed:

- Before touching a patient
- Before clean/aseptic procedures
- After body fluid exposure risk
- After touching a patient
- After touching a patient's immediate surroundings

Evidence shows that improving hand hygiene contributes significantly to the reduction of HCAIs [11]. Health care workers have the greatest potential to spread micro-organisms that may result in infection, due to the number of times they have contact with patients or the patient environment. Hands are therefore a very efficient vehicle for transferring micro-organisms.

Personal Protective Equipment

Before undertaking any procedure, staff should assess any likely exposure and ensure PPE is worn that provides adequate protection against the risks associated with the task. This may include gloves and aprons. Gloves should be worn whenever contact with blood and body fluids, mucous membranes or non-intact skin is a risk, they should not be considered a substitute for hand hygiene. Hand hygiene must always be performed following the removal of gloves.

Safe Management of Equipment

Local protocol will guide the conditions necessary for a particular procedure. The equipment may be:

- Single-use e.g. needles and syringes.
- Single patient use—equipment which can be reused on the same patient, e.g. oxygen mask, linen (if clean).
- Reusable invasive equipment—used once then decontaminated e.g. surgical instruments.
- Reusable non-invasive equipment (often referred to as communal equipment)—reused on more than one patient following decontamination between each use e.g. ultrasound couch and probe, mammography equipment. Cleaning of re-usable equipment with soap and water, or manufacturer recommended

agents, removes visible contamination but does not necessarily destroy micro-organisms, although it should reduce their numbers. The appropriate selection of disinfectant wipes is important as infection prevention efforts may be compromised (and equipment damaged) if the wipe is not fit for its intended purpose. Effective cleaning is an essential prerequisite to both disinfection and sterilisation.

Safe Management of Care Environment

The care environment must be:

- Visibly clean, free from non-essential items and equipment to facilitate effective cleaning
- Well maintained and in a good state of repair
- Routinely cleaned in accordance with local protocol for that environment and procedures undertaken, staff groups should be aware of their environmental cleaning schedules and be clear on their specific responsibilities

Cleaning protocols should include responsibility for; frequency of; and method of environmental decontamination.

Safe Management of Linen

Linen can be placed in routine laundry unless it has been used by a patient who is known or suspected to be infectious. In all cases, local protocol will guide correct management in selecting the correct technique. This may be:

- Clean—soap and water or wipes. These are increasingly being used to decontaminate low risk patient equipment or environmental surfaces. Currently there is little evidence to support the wide scale use of disinfectant wipes, as opposed to detergent only products, as an effective infection prevention beyond specific manufacturers decontamination instructions. Dirt removal should be considered the main

purpose of a detergent wipe, but antimicrobial activity as a result of the inclusion of a disinfectant may be of use in some circumstances. The appropriate selection of disinfectant wipes is important as infection prevention efforts may be compromised if the wipe is not fit for its intended purpose.

- Aseptic—aims to prevent transmission of infection.
- Sterile—make (something) free from bacteria or other living microorganisms.

Local protocols will define the circumstances for each [9].

Safe Management of Blood and Body Fluid Spillages

Spillages of blood and other body fluids may transmit blood borne viruses. Spillages must be decontaminated immediately by staff trained to undertake this safely. Responsibilities for the decontamination of blood and body fluid spillages should be clear within each area/care setting [12].

Safe Disposal of Waste (Including Sharps)

The Health and Safety (Sharp Instruments in Healthcare) Regulations 2013 outline the regulatory requirements for employers and contractors in the healthcare sector in relation to the safe disposal of sharps [12]. This includes:

- Arrangements for the safe use and disposal of sharps
- Provision of information and training to employees
- Investigations and actions required in response to work related sharps injuries

Sharps handling must be assessed, kept to a minimum and eliminated, if possible, with the use of approved safety devices. Manufacturers' instructions for safe use and disposal must be followed.

Sharps injuries are preventable and learning following incidents should be put in place to avoid repeat accidents. A significant occupational exposure is:

- A percutaneous injury e.g. injuries from needles, instruments, bone fragments, or bites which break the skin
- Exposure of broken skin (abrasions, cuts, eczema, etc.)
- Exposure of mucous membranes including the eye from splashing of blood or other high risk body fluids

There is a potential risk of transmission of a Blood Borne Virus (BBV) from a significant occupational exposure and staff must understand the actions they should take when a significant occupational exposure incident takes place. There is a legal requirement to report all sharps injuries and near misses to line managers/employers. Local protocols will guide the actions necessary. Disposal of non-sharps waste is categorised in terms of associated risk and local protocols will determine the correct method of disposal (usually colour coded) [12].

Compliance and Governance Monitoring and Audit

As an organisation training in IPC measures must be provided to all staff. In addition:

- Risk assessment(s) undertaken for any new procedures/areas of work. IPC practices must be monitored
- Resources in place to implement good IPC practice in all relevant areas and for all staff (permanent, agency and external contractors)
- Ensure local culture promotes incident reporting, including near misses, while focusing on improving systemic failures and encouraging safe working practices

Staff providing care must:

- Show their understanding by applying the infection prevention and control principles

- Maintain competence, skills and knowledge by completing training
- Have up-to-date occupational immunisations, health checks as appropriate
- Report to line managers and document any deficits in knowledge, resources, equipment and facilities or incidents that may result in transmitting infection including near misses
- Not provide care while at risk of transmitting infectious agents to others; if in doubt, they must take advice [13]

Infection Control Issues Specific to Mammography

Routes of Infection

All the aforementioned precautions apply to the breast imaging department, including some of the more involved procedures of screening assessment and post treatment review. However, breast screening often takes place in the community and the rapid throughput of clients brings a more specific set of infection control considerations. The mammographer must remain conscientious in the implementation of IC measures for both self and environment. Repeated hand hygiene means they should be aware of irritated or broken skin on their hands and use recommended barrier/therapeutic measures seeking advice from the IC team if necessary. They should also be aware of the integrity of the client skin, particularly in the under-breast area.

Under Breast Soreness: Intertrigo

The skin under the breasts can often be fragile, some clients can have a rash under the breast or breasts, between the folds of skin. It is usually caused by a skin condition called intertrigo. It is a very common condition that can occur throughout life. The main causes of intertrigo are moisture, heat, lack of air circulating and friction between skin folds (where skin rubs against skin). This can lead to a red or reddish-brown rash, raw, itchy or weeping skin with or without a smell, cracked skin and pain.

Intertrigo (sometimes called candida intertrigo) can occur anywhere on the body where skin rubs against skin, such as between the thighs or on the underside of the belly or armpit. A warm, moist environment encourages infection by either yeast, fungus or bacteria. Sometimes swelling, sores and blisters can also occur. Care must be taken when manipulating the breast during mammography to avoid tearing the skin, which is often fragile. By its nature, once broken, this type of skin can be difficult to heal [14]. Chapter 17 provides further information around this area.

Clinical Pearls
- Infection control is everyone's responsibility and an integral part of healthcare practice
- Prevention is better than cure
- National policy devolved to local guidance ensures standardisation
- Risk assessment, training and audit are important aspects of compliance

---

Chapter Review Questions
Review Questions

1. Name two ways in which an infection prevention protocol may be seen to be effective?
2. What is the most common way of healthcare workers transmitting infection?
3. Name one common skin condition which may be prone to/transmit infection in mammography?

Answers

1. (any two of three answers)
   (a) Reduce the risk of resistance to treatment
   (b) Reduce morbidity (and in some cases mortality) from infection
   (c) Minimise healthcare costs in treating infection and any associated complications
2. On the hands
3. Intertrigo

Appendix

Test your learning and check your understanding of this book's contents: use the "Springer Nature Flashcards" app to access questions using https://sn.pub/dcAnWL.

To use the app, please follow the instructions in Chap. 1.

Flashcard code:

48341-69945-ABCB1-2A8C7-CE9D2.

Short URL: https://sn.pub/dcAnWL.

References

1. National Institute for Health and Care Excellence (NICE). Healthcare-associated infections: prevention and control [PH36]. London: NICE; 2011. http://www.nice.org.uk/guidance/ph36. Accessed 15 Jan 2021.
2. Casewell MW. The nose: an underestimated source of Staphylococcus aureus causing wound infection. J Hosp Infect. 1998;40:S3–11.
3. NICE. Healthcare associated infections. London: NICE; 2016. www.nice.org.uk/guidance/qs113. Accessed 9 Feb 2022.
4. Guest JF, Keating T, Gould D, Wigglesworth N. Modelling the annual NHS costs and outcomes attributable to healthcare-associated infections in England. BMJ Open. 2020;10(1):e033367.
5. Public Health England. Healthcare associated infections (HCAI): guidance, data and analysis. London: PHE. www.gov.uk. Accessed 15 Jan 2021.
6. NHS England. Standard infection control precautions: national hand hygiene and personal protective equipment policy. Lonon: NHS. https://www.england.nhs.uk/publication/standard-infection-control-precautions-national-hand-hygiene-and-personal-protective-equipment-policy/. Accessed 15 Jan 2021.
7. PHE. Health Act 2009. London: PHE; 2009. https://www.legislation.gov.uk/.
8. Health & Care Professions Council. Standards of conduct, performance and ethics. London: HCPC. https://www.hcpc-uk.org/globalassets/resources/standards/standards-of-conduct-performance-and-ethics.pdf. Accessed 15 Jan 2021.
9. Society of Radiographers. Health Care Associated Infections (HCAIs): practical guidance and advice. London: Society of Radiographers; 2006.
10. Loveday HP, Wilson JA, Pratt RJ, Golsorkhi M, Tingle A, Bak A, Browne J, Prieto J, Wilcox M. epic3: national evidence-based guidelines for preventing healthcare-associated infections in NHS hospitals in England. J Hosp Infect. 2014;86:S1–70.

11. NHS England and NHS Improvement. Standard infection control precautions: national hand hygiene and personal protective equipment policy. London: NHS; 2019.

12. HSE. The health and safety (sharp instruments in healthcare) regulations. London: HSE; 2013. https://www. hse.gov.uk/pubns/hsis7.htm. Accessed 15 Jan 2021.

13. Wilson J. Infection control in clinical practice updated edition 3e. London: Bailliere Tindall; 2019.

14. O'Connell M, Curtis J. A study into under-breast soreness and its impact on breast screening. London: SoR. www.sor.org. Accessed 8 Feb 2022.

Repetitive Strain Injury

26

Claire Borrelli

Learning Objectives
- Promote best clinical practice to avoid/reduce injury and for identifying, reporting and resolving problems
- Develop a learning culture between staff to promote effective training and continual professional development (CPD)

Introduction

Work-related repetitive strain injury (RSI) and musculoskeletal disorders (MSKD) may encompass a wide range of inflammatory and degenerative disorders and are a major occupational hazard for practitioners. These conditions are caused by repetitive, forceful, or awkward movements that can result in injury to muscles, nerves, tendons, and ligaments and can include carpal tunnel syndrome, tendonitis, lower back pain and tension neck syndrome [1]. Common areas of the body to be affected by musculoskeletal pain for practitioners include the hands, wrists, elbows, neck, shoulders, and lower back, although this list is not exclusive. The repetitive nature of prac-

titioners' work, as well as the awkward postures used while working can cause significant stress on their bodies and the physical strain can cause, or exacerbate, these conditions.

It is not necessarily the nature of a person's movements that cause the musculoskeletal pain (they are often ordinary movements such as bending, straightening, gripping, holding, twisting, clenching and reaching). It is a fact that a person may make the same movements repetitively, often at speed, and using force with no recovery time between movements that makes them hazardous. This is a particularly important consideration within breast screening, as to maintain the throughput and meet the demands of numbers attending practitioners are likely to adopt unusual postures when pressed for time, although positioning should ideally be efficient and timely to reduce the risk of injury [2]. In some cases, the person's work environment may be poorly designed which may also mean that their work position or posture is awkward and yet avoidable had consideration been given at the planning stage.

The most common symptom associated with musculoskeletal disorders is pain, although some sufferers report joint stiffness, muscle tightness, 'pins and needles' and redness and swelling of the affected area. Musculoskeletal disorders can range from mild to severe and, as they are cumulative in nature, can be measured depending on the severity/longevity of the pain and the extent to which the pain affects a person's ability to work.

C. Borrelli (✉)
St George's National Breast Education Centre,
St George's University Hospital NHS Foundation
Trust, London, UK
e-mail: claire.borrelli@stgeorges.nhs.uk

The Risks of Musculoskeletal Disorder

A study conducted in 1997 sought to determine if practitioners experienced any musculoskeletal discomfort and, if so, the nature and extent of the problem [3]. The study was extended to investigate and determine the possible occupational, causal, or contributory factors, proposing a technique for practitioners to adopt to help alleviate discomfort caused by their repetitive actions. In 2007, the National Health Service Breast Screening Program (NHSBSP) in England conducted an ergonomic assessment of different mammography units, reporting that repetitive strain injuries affecting thumbs and wrists remains a particular problem [4].

Repetitive strain injuries in practitioners have more recently been described in a professional document published by the Society of Radiographers in the UK (SoR) [5]. This document includes a survey of radiographers, in which 62% indicated that they often or always have to manoeuvre into awkward positions [6]. This, combined with the inevitable time constraints of the job and ever-increasing workload, can lead to a range of symptoms such as pain, tenderness, swelling, and muscle weakness. These symptoms often result in conditions such as rotator cuff syndrome, carpal tunnel syndrome, tendinitis, and trigger finger or thumb. Ransom [1] states that the aforementioned conditions are progressive and can typically be classified into three stages: mild, moderate or severe. At the severe stage, sleep can be disturbed, sometimes leading to an inability to carry out even the most mundane tasks and can even result in permanent disability.

Equipment design is important in helping to reduce repetitive strain injury in practitioners, as different functions and workflows all play their part in either contributing to or limiting these risks. While the UK, NHSBSP have recommended equipment improvements specifically to address this issue, as yet no industry standards have been created. If the practitioner has concerns about any work-related injury, they should discuss this with their line manager to raise awareness and seek guidance. This may include completion of a risk assessment of your role and referral to occupational health for further investigation and support.

Equipment Considerations

The Column/Gantry

A second major reduction of fatigue and stress results from how rotation is configured on the equipment. Automatic tube angling is a feature that causes the tube head to move automatically into the oblique position to a pre-set angulation, reducing the amount of stretching required for each examination, and thus decreasing stress on the upper body. However, even with powered rotation, conventional systems require the practitioners to initiate the movement by pressing a button on the tube head and this upper body movement is repetitive during positioning.

On older imaging systems, this requires practitioners to raise their arms up to the button height, and to maintain finger pressure on the button as the tube head rotates. To maintain continuous pressure on the button, practitioners have to stretch their arms through the rotations, and if the mammographer did not have correct posture at the initiation of the rotation, this could result in inappropriate twisting.

An important ergonomic consideration for the manufacturers is to include automatic tube angulation in all designs and to ensure that movement buttons are strategically placed along the column e.g. tube head, breast platform and bottom of column, to suit practitioners' height and positioning stance. This will help to ensure ergonomic safety when rotating the gantry (Fig. 26.1).

Easy Height Adjustment of Equipment

Only a light touch should be required to depress buttons and reaching the buttons should be almost effortless. Buttons are replicated both on the tube head and side of the breast platform, so practitioners can use the set of controls that are easiest to access from their position, or alternate between controls, to help reduce repetitive movements and the risk of repetitive strain.

The NHSBSP guidelines indicate that it is good practice to offer a choice in how to manipulate the system, and ergonomic development will

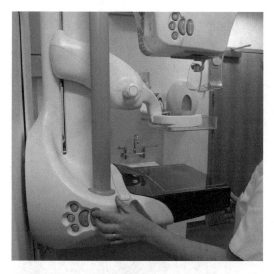

Fig. 26.1 Strategic placement of buttons on the gantry. (Source: BreastCheck, Ireland)

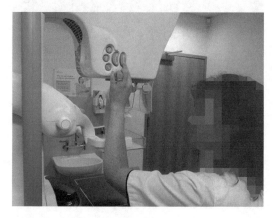

Fig. 26.2 Ease of reaching buttons on tube head. (Source: BreastCheck, Ireland)

help vary routine and reduce repetitive strain injuries [3, 4] (Fig. 26.2).

Motorised Compression

Breast compression is achieved by the use of a foot switch on the gantry, which allows practitioners to use their hands for positioning the breast. A number of features that may help to reduce injury include:

• Some mammography systems do not require practitioners to make physical changes to the

compression paddle between small and large women, thereby reducing the risk of strain.

• Some mammography systems now have client assisted compression where the client can assist in the application of compression.

• Where hand-controlled compression knobs, for fine-tuning the level of compression are avoided, the need for repeated twisting of the wrist is reduced.

• Use of a high-edge paddle pushes the contralateral breast back and supports it away from the field of view. This means that the practitioner does not need to ask (or assist) the client to do this during the oblique projections, thereby reducing the risk of injury.

Acquisition Workstation

Musculoskeletal injury can be associated with repetitive keyboard use and this can be reduced by limiting the number of steps requiring the use of a mouse or keypad, or by employing touchscreen technology, maintaining good posture and taking regular breaks.

Room Design

Careful design of the mammography room can also help to reduce musculo-skeletal strains and improve workflow. The working triangle should be as small as possible whilst including considerate choice of equipment. The design of the reporting room should also be considered as many practitioners are now involved in image interpretation as well as mammography practice. The same principles will apply to practitioners involved in extended roles, such as ultrasound.

Staff Rotation and Working Patterns

To avoid/reduce the risk of repetitive strain injury, consideration should be given to rotating staff between clinical practice and other work-related duties to minimise harm.

Positioning Considerations

Always adopt good communication skills with the client as this will enable them to move independently rather than being moved. The practitioner should be familiar with the full range of the equipment and its controls to adopt a positioning technique that is ergonomically safe and most convenient for repetitive use. Maintaining a good posture throughout the examination, reduce any requirements to overstretch, is important to minimise strain or injury.

Consider the use of a positioning stool for either the client or the practitioner. This will require the provision of suitable chairs and flooring and should be part of the design process for each room. Each practitioner must adjust their seat height and proximity to suit each client to avoid over-extension of their elbows and shoulders. The wheels on the stool must be selected to give the right level of grip for the type of floor (Fig. 26.3).

Practitioners' positioning practice should be observed regularly by an experienced colleague. The colleague should identify behaviour and practices that might lead to ergonomic injuries and advise on alternative approaches. This is a measure of best practice and could serve as CPD activity.

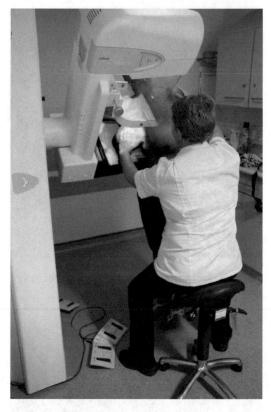

Fig. 26.3 Use of a saddle stool for positioning of the client/patient to improve ergonomic posture for the practitioner. (Source: The Rose Centre, St George's Hospital, London)

Some additional and beneficial positioning considerations [7]:
• Rather than using the thumb and forefinger to support the whole breast, use the whole hand, or as much of the hand as possible to position the breast.
• Consider the design of exposure control to enable the practitioners to use different fingers and therefore different movements to press the exposure button to avoid injury.
• Prior to imaging, ensure that the foot pedals are placed correctly so that there is no need to stretch extremities to reduce the risk of injury.

It is the responsibility of individuals for their own health and safety, and that of work colleagues, to ensure that safe practices are used when performing mammography and undertaking other imaging related duties. The health and safety of all practitioners performing mammograms are critically important, and the Employers' Liability Act makes it the employer's responsibility to care for the health and safety of their employees whilst at work [8].

The Health and Safety Executive [9] recommends that employees complete exercises before the start of the working day and during microbreaks. Employees may want to seek guidance from occupational health or physiotherapy colleagues for more advice.

Conclusion

Due to the repetitive nature of breast imaging and the fact that undertaking a mammogram is a notably physical activity, great care should be taken to support the well-being of staff. In deciding which equipment to use, consideration should be given to the ergonomic suitability of the systems. Staff should be familiar in using the equipment effectively and ensure that high image quality is obtained without compromising their own health.

> **Clinical Pearls**
> - Encourage staff to adopt best ergonomic practice early in their career to avoid or minimise harm from work-related injuries within their clinical practice.
> - Aim to drive continuous improvement in positioning techniques and promote the development of a learning culture and to share best practice.

Chapter Review Questions
Review Questions

1. Does the employer have a responsibility to ensure that employees are safe in their working practices?
2. If I start to experience signs of repetitive strain injury, what should I do?

Answers

1. This is a shared responsibility between the employer and the employee. The Management of Health and Safety at Work Regulations 1999 state that the employer must risk-assess the workplace and employees must co-operate with the employer so that legal requirements are met.
2. In the first instance, you should discuss this with your line manager to raise awareness and seek guidance. This may include completion of a risk assessment of your role and referral to occupational health for further investigation and support.

Acknowledgments To all colleagues that have kindly shared photographs where appropriate permissions are in place.

Appendix

Test your learning and check your understanding of this book's contents: use the "Springer Nature Flashcards" app to access questions using https://sn.pub/dcAnWL.

To use the app, please follow the instructions in Chap. 1.

Flashcard code: 48341-69945-ABCB1-2A8C7-CE9D2.

Short URL: https://sn.pub/dcAnWL.

References

1. Ransom E. The causes of musculoskeletal injury amongst sonographers in the UK. London: Society of Radiographers; 2002.
2. The Cancer Reform Strategy. Policy document. London: Department of Health; 2007.
3. Gale A, May JG. An evaluation of musculoskeletal discomfort experienced by radiographers performing mammography, vol. 36. London: NHSBSP Publication; 1997.
4. Gale A, Hunter N, Lawton C, Purdy K. Ergonomic assessment of radiographer units. NHSBSP equipment report 0708. Sheffield: NHS Cancer Screening Programmes; 2007.
5. Wigley L, Dixon A. Musculoskeletal disorders in mammography: a guide to tackling the issues in the workplace. London: Society of Radiographers Journal; 2009.
6. Breast Check Ireland and Musgove Park Taunton Breast Screening. Interviews with radiographers at Breast Check Ireland and Musgove Park Taunton Breast Screening by Miles, J. Breast Check Ireland (BCI): Joanne Hammond, National Radiography Manager, BreastCheck Ireland; Catherine Vaughan, Radiographer, Coventry and Warwickshire Breast Screening Centre; Sharon Hoffmeister, Deputy Superintendent Radiographer Musgove Park Taunton Breast Screening: Pat Middleton and her staff. Annemarie Dixon, Senior Lecturer, Leeds University; 2011.
7. Public Health England. Breast screening mammography: ergonomics good practice. London: PHE. https://www.gov.uk/government/publications/breast-screening-ergonomics-in-screening-mammography/breast-screening-mammography-ergonomics-good-practice. Accessed 4 Dec 2021.
8. HM Government. The Employers Liability Act 1969. London: HMG; 1969. https://www.legislation.gov.uk/ukpga/1969/57/contents. Accessed 4 Dec 2021.
9. Health and Safety Executive. n.d.. https://www.hse.gov.uk/. Accessed 4 Dec 2021.

Practical Mammography

27

Claire Mercer, Katy Szczepura, Catherine A. Hill, Lyndsay A. Kinnear, Allison Kelly, and Helen L. Smith

Learning Objectives
- Demonstrate knowledge and apply evidence-based practice for basic mammography positioning, with appropriate service-user adaptation as required
- Understand and apply the knowledge of compression application during imaging
- Evaluate the value of effective compression and its effect on the resultant images

C. Mercer (✉) · K. Szczepura
School of Health and Society, University of Salford, Manchester, UK
e-mail: c.e.mercer@salford.ac.uk;
k.szczepura@salford.ac.uk

C. A. Hill
DetectEd-X, Sydney, NSW, Australia
e-mail: cathy.hill@detectedx.com

L. A. Kinnear · A. Kelly
Nightingale Centre, Wythenshawe Hospital, Manchester University NHS Foundation Trust, Manchester, UK
e-mail: lyndsay.kinnear@mft.nhs.uk;
Allison.Kelly@mft.nhs.uk

H. L. Smith
Breast Care Unit, Royal Lancaster Infirmary, University Hospitals of Morecambe Bay NHS Foundation Trust, Lancaster, UK

Contextual Use

Positioning for a mammogram requires skill and expertise; undertaking mammography requires a high standard of accurate and reproducible positioning skills incorporating effective compression with a high level of communication. It is deemed essential that practitioners employ a systematic approach to positioning and compression to ensure consistent, high-quality imaging. For any screening and symptomatic service, successive mammogram images are compared to identify subtle changes, therefore practitioners need to ensure their images are of high quality, reproducible and comparable with their colleagues.

An initial observation of the breast tissue to check for sores or rashes (Chap. 17) should be completed and recorded in the appropriate format following your service procedures. In addition, some additional information may be required from your service-user prior to mammography acquisition, this is detailed in Chap. 24.

Remember, the service-user may feel vulnerable, putting them at ease is a priority to assist in the production of high-quality images. They should be asked to undress from the waist up, whilst doing so the appropriate paddle size for the equipment should be selected. The craniocaudal (CC) and medio-lateral oblique (MLO) views are then performed.

Effective Compression Force Application

Breast compression during mammography is a necessary requirement to produce an image of optimal diagnostic value [1]. Effective compression has multiple benefits to ensure optimisation of the imaging process, it [1]:

- Creates an even breast thickness to ensure equal contrast across the whole breast
- Spreads out overlapping tissues to enable better visualisation of breast structures
- Improves visualisation of tissues near the chest wall
- Holds the breast in place to reduce blur due to service-user movement
- Reduces breast thickness which will reduces scatter, and so improves image quality, but also allows a lower exposure to be used, therefore reducing radiation dose.

Although compression has benefits for optimisation it has the potential to cause the service-user discomfort (Chap. 16) which may ultimately deter them from subsequent mammography attendance [2, 3]. It is acknowledged that one of the most important factors in determining the success of a screening programme is screening uptake [4, 5]. The reasons for any non-attendance are multifactorial (Chap. 16); however, a systematic review undertaken by Whelehan and colleagues in 2013 [3] demonstrated that between 47,000 and 77,000 women in England do not re-attend for breast screening in a year due to pain directly related to a previous mammogram experience. It is therefore essential that every service-user has a similar experience at each attendance, ensuring consistency between examinations and visits [6–8].

Your goal, as a practitioner, is to achieve optimum image quality, with minimal radiation dose, and minimal discomfort to every service-user. This can be achieved by adopting an evidence based mammographic technique, which incorporates effective, but not excessive compression force which enables a balance of pressure between the image receptor (IR) and the compression paddle [9]. The following sections will help you achieve this.

Compression Force and Pressure

Research has demonstrated that there can be variations between practitioners in the compression force that they apply to the breast tissue during a mammographic procedure [6–8] which impacts on the both the service-users experience and the consistency of the images between successive attendances. As such, you should aim for a similar amount of applied compression and breast thickness *on each successive attendance*, to ensure consistency of the image and service-user experience. It is important to recognise that every individual is different; therefore, although compression force and thickness may vary between service-users, consistency for an individual at each attendance is important.

The amount of force needed to be applied for effective compression is dependent upon both the size and the composition of the breast. Applying a certain force on a small, dense breast has a different effect than applying the same force on a large, less dense breast. This is because the force is distributed over different areas of contact between the breast and the paddle, and the breast and the image receptor. This results in a different compression pressure being applied to the breast. This can be explained by the equation:

$$Pressure(Pa) = \frac{Force(N)}{Area(m^2)}$$

The *pressure* exerted on the breast is the amount of *force* divided by the *area* of the breast tissue. As such, for the same level of force applied, a smaller breasted individual will receive higher compression pressure than a larger breasted individual. The following chapter (Chap. 28) provides detailed information on the use of pressure to optimise breast compression [10, 11].

> *Applied pressure is inversely proportional to breast size if the applied compression force is constant* [10]

Achieving Compression Balance

The position of the image receptor (IR) has a considerable effect on the balance of compression between the IR and breast, and the compression paddle and breast. In turn, this also has a direct impact on the amount of breast in contact with the IR and the paddle [9]. It is important to balance compression force between the paddle and the IR to ensure that more force is not exerted from either above or below the breast. Balancing the force has the potential to minimise discomfort by equalising the force and therefore ensuring the applied pressure is more effective. One way to achieve a good balance is to optimise the position of the breast.

Pressure maps of the CC views have been created to assist in the understanding of this process, pressure mapping demonstrates the pressure applied across the area of contact between two surfaces, a colour scale has been applied where red demonstrates the highest pressure within that area.

The images demonstrate the pressure exerted on the breast by the image receptor on the left, and the paddle on the right, for the same applied compression force. Figure 27.1 demonstrates the pressure exerted on the breast when the IR is positioned at the infra mammary fold, whereas Fig. 27.2 demonstrates the pressure exerted when the IR is raised 2 cm above the level of the IMF. As can been seen from these images, raising the IR above the IMF creates a more balanced pressure exerted on the breast from the IR and the paddle. It also creates an increased contact area, demonstrating that the applied force is more effective.

Fig. 27.1 Left CC with IR at IMF

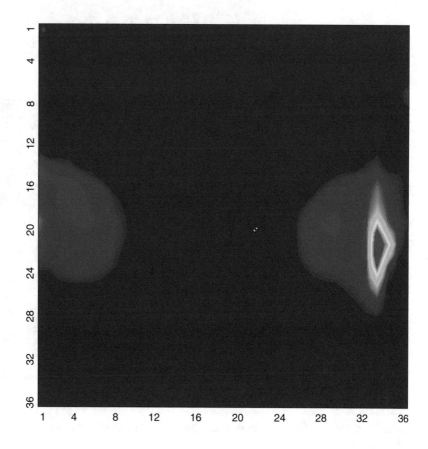

Fig. 27.2 Left CC with IR at IMF + 2 cm

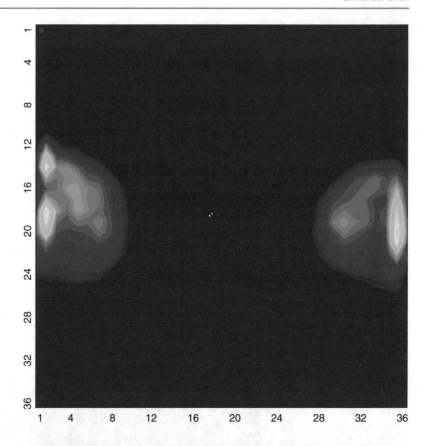

Fig. 27.3 CC Mammogram image

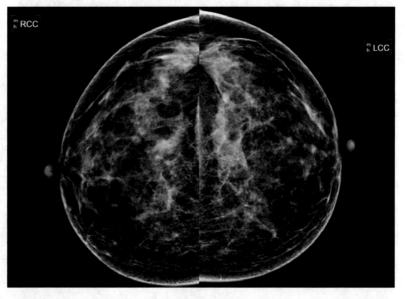

Cranio-Caudal (CC) View: A Step by Step Guide

The CC mammographic image (Fig. 27.3) should demonstrate the majority of the breast tissue with the exclusion of the axillary tail. To ensure this is achieved in the resultant image, the following positioning technique should be followed. Firstly, stand the service-user facing the mammography system about 10 cm away from the IR (Fig. 27.4). Ask them to stand with their feet facing the image receptor

(Fig. 27.5) with their hand (of the side being imaged) on their abdomen. Some may wish to stand with their feet a hips width apart for stability.

> You should always be aware of your own postural techniques during positioning to reduce any risk of repetitive strain injury.

Stand next to the service-user, on the contra-lateral side, and ask them to turn their head to face you and rest their cheek against the face guard (Fig. 27.6).

Following this, ask them to keep their feet in the same position and bend forwards slightly, pushing their hips back. Lift the breast being

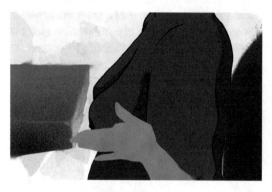

Fig. 27.4 CC Initial positioning

imaged, using its natural mobility, raising it with the palm of your hand. The extent to which the breast should be raised prior to positioning for the CC view is important. Adjust the height of the IR to allow the breast to sit at a 90° angle at the chest wall in the first instance. It is important to raise the IR by 1–2 cm above the level of the infra mammary fold (IMF) to achieve compression force balance to the top and bottom of the breast and achieve maximum contact area. The amount the IR can be raised above the IMF will be dependent on the mobility of the breast, additionally It is important to ensure that the IR is not raised too much as this could result in a loss of breast tissue on the image and cause the nipple to be inverted down (Fig. 27.7).

Using the breasts natural mobility, lift and guide their breast forwards onto the image receptor, ensuring that the nipple is centrally placed with lateral and medial borders pulled on and within the field of view. There are two ways to ensure adequate positioning is achieved; hands can be placed at the lateral and medial sides or above and below the breast (the sandwich approach).

It has been demonstrated, following correct positioning, the nipple will fall into profile in at least one view with almost all located along or close to the breast boundary [12, 13], adjust so that the nipple is centrally placed (Fig. 27.8). The

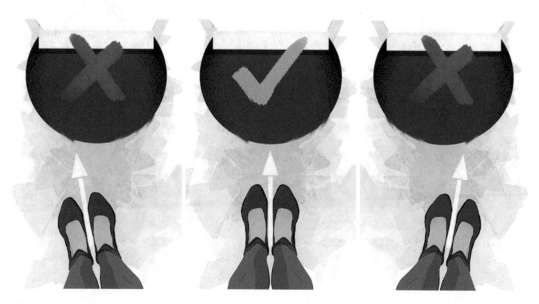

Fig. 27.5 CC Positioning

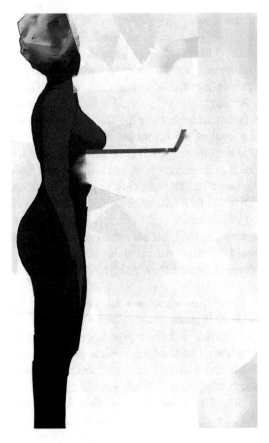

Fig. 27.6 CC head position

nipple is a standard and reliable landmark to ensure accurate breast positioning.

Now check for creases and air gaps and smooth the breast tissue. Ensure the nipple is centrally placed and in profile; but not at the expense of breast tissue being demonstrated. Whilst holding the breast securely with one hand, place one arm around the back of the service-user and gently guide their shoulder down, allowing relaxation of the lateral breast tissue. Placing your hand positively around the back of them will encourage a 'leaning forwards motion' followed by compression force application.

You can now alert that compression is about to commence. Apply compression force slowly and evenly using the foot pedal. At the same time, move your hand towards the nipple/away from the chest wall as the compression paddle takes over from the hand. If available on the equipment, hand-held compression (for the service-user to control) should be used to allow a slow, measured compression force application.

The breast should be compressed until it is immobilised, the breast surface may feel taut to the touch. Consistency between sequential atten-

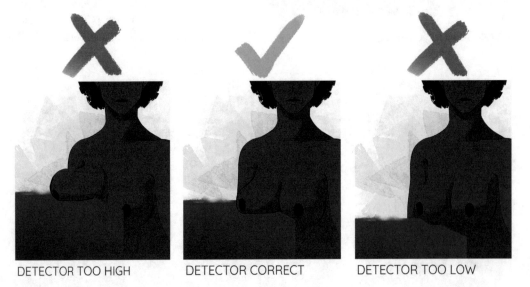

DETECTOR TOO HIGH   DETECTOR CORRECT   DETECTOR TOO LOW

Fig. 27.7 CC image detector position

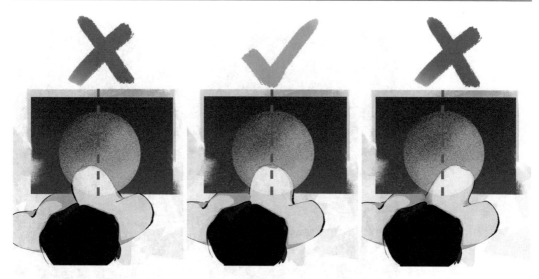

Fig. 27.8 CC Nipple position

dances for an individual service-user is imperative and the compression force could be standardised between 90 and 130 N of force [14]; it is important to apply lower forces if experiences of discomfort are perceived, and higher forces if the breast remains immobile. Remember if you have a paddle that indicates pressure, then aim for 10 kPa; with a range between 7 and 15 kPa [10, 11]; this is discussed in more detail within Chap. 28.

Now check the medial and lateral borders for skin folds, if present, smooth out with fingers ensuring not to disturb any breast tissue. Perform a last check to ensure no artefacts are present within the field of view and perform the exposure. Following automatic compression release, lower the height of the IR slightly prior to imaging the opposing side; this allows for correct breast uplift to be achieved on the other side.

Medio-Lateral (MLO) View: A Step by Step Guide

The MLO mammogram image should demonstrate all the breast tissue (Fig. 27.9), with the IMA, nipple in profile and pectoral muscle demonstrated.

Angle selection

Angle selection for the MLO view is a skill and refinement will be required. In the first instance, an observation of the body habitus of the service-user can provide an indication and enable you to select an appropriate angle. One way is to assess their sternal angle and aim to get this in parallel with the IR (Fig. 27.11).

Recent research which measured pectoral muscle length, width and shape of females in Norway demonstrated that 60° angulation may be suitable for those with a height of 163 cm or above, those with a shorter stature may benefit from an angle less than 60° [15]. In 2019, Bedene and colleagues [16] recommended 55° for those with longer thoraxes and smaller breasts and a very low angle of 35° for those with shorter thoraxes and larger breasts. In 2018, Agius [17] and colleagues determined that angulation techniques in the MLO should be altered according to the service-user; rotating the image receptor from 45° to 35° for those who are shorter with larger breasts up to around 55° for those who are taller with smaller breasts. Continued research is ongoing in this area within the UK incorporating a standardised positioning technique to assess pain and breast contact area with varying tube angulation.

The following positioning technique can then be followed:

For your initial set up, reduce the height of the IR slightly from the CC view and angle the tube head initially to around 50°. Now set the IR angle in accordance with the height and body habitus of your service-user; a good starting point is demonstrated within Fig. 27.10. Aim to have the top

Fig. 27.9 MLO
Mammogram image

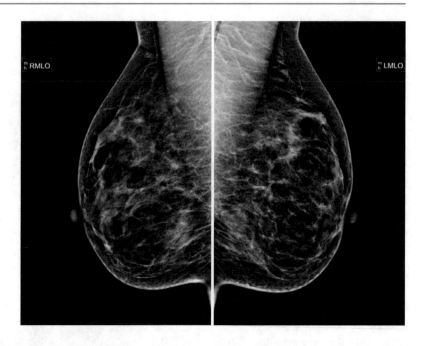

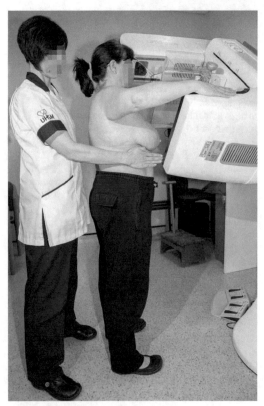

Fig. 27.10 MLO initial angle position

of the IR halfway between the shoulder and the axillary crease, it is important that the correct angle of the IR is selected. Suboptimal positioning and incorrect angle selection may result in excessive compression force being applied to the chest wall/axilla (Fig. 27.11).

For stability, ask the service-user to face the mammography machine with feet a hips width apart. Standing behind them, place your hand at the bottom of the rib cage of the side being imaged. Move them forwards until your fingertips are just touching the front and bottom aspect of the IR; they will be approximately 10 cm back from the IR (Fig. 27.12). Rest their arm along the top of the IR.

Standing at 90° to the service-user, place your hand to the lateral aspect of their breast and place your other arm, in a supportive position, around their back. Lift their breast with one hand, whilst supporting them with the other, and guide their movement to position the breast on the image receptor. Move around to the back of them and position their arm; lifting it upwards, gently reaching the shoulder over the IR. Adjust the height; the corner of the IR should be seated into

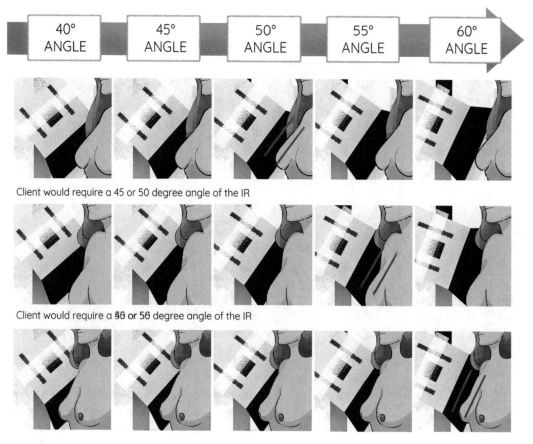

Client would require a 45 or 50 degree angle of the IR

Client would require a 50 or 50 degree angle of the IR

Fig. 27.11 IR angle selection

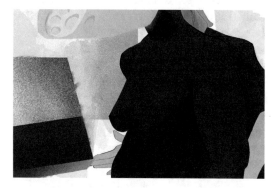

Fig. 27.12 Service-user position

the axilla (mid axillary line between the latissimus dorsi muscle and pectoral muscle), or in the space if the axilla is hollow. They can drape their

arm over the IR and rest their hand on the handle of the equipment; but not grasp too tightly as this will cause the pectoral muscle to tense. Ensure their arm is not higher than their shoulder and check that their pectoral muscle is flat and not over stretched.

Then return to the front of them and sit on an appropriate stool (Fig. 27.13) for correct ergonomic positioning (Chap. 26). Now ask them to relax down onto the IR and gently ease the shoulder backwards, carefully pulling their breast through onto the IR with both hands. Their breast should be centrally placed on the IR with the corner of the compression paddle seated just below the head of humerus—adjust the height accordingly if required.

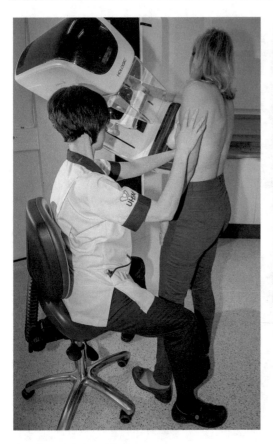

Fig. 27.13 MLO positioning

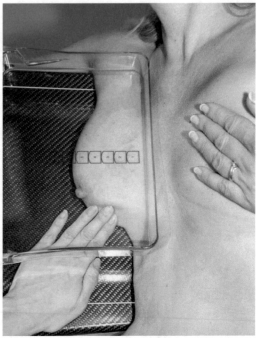

Fig. 27.14 MLO compression

Sweep your hand down the back of their breast from the axilla to the infra mammary angle, checking for creases and ensuring all breast tissue is pulled on. Ensure their hips are back, smooth the infra mammary angle. Ask them to push their hips back slightly if the abdomen is protruding. Using your hand, lift their breast up and away from the chest wall; the breast is to be imaged at 90° to the chest wall. Their nipple should be in profile with no air gaps between the breast and the IR.

Various methods of supporting their breast can be used to help minimise the risk of injury (Chap. 26). You can now alert them that compression is about to commence. Apply compression force slowly and evenly using the foot pedal. At the same time move your hand towards the nipple/away from the chest wall as the compression paddle takes over from the hand. If available on the equipment, hand-held compression (for the service-user) should be used to allow a slow, measured compression force application. The top of the compression paddle should sit just below the clavicle, head of humerus and the inner edge alongside the sternum. Ask them to hold the other breast away from the field of view, if required, and raise their chin slightly (Fig. 27.14).

The compression force could be standardised between 90 and 130 N of force [13]; it is important to apply a lower force if they experience discomfort and a higher force if the breast remains immobile. Remember if you have a pressure paddle then aim for 10 kPa; range between 7 and 15 kPa (Chap. 28).

Ensure the infra mammary angle is open and free from skin folds and perform a last check to ensure no artefacts are present on the image. Perform the exposure. Following automatic compression release, lower the height of the IR slightly prior to imaging the opposing side; this allows for effective breast and shoulder placement.

Checklists

Table 27.1 provides an aid for an overview image quality check.

> It is important that a decision to perform a repeat of an image is only taken following your departments' protocols and ionising radiation regulations. A repeat image should have perceived diagnostic improvements. You should never repeat an image for non-diagnostic reasons.

Continued professional development is essential for any practitioner and this is supported by the research conducted by Huppe and colleagues in 2017 [18] who noted that traditional positioning standards that were based on film screen technology can be improved with continued positioning training.

Clinical Pearls
- Successive mammographic images are compared for subtle changes and practitioners need to ensure their images are of consistent high quality and comparable with their colleagues.
- In the CC projection, to achieve maximum contact area and optimum compression force balance, aim to position the IR approximately 1–2 cm above the level of the infra mammary angle at 90°. This will have perceived image quality improvements and support the service-user experience.
- In the MLO projection, alter the angle of the IR to suit the body shape of your service-user, this could support their experience.

Table 27.1

View	Checklist
Both	Nipple in profile
	All breast tissue imaged
	Skin fold artefact free
	Symmetrical
	Free from blurring
	Correct exposure parameters used
CC	Back of breast imaged, within 1 cm of the MLO
MLO	Pectoral muscle to nipple level and appropriate width (correct height and angle of IR)
	Infra mammary angle demonstrated

Chapter Review Questions
Review Questions

1. Why is it important to raise the level of the IR when positioning for the CC view?
2. Why is compression, rather than force, important for optimised imaging?
3. Why is standardized compression advised for individual, but not between individuals?
4. What could be the possible consequences of incorrect angle selection of the IR in the MLO view?
5. What steps should be taken to ensure clear demonstration of the IMF in the MLO view?

Answers

1. To achieve the maximum amount of breast contact area on the IR and the paddle and to balance the compression between them
2. The applied force can vary between service-users as the applied pressure depends on the breast size and composition
3. (a) To ensure consistency for service-users between sequential visits
   (b) To aim to improve attendance for mammography on sequential visits

4. (a) Suboptimal positioning
   (b) Excessive compression pressure being applied to the chest wall/axilla
   (c) Unnecessary discomfort
   (d) Inadequate breast compression
5. (a) Sweep the hand down the back of the breast to ensure all breast tissue is imaged and creases are eliminated
   (b) Ensure the hips are pushed back and there is no abdomen protruding
   (c) Lift the breast up and out, away from the chest wall
   (d) Ensure the breast is in good contact with the IR to avoid airgaps
   (e) Adequately support the breast while compression is applied
   (f) Ensure the field of view is free from artefacts, including the contralateral breast

Acknowledgments The authors would like to pay particular thanks to Penelope Booth art.penelope.booth@gmail.com for the artwork contained within this chapter, and to Gill Brett, for the photographs within this chapter.

Appendix

Test your learning and check your understanding of this book's contents: use the "Springer Nature Flashcards" app to access questions using https://sn.pub/dcAnWL.

To use the app, please follow the instructions in Chap. 1.

Flashcard code:
48341-69945-ABCB1-2A8C7-CE9D2.

Short URL: https://sn.pub/dcAnWL.

References

1. Public Health England. Breast screening: guidance for breast screening mammographers. London: PHE; 2020. www.gov.uk. Accessed 19 Mar 2022.
2. Poulos A, McLean D. The application of breast compression in mammography: a new perspective. Radiography. 2004;10:131–7.
3. Whelehan P, Evans A, Wells M, Macgillivray S. The effect of mammography pain on repeat participation in breast cancer screening: a systematic review. Breast. 2013;22(4):389–94.
4. Marmot MG, Altman DG, Cameron DA, Dewar JA, Thompson SG, Wilcox M. The benefits and harms of breast cancer screening: an independent review. Br J Cancer. 2013;108(11):2205–40.
5. Weller DP, Campbell C. Uptake in cancer screening programmes: a priority in cancer control. Br J Cancer. 2009;101(Suppl 2):S55–9. https://doi.org/10.1038/sj.bjc.6605391.
6. Mercer CE, Hogg P, Lawson R, Diffey J, Denton ERE. Practitioner compression force variability in mammography: a preliminary study. Br J Radiol. 2013;86:20110596.
7. Mercer CE, Hogg P, Szczepura K, Denton ERE. Practitioner compression force variation in mammography: a 6-year study. Radiography. 2013;2013(19):200–6.
8. Mercer CE, Szczepura K, Kelly J, Millington SR, Denton ERE, Borgen R, Hilton B, Hogg P. A call for client consistency in compression. Bournemouth: Symposium Mammographicum; 2014.
9. Smith H, Hogg P, Maxwell A, Mercer CE, Szczepura K. An analysis of the compressed breast area and image receptor/compression paddle pressure balance in different mammographic projections. UKRC 2013 abstract. Manchester: UKRC; 2013.
10. De Groot JE, Broeders MJM, Branderhorst W, den Heeten GJ, Grimbergen CA. A novel approach to mammographic breast compression: improved standardization and reduced discomfort by controlling pressure instead of force. Med Phys. 2013;40(8):081901.
11. Branderhorst W, de Groot JE, Neeter LM, van Lier MG, Neeleman C, den Heeten GJ, et al. Force balancing in mammographic compression. Med Phys. 2016;43(1):518.
12. Pearl O. Breast imaging mammography. Mammography and breast imaging prep, program review and exam preparation. New York, NY: McGrawHill Medical; 2012.
13. Chuan Z, Chan HP, Paramagul C, Roubidoux MA, Sahiner B, Hadiiiski LM, Petrick N. Computerized nipple identification for multiple image analysis in computer aided diagnosis. Med Phys. 2004;31(10):2871–82.
14. Hogg P, Taylor M, Szczepura K, Mercer C, Denton E. Pressure and breast thickness in mammography—an exploratory calibration study. Br J Radiol. 2013;86(1021):20120222.
15. Moshina N, Bjørnson EW, Holen ÅS, Larsen M, Hansestad B, Tøsdal L, Hofvind S. Standardised or individualised X-ray tube angle for mediolateral oblique projection in digital mammography? Radiography. 2022;28:772.

16. Bedene A, Alukić E, Žibert J, Mekiš N. Mediolateral oblique projection in mammography: use of different angulation for patients with different thorax anatomies. J Health Sci. 2019;9(1):40–5.
17. Agius EC, Naylor S. Breast compression techniques in screening mammography –a Maltese evaluation project. Radiography. 2018;24(4):309–14.
18. Huppe AI, Overman KL, Gatewood JB, Hill JD, Miller LC, Inciardi MF. Mammography positioning standards in the digital era: is the status quo acceptable? Am J Roentgenol. 2017;209(6):1419–25.

Mammographic Compression: A Need for Mechanical Standardisation

28

Jerry E. de Groot, Woutjan Branderhorst,
Monique G. J. T. B. van Lier, Ralph Highnam,
Ariane Chan, Marcela Böhm-Vélez,
Mireille J. M. Broeders, Cornelis A. Grimbergen,
and Gerard J. den Heeten

Introduction

In mammography, image quality is of utmost importance. Good mechanical compression of the breast is one of the essentials of effective mammography. Potential benefits derived from good compression include [1–5]: (1) A more uniform breast thickness resulting in a better fit

J. E. de Groot · M. G. J. T. B. van Lier (✉)
W. Branderhorst · C. A. Grimbergen
Sigmascreening B.V. Enschede,
Amsterdam, The Netherlands
e-mail: jerry.degroot@sigmascreening.com;
monique.van.lier@sigmascreening.com

R. Highnam · A. Chan
Volpara Health Technologies Ltd,
Wellington, New Zealand
e-mail: ralph.highnam@volparahealth.com;
ariane.chan@volparahealth.com

M. Böhm-Vélez
Weinstein Imaging Associates, Pittsburgh, PA, USA

M. J. M. Broeders
LRCB Dutch Expert Centre for Screening,
Nijmegen, The Netherlands
e-mail: m.broeders@lrcb.nl

G. J. den Heeten
Sigmascreening B.V. Enschede,
Amsterdam, The Netherlands

Department of Radiology and Nuclear Medicine,
University of Amsterdam,
Amsterdam, The Netherlands

of the exposure into the dynamic range; (2) Reduced blurring from breast motion; (3) Reduced scattered radiation and improved contrast sensitivity; (4) Reduced radiation dose; (5) Better visualisation of tissues near the chest wall; and (6) Reduced superimposition of overlapping tissues.

However, there is an issue in clinical practice in the sense that "good compression" is not easily defined to be followed routinely. The natural shape of the breast results in varying thickness from the nipple to the chest wall and is a general deterrent to achieving good contrast and visibility without compression. "Good compression" transforms the breast into a more uniform thickness and makes the breast tissue somewhat thinner for better imaging.

All aspects of the mammographic image acquisition process are subject to quality standards (European Guidelines [1], Mammography Quality and Standards Act (MQSA) [2]), but the instructions for compression are too vague to provide any sort of standardisation. To cite the European guidelines literally:

The compression should be firm but tolerable. There is no optimal value known for the force, but attention should be given to the applied compression and the accuracy of the indication.

The MQSA only mentions requirements for testing compression devices and provides no indication on how much force to use in clinical practice. Both guidelines do state an upper limit of 20 decanewton (daN) and all mammographic machines restrict the motor drive to this level. In practice, the amount of compression is guided by approximating the individual pain threshold of the patient and the individual performance of mammographers. For that reason, breast compression is patient and operator dependent [6, 7].

Since little is known about compression standardisation, we tried to find information in the literature about compression parameters in the DICOM headers like force and breast thickness. We found that considerable variations exist, especially in the force at exposure [8–12].

It came to our attention that in different countries different policies are maintained. For example, in the Dutch screening a minimum force of 12 daN is maintained, while in the U.S. there seems to be no target force at all.

The Mechanics of Compression

Mechanical compression makes the breast flatter by applying force. One decanewton (daN) of force is equivalent to the weight of approximately 1 kg. Applying a certain force on a small breast has a different effect than applying the same force on a large breast. This is because the force is distributed over different areas of contact. A better comparison is obtained by dividing the applied force by the total breast contact area. This value gives force per unit contact area, also known as contact pressure, which is measured in kilopascal (kPa; $1 \text{ kPa} = 1 \text{ daN/}dm^2 \approx 7.5 \text{ mmHg}$). Applying the same pressure on small or large breasts has the same effect on the tissue because the force is proportional to the breast contact area. This might be relevant because the middle 95% of breast volumes in the sample of this chapter vary by a factor 10 (ca. $0.22–2.2 \text{ dm}^3$). Furthermore, individual breast mechanical properties can differ significantly depending on tissue composition, age and properties of the skin [13].

Research in this field showed that it is feasible to use a pressure-standardised compression approach. In addition, a study found that contact area is a significant predictor for pain while compression force itself is not [14]. This makes contact pressure, being the ratio of force and contact area, a better predictor for pain. Pain during and after mammographic compression is a common complaint [15–17] and for some women a reason to avoid screening [18].

Mammographic Monitoring Software

Software for the evaluation of mammogram DICOM information is available (VolparaAnalytics, Volpara Health Technologies Ltd., Wellington, New Zealand) enabling cross-comparison of populations. For the first time, this allows for large scale and comprehensive analysis of some of the mechanical parameters of compression of the breast that occur in daily practice in different countries.

The purpose of this chapter is to compare, analyse and visualise the current mammographic compression practice in the Netherlands and the U.S. from a mechanical point of view, and to hypothesise if mechanical standardisation could lead to a more reproducible procedure.

Methods

The analysis software (VolparaAnalytics (version 1.0) and VolparaDensity (algorithm version 1.5.0), Volpara Health Technologies Ltd., Wellington, New Zealand) calculates breast volume and density, as well as contact area for contact pressure estimates. It also calculates absorbed glandular dose (AGD) using a comprehensive dose model [19–22] that incorporates a patient's own breast density, which enables AGD-comparison between DICOM data from different mammography device manufacturers.

Two large, anonymised data sets were available, one from the Dutch breast cancer screening programme ($n = 13,610$, August 2012–September 2013), and one from an imaging centre in Pittsburgh, PA, U.S. ($n = 7179$, January 2008–March 2014). Figure 28.1 gives an impression of

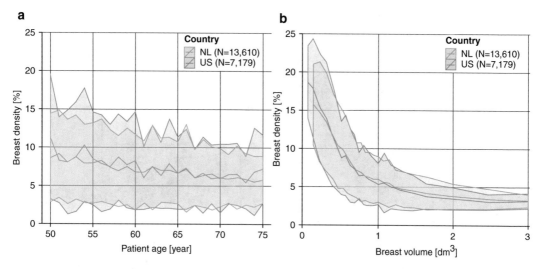

Fig. 28.1 (**a**) Breast density (%) versus patient age (years); mean ± standard deviation. (**b**) Breast density (%) versus breast volume (dm³) mean ± standard deviation

the comparability of breast densities and volumes of women aged 50–75 in both data sets.

Since contact area is the parameter that links force to pressure (P = F/A), we compared parameters as a function of contact area. It is worth mentioning that contact area is strongly correlated with breast volume (Pearson's rho = 0.82, $p < 0.001$). This enabled us to compare the variation in compression forces and pressures as function of breast size, as performed by practitioners in two different countries, one with a 12 daN minimum force (The Netherlands) and one without a specific target compression force (U.S.).

Results

Figure 28.2a shows compression force (daN) versus contact area (dm²) for both data sets. In this figure, four pressure values (5, 10, 15, 20 kPa) are indicated as straight lines: Force (daN) = Pressure (kPa) × Contact area (dm²). Figure 28.2b shows contact pressure (kPa) versus contact area (dm²) for the same data. In this figure four force values (5, 10, 15, 20 daN) are indicated as hyperbolas: Pressure (kPa) = Force (daN)/Contact area (dm²).

It is clearly visible that the applied forces and pressures were considerably higher in the Netherlands; however, in both countries similar trends existed as a function of contact area: Smaller breasts received lower forces than larger breasts in both countries, and pressures were higher for smaller breasts compared to larger breasts.

Comparing the number of high compression forces in both data sets, we saw that 18.6% (n = 2528) compressions in the Dutch set were greater than 15 daN, versus 1.9% (n = 139) in the U.S. In terms of high pressures, we found 10.7% (n = 1458) of compressions were greater than 20 kPa in the Netherlands, versus 1.7% (n = 119) in the U.S. At the other end of the spectrum, we compared the number of low compression forces. The U.S. data set contained 23.5% (n = 1688) of compressions acquired with less than 5 daN versus practically none, 0.04% (n = 6), in the Netherlands. Lastly, we found 21.7% (n = 1555) of compressions below 5 kPa of pressure in the U.S., versus only 0.8% (n = 114) in the Netherlands.

Figure 28.3a shows breast thickness (mm) versus contact area (dm²) for both datasets. The average thickness was nearly identical for both datasets, but the standard deviation in the U.S. data was on average 16% larger. Figure 28.3b shows AGD (mGy) versus contact area (dm²). All dose values were recalculated with Volpara's comprehensive dose model, which enables intermanufacturer comparison. The U.S. data had a higher mean AGD value and a much larger

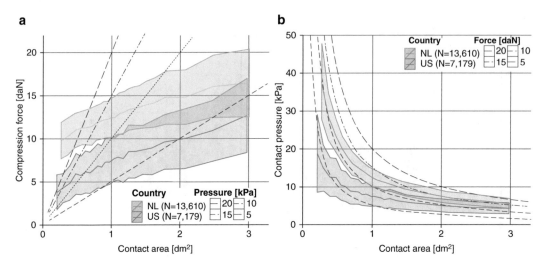

Fig. 28.2 (**a**) Compression force (daN) versus contact area (dm²); mean ± standard deviation. (**b**) Contact pressure (kPa) versus contact area (dm²); mean ± standard deviation

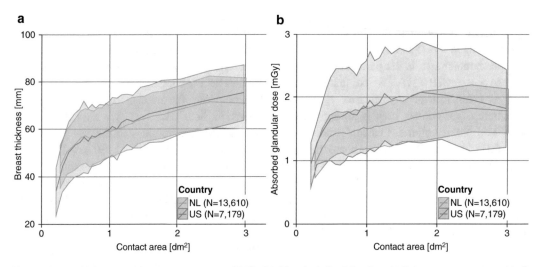

Fig. 28.3 (**a**) Thickness (mm) versus contact area (dm²). (**b**) Absorbed glandular dose (mGy) versus contact area (dm²)

standard deviation compared to the Dutch data. These differences are possibly influenced by the larger variation of the breast thickness in the U.S. set. Another source of variation is that U.S. images were acquired on mammography machines with various target- and filter materials, whereas the Dutch screening only used machines with Tungsten target and Rhodium or Silver filter.

Figure 28.4 illustrates modelled compressions following a strict force protocol ($F = 14$ daN ± 5% standard deviation) and a strict pressure protocol ($P = 10$ kPa ± 5% standard deviation). In Fig. 28.4a, the force values for the 10 kPa-protocol were proportional to the contact area until reaching the 20 daN guideline upper limit. The modelled 14 daN-protocol was constant around 14 daN. In Fig. 28.4b the pressure values for the 10 kPa-protocol were constant around the target value of 10 kPa, and again limited to 20 daN of force for contact areas larger than 2.0 dm². The strict 14 daN-protocol extends far beyond the scale with a maximum pressure of 120 kPa (900 mmHg) for the smallest breast found in these data sets.

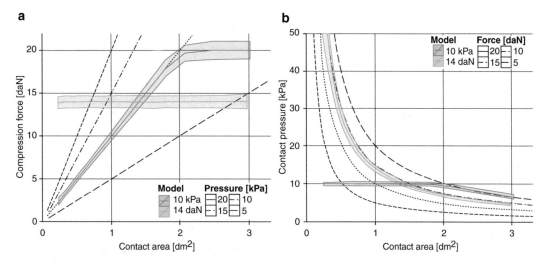

Fig. 28.4 (**a**) Modelled compression force (daN) versus contact area (dm²) for a strict pressure (10 kPa) and force (14 daN) protocol. (**b**) Modelled pressure (kPa) versus contact area (dm²) for a strict pressure (10 kPa) and force (14 daN) protocol

Discussion

The results obtained from this study show that current mammographic compression policies in the Netherlands and in the United States lead not only to a wide range of applied forces but also to a wide range of pressures. We found a large difference between the countries, but also large standard deviations for women with the same breast size within each population. This implies that from the individual woman's point of view, the procedure is far from reproducible, and the amount of applied pressure is unpredictable.

This is the first study on breast compression in which not only the applied force, but also the contact pressure, is compared between two large data sets from different countries. Large variations in applied forces in mammography have been reported between and within counties, imaging centers and screening participants [8–12, 23] and are a logical result of current compression policies in which practitioners are expected to fixate the breast based on experience, observation of the patient and tautness of the breast tissue [1, 2]. The practitioners thereby subjectively adjust the force to a certain extent compensating for breast size, composition and pain. Since these parameters are highly variable over the population, a large variation in applied forces can be expected. However, if the compression force would be objectively adjusted to breast size and composition (elasticity), this would lead to a similar pressure in all breasts [14].

In the results of this study, we observed that the applied average pressure is highly variable in current mammographic compression practice. The compression force chosen by the practitioner must therefore be predominantly determined by factors other than the breast size and elasticity. In other words, at least from a mechanical point of view, mammographic compression is not standardised. There seems to be only a very weak relation between the biomechanical parameters involved.

On the other hand, mammography has already been employed successfully for decades [24, 25]. Our data shows that current clinical practice leads to strikingly high pressures for women with smaller breasts, particularly in The Netherlands. Besides, in another publication, it was concluded that small-breasted women experience more pain [14]. At the other extreme, in the U.S., a large number of women received alarmingly low pressures, which could be associated with an increased risk of image quality issues and receiving higher dose. In both countries, women will likely endure wide variations in compression over the course of repeated examinations, depending on the performance and training of the practitioners [6]. In addition, the accuracy of automated volumetric assessment of mammographic density may be affected by breast compression [24].

The absence of compression guidelines, especially in the U.S., may have led to a gradual decrease of applied compression forces as a measure to avoid pain complaints. This so-called compression creep may unnoticeably affect image quality and dose. We believe that pressure-standardised compression protocols, as part of a more personalized examination, might improve this unwanted situation and may contribute to improve patient comfort [25–27] and screening reattendance [28]. However, further research is necessary.

Conclusion

Comparing mammographic compression in the Netherlands (maintaining only a 12 daN minimum force) and the U.S. (without a specified target force), forces and pressures are considerably higher in the Netherlands. Variations between women with the same breast size (contact area) are large in both countries.

Standardising with a target force will still lead to large differences between individuals with different breast sizes and is therefore not an effective standardisation. Standardising with a target pressure, which objectively takes the size of the breast into consideration, effectively leads to a standard tissue pressure and probably less variation in thickness reduction.

Implementation of Mechanical Standardisation; Pressure-Assisted Compression

In this chapter, an example of the large variability in compression practice was given and a potential new approach of standardising with a target pressure instead of a target force was suggested. As mentioned before, breast contact area is the parameter that links force to pressure (P = F/A). As this parameter is not present in current mammography systems, de Groot et al. equipped a rigid compression paddle with a radiolucent and calibrated detector sheet to measure in real-time this contact area of the breast with the paddle [29]. This calculation of the ratio of the applied force and the breast contact area represents the mean contact pressure, or interface pressure, enabling pressure-information-assisted compression during mammography.

In the recent years, several studies have appeared in which the impact of using this new approach was studied using conventional two-dimensional (2D) mammography in, for example, clinical practice [30, 31] and screening environments [26, 32]. In a review by Serwan et al., aiming to assess the feasibility of mechanically standardised compression, it was concluded that;

[…] a compression pressure approximately 10kPa was found to decrease pain, with a negligible effect on breast thickness, AGD and resultant image quality. This also aids the reproducibility of image acquisition between and within women, whilst offering suggested guidelines for mammographers. It is therefore suggested that patient compliance would increase in accordance with the perceived benefits of a standardised technique, which would ultimately aid in the detection of early-stage breast cancer. [33].

These earlier studies were predominantly conducted in Europe and in 2D mammography. Recently, this approach was also studied in digital breast tomosynthesis in the US [34]. In addition, a flexible paddle (deflecting more towards the nipple during compression, compared to a rigid paddle) was used instead of a rigid paddle. In that study, the compression pressure variability as well as the mean breast thickness, and glandular dose decreased, while at the same time, both the participant and technician experience improved. The impact on image quality and breast positioning was not studied. A study by Broeders et al. comparing the performance of a flexible versus a rigid compression paddle in 2D mammography, showed that the projected breast area decreased when using a flexible paddle. As the compression forces used were much higher in the study of Broeders at al. (128 N) [35] compared to the study by van Lier et al. (86 N for craniocaudal views and 103 N for mediolateral oblique views) [34], the impact may be different.

The first studies using this new technique show positive results for compression reproducibility and patient and technician experience. However, a prospective randomised study to investigate the effects of this intervention has not been performed yet. Nevertheless, studies have suggested that there is an association between compression forces (whether excessive high or low), the resulting pressures, and impaired screening performance in 2D mammography [36, 37]. A recent study showed that no association was found between force and pressure levels and screening performance in digital breast tomosynthesis [38].

Appendix

Test your learning and check your understanding of this book's contents: use the "Springer Nature Flashcards" app to access questions using https://sn.pub/dcAnWL.

To use the app, please follow the instructions in Chap. 1.

Flashcard code:

48341-69945-ABCB1-2A8C7-CE9D2.

Short URL: https://sn.pub/dcAnWL.

References

1. Perry N, Broeders M, de Wolf C, Törnberg S, Holland R, von Karsa L. European guidelines for quality assurance in breast cancer screening and diagnosis. 4th ed. Luxembourg: Office for Official Publications of the European Communities; 2006.
2. USC. Mammography Quality Standards Act of 1992. Washington, DC: USC; 1992. Pub. L. No. 102-539.
3. Saunders RS Jr, Samei E. The effect of breast compression on mass conspicuity in digital mammography. Med Phys. 2008;35(10):4464–73.
4. Pisano ED, Yaffe MJ. Digital mammography. Radiology. 2005;234(2):353–62.
5. Heine JJ, Cao K, Thomas JA. Effective radiation attenuation calibration for breast density: compression thickness influences and correction. Biomed Eng Online. 2010;9(1):1–26.
6. Mercer CE, Hogg P, Lawson R, Diffey J, Denton ER. Practitioner compression force variability in mammography: a preliminary study. Br J Radiol. 2013;86(1022):20110596.
7. Mercer CE, Hogg P, Szczepura K, Denton ERE. Practitioner compression force variation in mammography: a 6-year study. Radiography. 2013;19:200–6.
8. Hendrick RE, Pisano ED, Averbukh A, Moran C, Berns EA, Yaffe MJ, Herman B, Acharyya S, Gatsonis C. Comparison of acquisition parameters and breast dose in digital mammography and screen-film mammography in the American College of Radiology Imaging Network digital mammographic imaging screening trial. AJR Am J Roentgenol. 2010;194(2):362–9.
9. Sullivan DC, Beam CA, Goodman SM, Watt DL. Measurement of force applied during mammography. Radiology. 1991;181(2):355–7.
10. Ng KH, Mill ML, Johnston L, Highnam R, Tomal A. Large variation in mammography compression internationally. ECR. 2017;
11. Lau S, Abdul Aziz YF, Ng KH. Mammographic compression in Asian women. PLoS One. 2017;12(4):e0175781.
12. Waade GG, Sanderud A, Hofvind S. Compression force and radiation dose in the Norwegian Breast Cancer Screening Program. Eur J Radiol. 2017;88:41–6.
13. Gefen A, Dilmoney B. Mechanics of the normal woman's breast. Technol Health Care. 2007;15(4): 259–71.
14. de Groot JE, Broeders MJ, Branderhorst W, den Heeten GJ, Grimbergen CA. A novel approach to mammographic breast compression: improved standardization and reduced discomfort by controlling pressure instead of force. Med Phys. 2013;40(8):081901.
15. Poulos A, Rickard M. Compression in mammography and the perception of discomfort. Australas Radiol. 1997;41(3):247–52.
16. Keemers-Gels ME, Groenendijk RP, van den Heuvel JH, Boetes C, Peer PG, Wobbes TH. Pain experienced by women attending breast cancer screening. Breast Cancer Res Treat. 2000;60(3):235–40.
17. Sharp PC, Michielutte R, Freimanis R, Cunningham L, Spangler J, Burnette V. Reported pain following mammography screening. Arch Intern Med. 2003;163(7):833–6.
18. Whelehan P, Evans A, Wells M, Macgillivray S. The effect of mammography pain on repeat participation in breast cancer screening: a systematic review. Breast. 2013;22(4):389–94.
19. Dance DR. Monte Carlo calculation of conversion factors for the estimation of mean glandular breast dose. Phys Med Biol. 1990;35(9):1211–9.
20. Dance DR, Skinner CL, Young KC, Beckett JR, Kotre CJ. Additional factors for the estimation of mean glandular breast dose using the UK mam-

mography dosimetry protocol. Phys Med Biol. 2000;45(11):3225–40.

21. Dance DR, Young KC, van Engen RE. Further factors for the estimation of mean glandular dose using the United Kingdom, European and IAEA breast dosimetry protocols. Phys Med Biol. 2009;54(14): 4361–72.

22. Dance DR, Young KC, van Engen RE. Estimation of mean glandular dose for breast tomosynthesis: factors for use with the UK, European and IAEA breast dosimetry protocols. Phys Med Biol. 2011;56(2): 453–71.

23. Waade GG, Sebuodegard S, Hogg P, Hofvind S. Breast compression across consecutive examinations among females participating in BreastScreen Norway. Br J Radiol. 2018;91(1090):20180209.

24. Moshina N, Roman M, Waade GG, Sebuodegard S, Ursin G, Hofvind S. Breast compression parameters and mammographic density in the Norwegian Breast Cancer Screening Programme. Eur Radiol. 2018;28(4):1662–72.

25. Moshina N, Sagstad S, Sebuodegard S, Waade GG, Gran E, Music J, Hofvind S. Breast compression and reported pain during mammographic screening. Radiography. 2020;26(2):133–9.

26. Moshina N, Sebuodegard S, Evensen KT, Hantho C, Iden KA, Hofvind S. Breast compression and experienced pain during mammography by use of three different compression paddles. Eur J Radiol. 2019;115:59–65.

27. Feder K, Grunert JH. Is Individualizing Breast Compression during Mammography useful? - Investigations of pain indications during mammography relating to compression force and surface area of the compressed breast. RöFo. 2017;189(1):39–48.

28. Moshina N, Sebuodegard S, Holen AS, Waade GG, Tsuruda K, Hofvind S. The impact of compression force and pressure at prevalent screening on subsequent re-attendance in a national screening program. Prev Med. 2018;108:129–36.

29. de Groot JE, Branderhorst W, Grimbergen CA, den Heeten GJ, Broeders MJM. Towards personalized compression in mammography: a comparison study between pressure- and force-standardization. Eur J Radiol. 2015;84(3):384–91.

30. den Boer D, Dam-Vervloet LAJ, Boomsma MF, de Boer E, van Dalen JA, Poot L. Clinical validation of a pressure-standardized compression mammography system. Eur J Radiol. 2018;105:251–4.

31. Jeukens C, van Dijk T, Berben C, Wildberger JE, Lobbes MBI. Evaluation of pressure-controlled mammography compression paddles with respect to force-controlled compression paddles in clinical practice. Eur Radiol. 2019;29(5):2545–52.

32. Christiaens D, van Lier MG, Goris HK, Claikens B. Mammographic examination cycle time decreased after introducing a real-time pressure indicator in two independent radiology departments. EUSOBI. 2019;

33. Serwan E, Matthews D, Davies J, Chau M. Mammographic compression practices of force- and pressure-standardisation protocol: a scoping review. J Med Radiat Sci. 2020;67(3):233–42.

34. van Lier MGJTB, de Groot JE, Muller S, den Heeten GJ, Schilling KJ. Pressure-based compression guidance of the breast in digital breast tomosynthesis using flexible paddles compared to conventional compression. J Breast Imag. 2020;2(6):541–51.

35. Broeders MJ, Ten Voorde M, Veldkamp WJ, van Engen RE, van Landsveld-Verhoeven C, NL't Jong-Gunneman M, de Win J, Broogh-de Greve K, Paap E, den Heeten GJ. Comparison of a flexible versus a rigid breast compression paddle: pain experience, projected breast area, radiation dose and technical image quality. Eur Radiol. 2015;25(3):821–9.

36. Moshina N, Sebuodegard S, Hofvind S. Is breast compression associated with breast cancer detection and other early performance measures in a population-based breast cancer screening program? Breast Cancer Res Treat. 2017;163(3):605–13.

37. Holland K, Sechopoulos I, Mann RM, den Heeten GJ, van Gils CH, Karssemeijer N. Influence of breast compression pressure on the performance of population-based mammography screening. Breast Cancer Res. 2017;19(1):1–8.

38. Moshina N, Larsen M, Holen AS, Waade GG, Aase HS, Hofvind S. Digital breast tomosynthesis in a population based mammographic screening program: breast compression and early performance measures. Eur J Radiol. 2021;139:109665.

Supplementary Projections

29

Judith Kelly, Hannah Kearsley, Lyndsay A. Kinnear, and Sheetal Ruparelia

Learning Objectives
- Understand different techniques used within mammography to demonstrate all regions of breast tissue
- Demonstrate knowledge to apply evidence-based practice adaptations in supplementary techniques to improve both the client and practitioner outcomes
- Evaluate current radiographic practice against the gold standard techniques for supplementary projections

Introduction

Some breast abnormalities are located in the extreme medial or lateral aspects of the breast. The techniques described in Chap. 27, the practical mammography chapter, for the standard craniocaudal (CC) and mediolateral-oblique (MLO) projections do not image all the breast tissue in its entirety since these extreme aspects are usually not routinely included. In such cases supplementary projections are necessary to ensure significant abnormalities are not overlooked or misinterpreted in any assessment process. Examples include clinical presentation of a mass which is not seen on the standard projections or a partially demonstrated perceived abnormality in asymptomatic clients seen on a standard projection, but not on the corresponding projection [1]. Furthermore, a fictitious appearance may be created by overlapping breast tissue, simulating the appearance of a mass or architectural distortion [2]. Occasionally a perceived mammographic abnormality lies within the superficial skin layers or on the skin surface and projections utilising correlative radiopaque skin markers are required for confirmation of their location.

The availability of various additional supplementary projections is invaluable in assisting to solve some of these diagnostic dilemmas. Although more recently, we are seeing a significant increase in the use of Digital Breast Tomosynthesis (DBT) which is replacing some of the conventional supplementary mammography

J. Kelly (✉)
The Countess of Chester Hospitals NHS Foundation Trust, Chester, UK
e-mail: judith.kelly2@nhs.net

H. Kearsley
School of Health and Society, University of Salford, Manchester, UK
e-mail: H.S.Kearsley1@salford.ac.uk

L. A. Kinnear
Nightingale Centre, Wythenshawe Hospital, Manchester University NHS Foundation Trust, Manchester, UK
e-mail: lyndsay.kinnear@mft.nhs.uk

S. Ruparelia
Credit Valley Hospital, Mississauga, ON, Canada

views in non-calcific, screen-detected mammographic abnormalities [3]. This section describes
techniques to perform the most frequently
employed supplementary projections. The positions for the client are likely to be difficult to
maintain and therefore accuracy and efficiency
are particularly important practitioner skills.

The ability to decide which supplementary
views are appropriate and when to utilise them
are important skills that all practitioners should
develop under the direction of a healthcare professional trained in mammographic image
interpretation [4]. Please note, when performing
supplementary projections practitioners are
advised to refer to the comprehensive general
guidance on positioning, AEC considerations,
application of compression force and repetitive
strain risk reduction techniques described earlier
within this book.

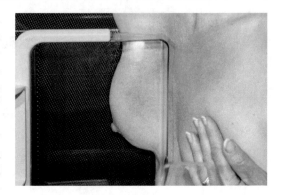

Fig. 29.1 Correct mediolateral positioning

wards until the lateral aspect is fully resting against
the image receptor and the corner is in the axilla.
Compression is applied and exposure performed,
ensuring the inframammary angle is well demonstrated and nipple in profile. Figure 29.1 illustrates
positioning technique for this projection.

Lateral Images: Mediolateral Approach

Contextual Use

A true lateral is likely to be performed to give a
more accurate indication of the location of an
abnormality (especially the actual depth); clarify
the presence/absence of a possible abnormality
seen on one or both standard CC/MLO projections. It can also give clearer visualisation of the
inframammary angle and inferior border; provide
post image-guided localisation of a radiopaque
marker or wire [5].

Positioning Technique

The mammography machine should be in a vertical position so the breast will be imaged at a true
90° to the horizontal. Positioning should commence with the client standing (or seated) facing
the machine and the lateral edge of the chest (left
or right, depending on which breast is to be
imaged) parallel to the image receptor. The ipsilateral arm should be raised and rested across the
machine. The breast is then lifted upwards and for-

Lateral Images: Lateromedial Approach

Contextual Use

To demonstrate a particular lesion that is closer to
the lateral aspect than the medial aspect. This
view can often be performed during a stereotactic
biopsy procedure, to clarify the presence/absence
of a possible abnormality seen on one or both
standard CC/MLO projections, including the
same depth as demonstrated on the CC projection. It can provide clearer visualisation of the
inframammary angle and inferior border [5].

Positioning Technique

The machine is positioned as for the lateral
image - mediolateral approach. The client is positioned again facing the machine with the image
receptor outer edge in line with the sternum. The
ipsilateral arm is raised and rested across the
machine with the elbow slightly flexed. The
breast should be lifted upwards and forwards
away from the chest wall until the sternum is rest-

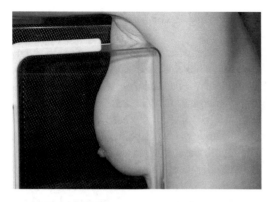

Fig. 29.2 Correct lateromedial positioning

ing against the machine and the medial breast in contact with the image receptor. Position the nipple in profile, bearing in mind this can be more difficult to achieve in the lateromedial projection. Figure 29.2 illustrates positioning technique for this projection.

Laterally Extended Cranio Caudal Projection

Contextual Use

To demonstrate a lesion that is located within the upper/lower outer aspect of the breast, where a large proportion of breast carcinomas can develop.

Region Demonstrated

This maximises visualisation of lateral, axilla and axillary tail breast tissue. The medial breast will be excluded. Pectoral muscle should be demonstrated in the lateral aspect of the image and the nipple will point towards the medial [5].

Positioning Technique

The machine angle should be raised from the horizontal approximately 5–10° laterally. Positioning should commence as for a standard CC projection (Chap. 27) with the breast lifted onto the image receptor and the nipple in pro-

file. The client is then rotated approximately 60° away from the right or left side (depending on which breast is being imaged). Keeping their arm and shoulder as relaxed as possible the lateral breast and axillary region are moved into the imaging field and compression applied whilst ensuring the elimination of any skin folds. Care should be taken not to include any aspect of the shoulder or other body part within the region of interest before performing the exposure.

Medially Extended Craniocaudal Projection

Contextual Use

To demonstrate a lesion that is located within the most medial portion of the breast.

Region Demonstrated

This maximises visualisation of medio-posterior part of the breast tissue, demonstrating lesions in the medial portion. The lateral breast will be excluded [5].

Positioning Technique

Positioning commences as for a standard CC projection (Chap. 27) and the breast is lifted onto the image receptor with the nipple in profile. If the left breast is being imaged the breast should be aligned marginally right of centre on the image receptor (the opposite applies for imaging the right breast). The medial aspect of the right breast should be lifted onto the image receptor to prevent pulling of the left breast and to assist visualisation of the cleavage. Ensure the maximum amount of medial breast tissue is included in the imaging field and eliminate all folds before applying compression and performing the exposure. For the contralateral breast a mirror image of this technique should be performed. Difficulty may be encountered with this projection in moving the client's head around the X-ray tube housing and careful manipulation is therefore required.

Mediolateral Axillary Tail Projection

Contextual Use

To demonstrate a lesion that is only shown in the axillary tail of the MLO projection, to demonstrate the most lateral portion of the breast. This view is also beneficial when locating axillary clips/magnetic seeds.

Region Demonstrated

This maximises visualisation of the axillary tail, pectoral muscle and low axilla, where lymph gland involvement is suspected, as it demonstrates tissue high up into the axilla [5].

Positioning Technique

Set the mammography machine and commence positioning initially for a standard mediolateral oblique projection as described earlier in Chap. 27. The machine is then raised higher to include more of the breast axillary tail and lower axilla regions. The affected shoulder should be as relaxed as possible and compression applied, making sure the humeral head and clavicle are not caught by the compression paddle.

Extended Craniocaudal (Cleopatra) Projection

Contextual Use

To demonstrate a lesion that is more laterally orientated.

Region Demonstrated

This maximises visualisation in the extreme outer quadrant and axillary tail.

Positioning Technique

Commence as for a standard CC projection and then rotate the client medially to demonstrate the lateral outer quadrant (of whichever breast is under examination). The image receptor may be angled 5–10° laterally to help facilitate the positioning and avoid including the humeral head. The nipple should be placed at the medial aspect of the image receptor as this enables the client to be leaned back onto the lateral aspect, allowing maximum demonstration of the outer breast tissue. Lift the breast onto the image receptor and manipulate into position, eliminate skin creases and apply compression as usual [2].

Digital Breast Tomosynthesis

The introduction of Digital Breast Tomosynthesis (DBT) into many breast imaging units in recent years has inevitably led to a decline in the need to perform some of the supplementary views described in this chapter. DBT reduces the effect of superimposition of breast tissue and can be used for assessment of perceived abnormalities and is also able to clarify whether an abnormality lies within the superficial skin layers [5, 6]. DBT is described in more detail in Chap. 37.

Studies have shown that DBT is at least as accurate as coned compression projections in the assessment of non-calcified abnormalities and that it significantly improves diagnostic accuracy by clearer characterisation of lesions in comparison to other supplementary mammographic projections [7].

Contextual Use

To locate accurately the depth of a lesion and remove the visually obstructive effect of breast tissue superimposition.

Region Demonstrated

The region demonstrated will be dependent on the location/area of interest. DBT can be performed in the standard CC or MLO projections or in one of the supplementary projections discussed in this chapter. DBT will be discussed in more detail in Chap. 38.

Equipment

A fixed DBT face guard allows the client to rest their head/face while the X-ray tube moves in an arc. This may be used for all imaging or attached just for DBT projections (please check the manufacturers recommendations). Ensure the exposure settings are correct as per local departmental protocol before positioning. There are generally three options available:

Exposure setting	Imaging acquired
DBT	Slices (± slabs dependent on manufacturer)
DBT + Synthetic View	Slices (± slabs dependent on manufacturer) and a 2D synthetic view, reconstructed from DBT data
DBT + 2D	Slices (± slabs dependent on manufacturer) and 2D image, additional exposure for 2D view required

Select the appropriate paddle size. Be mindful of lateral or medial 'cut off' as the X-ray tube moves in an arc as the images/slices are acquired.

Positioning Technique

Position the client as normal for the projection being performed. Some literature suggests using a compression force sufficient to retain the breast securely in position during the procedure. However, to date there is no evidence-based research to support using any alternative to the compression force recommended in Chaps. 27 and 28 for standard mammographic projections [8].

Cleavage Projection

Contextual Use

To be used in the most medial and midline lesions that cannot be seen when performing the standard MLO.

Region Demonstrated

Maximises the volume of medioposterior breast tissue bilaterally and clearly shows the cleavage.

Positioning Technique

Commence positioning as for a CC projection but keep the client centralised rather than off set to one side as is the case when performing separate right or left breast imaging. Lift both breasts forwards separately and rest them onto the image receptor. Lean the client inwards to maximize visualisation of the inner breast. Place a thumb on each medial aspect and rotate the breasts laterally to demonstrate fully the medial regions while applying compression. Figures 29.3 and 29.4 illustrate ideal positioning technique for this projection. It is important that a manual exposure is selected (guided by a previously recorded CC projection) to avoid the AEC delivering a suboptimal exposure.

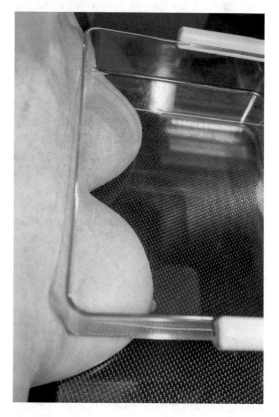

Fig. 29.3 Correct cleavage view positioning

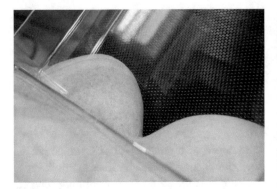

Fig. 29.4 Correct cleavage view positioning

Nipple in Profile Projection

Contextual Use

To be used when the nipple is not in profile on at least one of the images during standard CC and MLO projections. The nipple needs to be in profile so that the ducts are parallel to the image receptor and thus can be visualised adequately. Ducts that are *en face* or perpendicular to the image receptor are not able to be evaluated correctly.

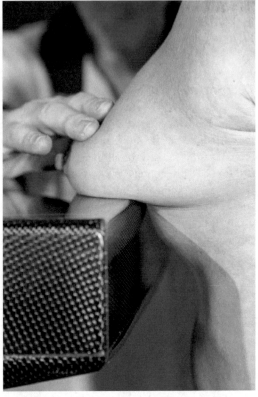

Fig. 29.5 Positioning for nipple in profile

Region Demonstrated

The nipple should be in perfect profile to demonstrate the subareola structures. This provides clarification that a perceived mass on a standard CC view (where the nipple was not in profile) is in fact the nipple superimposed onto the adjacent breast tissue. This also facilitates accurate orientation, allowing measurement of the location of a perceived abnormality in relation to the nipple.

Positioning Technique

Technique should mirror the standard CC (or MLO/ML) positioning initially but concentration should focus on ensuring the nipple is projected in profile. Demonstration of the breast posterior aspect is of lesser importance. Apply compres-

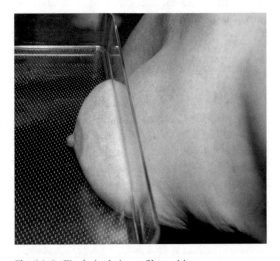

Fig. 29.6 Final nipple in profile position

sion as described for the standard projections earlier in this chapter. Figures 29.5 and 29.6 illustrate ideal positioning technique for this projection in the CC view.

Inverted Craniocaudal Projection

Contextual Use

Can be used when the client is kyphotic, whereby the head and chin would cause artefact on the standard CC projection. This is also known as the FB view ('from below').

Region Demonstrated

Demonstrates an inverted CC image of inferior technical quality to a standard CC due to the difficulties involved in physically performing this projection. The posterior aspect of the breast and pectoral muscle are unlikely to be imaged. It is imperative that the image is orientated accurately for image readers to enable the location of perceived abnormalities to be correlated with precision in relation to the other projections performed (i.e. MLO).

Positioning Technique

This technique is seldom used in practice yet indications to perform it are for clients with extreme kyphosis whose head and shoulders would superimpose the breast on a standard CC projection. The ability of the mammography machine to accommodate this positioning should be ascertained prior to any attempt at positioning. Commence positioning as for a standard CC view but the breast weight will be supported by the compression paddle therefore careful manipulation is required. This projection requires the involvement of two practitioners due to the technical challenges and the fact that the client may have limited mobility. Aim to maximize the volume of breast tissue included in the imaging field and apply the compression force appropriately whilst supporting the breast. Care should be taken not to trap practitioner hands within the equipment. Figures 29.7 and 29.8 illustrate ideal positioning technique for this projection. It is important to note that this position is unlikely to be feasible in large breasted clients.

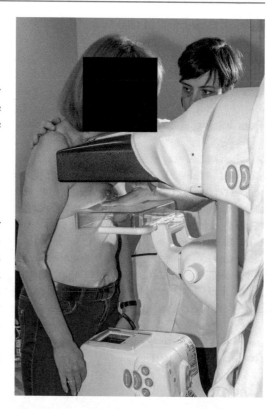

Fig. 29.7 Positioning for inverted craniocaudal projection

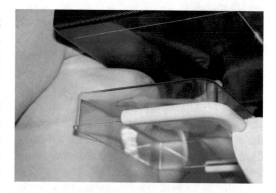

Fig. 29.8 Final inverted craniocaudal position

Projections Using Skin Markers to Localise Skin Lesions/ Tangential View

Contextual Use

To try and distinguish if a lesion is on the skin or within the breast; to save unnecessary biopsy attempts.

Region Demonstrated

To distinguish or prove skin lesion, palpable mass or dermal calcifications.

Positioning Technique

A suitable radiopaque marker (there are multiple varieties available commercially) should be placed on the skin over the lesion in question and an appropriate projection selected to demonstrate best the abnormality which correlates with the original mammogram. Position the breast so the radiopaque marker is tangential to the beam by either angling the tube, the client or the breast, alternatively position radiopaque marker to appear as a nipple in profile view.

Rolled Projection

Contextual Use

To avoid superimposition of lesions and overlying structures.

Region Demonstrated

These projections are adapted from the standard CC and MLO positions and are an alternative, effective way to solve equivocal mammography findings by separating overlapping structures from each other and differentiating summation artefacts from genuine lesions [9]. Such projections should be performed under the direction of an individual qualified to interpret mammograms and in conjunction with other additional projections such as coned compression views.

Positioning Technique

The rolled view changes the breast positioning but not the obliquity of the X-ray beams. From the CC position, the breast is rolled in either the medial or lateral direction. For example, while the upper part of the breast is rolled medially (from lateral to medial), the inner part changes its position laterally along the X-axis of the breast. In the MLO position, the breast is rolled in either the inferior or superior direction. The lateral aspect is rolled inferiorly (from superior to inferior) whilst the medial aspect changes its position in the opposite direction. Compression should then be applied as described for the standard projections.

Clinical Pearls
- As a practitioner it is important to understand the contextual uses of all of the different supplementary projections adopted in mammography
- As a practitioner it is important to be able to apply the radiographic principles and positioning techniques demonstrated in this chapter into clinical practice

---

Chapter Review Questions
Review Questions

1. Why are supplementary mammographic projections sometimes required?
2. Which supplementary mammographic projection(s) maximise the visualisation of the lateral and axillary tail breast tissue?
3. What is the mediolateral projection used to demonstrate?

Answers

1. The standard mammographic projections do not image the breast tissue in its entirety, as the extreme medial and lateral aspects are not routinely included.
2. The laterally extended CC projection and the extended CC (Cleopatra) projection.
3. The presence/absence of a possible abnormality seen on a standard projection; An accurate indication of the depth of an abnormality; Clearer visualisation of the inframammary angle; To confirm the position of a radiopaque marker or wire.

Acknowledgments The author is most grateful to the professional photographer Gill Brett for her photographic skills and the team from the Nightingale Centre, Manchester University NHS Foundation Trust, for directing and arranging the production of the photographs in this chapter.

Appendix

Test your learning and check your understanding of this book's contents: use the "Springer Nature Flashcards" app to access questions using https://sn.pub/dcAnWL.

To use the app, please follow the instructions in Chap. 1.

Flashcard code:

48341-69945-ABCB1-2A8C7-CE9D2.

Short URL: https://sn.pub/dcAnWL.

References

1. Feig S. The importance of supplementary mammographic views to diagnostic accuracy. Am J Roentgenol. 1988;151(1):40–1.

2. Barbarkoff D, Gatewood MD, Brem RF. Supplemental views for equivocal mammographic findings: a pictorial essay. Breast J. 2000;6(1):34–43.

3. Whelehan P, Heywang-Köbrunner SH, Vinnicombe SJ, Hacker A, Jaensch A, Hapca A, Gray R, Jenkin M, Lowry K, Oeppen R, Reilly M. Clinical performance of Siemens digital breast tomosynthesis versus standard supplementary mammography for the assessment of screen-detected soft-tissue abnormalities: a multi-reader study. Clin Radiol. 2017;72(1):95–e9.

4. Sickles EA. Practical solutions to common mammographic problems: tailoring the examination. Am J Roentgenol. 1988;151(1):31–9.

5. Whitley AS, Jefferson G, Holmes K, Sloane C, Anderson C, Hoadley G. Clark's positioning in radiography 13E. CRC Press; 2015.

6. Helvie MA. Digital mammography imaging: breast tomosynthesis and advanced applications. Radiol Clin North Am. 2010;48(5):917–29.

7. Michell MJ, Batohi B. Role of tomosynthesis in breast imaging going forward. Clin Radiol. 2018;73(4):358–71.

8. Agasthya GA, D'Orsi E, Kim YJ, Handa P, Ho CP, D'Orsi CJ, Sechopoulos I. Can breast compression be reduced in digital mammography and breast tomosynthesis? AJR. 2017;209(5):W322.

9. Alimoglu E, Ceken K, Kabaalioglu A, Cassano E, Sindel T. An effective way to solve equivocal mammography findings: the rolled views. Breast Care (Basel). 2010;5(4):241–5.

Magnification and Compression Views

30

Victoria L. Ebanks

Learning Objectives
- Explain why further mammographic views are needed and justify which views are specific to each abnormality
- Analyse the difference between equipment set up for coned compression views versus magnification views
- Describe the positioning for further mammographic views in the craniocaudal and lateral views with and without magnification

Introduction

Following initial mammography imaging (craniocaudal and mediolateral oblique views), an abnormality may be perceived which requires further analysis. Clear mammographic presentation of a lesion or microcalcification is crucial for accurate assessment. Identifiable masses such as cysts, fibroadenomas and larger carcinomas usually proceed to an ultrasound examination without the requirement for further mammographic

V. L. Ebanks (✉)
Breast Imaging, Whipps Cross Hospital, Barts Health NHS Trust, London, UK
e-mail: victoria.ebanks@nhs.net

views [1–3]. Many masses demonstrated as microcalcification or an asymmetrical density may not be instantly identifiable on the initial mammograms and will need further assessment with specialised mammography [2]. The location of the abnormality in the breast can be confirmed by obtaining a lateral view, particularly in the case of microcalcification, which enables the microcalcification to be characterised [3]. Conventional imaging using magnification views to fully evaluate microcalcification remains the gold standard over tomosynthesis [3, 4].

Magnification Views

Magnification views are used mainly for the mammographic analysis of microcalcification produced by very tiny deposits of calcium phosphate, or calcium oxalate, resulting from a secretory lesion or malignancy [3]. Microcalcification is minute (50–300 µm) and for an accurate radiological examination, the image must be as sharp as possible. Magnification views allow morphological evaluation and assessment of the extent of the microcalcification [3, 5].

Magnification views facilitate the interpreting practitioner to assess the area of microcalcification for size, shape and distribution of the particles. This informs the next stage of the diagnostic workup process. Digital mammography allows the images to be manipulated post acquisition. Acquiring geometrically magnified images is preferable to the use of an electronic zoom function because the initial mammograms do not always demonstrate all the microcalcification present [6, 7]; the initial mammogram is simply increased in size (zoomed) and may not demonstrate subtle microcalcification, which may be better detected on the geometrically magnified views.

A magnification table is used to create a distance between the breast and the detector, creating a geometrically magnified image. This is attached to the mammography equipment in exchange for the regular platform. The magnification board may be constructed of carbon fibre or polycarbonate and is therefore lightweight; the anti-scatter grid is excluded in this set up.

Magnification views are subject to some compounding issues. The distance created between the breast and the detector results in increased geometric unsharpness, which may affect the resultant image. In conventional radiography, the X-Ray tube focus can be moved further from the object, decreasing the effect of geometric unsharpness; but this is not possible in mammography due to the fixed height of the tube. As a result, there would be increased dose to the breast, therefore a grid is not used. High image resolution is maintained, despite the absence of an anti-scatter grid in the magnification table caused by the air gap between the breast and the detector [8]. The use of a fine focal spot size and the high resolution of the detector also maximises image resolution for this, along with a limited range of magnification factors [7]. These can vary between manufacturers but are usually ×1.5 (Fig. 30.1) to ×2.0 (Fig. 30.2) [9]; a difference in object to detector difference is clearly demonstrated.

When selecting the paddle for magnification views, the practitioner should be aware that they are sometimes different to those used for coned compression views. For some manufacturers, the paddle for the magnification view has a *straight arm*. There are different sized paddles available which allows small and large areas to be focused on appropriately. A small paddle should be chosen for smaller abnormal areas, whilst a larger one is reserved for a more extensive abnormality.

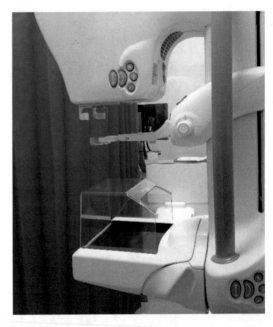

Fig. 30.1 Mammography equipment set up for ×1.5 magnification view

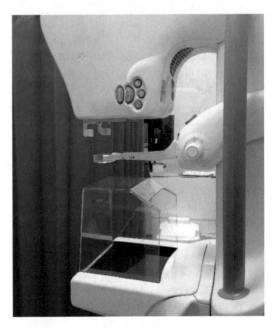

Fig. 30.2 Mammography equipment set up for ×1.8 magnification view

A larger paddle is used with a lower magnification table, utilising a greater field of view (FOV). An example of the choice of paddles for magnification views is illustrated in Fig. 30.3.

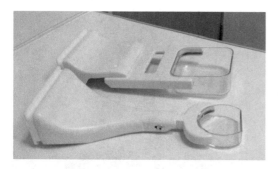

Fig. 30.3 A choice of paddles for magnification views (General Electric)

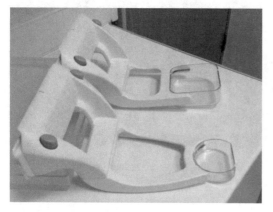

Fig. 30.4 A choice of paddles for coned compression/paddle views (General Electric)

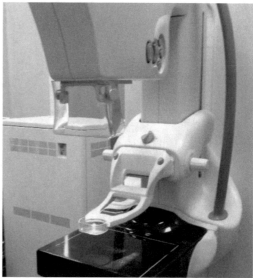

Fig. 30.5 Mammography equipment setup for coned compression/paddle views

which allow a smaller or larger area to be focused on. The image is acquired with the breast positioned directly on the usual contact surface (Fig. 30.5).

Coned Compression Views

Coned compression views, or paddle views, are another tool for evaluating an abnormality in the breast following initial mammography. This technique is used typically to facilitate characterisation of a mass, an asymmetrical density, or a parenchymal distortion demonstrated on initial imaging. The main tool for compression views is the focal compression paddle. These may differ from those used for magnification views in that the *arm of the paddle is curved* (Fig. 30.4).

This allows the paddle to apply focal pressure concentrated on the abnormal area. As with the magnification paddle, there are different sized paddles for coned compression views

Mammographic Technique

The same mammography procedure applies to both techniques, but the equipment set up utilised is different. Using the initial mammograms for reference, a measurement using the integrated digital caliper from the nipple to the abnormality should be taken, which will need to be done for each orientation. It is useful to document these details. Measurements obtained, for example, may be as follows: 4 cm deep to the nipple and 2 cm laterally. This is then transferred back to the client to obtain the same location as that seen on the mammograms. If possible, display the images in the imaging room for reference purposes. (NB This measurement process is more complex if the nipple is not demonstrated in profile on the original mammograms).

Localising the Abnormal Area:

- Each contact view is uploaded in turn on to the mammographic workstation.
- The abnormal area is confirmed by the reporting practitioner.
- The linear measuring tool is selected.
- A horizontal line is drawn from the nipple posteriorly to the level of the abnormal area.
- A vertical line (on the image) is then drawn to the abnormality.
- Two measurements will be presented on the screen which should be documented for reference (Figs. 30.6 and 30.7).
- If two separate further views are required, this procedure should then be repeated for the other projection.

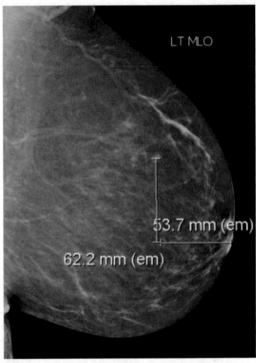

Fig. 30.7 Illustration of lesion localisation measurements in MLO projection

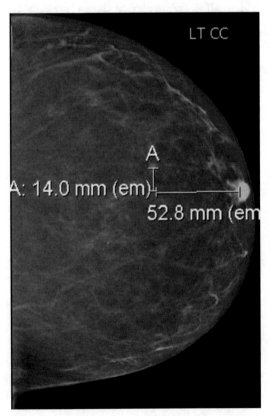

Fig. 30.6 Illustration of lesion localisation measurements in CC projection

The positioning for coned compression and magnification views is similar to that used for routine mammograms (Chap. 27). The technique used for the magnification views will require adaptation due to the height of the magnification table and X-Ray tube head. The practitioner should prepare the imaging room and should select the correct identifying details from the work list at the acquisition station. Digital mammography equipment usually acknowledges the magnification table and the specific compression paddles, therefore preselecting an automatic exposure, but this should be confirmed.

The vast majority of clients attending for assessment of a perceived abnormality will be anxious and will require sensitive communication. A member of the breast imaging team will need to explain to the client the reason why further imaging is required; this should not provoke anxiety or be over reassuring, as this is not in the best interests of the client [10] (Refer to Chaps. 12 and 13 for additional information).

The client should be asked to undress to the waist and the positioning directed as follows:

- Position the client in front of the mammography machine in the same way used for a routine mammogram (Chap. 27), with their feet hips width apart.
- Their head should be turned away from the affected side, ensuring that there is no superimposition of their ears or hair over the area of interest.
- The light beam diaphragm should be turned on.
- The practitioner should raise the affected breast on to the contact surface or magnification table (for magnification views) using their opposing hand.
- Locate the abnormal area on the corresponding skin surface of the breast using the previously obtained measurements. It is often useful to identify this with an inked skin mark, but client consent should be sought first. The practitioner should adjust the position of the breast to align the area of interest within the field of view.
- Apply a small amount of compression to the breast just to hold it taught in place.
- Re-check the position using the original measurements.
- Once an accurate position has been achieved, the breast can then be compressed for imaging. The breast will feel tense when pressed adjacent to the paddle. This can feel uncomfortable due to the focal pressure, so this should be explained to the client.
- The exposure is completed using an automatic selection and not a manual exposure. This is to ensure that the most accurate exposure is given to allow image interpretation, and to avoid repeat X-Ray exposures.

Case Studies

The mammographic positioning is illustrated in the following case studies. These cases demonstrate how the practitioner would identify the location of the abnormality on the mammograms, apply this to the client, and position for each image.

Case A: Paddle Views

An asymmetrical density is seen in the upper outer quadrant of the left breast as shown above. The integrated digital caliper is used to measure the distance from it to the nipple. This is so that the practitioner can position the client accurately for imaging. The same procedure is used for each view required; though it is often only necessary to image the asymmetrical density in one projection.

The breast is manoeuvred so that the correct area of interest (as marked on the skin) is positioned centrally within the field of view (Figs. 30.8 and 30.9). The compression paddle is first applied gently and, once satisfactory positioning is achieved, additional compression force can be applied.

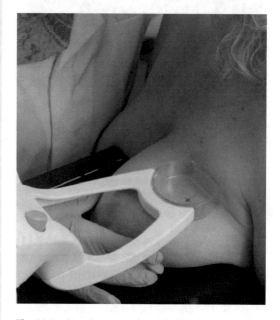

Fig. 30.8 Coned compression CC view

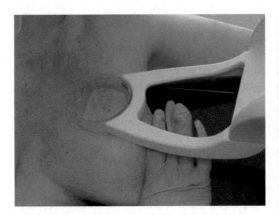

Fig. 30.9 Coned compression MLO view

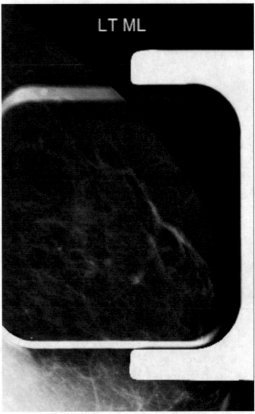

Fig. 30.11 Coned compression image in the MLO position with spiculate mass shown centrally

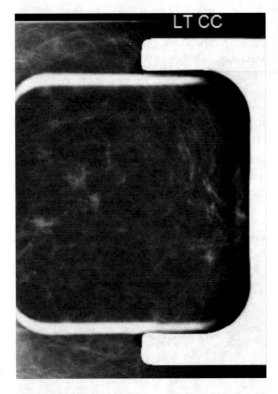

Fig. 30.10 Coned compression craniocaudal image with spiculate mass shown centrally

during compression with no smooth margins visualised.

Case B: Magnification Views

A focus of pleomorphic microcalcification is demonstrated in the lower inner quadrant of the right breast. A lateral view was completed as an additional view. Measurements were then taken from the nipple to the focus of microcalcification, using the CC and lateral views (Figs. 30.12 and 30.13).

The client is then positioned accurately for each projection using the measurements. The height of the mammography machine will require adaptation once the magnification table is

The resulting images (Figs. 30.10 and 30.11) should include the area of interest in the centre of the image. It can be demonstrated from this case that the density is a spiculate mass (Figs. 30.10 and 30.11); as this remains visible

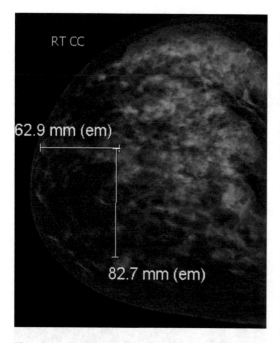

Fig. 30.12 The digital caliper is used on the craniocaudal view to identify the location of the abnormal microcalcification

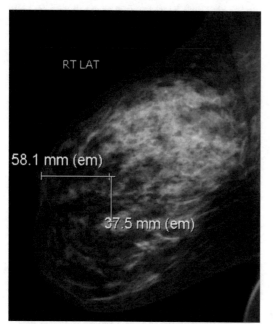

Fig. 30.13 The digital caliper is again used to localise the area of the microcalcification in the lateral position

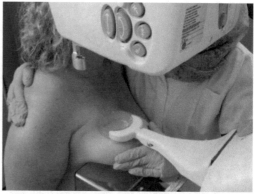

Fig. 30.14 Position for craniocaudal magnification view

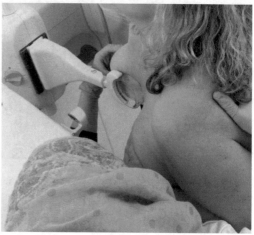

Fig. 30.15 Position for lateral magnification view

attached. The breast is maneuvered so that the area of interest, as marked on the skin, can be positioned centrally within the field of view (Figs. 30.14 and 30.15). The compression paddle is firstly applied gently and, once satisfactory positioning is achieved, additional compression is then applied.

An MLO image should not be used to obtain measurements which are then transferred to a client who is positioned for a lateral view.

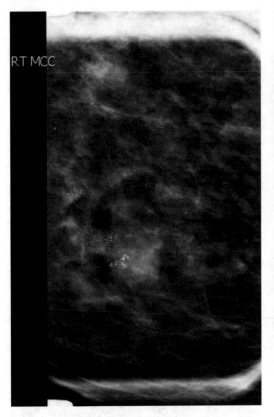

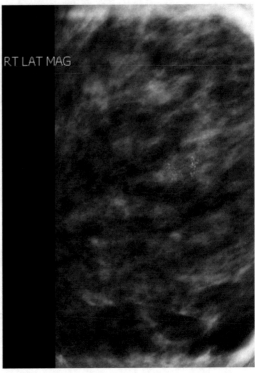

Fig. 30.17 Resultant lateral magnification image showing the abnormal microcalcification positioned centrally within the field of view

Fig. 30.16 Resultant craniocaudal magnification image showing the abnormal microcalcification positioned centrally within the field of view

The shape and distribution of the focus of microcalcification can now be seen with greater clarity on the resulting images (Figs. 30.16 and 30.17). A larger extent of this calcification can be visualised in these two views, due to magnification of the area and the high resolution of the resultant images. Often only one view is requested for additional imaging.

Sometimes the abnormality will lie deep in the breast and it may be difficult to place the abnormality within the field of view using the typical positioning. In these cases, reversing the angle of the mammography machine (as if you were positioning for the other breast) and then positioning the client so that the medial aspect of the breast is closest to the detector, may assist in this.

Clinical Pearls
- Conventional magnification views remain the gold standard for the assessment of foci of microcalcification over tomosynthesis.
- Digital zooming of mammograms does not provide the same quality of image to allow accurate morphological assessment and area of extent in the same way magnification views demonstrates them.
- Coned compression views are used to confirm the presence of an asymmetrical density or further assess architectural distortion and mass lesions.
- The mammographic technique for both magnification views and coned compression views is the same, but the equipment configuration differs.

Chapter Review Questions
Review Questions

1. What possible effect is caused by performing magnified X-Rays and how is this specifically overcome in mammography to maintain the quality of the image?
2. What should practitioners be aware of when performing coned compression versus magnification views in terms of paddle selection?
3. How would practitioners locate the abnormal area to perform magnification or coned compression views from the contact views?

Answers

1. Geometric unsharpness is a degrading effect caused by performing magnification views. In general radiography, the X-Ray tube can be moved further back away from the object. However, in mammography this is not possible, so the anti-scatter grid is removed to minimise radiation dose to the breast and improve image sharpness.
2. The paddles for magnification views may differ to those for coned compression views. The ones for coned compression may have a curved arm.

   There are smaller paddles for smaller abnormal regions and larger paddles for more diffuse change. The smallest paddle for the abnormal region should be used to minimize radiation exposure to the glandular breast tissue, as the field is focused to the paddle size.
3. Each contact view is uploaded in turn on to the mammographic workstation.

   The abnormal area is confirmed by the reporting practitioner.

   The linear measuring tool is selected.

   A horizontal line is drawn from the nipple posteriorly to the level of the abnormal area.

   A vertical line (on the image) is then drawn to the abnormality.

   Two measurements will be presented on the screen which should be documented for reference.

If two separate further views are required, this procedure should then be repeated for the other projection.

Write each location down on paper so that these details can be easily transferred to the patient when in the mammography room.

Appendix

Test your learning and check your understanding of this book's contents: use the "Springer Nature Flashcards" app to access questions using https://sn.pub/dcAnWL.

To use the app, please follow the instructions in Chap. 1.

Flashcard code:

48341-69945-ABCB1-2A8C7-CE9D2.

Short URL: https://sn.pub/dcAnWL.

References

1. Harris JR, Lippman ME, Morrow M, Osborne CK. Diseases of the breast. 5th ed. Philadelphia: Wolters Kluwer Health; 2014.
2. Michell MJ. Breast cancer. 1st ed. Cambridge: Cambridge University Press; 2010.
3. Wallis M, Borrelli C, Cohen S, Duncan A, Given-Wilson R, Jenkins J, Kearins O, Pinder S, Sharma N, Sibbering M, Steel J. Clinical guidance for breast cancer screening assessment - Publication No. 49. 4th ed. London: Public Health England; 2016.
4. PHE (Public Health England). Guidance breast screening: digital breast tomosynthesis. Available from: https://www.gov.uk/government/publications/breast-screening-digital-breast-tomosynthesis/breast-screening-digital-breast-tomosynthesis. Accessed 7 July 2021.
5. Haghayeghi K, Najibi M, Wang H, Donegan L, Wang Y. Clinicopathologic update of calcium oxalate in breast: a 15-year retrospective review. Breast J. 2020 Sep;26(9):1736–41.
6. Kim MJ, Youk JH, Kang DR, Choi SH, Kwak JY, Son EJ, Kim E-K. Zooming method (x2.0) of digital mammography vs digital magnification view (x1.8) in full-field digital mammography for the diagnosis of microcalcifications. Br J Radiol. 2010;83(990):486–92.
7. Koutalonis M, Delis H, Pascoal A, Spyrou G, Costaridou L, Panayiotakis G. Can electronic zooming replace magnification in mammography?

A comparative Monte Carlo study. Br J Radiol. 2010;83(991):569–77.

8. McParland BJ. Image quality and dose in film-screen magnification mammography. Br J Radiol. 2000;73(874):1068–77.

9. Park HS, Oh Y, Kim ST, Kim HJ. Effects of breast thickness and lesion location on resolution in digi-tal magnification mammography. Clin Imaging. 2012;36(4):255–62.

10. Harvey JA, Cohen MA, Brenin DR, Nicholson BT, Adams RB. Breaking bad news: a primer for radiologists in breast imaging. J Am Coll Radiol. 2007;4(11):800–8.

Specimen Imaging

Amanda Coates and Rachel Reilly

Learning Objectives
- Understand the requirements of specimen imaging in mammography
- Describe and appreciate the different methods of obtaining images
- Report content of specimen imaging

Introduction

Imaging of specimens forms an important part in the diagnostic pathway and provides important information on accurate lesion sampling and radiologic and pathologic correlation [1]. Such imaging is performed using mammography imaging equipment or dedicated specimen cabinets. By using a magnification table or the compression paddle on a mammography machine, appearances of small lesions can be made clearer [2]. Updated mammography machines have a built-in facility to image biopsy specimens without removing the client from the biopsy device first. This system uses an attachment to collimate the X-Ray beam, shielding the client, combined with angulation of the tube head to enable the specimens to be placed on the image detector away from the client's breast (Fig. 31.1a, b). A dedicated specimen cabinet houses an X-Ray tube with either an adjustable transparent shelf to place the specimen on, or a tray to place the specimen samples in (Fig. 31.2). Specimen cabinets should be subjected to routine testing by Medical Physics. Image quality is of paramount importance and all specimen images should contain correct client information along with breast laterality.

A. Coates (✉) · R. Reilly
Breast Imaging, Mid Yorkshire Hospitals Trust,
Pinderfields Hospital, Wakefield, UK
e-mail: amanda.coates2@nhs.net

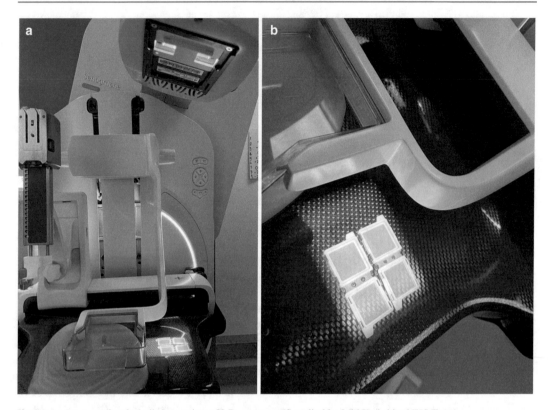

Fig. 31.1 An example of a built-in specimen X-Ray system (Supplied by Mid Yorkshire NHS Trust)

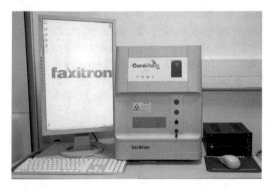

Fig. 31.2 An example of a dedicated specimen cabinet (Supplied by Nightingale Centre, University Hospital, South Manchester)

Types of Specimen Imaging and Reporting

There are three main types of breast specimen imaging:

- Diagnostic biopsy specimens
- Surgical excision specimens
- Fixed pathological specimens

Biopsy Specimen Imaging

The imaging of biopsy specimens, either 14 gauge or larger vacuum assisted biopsies, is usually to determine the presence of microcalcifications following stereotactic guided biopsies. This should be carried out prior to removal of the client from the mammography biopsy machine so further sampling can take place if calcification retrieval is inadequate (Fig. 31.3). Adequacy will be determined by the amount of calcification present before biopsy and local protocol. It has been suggested [3] that three or more samples containing calcification, or five flecks or more calcification in total, increases the likelihood of a successful biopsy and a definitive pathological diagnosis. Some pathologists prefer the separation of biopsy samples containing calcification from those without calcification. This allows the pathologist to concentrate and sample more comprehensively the tissue with known calcifications [4].

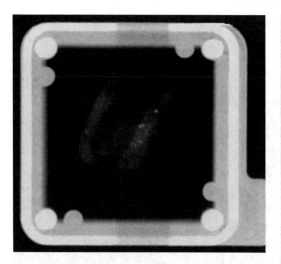

Fig. 31.3 Calcification identified in magnified core biopsy specimens

Within biopsy specimen reports, good practice would include the following:

- The number of samples obtained
- The number of samples which contain calcification
- If a marker clip was deployed
- The relationship between the marker clip and the area of calcification.

The report should be available to the pathologist before any multi-disciplinary team meeting (MDT) discussion takes place on future management, in order to correlate radiologic and pathologic findings.

Surgical Excision Specimen Imaging

Specimen radiography of non-palpable lesions excised during breast conservation surgery should take place before skin closure and be available to the surgeon so that determination of total lesion removal can be achieved. Surgical clips, sutures or colour coded inking are often used to orientate the specimen [5]. If the lesion appears to extend to a margin, the surgeon can make an appropriate further excision [6, 7]. An advantageous use of a specimen cabinet located in theatre would allow almost immediate results, reducing theatre/anaesthetic time.

As imaging of a specimen is a two-dimensional image of a three-dimensional object, imaging in more than one plane can be useful but not always easy to do, due to the shape of the specimen. If using mammography equipment, careful and slow use of the compression paddle, can often achieve this (Fig. 31.4a, b).

When reporting excision specimens, a description of whether good radiological margins have been achieved is important, and if this appears not to be the case, a description of which margin/s is thought to be involved. It is useful to indicate whether a wire, Magseed and or biopsy marker clip can be seen in the specimen and its relationship to the lesion excised. Lesion/abnormality size should be included and correlated with the original diagnostic imaging. This information will aid the pathologist to verify complete lesion excision and correlate radiological/pathological size. A radiological margin of <5 mm is reported as a risk factor for margin involvement [8] however, other research [9] demonstrates that a radiological margin of <11 mm is 58% likely to have histologically involved margins.

Often it is necessary to contact the operating theatre and speak to the surgeon to describe the findings. If this takes place, a notation on the radiology report of '*Theatres informed*' or '*Discussed with…*' can be useful, in case there is any uncertainty expressed later.

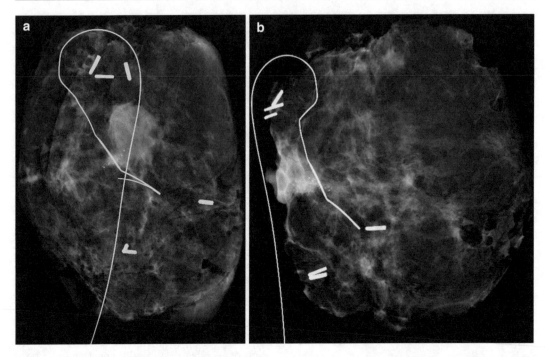

Fig. 31.4 Demonstration of a lesion appearing centrally in the excision (**a**) yet at the margin when an orthogonal view is obtained (**b**)

Fixed Pathology Specimen Imaging

Fixed pathology specimens are usually samples from a mastectomy where perhaps a small lesion in multifocal disease or calcifications cannot be located by pathologist observation [1]. Each slice will be labelled by the pathologist, numerical labelling being common. This may appear on the container the slice arrives in or alternative packaging. In order to match the slice to the image, this identification must be on the image itself, for example, numeric identification, slice 1, slice 2. This by far is the easiest form of identification, and lead numbers or pieces of lead shot of corresponding amount can be adhered to the image receptor before X-Ray exposure. Alternatively, free text can be annotated to the image before or after image storage, depending on equipment.

The reporting of fixed specimens usually requires a description of the findings in each slice. This will be determined by the information required, for example '*calcification seen in slices 5 and 6*' or '*5 mm spiculate mass seen in slice 3*' (Fig. 31.5).

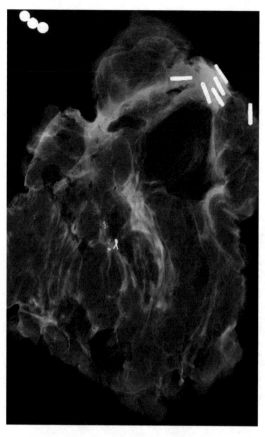

Fig. 31.5 Calcifications and biopsy marker clip demonstrated in fixed pathology sliced specimen. Lead shot used to indicate slice number

Clinical Pearls

Specimen imaging provides:

- Information on accurate lesion sampling
- Correlation between radiographic and pathologic findings

Chapter Review Questions
Review Questions

1. How are specimen images performed?
2. When should specimens be imaged?

Answers

1. Using dedicated mammography equipment and/or specimen X-Ray cabinets
2. Core biopsy specimens at the time of biopsy to ensure adequate lesion sampling

During surgical procedures to ensure complete excision and disease margin status.

Appendix

Test your learning and check your understanding of this book's contents: use the "Springer Nature Flashcards" app to access questions using https://sn.pub/dcAnWL.

To use the app, please follow the instructions in Chap. 1.

Flashcard code:

48341-69945-ABCB1-2A8C7-CE9D2.

Short URL: https://sn.pub/dcAnWL.

References

1. England PH. Quality assurance guidelines for breast pathology services, vol 2. Available from: https://www.gov.uk/government/publications/breast-screening-quality-assurance-guidelines-for-breast-pathology-services/breast-screening-quality-assurance-guidelines-for-screening-pathology-services. Accessed 4 Dec 2021.
2. Morrow M, Strom EA, Bassett LW, Dershaw DD, Fowble B, Harris JR, O'Malley F, Schnitt SJ, Singletary SE, Winchester DP. Standard for the management of ductal carcinoma in situ of the breast (DCIS). CA Cancer J Clin. 2002;52(5):256–76.
3. Bagnall M, Evans A, Wilson A, Burrell H, Pinder S, Ellis I. When have mammographic calcifications been adequately sampled at needle core biopsy? Clin Radiol. 2000;55(7):548–53.
4. Margolin FR, Kaufman L, Jacobs RP, Denny SR, Schrumpf JD. Stereotactic core breast biopsy of malignant calcifications: diagnostic yield of cores with and cores without calcifications on specimen radiographs. Radiology. 2004;233(1):251–4.
5. Volleamere AJ, Kirwan CC. National survey of breast cancer specimen orientation marking systems. Eur J Surg Oncol. 2013;39(3):255–9.

6. Amendoeira I, Perry N, Broeders M, de Wolf C, Törnberg S, Holland R, von Karsa L. European guidelines for quality assurance in breast cancer screening and diagnosis. European Commission; 2013.

7. Ihrai T, Quaranta D, Fouche Y, Machiavello JC, Raoust I, Chapellier C, Maestro C, Marcy M, Ferrero JM, Flipo B. Intraoperative radiological margin assessment in breast-conserving surgery. Eur J Surg Oncol (EJSO). 2014;40(4):449–53.

8. Mazouni C, Rouzier R, Balleyguier C, Sideris L, Rochard F, Delaloge S, Marsiglia H, Mathieu C, Spielman M, Garbay JR. Specimen radiography as predictor of resection margin status in non-palpable breast lesions. Clin Radiol. 2006;61(9):789–96.

9. Britton PD, Li S, Yamamoto AK, Koo B, Goud A. Breast surgical specimen radiographs: how reliable are they? Eur J Radiol. 2011;79(2):245–9.

Imaging the Augmented Breast

32

Claire Borrelli

Learning Objectives
- Understand how to perform the Eklund technique in mammography for clients presenting with breast augmentation to improve breast tissue visualisation.
- Recognise and understand the importance of breast awareness and signpost clients if they have concerns:
- about new symptoms
- following mammography
- regarding implant integrity

Introduction

Whilst mammography remains the gold standard for breast cancer imaging [1], the presence of breast implants in clients who have undergone breast augmentation represents an important imaging challenge. Breast implants may interfere with the accurate imaging of breast tissue and could also expose clients to risk factors such as implant rupture during the mammography procedure. Mammography performed by an experienced practitioner reduces the likelihood of rupture and other complications during the mammogram procedure. In addition, techniques are available to achieve successful breast imaging in clients with implants.

Consideration for Practitioners

Prior to mammography, clients with implants should be advised of the lack of efficacy of breast imaging due to the opaque nature of the implant and the possibility of reduced sensitivity with mammography. This is because the amount of compression force required for an optimal mammography study reduces the likelihood of adequately imaging the breast parenchyma [1].

A relevant breast history should be taken prior to undertaking the mammogram and information on the type of implant in situ should be obtained from the client, if possible. The practitioner should observe and record anything considered unusual, including differences in the size of the breasts, position of the nipple, skin colour of the breast and contour of the breast. Any differences should be discussed with the client prior to mammography. If a ruptured implant is suspected, it is advisable that mammography is not undertaken and local procedures should be followed [1].

C. Borrelli (✉)
St George's National Breast Education Centre, St George's University Hospital NHS Foundation Trust, London, UK
e-mail: claire.borrelli@stgeorges.nhs.uk

It is important to gain and record consent when imaging clients with implants. The practitioner must explain the use of minimum compression force and the likelihood that this would not damage the implant. In addition to routine views, the Eklund technique may be used to pull the breast tissue forward from the implant and improve breast tissue visualisation – a full explanation of the imaging technique should be given prior to undertaking the mammogram [1].

Despite the best efforts to maximise the amount of breast tissue visualised free of the implant, in most clients who have breast implants there will be some compromise in visualisation of all breast tissue. The practitioner should record all details of the examination, for example, views taken, exposure, breast thickness and compression force. A routine post mammography clinical observation should be undertaken. If any changes have occurred, local policy should be followed. Clients should be informed that they should contact the imaging department for advice if they have any concerns following mammography. As with all clients, it is important to emphasise breast awareness and advise them that they should contact their General Practitioner immediately if they have any concerns about new symptoms or are concerned about implant integrity [1].

Visual Observation of the Breasts

The practitioner should observe the breast tissue both before and after the examination and record if any changes are observed. No specific training is required to undertake this observational check; this is not a breast examination. If any change is noted, follow local protocols. Unusual breast changes that may alert a change to the implant may include:

- Contour of the breast
- Position of the nipple
- Differences in the size and shape of the breast/s

Any differences observed should be pointed out to the clients with a high level of sensitivity and care prior to undertaking the examination.

Mammographic Imaging

Local protocols on the views to be undertaken should be written. Following a national audit [1, 2], it is recommended that these include:

- Standard MLO views first to establish the position of the implant (subglandular or subpectoral). This will help with decisions about imaging of that client.
- Standard CC views to get as far back onto the chest wall as possible and demonstrate both medial and lateral borders.
- Eklund CC views to demonstrate the anterior breast tissue with the implant displaced posteriorly or
- If the implant is immobile (encapsulated), consider the value of a true lateral view. This additional image will be a local decision following local discussion and agreement.

Breast Implant Placement

The exact anatomical placement of breast implants can vary, but the location of the implant is typically subglandular or subpectoral (Fig. 32.1). Should the placement site be known by the client or from previous imaging, this should be documented by the practitioner. Incision sites for implants are usually periareolar, inframammary, or transaxillary [1]. Considerations are taken when determining the best incision site and implant placement [3]. Implants that are placed below the pectoral muscle may be less likely to interfere with mammography imaging [4]. After breast reconstruction surgery, clients are encouraged to maintain a normal mammography schedule. Whilst there is no published guidance on compression force used, typically, a reduced force in this context could be approximately 6–8daN.

Fig. 32.1 Breast Anatomy demonstrating implant positioning Subglandular implant placement (*left image*) and subpectoral implant placement (*right image*) are options for breast augmentation

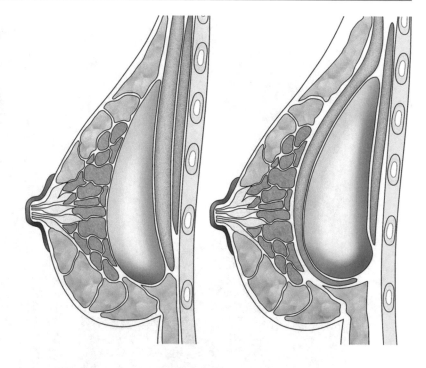

Fig. 32.2 Subglandular implant obscuring breast tissue in the medio-lateral oblique view

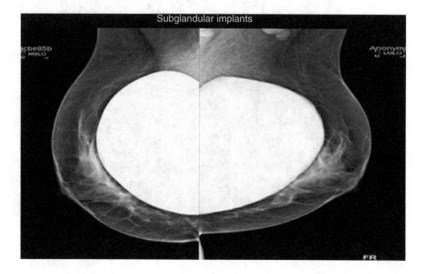

Subglandular Placement

In subglandular placement, the implant is positioned posterior to the breast parenchyma and superficial to the pectoral muscle [3]. Subglandular placement can make breast augmentation surgery shorter and reduce recovery time [3]. A possible disadvantage could be having breast implant edges more visibly noticeable under the skin. Imaging during a mammogram can also be more difficult when breast implants are placed by this method (Figs. 32.2 and 32.3a, b).

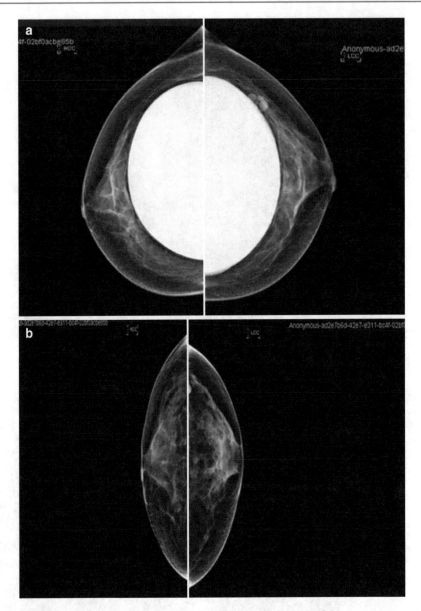

Fig. 32.3 (a) Subglandular implant obscuring breast tissue in the cranio-caudal view but demonstrating both medial and lateral borders as far back onto the chest wall as possible. (b) Subglandular implant with the Eklund view employed to displace the implant posteriorly onto the chest wall and apply compression to the anterior breast tissue to demonstrate this glandular tissue in more detail

Subpectoral Placement

In subpectoral placement, the implant is placed under the pectoralis major muscle and over the pectoralis minor muscle [3]. This technique is most commonly used for maximal coverage of implants used in breast reconstruction. Subpectoral placement may reduce the chances of breast implants being felt through the skin, and it may help reduce the chance of scar tissue hardening around breast implants. It will also make it easier to image breast tissue during a mammogram. Possible disadvantages of this placement choice could be a longer surgery and recovery period [3] (Figs. 32.4 and 32.5).

Fig. 32.4 Subpectoral implant seen in the medio-lateral view with minimal breast tissue obscured

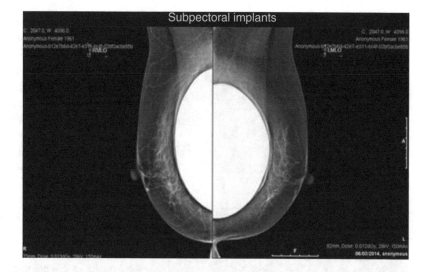

Fig. 32.5 Subpectoral implant seen in the cranio-caudal view at the posterior margin of the breast with minimal breast tissue obscured

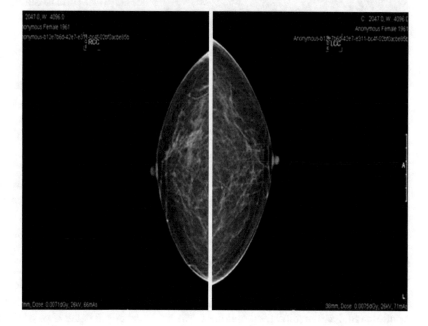

Implant Displacement: Eklund Views

Standard mammography views are taken first using minimum compression. Eklund views are performed with the implant pushed back against the chest wall. Implant displacement views, or Eklund views (Fig. 32.6), are used to adequately image breast tissue in clients with implants. These views are achieved by pulling breast tissue forward, away from the implant. At the same time, the implant is displaced posteriorly against

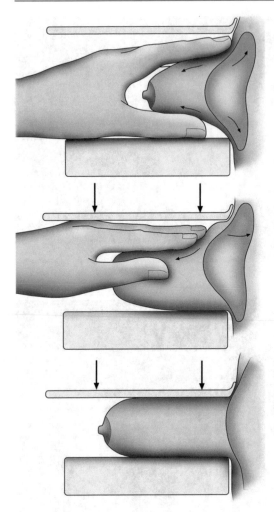

Fig. 32.6 Eklund technique

the chest wall so that it is out of the field of view. The practitioner then applies compression force to the tissue in front of the implant [5, 6]. Standard cranio-caudal and mediolateral oblique views are typically taken first. The implant displacement view provides improved imaging of the tissue at the front of the implant, while the standard views provide images of the tissue behind and underneath the implant, as well as the lower axillary area [3]. However, implant displacement views increase the amount of radiation that is delivered during a mammogram procedure and may increase the risk of implant rupture [1, 7].

The quality of imaging studies with implant displacement views and the amount of breast tissue imaged can be impacted by client factors such as breast size, glandularity, and fat content, as well as implant factors such as size, position, and implant-associated complications. Implant position and capsular contracture have the greatest impact on mammography success in clients with implants [3]. Implants placed below the pectoral muscle are less likely to interfere with imaging, resulting in almost twice the amount of breast tissues imaged compared with subglandular breast implants [3, 4].

Implant Complications

Aside from breast cancer screening, imaging of the breasts in clients with implants may be necessary over time to diagnose common complications associated with implants, including implant rupture, silicone extravasation (leakage), gel bleed, polyurethane breakdown, and peri-implant fluid collections. Although imaging with ultrasound and mammography have both been used successfully to evaluate the integrity of implants and detect possible problems over time, MRI is the preferred modality to detect implant rupture [8].

Realistic Client Expectations

While clients with implants may be concerned about their implants interfering with adequate breast cancer imaging, the available evidence suggests that implants do not greatly impact clinical outcomes in patients who do develop breast cancer, despite a possible delay in diagnosis [7, 9]. Clients should be aware that the presence of implants will increase the length of their mammography visits and may require breast manipulations to improve the visualisation of the breast parenchyma in a small number of cases.

Injectable Enhancements

An alternative to breast augmentation with the use of implants is the option for injectable fillers that may be used for volume restoration and body contouring. A number of products have been offered over the years with varying levels of success. Prior to breast imaging, it is helpful for the practitioner to know in advance if breast fillers or fat transfer have been used, as some products may compromise the visualisation of breast tissue and could present as cysts or round masses. This can significantly reduce the diagnostic quality of the mammograms, which may in turn lead to misdiagnosis [10].

Breast Awareness

Breast awareness is about encouraging all clients to become more aware of their bodies and to generally get to know their own breasts. This is an important message for all clients as only by knowing what is 'normal' for them might they then recognise any changes. Clients should be advised that if they ever notice any changes, they should contact their GP immediately to seek guidance.

Training and Education

Practitioners have a professional responsibility to ensure that they seek education and training to undertake imaging clients with breast implants. In line with IRMER regulations and clinical governance, evidence of internal training records must be kept for those undertaking this technique [11].

Conclusion

Clients who have undergone breast augmentation present an important imaging challenge for the practitioner as the breast implant obscures the breast tissue. Additional mammographic views are required in clients with implants to ensure an effective imaging study, to demonstrate maximum breast tissue and enable an accurate diagnosis, but adequate screening is still possible. Despite the challenges for mammography posed by breast implants, clinical outcomes in clients

who do develop breast cancer are not noticeably affected in those who have undergone breast augmentation or reconstructive surgery.

Clinical Pearls
- It is important to clearly explain to clients the need for additional images to be able to visualise as much breast tissue as possible to increase sensitivity. Understanding the need for additional imaging will promote informed consent.
- Do consider the importance of communication. Perhaps consider saying "I will ease the breast tissue forward and away from the implant" rather than "I will push the implant back against your chest wall". Consider the impact that the choice of terminology may have on the client.

Chapter Review Questions
Review Questions

1. Does undertaking mammography on a client with breast implants cause a rupture?
2. Is mammography the best modality to detect implant rupture?

Answers

1. This is a very common question and understandably may cause a level of anxiety for the individual prior to imaging. Whilst there is not a wealth of evidence to support that mammography causes rupture, there is always a small risk. A clear explanation that minimal compression is used for the examination and that care will be taken throughout is an important message to convey.
2. Mammography is not the best imaging modality to review implant integrity. Magnetic Resonance Imaging (MRI) or Ultrasound would be the modalities of choice under these circumstances.

Acknowledgments To all colleagues that have kindly shared photographs where appropriate permissions are in place.

Appendix

Test your learning and check your understanding of this book's contents: use the "Springer Nature Flashcards" app to access questions using https://sn.pub/dcAnWL.

To use the app, please follow the instructions in Chap. 1.

Flashcard code:

48341-69945-ABCB1-2A8C7-CE9D2.

Short URL: https://sn.pub/dcAnWL.

References

1. Public Health England. NHS Breast Screening Programme Screening women with breast implants. Available from: https://assets.publishing.service.gov.uk/government/uploads/system/uploads/attachment_data/file/624796/Screening_women_with_breast_implants_guidance.pdf. Accessed 6 Dec 2021.
2. Curtis J, Borrelli C. Developing a national standard. SoR Imaging & Therapy Practice. 2013. ISSN: 1360-5518. 2013. http://www.sor.org
3. Smalley SM. Breast implants and breast cancer screening. J Midwifery Womens Health. 2003;48:329-37.
4. Handel N, Silverstein MJ, Gamagami P, Jensen JA, Collins A. Factors affecting mammographic visualization of the breast after augmentation mammaplasty. JAMA. 1992;268:1913-7.
5. Gorczyca DP, Brenner RJ. The augmented breast: radiologic and clinical perspectives. New York: Thieme; 1997.
6. Eklund GW, Busby RC, Miller SH, Job JS. Improved imaging of the augmented breast. AJR Am J Roentgenol. 1988;151:469-73.
7. Brinton LA, Lubin JH, Burich MC, Colton T, Brown SL, Hoover RN. Breast cancer following augmentation mammoplasty. Cancer Causes Control. 2000;11:819-27.
8. O'Toole M, Caskey CI. Imaging spectrum of breast implant complications: mammography, ultrasound, and magnetic resonance imaging. Semin Ultrasound CT MR. 2000;21:351-61.
9. Brinton LA. The relationship of silicone breast implants and cancer at other sites. Plast Reconstr Surg. 2007;120(7):94S-102S.
10. Ishii H, Sakata K. Complications and management of breast enhancement using hyaluronic acid. Plast Surg. 2014;22(3):171-4.
11. Smathers RL, Boone JM, Lee LJ, Berns EA, Miller RA, Wright AM. Radiation dose reduction for augmentation mammography. AJR Am J Roentgenol. 2007;188:1414-21.

Imaging the Male Breast

33

Sue Garnett and Zebby Rees

Learning Objectives

Learning Objectives
- Identify and state the signs and symptoms of male breast cancer
- Demonstrate knowledge to apply evidence-based practice adaptations when performing male mammography
- Define the term gynaecomastia
- Demonstrate knowledge of the male breast cancer treatment pathway

The signs and symptoms of male breast cancer can be defined as [3]:

- Lump in breast or axilla
- Ulceration of the skin
- Skin puckering or dimpling
- Redness, scaling or itching of the nipple
- Retraction (inversion) of the nipple
- Nipple discharge—blood stained
- Breast cancer can occur in males at any age, but is more common in men aged 50 or over

Overview

Male breast cancer is rare compared to female breast cancer, with less than 1% of all breast cancer patients being male [1]. However, the incidence of male breast cancer is increasing [2]. All breast pathologies found in the female breast may also be seen in the male breast, and treatments are similar.

Factors that increase the risk of male breast cancer are as follows [4]:

- Older age—the risk of male breast cancer increases with age
- Exposure to oestrogen—oestrogen related drugs either for sex change procedures or hormone therapy for prostate cancer
- BRCA gene mutation—men with a BRCA gene mutation have a higher risk of breast cancer, prostate cancer and skin cancer (Melanoma). Also an increased risk of lymphoma, melanoma and cancers of pancreas and bile duct
- Exposure to radiation
- Chronic liver conditions
- Obesity—more oestrogen is produced
- Family history

S. Garnett (✉)
Breast Unit, University Hospital, Coventry, UK
e-mail: sue.garnett@uhcw.nhs.uk

Z. Rees
Bronglais and Singleton Hospitals,
Aberystwyth, West Wales, UK
e-mail: zebby.rees@wales.nhs.uk

© The Author(s), under exclusive license to Springer Nature Switzerland AG 2022
C. Mercer et al. (eds.), *Digital Mammography*, https://doi.org/10.1007/978-3-031-10898-3_33

When diagnosing breast abnormalities in men, investigations can include: a clinical breast examination, mammography and ultrasound imaging, and biopsy. If these tests prove the presence of breast cancer, the specialist may consider magnetic resonance imaging (MRI), a bone scan and a CT scan.

Mammography

When performing male mammography, practitioners must be aware of the sensitivities of the individual in an essentially female environment. Using terms such as 'X-raying the chest wall', giving reassurance and addressing the man's anxiety assists positioning and encourages relaxation. This allows the entire length of the soft tissue region over the muscle down to the lower chest wall to be lifted onto the image receptor.

Mammography in the male is a straightforward procedure because the pectoral muscle is positioned easily in the Medio-Lateral Oblique (MLO) projection. Care must be taken not to position the image receptor too high into the axilla for the MLO projection. The Cranio-Caudal (CC) projection is more challenging as the soft tissue behind the nipple can slip off the image receptor (IR) before compression force can be applied. This is especially true if the receptor is placed too high on the chest wall. The retro areolar region must be adequately visualised to assess all the glandular tissue. Tall men can present technical positioning difficulties for the female operator if there is a significant height difference. Seating the client will help positioning of the upper chest wall across the IR and the better developed pectoral muscle aids imaging of the overlying soft tissue.

The resultant mammogram image should demonstrate the pectoral muscle across two-thirds of the soft tissue image and well below the nipple with a fatty background density. The nipple is easy to image in profile, thereby clearly demonstrating the rudimentary ductal system in the subareolar region.

Gynaecomastia

Gynaecomastia is the most common condition in males [1]. An oestrogen surge in young men, or a drop in testosterone in men older than 60 years can influence development of the rudimentary ducts and lobules behind the nipple, producing a symmetrical or asymmetrical lump. Pseudo-gynaecomastia is breast enlargement in men mainly due to fatty tissue and with no increased glandular or stromal tissue [5].

Gynaecomastia is usually assessed by ultrasound to determine its dendritic nature. More asymmetric and harder masses can also be assessed by ultrasound, although mammography is useful for excluding calcifications and secondary lesions. Fentiman et al. [4] in a review study, concluded that most male symptoms are benign. However, some radiological features that are considered benign in a female are more uncertain in males, such as well circumscribed masses or larger rounder and scattered calcifications. In males, breast cancer often presents as a firm subareolar mass eccentric to the nipple [1].

Mammography is not the first imaging modality indicated for assessing male breast symptoms. If clinical breast examination suggests benign gynaecomastia, imaging is not essentially required [6], however ultrasound is often routinely undertaken in symptomatic clinics. A suspicion of breast cancer on clinical examination and ultrasound should be followed with bilateral mammograms.

Ductal Carcinoma In Situ (DCIS)

Ductal carcinoma in situ has not been well documented in males, but DCIS can present as a palpable nodularity mimicking gynaecomastia [4]. With continuously improving ultrasound technology, calcification can more easily be identified in such rare cases.

Invasive Carcinoma

Invasive ductal carcinoma is the most common form of breast cancer in males [7]. Invasive lobular carcinoma is rarely seen due to very few lobule formations compared to female breast tissue [2]. Male breast cancers will rapidly metastasise as breast tissue is minimal and the lymph nodes proximal. Risk factors for invasive breast cancer are similar to female breast cancer but are gender specific risks. These include Klinefelter's syndrome [8] and oestrogen-based drug treatment for prostate cancer.

Treatment is identical to female disease, although it is uncertain if risk, genetic and biological characteristics are gender specific [4]. Due to small breast size in males, mastectomy is commonly performed, with some lymph nodes removed, and hormone treatment given as appropriate.

If the cancer has spread beyond the breast the oncologist may recommend [9]:

- Hormone Treatment—if the cancer cells have hormone-receptor positivity, the oncologist may prescribe hormone therapy to reduce the chance of the cancer returning. Usually taken for up to 5 years
- Chemotherapy—helps to reduce the chance of systemic metastases developing
- Targeted cancer drug therapy
- Radiotherapy—to lower the risk of cancer cells growing back in the area of the breast [10]
- A combination of treatments

International Male Breast Cancer Program

Male breast cancer is still a relatively rare disease for which there is limited understanding of treatment patterns and prognostic factors [10]. A multinational program [11] has been established which looked at:

- Risk factors for male breast cancer
- Types of cancer
- The protein marker on the cancer
- Treatment
- How well treatments work
- Quality of life and well being

The program is running clinical trials for men with breast cancer, to improve standard treatments for male breast cancer as well as looking at new treatments [11]. It is a global effort to obtain meaningful data from this rare disease; the initial findings were published in 2018. It also highlighted poor treatment pathways for men due to lack of guidelines and the assumption treatment is identical to female disease.

Clinical Pearls
- Practitioners need to consider male sensitivity when performing a mammogram
- When positioning it is often easier to sit your client down if they are tall
- Ultrasound for gynaecomastia—It is often helpful to compare both nipple areas to confirm increased density behind the symptomatic nipple area

Chapter Review Questions
Review Questions

1. What are the sensitivities to be considered when performing a male mammogram?
2. What is the difference between gynaecomastia and pseudogynaecomastia?

Answers

1. Consider anxieties, and possible embarrassment of investigations in a mainly female environment.

   Communicate with empathy and understanding. Refer to chest wall soft tissue area, posterior nipple region.
2. Gynaecomastia is the formation of rudimentary ducts and lobules in the retro areolar area in a male, which is often tender.

Pseudogynaecomastia is mimicking gynaecomastia in the retroareolar area with a fatty soft tissue mound.

Appendix

Test your learning and check your understanding of this book's contents: use the "Springer Nature Flashcards" app to access questions using https://sn.pub/dcAnWL.

To use the app, please follow the instructions in Chap. 1.

Flashcard code:

48341-69945-ABCB1-2A8C7-CE9D2.

Short URL: https://sn.pub/dcAnWL.

References

1. Cardoso F, Kyriakides S, Ohno S, Penault-Llorca F, Poortmans P, Rubio IT, Zackrisson S, Senkus E. Early breast cancer: ESMO clinical practice guidelines for diagnosis, treatment and follow-up. Ann Oncol. 2019;30(8):1194–220.
2. Giordano SH. Breast cancer in men. New Engl J Oncol. 2018;378(24):2311–20.
3. National Institute for Health and Care Excellence (NICE). Early and locally advanced breast cancer: diagnosis and treatment. Nice Guideline [NG101]. 2018. Available from https://www.nice.org.uk/guidance/ng101. Accessed 3 December 2021.
4. Fentiman IS, Fourquet A, Hortobagyi GN. Male breast cancer. Lancet. 2006;367(9510):595–604.
5. Billa E, Kanakis GA, Goulis DG. Imaging in gynaecomastia. Andrology. 2021;9(5):1–13.
6. Grimm LJ. Male breast cancer imaging questions & answers. Available from https://emedicine.medscape.com/article/345979-overview#showall. Accessed 16 August 2021.
7. Brierley JD, Gospodarowicz MK, Wittekind C. TNM classification of malignant tumours. 8th ed. Hoboken: Wiley; 2017.
8. Evans DB, Crichlow RW. Carcinoma of the male breast and Klinefelter's syndrome: is there an association? CA Cancer J Clin. 1987;37(4):246–51.
9. Yadav S, Karam D, Bin Riaz I, Xie H, Durani U, Duma N, Giridhar KV, Hieken TJ, Boughey JC, Mutter RW, Hawse JR. Male breast cancer in the United States: treatment patterns and prognostic factors in the 21st century. Cancer. 2020;126(1):26–36.
10. Matuschek C, Bölke E, Haussmann J, Mohrmann S, Nestle-Krämling C, Gerber PA, Corradini S, Orth K, Kammers K, Budach W. The benefit of adjuvant radiotherapy after breast conserving surgery in older patients with low risk breast cancer-a meta-analysis of randomized trials. Radiat Oncol. 2017;12(1):1–8.
11. Cardoso F, Bartlett JM, Slaets L, Van Deurzen CH, van Leeuwen-Stok E, Porter P, et al. Characterization of male breast cancer: results of the EORTC 10085/TBCRC/BIG/NABCG International Male Breast Cancer Program. Ann Oncol. 2018;29(2):405–17.

Imaging Bariatric, Post-Surgical and Limited Mobility

34

Lyndsay A. Kinnear, Elizabeth G. Harrison, Allison Kelly, and Lisa Bisset

Learning Objectives
- Understand how to adapt mammography positioning for bariatric clients, those with post-surgical changes and limited mobility to achieve high-quality images
- Appreciate the importance of individualised care and communication
- Demonstrate knowledge of post-surgical appearances

Introduction

A proportion of clients have additional requirements that a practitioner must consider and adapt their technique accordingly. Practitioners should endeavor to produce the best possible images whilst maintaining appropriate care and this requirement is reflected in many professional codes of conduct, one example is reflected in the College and Society of Radiographers [1].

Bariatric Imaging

According to the National Cancer Institute (NCI) [2] obesity is associated with an increased risk in breast cancer. There is also a link between obesity and increased rates of recall, biopsy and stage of cancer at diagnosis [3]; therefore, high quality imaging is essential [4]. Some studies have demonstrated that these clients are less likely to attend screening [5, 6]. Further studies have demonstrated that there is a higher morbidity rate in those who are obese [7]. Training in bariatric imaging, to encompass a sensitive approach to the needs of the individual, should be encouraged to increase re-attendance rates and attendance to symptomatic units when appropriate [8].

Some of the barriers to bariatric clients attending screening are found to include insensitive comments about weight and equipment, along with gowns and changing facilities that were too small [8]. These factors should be considered by the practitioner, as they play a primary role in ensuring that those who do attend have a positive experience, and a continued acceptance of the screening service [9]. A relaxed client is also more likely to be co-operative and tolerate the examination. The needs of individuals must be recognised [9] and studies have found that

L. A. Kinnear (✉) · E. G. Harrison · A. Kelly
Nightingale Centre, Wythenshawe Hospital,
Manchester University NHS Foundation Trust,
Manchester, UK
e-mail: lyndsay.kinnear@mft.nhs.uk;
Elizabeth.Harrison@mft.nhs.uk;
Allison.Kelly@mft.nhs.uk

L. Bisset
Dorset Breast Screening Unit,
Poole General Hospital, Dorset, UK
e-mail: lisa.bisset@poole.nhs.uk

© The Author(s), under exclusive license to Springer Nature Switzerland AG 2022
C. Mercer et al. (eds.), *Digital Mammography*, https://doi.org/10.1007/978-3-031-10898-3_34

practitioners being sensitive and reactive to the needs of the client have helped make an uncomfortable examination more bearable [8].

Positioning and visualisation of the large breast can be challenging. However, a bariatric client with small breasts can pose additional imaging challenges for the practitioner [10].

Imaging Bariatric Clients with Larger Breasts

An increased body mass index (BMI) has been associated with greater compressed breast thickness which results in increased geometric unsharpness, decreased image contrast and possibly blurring of the image [11, 12]. It is essential that technique is adapted to ensure images of the highest quality are produced to enable cancer detection rates to be maximised [9]. Reducing the angle of the IR in the MLO view

will help support the weight of the breast and distribute the compression force more evenly, making the examination more comfortable for the client [13].

Standard imaging (Chap. 27) involves a single cranio caudal (CC) view and a single medio lateral oblique (MLO) view of each breast. Whilst these four views are the aim, it must be accepted that sometimes standard views are not adequate and additional imaging may be required. Mosaic (or tiling) imaging may be appropriate to ensure the medial, lateral, posterior, and anterior breast tissue is adequately visualised [14] (Fig. 34.1). Where additional exposures are necessary to image the entire breast, departmental protocols should be followed along with any statutory regulations [15].

An example of an imaging protocol for larger breasts may include:

- For craniocaudal views, image from the nipple back.

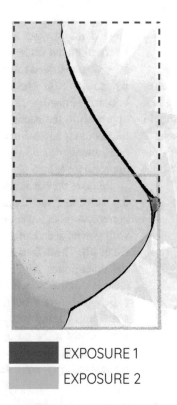
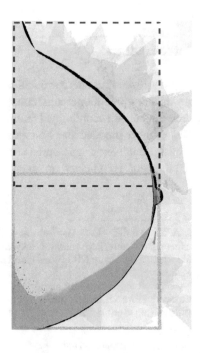

Fig. 34.1 An example of mosaic (tiling) imaging

EXPOSURE 1
EXPOSURE 2

- For the medio lateral view, image from the chest wall forward.
- If additional exposures are taken, ensure they overlap to confirm all breast tissue is imaged.

A large breast is generally extremely mobile making it easy to alter its true anatomic orientation. Ensure the breast is pulled straight forward and not rolled; it is important that any detected abnormalities can be accurately localised [10]. It can be difficult to maintain the nipple in profile and an additional view may be required if not achieved in one or both views. Departmental protocol should be followed.

Learning Points
- Employ appropriate manual handling techniques. Two practitioners may be required.
- Always review previous images if available.
- For heavier breasts a shallower IR angle can be useful to support the weight and even out compression force.
- Mosaic/tiling of images may be necessary. Departments should have a protocol for imaging those with larger breasts to aid consistency and comparison with subsequent examinations.
- Ensure breast tissue is not rolled and anatomical orientation is maintained.
- When lifting and pulling the breast be careful not to tear skin in the IMF (Chap. 17).

Imaging Bariatric Clients with Smaller Breasts

It is essential the client is stood back from the IR to allow an adequate lean in, encouraging the hips and abdomen back. Additional craniocaudal (CC) images, such as an extended craniocaudal (CC), may be required if the breast tissue wraps around laterally [10]. Reducing the angle of the IR in the MLO and using the small (18 × 24 cm) compression paddle may help to avoid the abdomen, improving and aiding a more even compression force to be applied.

Learning Points
- Stand the client back from the IR to aid an adequate lean in and manipulation of the abdomen.
- For small breasts a shallower IR angle and small paddle can help positioning and application of compression.
- When lifting and pulling the breast be careful not to tear skin in IMF (Chap. 17).

Post-surgical Imaging

All those who have had breast conserving surgery (BCS) should be offered surveillance mammography. This has been shown to improve survival rates by the early detection of local recurrence [16, 17]. Current UK NICE Guidelines (NG101) [18] state:

- Offer annual mammography to those with early breast cancer, including DCIS, until they enter the NHSBSP/BTWSP. Those diagnosed with early breast cancer that are already eligible for screening should have annual mammography for 5 years.

This guidance is open to interpretation and therefore differing breast screening programmes could have different protocols. Postsurgical changes can often overlap with malignant mammographic features. High quality images are essential, though imaging the surgically altered breast poses challenges to the practitioner and the image reader. There are several benign post-surgical features that make both performing and interpreting the mammogram challenging. These include scar formation that can mimic cancer, post irradiation changes, oedema, skin thickening, fat necrosis, and seromas [19].

Post-surgical calcification develops in about a third of cases, which is caused by trauma to breast fat; this can develop 2–5 years after treatment. Skin

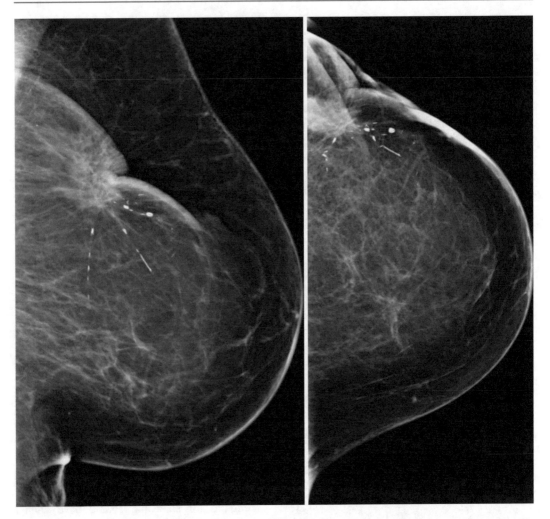

Fig. 34.2 Post surgery mammogram with benign macro calcification and distortion. The left image is a left medio lateral oblique, the right is a left CC

thickening is the most common finding [19]. Breast oedema gradually diminishes and resolves for many patients by the second-year mark, but in the interim period this can make mammography uncomfortable as the breast is enlarged and compression may be difficult [20]. It is important the practitioner is aware of these normal post-operative changes that occur, so they approach the patient in an empathetic manner allowing for the production of best quality images.

If reduced compression is required it is essential to communicate the importance of minimising movement and an instruction to pause breathing may be given, expressing that a large intake of breath could be detrimental (cause movement due to limited compression or blur). Be aware of ANC surgery, extra care should be given when position-

ing the arm in the MLO view. Where possible, eliminate creases and ensure good contact with the IR, adjusting the angle to suit the individual.

The post-surgical changes demonstrated in the left upper outer quadrant in Fig. 34.2 have features which overlap with a carcinoma. There is a clear distortion and skin puckering.

Post-surgical changes can create difficulties in positioning the breast with the nipple in profile. There appears to be a well-defined mass on the right medio-lateral oblique (MLO) projection in Fig. 34.3, but this represents the nipple. Skin thickening and oedema are also present on these images.

A common feature seen on post-surgical mammography is fat necrosis, as seen in the left upper outer quadrant in Fig. 34.4.

The patient in Fig. 34.5 has a distortion at the site of previous surgery. It is important that the practitioner records accurate clinical information and surgical procedures with dates and marks the scars for the image reader (only in screening). The distortion has similar features to a carcinoma. Previous images are paramount for comparison in such cases.

Learning Points
- It is essential that the practitioner records all scars and takes a brief history so that the image reader is aware of the scars precise location when reporting the mammogram.

- A thorough explanation of the procedure, particularly compression force, is important as this can reduce anxiety.
- Review previous images if available.
- If the breast is distorted, a separate projection with the nipple in profile may be required.
- Some clients experience tenderness and discomfort longer than others, so an empathetic and professional manner is important.
- Large posterior seromas can make adequate compression of the breast difficult and additional projections of the anterior of the breast may be required.

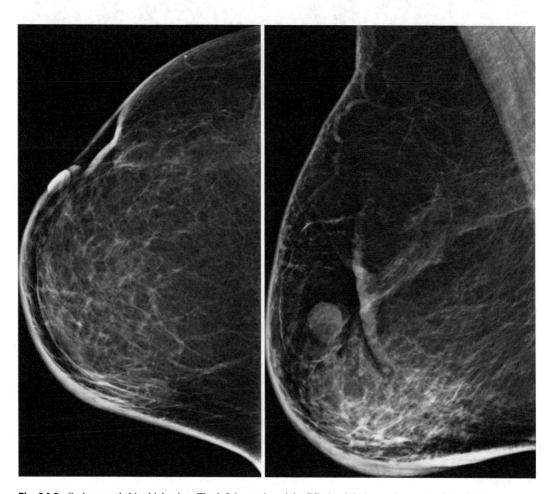

Fig. 34.3 Oedema and skin thickening. The left image is a right CC, the right image is a medio lateral oblique

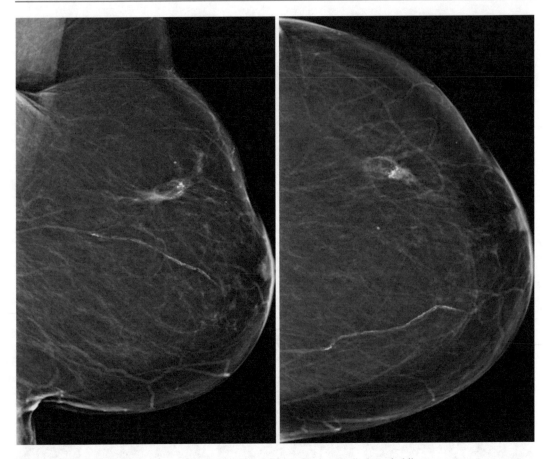

Fig. 34.4 Fat necrosis. The left image is a right CC, the right image is a medio lateral oblique

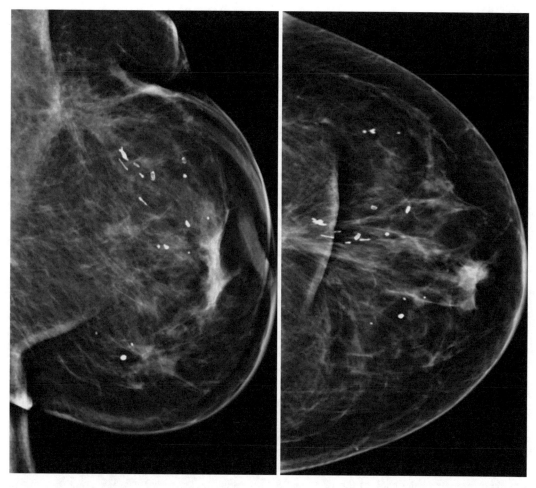

Fig. 34.5 Post surgical changes causing distortion. The left picture is a left medio lateral oblique, the right picture is a left CC

Imaging Clients with Limited Mobility

Imaging clients that present with limited mobility or a disability can be challenging. A disability can be defined under the Equality Act 2010 if 'you have a physical or mental impairment that has a 'substantial' and 'long-term' negative effect on your ability to do normal daily activities' [21]. This definition covers a wide spectrum of disabilities.

Those with disabilities are at increased risk of breast cancer mortality [22]; there is also low screening uptake amongst clients with limited mobility. Recurring themes that prevent these clients attending breast screening include previous

poor experience, factors related to the environment, finance, lack of knowledge, physical limitations, and carers lack of knowledge [23, 24]. Further barriers have been identified as explanation of the procedure, accessible changing facilities, and the availability of disabled parking [25].

Producing high quality images whilst ensuring a positive experience for these clients is a challenging task. The procedure itself is physically demanding, requiring the practitioner to manipulate the client, and often a wheelchair, into the correct position. The use of manual handling aids is essential; these include an appropriate imaging chair and support pads. The overall quality of the screening imaging experience is a significant determinant of re-attendance. The interaction between practitioner and client contributes significantly to how the examination is perceived [26–28].

Whilst equal access to services is important for clients with limited mobility, it must also be accepted that breast screening is not possible for all and there is a balance to be found between the potential benefits and harm. Within the UK, there is currently no alternative screening method for those unable to have a mammogram available through National Health Service screening programmes.

Impaired client mobility such as reduced neck and arm movements, kyphosis and inability to stand require practitioners to adapt their mammography positioning and techniques to achieve the best quality images. For those who are unable to turn their head a reverse CC view should be considered. Alternatively, separate medial and lateral views (like mosaic imaging of the larger breast) may be more appropriate [14]. In the MLO view every effort should be made to ensure the chin is raised or positioned so that it is not within the field of view. Alternatively, a LM view could be performed.

A frozen shoulder or stroke are common causes of reduced arm and shoulder movement. For MLO positioning, consider lowering the IR before positioning the arm, slowly increasing the height to achieve a satisfactory position. The arm can hang freely over the back of the IR to avoid over stretching and associated pain in the shoulder. If the arm cannot be raised/moved at all, the client may be reluctant to lean for MLO positioning for fear of falling. In this instance a steeper IR angle may aid positioning while the client remains in a more upright position [14].

Seated Imaging

Two practitioners are required for all wheelchair and seated imaging. Safe manual handing is essential to avoid any harm to the practitioners and client.

If the arm supports cannot be removed from the wheelchair, it is reasonable to ask whether they are able to transfer to a dedicated imaging chair. The wheelchair design must allow the client to be positioned close enough to the IR for the CC view.

Aids such as support pads should be used when necessary to support the client and assist positioning. For the MLO view, use an IR angle that will help the client feel supported, being mindful of contact with the client's lower body. Using a small paddle, when appropriate, can help with positioning, avoiding the abdomen and allowing for application of even compression force. If the client is distressed and is unable to cooperate, the examination may have to be abandoned.

Some conditions, such as multiple sclerosis (MS), can have good and bad phases. It could be that the client can be encouraged to re-book an appointment at a better time for themselves.

A full explanation is essential before the examination. Ensure the examination requirements are fully understood and gain informed consent, their trust and assistance. Give opportunity to ask any questions. Use supportive aids such as pads or pillows and avoid any part of the machine digging in to prevent unnecessary discomfort to the client. Ensure that the client knows when and how they will get their results.

> **Learning Points**
> - Employ safe manual handling techniques at all times with two practitioners in the imaging room.
> - Discuss with the client if they are able to stand, however it is perfectly acceptable to perform mammography in an imaging chair or a wheelchair.
> - Aim to image as much of the breast as possible in two views. Additional projections may be required to achieve this. Follow departmental protocol.
> - If standard projections are not possible, consider other views such as reverse cranio-caudal (CC) and Latero-medial oblique (LMO). These are described in Chap. 27.
> - Be prepared to adapt angles in line with body habitus and ability to move mobility. A change of angle may help the client feel supported.

Clinical Pearls
- Mammogram images are reviewed for subtle changes and practitioners must strive to ensure images produced are of the highest quality in all client groups
- Adapting mammography technique to meet the needs of each individual client is essential
- The interaction between the practitioner and client contributes significantly to how the examination is perceived and can have a direct impact on the decision to reattend

Acknowledgments The authors would like to pay particular thanks to Penelope Booth art.penelope.booth@gmail.com for the artwork contained within this chapter.

Chapter Review Questions
Review Questions

1. When would mosaic imaging be appropriate?
2. What positioning adaptations can be used to ensure adequate visualisation of the IMA in bariatric clients?
3. When would a nipple view be appropriate?
4. What are the potential quality issues encountered when imaging the larger breast?
5. Why is adapting technique and providing client centered care essential?

Answers

1. For larger breasts, when all breast tissue cannot be visualised in the standard CC and/or MLO view. Departmental protocol should be followed.

   If a reverse CC cannot be performed, mosaic imaging may be required to cover both the lateral and medial aspects in the CC view for clients with limited neck movement and/or kyphosis.
2. Adjusting the angle of the IR; a shallower angle can help support the breast of clients with larger breasts and help to open the IMA.

3. When the nipple is not in profile in at least one of the views (follow departmental protocol). Note: This can be difficult in post-surgery imaging.
4. Increased breast thickness can result in increased geometric unsharpness, decreased image contrast and image unsharpness.
5. The overall quality of the screening/imaging experience is a significant determinant of re-attendance. The interaction between practitioner and client contributes significantly to how the examination is perceived.

Appendix

Test your learning and check your understanding of this book's contents: use the "Springer Nature Flashcards" app to access questions using https://sn.pub/dcAnWL.

To use the app, please follow the instructions in Chap. 1.

Flashcard code:

48341-69945-ABCB1-2A8C7-CE9D2.

Short URL: https://sn.pub/dcAnWL.

References

1. Society of Radiographers. Society of Radiographers Code of Conduct 2013. Available from: http://www.sor.org/learning/document-library/code-professional-conduct. Accessed 1 September 2014.
2. National Cancer Institute. Breast Cancer Prevention (PDQ®)–Health Professional Version. Available from https://www.cancer.gov/types/breast/patient/breast-prevention-pdq. Accessed 3 February 2022.
3. Hunt K, Sickles E. Effect of obesity on screening mammography: outcomes analysis of 88,346 consecutive examinations. AJR Am J Roentgenol. 2000;174(5):1251–5.
4. Gayde C, Goolam I, Bangash H. Outcome of mammography on women with large breasts. Breast. 2012;21(4):493–8.
5. Atkins E, Madhavan S, LeMasters T. Are obese women more likely to participate in a mobile mammography program? J Community Health. 2013;38(2):338–48.
6. Friedman A, Hemler J, Rossetti E. Obese women's barriers to mammography and pap smear: the possible role of personality. Obesity. 2012;20(8):1611–7.

7. Maruther N, Bolen S, Brancati F, Clark J. Obesity and mammography: a systematic review and meta-analysis. J Gen Intern Med. 2009;24(5): 665–77.
8. Peters K, Cotton A. Environmental, structural and process barriers in breast cancer screening for women with physical disability: a qualitative study. Radiography. 2016;22(3):184–9.
9. Public Health England. Guidance for breast screening mammographers 2020. Available from: https://www.gov.uk/government/publications/breast-screening-quality-assurance-for-mammography-and-radiography/guidance-for-breast-screening-mammographers. Accessed 3 February 2022.
10. Destounis S, Newell M, Pinsky R. Breast imaging and intervention in the overweight and obese patient. Am J Roentgenol. 2011;196(2):296–302.
11. Guest A, Helvie M, Chan H, Hadjiiski L, Bailey J, Roubidoux M. Adverse affects of increased body weight on quantitative measures of mammographic image quality. AJR Am J Roentgenol. 2000;173(5):805–10.
12. Mercer C, Hogg P, Lawson R, Diffey J, Denton E. Practitioner compression force variability in mammography: a preliminary study. Br J Radiol. 2013;86(1022):20110596.
13. Smith H, Szczepura K, Mercer C, Maxwell A, Hogg P. Does elevating image receptor increase breast receptor footprint and improve pressure balance. Radiography. 2015;21(4):359–63.
14. Jenkin M. Challenging scenarios in breast screening. Available from: https://portal.e-lfh.org.uk/LearningContent/Launch/61626. Accessed October 20, 2021.
15. Department of Health. The ionising radiation (medical exposure) regulations 2017. Available from: https://www.legislation.gov.uk/uksi/2017/1322/contents/made. Accessed 3 February 2022.
16. Robertson C, Arcot Ragupathy S, Boachie C. The clinical effectiveness and cost-effectiveness of different surveillance mammography regimens after the treatment for primary breast cancer: systematic reviews registry database analyses and economic evaluation. Health Technol Assess. 2011;15(34):1366.
17. McNaul D, Darke M, Garge M, Dale P. An evaluation of post-lumpectomy recurrence rates: is follow up every 6 months for 2 years needed? J Surg Oncol. 2013;107(6):597–601.
18. NICE guideline [NG101]. Early and locally advanced breast cancer: diagnosis and management. Available from: https://www.nice.org.uk/guidance/ng101/chapter/Recommendations#followup. Accessed 3 February 2022.
19. Dershaw D. Mammography in patients with breast cancer treated by breast conservation (lumpectomy with or without radiation). Am J Roentgenol. 1995;164(2):309–16.
20. Mendelson E. Evaluation of the post-operative breast. Radiol Clin N Am. 1992;30(1):107–38.
21. The National Archives. Legislation.gov.uk. The Equality Act 2010. https://www.legislation.gov.uk/ukpga/2010/15/section/6. Accessed 3 February 2022.
22. McCarthy E, Ngo L, Roetzheim R. Disparities in breast cancer treatment and survival for women with disabilities. Annu Int Med. 2006;145(9):637–45.
23. Todd A, Stuifbergen A. Breast cancer screening barriers and disability. Rehabil Nurs. 2012;37(2):74–9.
24. Lopez E, Vasudevan V, Lanzone M. Florida mammographer disability training vs needs. Radiol Technol. 2012;83(4):337–48.
25. Jarman M, Bowling J, Dickens P. Factors facilitating acceptable mammography services for women with disabilities. Women's Health Issues. 2012;22(5):1049–3867.
26. Sze Y, Liu M, Clark M. Breast and cervical cancer screening practices among disabled women aged 40–75: does quality of the experience matter? J Women's Health. 2008;17(8):1321–9.
27. Whelehan P, Evans A, Wells M, Macgillivray S. The effect of mammography pain on repeat participation in breast cancer screening: a systematic review. Breast. 2013;22(4):389–94.
28. Poulos A, Balandin S, Llewellyn G. Women with physical disability and the mammogram: an observational study to identify barriers and facilitators. Radiography. 2010;17:14–9.

Imaging Persons Living with Dementia

35

Adam Spacey, Rob Higgins, and Beverley Scragg

Learning Objectives
- Identify and state the main symptoms and behavioural changes associated with persons living with dementia (PLWD)
- Identify the different types and stages of dementia and the potential impacts on practice for both practitioner and client
- Demonstrate knowledge to apply evidence-based practice adaptations to improve both the client and practitioner experience
- Apply knowledge in how to obtain informed consent when imaging clients living with dementia
- Identify resources or organisations to support future development or raise awareness of dementia in the department

Introduction

The incidence of breast cancer and dementia increases with age [1]. Research has demonstrated that clients with cancer and comorbid dementia are less likely to receive cancer treatment, have increased complex care needs, and are more likely to experience adverse health outcomes and poorer survival rates in comparison to clients with solely a cancer diagnosis [2–4].

A significant number of research studies, government reports, audits, and enquiries published over the last decade have established that persons living with dementia (PLWD) (in England) are more likely to receive poor care at some point during their hospital admission [5–7]. There is currently very little published guidance to assist practitioners to manage and support PLWD who attend for breast imaging. This chapter will collate current evidence to provide guidance for practitioners to support them when caring for and imaging PLWD.

Dementia: Statistics and Symptoms

Worldwide approximately 50 million people are living with dementia and its prevalence is increasing internationally [8]. The increasing prevalence of dementia is particularly acute across European counties with rapidly ageing populations such as Italy, Germany, Spain and the UK [9, 10]. Specifically, in the UK, it is estimated that

A. Spacey (✉) · R. Higgins · B. Scragg
School of Health and Society, University of Salford,
Manchester, UK
e-mail: a.spacey@salford.ac.uk;
r.n.higgins@salford.ac.uk; b.c.scragg1@salford.ac.uk

approximately 850,000 people are currently living with dementia, with this number expected to surpass one million by 2025 [10]. Although dementia can affect people of all ages, the biggest risk factor is age, with a person's risk of developing dementia rising from 1 in 14 over the age of 65 to 1 in 6 over the age of 80 [10]. Thus, given women on average tend to live longer than men, worldwide women with dementia will outnumber men 2 to 1 [11]. As well as dementia, age is also a risk factor for cancer and by 2040 it is projected that nearly a quarter of people aged 65 and over in the UK will have a cancer diagnosis [12]. This increasing prevalence of comorbid cancer and dementia has led to greater numbers of women living with dementia attending mammography services across the UK [13].

Dementia is a multicausal syndrome which causes the progressive loss of brain function and cognitive abilities [14]. PLWD often present with a range of complex symptoms which vary depending on the type (Table 35.1) and stage of the condition as well as the individual themselves and their personality and life experiences [15]. Table 35.1 details the main symptoms associated with each type of dementia; these can be used to help tailor care to best meet the needs of the individual. For example, whilst a person living with late-stage Alzheimer's disease may present with communication difficulties, a person living with vascular dementia may still have strong communicative abilities. Similarly, whilst a client living with Lewy body dementia may present with confusion in the morning, they may be more relaxed and have more cognitive ability in the afternoon [10, 15].

Although symptoms vary depending on the type of dementia, it is recognised that many of these symptoms can overlap. The main symptom associated with dementia is progressive loss of cognitive functionality, which can inhibit a person's ability to retain and understand information, communicate and behave [15]. Given the progressive nature of the condition these symptoms can also become more pronounced over time [10]. However, as well as stage, symptoms can also become more pronounced in unfamiliar environments such as hospitals or mobile screening units [16]. The following section will detail how the environment can be adapted the meet the needs of PLWD.

Table 35.1 The main types of dementia and associated symptoms

Type	Main symptoms[a] [10]
Alzheimer's disease	Presents with increased memory loss, inability to learn new things and difficulty with language, reading and writing
Vascular dementia	Presents with slowness of thought and concentration problems, difficulty planning and changes in mood and behaviour
Lewy body dementia	Can present with confusion and alertness which can significantly vary from one time of the day to another, slowness and gait imbalances, visual hallucinations as well as delusions
Frontotemporal dementia	Behavioural and dramatic personality changes which often include swearing, impaired judgment, stealing and increased interest in sex

[a] Although each type of dementia can present with varying symptoms these often overlap, such as language/communication difficulty, memory loss and behavioural changes

Environment

A busy, noisy imaging department environment is often ill-suited to those with dementia and should be considered a stressor. This has the potential to cause distress and a deterioration in demeanor prior to the examination, which may result in sub-optimal preparation for a mammogram examination [17]. Environments can be altered for the better, not just for PLWD but for all users, with a little preparation.

When considering dementia friendly environmental factors, PLWD and staff want safe environments which support the client with navigation and orientation. The use of wall murals and wall art can stimulate or calm. Wall murals offer an excellent and cost-efficient way to provide comforting care environments. However, PLWD express a predilection for scenes that use nature and the outdoors [18]. When considering safety, it should be considered that PLWD can have visual disturbance or hallucinations and their proprioception and perception of the environment is affected by this.

Primarily, a well-lit department will assist in safe navigation. X-ray rooms are historically dimly lit but this should be altered if a PLWD is being examined. Doormats upon excessively shiny floors often appear like dark holes, as PLWD will walk around these [19] (so it should be considered that the appearance of the imaging detector could appear similarly, when we are asking them to place their breast upon it).

Additionally, it is recommended that the department has a clear entrance, is kept clean and decluttered [20]. A cluttered environment has been found to be a stressor for those working within it [21], it also promotes an unhygienic environment generally and thus should already be kept to a minimum; if this is the case then it has the added benefit of removing visual confusion for the PLWD. Waiting rooms can be noisy and over stimulative, so the use of televisions is not recommended, but music can be beneficial to all users.

A recent trend in using biophilic design (connectivity to the natural environment) and natural lighting in hospital environments can also work in harmony with PLWD preferences for nature. Biophilic design in healthcare can be seen as a positive therapeutic support that improves outcomes for everyone and is supported by a growing body of research [22]. In the breast screening department, simulated elements of nature can be incorporated into new and existing examination rooms, the simplest of which can be full wall murals of local nature scenes which have been shown also to have a positive effect on staff as well as clients [23].

Improved signage both to the department and around it will assist PLWD greatly and lessen anxiety. For example, signs to the toilets, changing room and the department itself should be designed to enable PLWD to read and understand [20]. High contrast signage with a consistent style will assist those with visual problems, colours can also be used to differentiate area/departments. Also, any signage should aim to minimise medical jargon as much as possible and be placed at a height

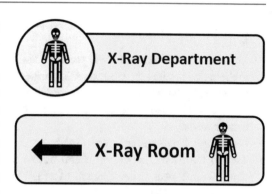

Fig. 35.1 Examples of dementia friendly signage

that is readable [20]. Figure 35.1 below provides an example of what dementia friendly signage could look like.

The King's Fund provide an evaluation tool for Hospitals wishing to look at improving their environments to better support the care needs of PLWD which can also translate to the imaging department [20]. Although the tool is mainly aimed at care homes, many of the design recommendations are transferable to hospital environments, including breast imaging departments, and support the recommendations made within this section.

Communication Adaptations

A PLWD in distress is likely to display behaviours that may be considered as 'challenging', however it is more correct to accept that these behaviours are merely symptomatic of distress in some way. If the distress can be lessened, then any behavioural 'challenges' are also lessened, and this should be the practitioner's aim.

Simple adaptations to communication have been shown to ease distress of PLWD and thus 'challenging' behaviours and poor experiences in unfamiliar environments [24]. Although adaptations to communication will vary depending on the type and stage of dementia, there are a number of common adaptations which have been shown to greatly improve interactions, these include:

- Always access the PLWD from the front. Try not to stand over them to communicate – it can feel intimidating. Instead, respect their personal space and try to sit or stand at eye level.

- Make sure you look at a PLWD when you talk to them and not just the carer or care partner.
- Give the PLWD some signs, as touching hand, or use their name before you start the conversation.
- Use simple language and speak slowly.
- Talk to the PLWD as an adult and not as a child. Do not speak in the presence of a PLWD as if they are not present.
- Give the PLWD enough time to process information and to respond.

However, it should be recognised that the time prior to the appointment is just as important in reducing distress as at the time of the examination. PLWD can bring their 'This is me' passport to the appointment and practitioners should view this as

part of examination preparation. This documents PLWD's preferences and which factors may cause distress and is an effective way of facilitating communication with the practitioner [25].

Additionally, when attending mammography services, PLWD often need to understand written as well as verbal communication [26, 27]. For example, information leaflets pertaining to the benefits and negatives of breast screening, as well as letters detailing the appointment information. To help address the need for dementia friendly written communication, the Dementia Engagement and Empowerment Project (DEEP) recommend that written as well as verbal communication is adapted [28]. Recommendations include using pictures, different colours to differentiate sections and large front sizes. Figure 35.2 synthesises current evidence to help support practitioners to adapt both their written and verbal communication.

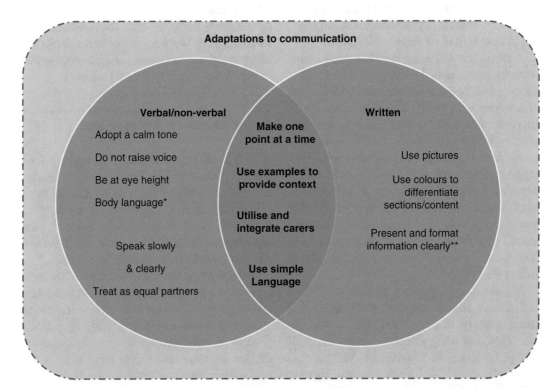

* Give eye contact, adopt open body language (i.e do not cross arms), keep facial expressions friendly i.e. try not to frown.
** Use bullet points, front size of at latest 12pt, one column of text, use simple front such as Arial and split information up into short paragraphs.

Fig. 35.2 Adaptations to communication

Carer and Care Partner Integration

Carers and care partners can also be integrated into examinations to support care, particularly in relation to communication. Studies are unanimous in their verdict that carers and care partner relatives need to be consulted and incorporated into episodes of care, as PLWD exhibit less signs of distress if they do so [17, 19]. For instance, a carer or care partner may know the PLWD's preferred communication style; this can assist in not only ascertaining consent [19] but also contribute to the success of the examination, as poor communication in mammography can affect the resultant image quality. Consulting both the PLWD and the carer or care partner regarding how the examination will proceed should be normalised and practitioners should approach this as a collaborative venture; both PLWD and the carer or care partner are the experts in the needs of the PLWD, not the healthcare professional, and this should be respected [29].

Excluding the carer or care partner from the examination has been shown to have a negative effect on the PLWD experiences which may prevent reattendance for follow up imaging [17]. However, the mammogram is classed as an intimate examination [30] and if the carer or care partner is not involved with the PLWD personal care then this may be inappropriate. The practitioner should consult with each party to ensure best practice, with the client's needs and preferences remaining paramount to ensure values-based practice [26].

Justification and Consent

Carers/care partners and staff have been known to question whether imaging examinations, specifically to exclude pathologies (as is the case in screening) are justified for PLWD [17], as dementia is a fatal condition with a shortened life expectancy; and the effects upon mortality from screening are not apparent until after 4 years [31]. The risk benefit ratio depends upon the life expectancy, level of understanding and any significant co-morbidities and should be discussed with the PLWD prior to the examination, rather than by a practitioner at the time of the examination. However, as screening programmes may not distinguish PLWD, this can still occur, which is essential in obtaining informed content.

As with every episode of care, informed consent needs to be obtained. For consent to be valid, the client must [27]:

- Have capacity
- Make an informed decision
- Not be under duress
- Know that they can refuse

Impairment of the memory process associated with dementia therefore raises issues regarding consent. Nonetheless, PLWD cannot be assumed to be incapable of making decisions. PLWD with mild to moderate dementia can evaluate, interpret, and derive meaning in their lives. The law assumes that all adults have capacity unless there is contrary evidence [32]. For consent to be valid, it must be voluntary and informed, and the person being consented must have the capacity to make the decision [33]. Consent can be given:

- Verbally—for example, a person saying they are happy to have the procedure
- In writing—for example, signing a consent form for surgery

The Mental Capacity Act (MCA) [34] provides guidance on how practitioners might proceed with investigations where a client might lack competence, for example those living with dementia. A key point to note is that the aim of mental capacity legislation is to empower those with impaired mental capacity. However, the dynamics between carer and client could possibly make it difficult to establish a person with dementia's capacity to consent. Mental capacity is both time and decision specific; capacity to consent can fluctuate. An individual may lack capacity in some areas but still be able to make a decision about their procedures in clinical imaging or radiotherapy. Examples of ways in which PLWD can be supported to make informed decisions include providing information in different, tailored formats such as pictures and short written summaries and including families or care partners (with permission) in consultations so they can support discussion and decision-making processes [19].

Assumptions about consent cannot be made, as understanding, values and perspectives will change over time. Public Health England have produced a simplified leaflet explaining the issues that should be available in screening departments for the PLWD prior to the appointment, and it may be more appropriate to ask the PLWD to look through this with their carer or care partner prior to the examination rather than discussion this within the examination room [27]. If a PLWD is already flagged on the system, this information should be sent with the invitation letter so that the PLWD is able to process the information without feeling under duress if they are already at the department.

Pre-appointment Adaptations

Imaging is secondary care and, as such, relies upon primary care to provide information about the client. Clinical information provided upon an imaging request does not have to include a diagnosis of dementia or cognitive impairment, as this is dependent upon the referring guidelines or the set-up of the Radiology Information System (RIS) requesting algorithm; both of which can be altered to include a question about dementia/cognitive impairment that can be made mandatory for clinicians before a request is able to be submitted.

A screening programme database may not have a specific field for identifying additional needs when arranging client appointments to attend for screening and is reliant on the client's positive action in order to inform the department. Therefore, it is not unusual for a client to attend at a satellite location with no prior indication of dementia or cognitive

impairment. This may prove unsuitable and practitioners should ensure that the client is identified on the system in some way as having dementia or cognitive impairment, so that they are called to the best location for their needs to be met—for example a breast screening unit located within the hospital rather than mobile mammography unit. The type of dementia should also be recorded as this influences the care needs—for example, vascular dementia is more likely to cause visual hallucinations and recording this may help the practitioner adapt their care towards the client [25].

Contextual Barriers and Training

The needs of PLWD add complexity to a mammographic examination and to the pressures that staff face in running a busy clinic environment. Whilst health professionals intend to provide person-centred care, the practicalities of doing so within a task-based organisation can often feel an insurmountable hurdle. Practitioners should avoid using organisational tropes such as routine, efficiency and safety as barriers to providing person-centred care to PLWD and should remain flexible and open in their attitudes; but this requires a departmental cultural shift and training [35].

The dementia champion system was developed as an organisational change mechanism, so that those individuals who had been trained would then effect change throughout the acute setting by influencing practice on the front line [36]. While this is a cost effective means of producing change agents, only having small numbers of staff trained to this standard will slow the pace of change and possibly not provide the cultural shift that is needed. As the type of dementia experienced also influences the care needs [25], it can be argued that a greater knowledge of the condition is required by all healthcare staff for person-centred care to be achieved.

Practitioners are required by their professional body to practice continuing professional development [37] and this could be the avenue that is used to promote awareness of the issues, leading on to a more cohesive training involving all the departmental staff. One-off training does not lead to the necessary cultural shift, and training needs to be re-affirmed to be successful [17, 19].

Summary

Ultimately, to successfully image PLWD, systemic changes and flexibility are a requirement from breast imaging departments; these changes need not be expensive but should be extensive.

Useful Resources and Websites for Further Information

- **The Alzheimer's Society:** Alzheimer's Society is a United Kingdom care and research charity for people with dementia and their carers.
- **Dementia Friends UK:** A Dementia Friends Champion is a volunteer who encourages others to make a positive difference to people living with dementia in their community. Dementia champions are staff members that have a special interest in dementia and improving the care and experience of dementia persons in the area where they work. The dementia champions have/are encouraged to attend the Tier 2 training and attend the dementia champion meetings/teaching on a regular basis.
- **Dementia UK**: Provide the specialist and compassionate support for all families, through their Admiral Nurse service. They also publish research on dementia.
- **John's Campaign:** Campaigns for extended visiting rights for family carers of patients with dementia in hospitals in the United Kingdom.

- **The Kings Fund:** This an independent think tank, which is involved with work relating to the health system in England which includes dementia and dementia environments.

Clinical Pearls
- Dementia is an umbrella term to describe the loss of cognitive functioning, thus different types and stages can produce differing symptoms
- Pre-examination preparation can have a large influence on the success of the imaging outcomes and client compliance: this however requires systemic change
- Capacity fluctuates, thus informed consent can depend on time of day (e.g. sun downing), the condition and the environment (e.g., clear signage)
- Integrating carers/relatives into the process can improve the experience for the person living with dementia and assist the practitioner in successfully optimising 'patient-centred care' and imaging outcomes

Chapter Review Questions
Review Questions

1. What are the key adaptations when caring for persons living with dementia attending for breast imaging?
2. What are the key considerations when obtaining informed consent from persons living with dementia and their care partners?

Answers

1. Key adaptations when caring for persons with dementia include integrating the carer in the examination (if deemed appropriate), ensuring you communicate effectively (e.g. no use

of medical jargon, speaking slowly and clearly), minimise stressors in the hospital environment (e.g. well-lit with a clear entrance way and navigation), and lastly ensure you have shared information on the hospital network to ensure future care can be tailored.

2. Key considerations when obtaining informed consent include always assuming that the client can consent and understand what is expected and why they are undergoing breast imaging. Be clear and provide sufficient information to the person living with dementia and their care partner by allowing them time to ask questions and take in the information shared with them. Appointment times should also be adapted to potential fluctuations in capacity, most persons living with dementia tend to have greater capacity in the late morning/early afternoon.

Appendix

Test your learning and check your understanding of this book's contents: use the "Springer Nature Flashcards" app to access questions using https://sn.pub/dcAnWL.

To use the app, please follow the instructions in Chap. 1.

Flashcard code:

48341-69945-ABCB1-2A8C7-CE9D2.

Short URL: https://sn.pub/dcAnWL.

References

1. Smyth KA. Current practices and perspectives on breast cancer screening and treatment in older women with dementia. J Am Geriatr Soc. 2009;57(2):272–4.
2. Hopkinson JB, Milton R, King A, Edwards D. People with dementia: what is known about their experience of cancer treatment and cancer treatment outcomes? A systematic review. Psycho-Oncology. 2016;25(10):1137–46.
3. Kedia SK, Chavan PP, Boop SE, Yu X. Health care utilization among elderly medicare beneficiaries with coexisting dementia and cancer. Gerontol Geriatr Med. 2017;3:2333. https://doi.org/10.1177/2333721416689042.
4. Ashley L, Kelley R, Griffiths A, Cowdell F, Henry A, Inman H, Hennell J, Ogden M, Walsh M, Jones L, Mason E. Understanding and identifying ways to improve hospital-based cancer care and treatment for people with dementia: an ethnographic study. Age Ageing. 2021;50(1):233–41.
5. Care Quality Commission. The state of health care and adult social care in England in 2013/14. London: The Stationery Office; 2014.
6. Fogg C, Griffiths P, Meredith P, Bridges J. Hospital outcomes of older people with cognitive impairment: an integrative review. Int J Geriatr Psychiatry. 2018;33(9):1177–97.
7. Martin A, O'Connor S, Jackson C. A scoping review of gaps and priorities in dementia care in Europe. Dementia. 2020;19(7):2135–51.
8. World Health Organisation (WHO). Dementia. Available from: https://www.who.int/news-room/fact-sheets/detail/dementia. Accessed 6 August 2021.
9. Alzheimer Europe. Dementia in Europe Yearbook. 2019. Available from: https://www.alzheimer-europe.org/Publications/Dementia-in-Europe-Yearbooks. Accessed 6 August 2021.
10. Alzheimer's Research UK. Prevalence. Available from: https://www.dementiastatistics.org/statistics-about-dementia/prevalence/. Accessed 21 April 2021.
11. Kiely A. Research blog: why is dementia different for women? Available from: https://www.alzheimers.org.uk/blog/why-dementia-different-women. Accessed 21 April 2021.
12. Cancer Research UK. Cancer incidence by age. Available from: https://www.cancerresearchuk.org/health-professional/cancer-statistics/incidence/age. Accessed 20 June 2021.
13. NHS Breast Screening Programme. Breast screening programme, England. Available from https://webarchive.nationalarchives.gov.uk/20180328133633/; http://digital.nhs.uk/catalogue/PUB23376. Accessed 7 May 2021.
14. World Health Organisation (WHO). Dementia. Available from: https://www.who.int/news-room/fact-sheets/detail/dementia. Accessed 10 May 2021.
15. Duong S, Patel T, Chang F. Dementia: what pharmacists need to know. Can Pharm J. 2017;150(2):118–29.
16. Riley J, Burgener S, Buckwalter C. Anxiety and stigma in dementia: a threat to aging in place. Nurs Clin North Am. 2014;49(2):213–31.
17. Challen R, Low F, McEntee F. Dementia patient care in the diagnostic medical imaging department. Radiography. 2018;24(1):33–42.
18. Fisher H, Edwards J, Pärn A, Aigbavboa O. Building design for people with dementia: a case study of a UK care home. Facilities. 2018;36(7/8):349–68.
19. The Society and College of Radiographers (SCoR). The Society and College of Radiographers practice guideline document. Available from https://www.sor.org/getmedia/db2b70ad-2771-42f1-a204009fde177071/sor_dementia_academic_doc_llv2.pdf. Accessed 21 May 2021.

20. The Kings Fund. Is your ward dementia friendly? EHE environmental assessment tool. 3rd ed. London: The Kings Fund; 2014.
21. Roster A, Ferrari R. Does work stress lead to office clutter, and how? Mediating influences of emotional exhaustion and indecision. Environ Behav. 2020;52(9):923–44.
22. Totaforti S. Applying the benefits of biophilic theory to hospital design. City Territory Archit. 2018;5(1):1.
23. McCunn L, Frey C. Impacts of large-scale interior murals on hospital employees: a pharmacy department case study. J Facil Manag. 2020;18(1):53–70.
24. Banovic S, Zunic J, Sinanovic O. Communication difficulties as a result of dementia. Mater Socio-med. 2018;30(3):221–4.
25. Marlowe F. Dementia care in radiography and the role of the dementia champion. Synergy. 2014;1:13–6.
26. The Association of Radiography Educators. Values-based practice in diagnostic and therapeutic radiography: a training template. Available from https://www.sor.org/sites/default/files/document-versions/2018.10.03_radiography_vbp_training_manual_-_final.pdf. Accessed 9 August 2021.
27. Public Health England. Breast screening: an easy guide about a health test for women aged 50 and over. Public Health England; 2018.
28. The Dementia Engagement and Empowerment Project (DEEP). Writing dementia-friendly information. Available from: http://dementiavoices.org.uk/wp-content/uploads/2013/11/DEEP-Guide-Writing-dementia-friendly-information.pdf. Accessed 21 April 2021.
29. Clissett P, Porock D, Harwood H, Gladman F. Experiences of family carers of older people with mental health problems in the acute general hospital: a qualitative study. J Adv Nurs. 2013;69(12):2707–16.
30. Society and College of Radiographers. Intimate examinations and chaperone policy. London: Society & College of Radiographers; 2016.
31. Raik L, Miller G, Fins J. Screening and cognitive impairment: ethics of forgoing mammography in older women. J Am Geriatr Soc. 2004;52(3):440–4.
32. Hegde S, Ellajosyula R. Capacity issues and decision-making in dementia. Ann Indian Acad Neurol. 2016;19(1):34–9.
33. National Health Service. Assessing capacity: consent to treatment. Available from https://www.nhs.uk/conditions/consent-to-treatment/capacity/. Accessed 21 June 2021.
34. Department of Health. Mental capacity act. London: HMSO; 2005.
35. Featherstone K, Northcott A, Bridges J. Routines of resistance: an ethnography of the care of people living with dementia in acute hospital wards and its consequences. Int J Nurs Stud. 2019;96:53–60.
36. Banks P, Waugh A, Henderson J, Sharp B, Brown M, Oliver J, Marland G. Enriching the care of patients with dementia in acute settings? The Dementia Champions Programme in Scotland. Dementia. 2014;13(6):717–36.
37. Health & Care Professions Council. Standards of conduct, performance and ethics. London: Health & Care Professions Council; 2016.

Stereotactic Image Guided and Tomosynthesis Guided Interventional Techniques

36

Rita M. Borgen, Susan E. Garnett, and Samantha West

Learning Objectives
- Develop an understanding of the principles and primary use of stereotaxis in the pre-operative diagnosis of non-palpable breast abnormalities
- Evaluate the use of DBT to aid stereotactic interventions
- Discuss the value of VAB in patient management pathways
- Distinguish between the different types of localisation techniques

Introduction

Stereotactic image guided interventional techniques are well established procedures incorporated as part of the diagnosis and treatment of breast disease. These techniques offer high levels of diagnostic accuracy in a timely manner, providing a definitive diagnosis in the majority of cases. The primary use of stereotaxis is the location of non-palpable lesions to aid intervention.

R. M. Borgen (✉) · S. West
Breast Screening Service, East Lancashire Hospitals NHS Trust, Burnley, UK
e-mail: Rita.borgen@elht.nhs.uk

S. E. Garnett
Breast Unit, University Hospital, Coventry, UK

Areas of calcification, deep lesions and lesions in mammographically demonstrated abnormalities not seen on ultrasound are ideal for stereotactic mammographic guidance [1]. The design of stereotactic equipment works on the principle of parallax—this is the distance of shift of a lesion on the image relative to a fixed point—which allows calculation of the depth or distance from that fixed point [2]. The computer within the equipment calculates this depth using two 2D images taken at the same angulation (15°or 20°) each side of the vertical plane (Fig. 36.1).

This method of imaging is used for a variety of procedures including 14gauge (g) core needle and 10g probe (vacuum-assisted) biopsy devises, wire marker and clip placements, and small lesion removal (vacuum-assisted). It is available for upright, lateral arm approaches and prone table systems and is also compatible with tomosynthesis-guided systems (DBT).

DBT guided biopsy negates the need for angled pair images and accurately defines lesion depth. The procedure is quicker and more accurate for lesion targeting, and the radiation dose is less than a stereotactic-guided procedure. However, some fine calcifications may not be easily visualised, so conventional stereotactic guidance must be used. The procedure is similar for either stereotactic or tomosynthesis systems once the lesion has been successfully targeted. Patient comfort, cooperation and tolerance are

Principle of Stereotactic localisation

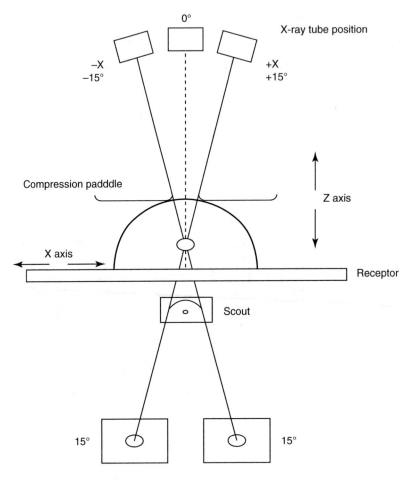

Shift in position of lesion from one image to the other.
The computer calculates the depth (Z)

Fig. 36.1 Principle of stereotactic localisation

paramount for successful harvesting of representative cores of tissue.

Stereotactic biopsy (SCB) is well established with 14g core needle and can be technically challenging for retrieving calcium. 10g vacuum assisted procedures have a higher success rate of sampling any invasive component. Procedural technique must be firmly established in the practitioners' approach. This includes a protocol that emphasises procedure explanation and patient consent. Patient comfort and compliance are imperative to success.

Appropriate positioning, ensuring the shortest targeting distance is used and safe posterior lesion thickness must be efficiently achieved in a timely and empathetic manner. Various innovative devices are now being trialed for lesion marking and visualisation. If ultrasound guidance is not possible then these Xray guided methods can be used with a high degree of success. The practitioner needs to be technically proficient and sympathetic to clients to achieve a successful outcome to both stereotactic and tomosynthesis guided methods. Table 36.1, outlines the available techniques and procedures utilised in current clinical practice to provide stereotactic image guided intervention.

Table 36.1 Principles of Stereotactic localization

Upright stereotactic biopsy	Prone table stereotactic biopsy	Tomosynthesis guided procedures
Vacuum assisted systems using a variety of different needle gauges	Vacuum assisted systems using a variety of different needle gauges	Vacuum assisted systems using a variety of different needle gauges
Conventional non vacuum assisted biopsy technique	Conventional non vacuum assisted biopsy technique	Conventional non vacuum assisted biopsy technique
Wire lesion localisation placement	Wire lesion localisation placement	Wire lesion localisation placement
Marker clip placement	Marker clip placement	Marker clip placement
Small lesion removal (vacuum assisted excision—VAE)	Small lesion removal (VAE—usually <20 mm)	Small lesion removal (vacuum assisted excision—VAE)
Lateral arm approach procedures		

3D Perception

Practitioners are required to perform stereotactic procedures efficiently and precisely. The area to be biopsied needs locating accurately to ensure the radiation dose is minimal. Developing a perception of the three-dimensional appearance of the mass or cluster of calcifications, by calculating its shape from two orthogonal projections, will aid effective positioning and targeting of the lesion. A co-ordinate system of x, y, and z is used to describe the position of the lesion. Although the computer system calculates where the lesion is within the field of view, the practitioner must understand how the equipment is acquiring the image and make adjustments to enable accurate targeting.

All breast types in respect of size, shape and glandular density are encountered and challenge positioning skills, whilst maintaining client acceptance and comfort. Small breasts with limited depth of breast tissue can be positioned with a 'standoff' device to protect the image receptor surface and provide client comfort. Large breasts will require accurate localisation and positioning

on the image receptor to target the lesion for adequate biopsy sampling.

Digital Breast Tomosynthesis (DBT) Guided Biopsy

The use of DBT in breast imaging has also enabled the development of DBT-guided biopsy. DBT guided biopsy may have a higher success rate than that of a conventional stereotactic core biopsy, with a shorter procedure time [3]. The implementation of this procedure is similar to that of a conventional stereotactic biopsy, but DBT allows for the use of the full detector size, which may facilitate improved lesion localisation [3].

Triangulation is not necessary at DBT for depth localisation. Conventional stereotactic biopsy is still needed if calcifications are too fine to be depicted with DBT. Also, if artefacts are visible this would jeopardize lesion visualization [3]. Studies in 2015 observed 100% success rate of DBT guided biopsies compared with 93% success rate of prone conventional stereotactic biopsies [4, 5]. Both studies demonstrated a reduction in the average procedure time, by up to 8 min. In addition, the clinical performance of DBT vacuum assisted biopsy (VAB) was significantly superior to prone stereotactic biopsy [5].

The initial step in the work up of an abnormality detected on DBT should be ultrasound correlation. If this is apparent, then management of this abnormality is similar as when seen on conventional two-dimensional digital mammography [6]. Tomosynthesis guided core biopsy is becoming more readily available, replacing traditional prone stereotactic biopsy.

Procedure

The procedure for digital breast tomosynthesis guided biopsy is similar to conventional two-dimensional stereotactic guided biopsy. Once the client is in the correct position under compression, tomosynthesis is performed. The most significant difference is lesion target, in that a slice is selected through the collected images of tomosynthesis, and the best visualised area of the lesion is targeted. This replaces the scout and 15-degree stereo pair images obtained in two-dimensional mammography guided stereotactic core biopsy.

The following steps best describe a DBT biopsy process [6]:

- The abnormality is targeted on the image slice that best shows the abnormality
- The machine allows targeting to be performed safely by displaying a line box on the images. If this is not displayed, the machine will not allow the operator to target.
- Once the target has been established, the remaining steps are essentially the same in that pre-fire images are taken prior to sampling.
- Samplings of the abnormality are taken, following local protocol, and a clip marker can be deployed post biopsy with check images taken to demonstrate the marker position.

The most significant challenge with tomosynthesis guided stereotactic biopsy is obtaining safe clearance from the client. The movement of the tube head must be clear of any obstruction, for example the client's head or other body parts. This may also interfere with image acquisition. With the machine having moving parts, client cooperation is paramount when positioning for the biopsy [6]. Subtle calcifications may be difficult to visualise on the tomosynthesis targeting images. Reverting to the conventional two-dimensional stereotactic guided biopsy would then be the solution. Calcifications may also cause artefactual appearances on the image and artefacts can obscure lesion visualisation during tomosynthesis. The most frequent artefacts related

to calcifications are shadowing and zipper artefacts [3]. Shadowing corresponds to dark lines, resembling shadows adjacent to large calcifications, while zipper artefacts represent repetition of dense calcifications or metallic material out of plane on the DBT image stack. Although the image processing algorithms reduce these artefacts, they may still impair lesion visualisation [7].

Overall, several studies have found that digital breast tomosynthesis breast biopsies are far more superior to conventional two-dimensional core biopsy. Tomosynthesis affords a more efficient biopsy time, therefore the breast under examination is not compressed as long, which leads to better tolerance of procedure and visualisation of breast lesion.

Indications for stereotaxis

- Indeterminate calcification not visualised on ultrasound
- Lesions demonstrated in only one mammographic view
- Lesion in the posterior aspect of the breast or deep in the breast at ultrasound examination

Stereotactic Core Biopsy

Image guided breast SCB became well established into clinical practices from the early 1990s [8, 9] and was the primary method used to sample mammographically impalpable lesions and areas of microcalcification. SCB has been highlighted as a technically challenging procedure [10, 11]. Failure rates of calcium retrieval following SCB have been reported between 0–16% with a 14-gauge core biopsy. This figure is reduced considerably to between 0 and 5% with a lower gauge vacuum assisted biopsy needle [12]. However, a number of studies have indicated that the presence of an invasive component may be underestimated by needle core biopsy with a diagnosis of pure Ductal Carcinoma in situ

(DCIS) in up to 25% of cases, which may be reduced again by the utilisation of a vacuum assisted biopsy [13].

Ultimately the success of SCB is multi-factorial, with equal weight given to planning both before and during the procedure. Pre SCB all patients should undergo a thorough evaluation which should include clinical examination and additional imaging [14]. Additional imaging techniques including coned/focal compression views, magnification techniques, digital breast tomosynthesis (DBT), and ultrasound evaluation will aid the practitioner to a full lesion evaluation prior to the core biopsy.

The majority of SCB procedures are undertaken using a conventional upright digital stereotactic add on device. An example is demonstrated in Fig. 36.2.

An alternative to the upright stereotactic system is the prone biopsy system. This incorporates all the components of the upright unit with the addition of a support table with a circular aperture onto which the client lies. The breast is positioned through the aperture and accessed from beneath the table. A thorough outline of the use of prone biopsy system in practice is well documented in the published literature [2].

Explanation of the Procedure

Prior to the commencement of the SCB it is important that a full explanation is given to the client, including a description of any likely risks associated with the procedure; these may include bleeding, haematoma, infection and pain. All staff in attendance should be introduced to the client and consent for the procedure should be gained. Informed consent is required for any procedure, but written consent is not essential for image guided core biopsy within the UK. Policies regarding obtaining written consent for breast interventional procedures are produced locally in accordance with hospital policy [14]. Obtaining medical history and other contraindications, for example anticoagulation, is essential prior to carrying out the procedure [15].

Client and Breast Positioning

Prior to the commencement of a SCB, an approach should be planned. The approach should enable the practitioner to position the client and facilitate accurate lesion targeting within the parameters of the stereotactic device. Appropriate positioning should ensure the shortest distance to the lesion is achieved by the biopsy needle. In general, most stereotactic units require a minimum amount of tissue beneath the lesion to accommodate the firing mechanism of the biopsy device and prevent damage to the image receptor. If the breast thickness is found to be insufficient for SCB to be undertaken, methods to increase the thickness of the breast can be carefully attempted.

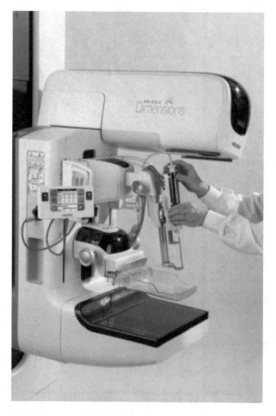

Fig. 36.2 Image provided courtesy of HOLOGIC®

This is usually undertaken by the addition of a spacer bar or platform sited between the breast and the image receptor, artificially increasing the breast thickness. Alternatively, the procedure may be performed via the horizontal approach [16]. This is achieved with the addition of a lateral arm to the stereo unit.

Appropriate client positioning prior to biopsy is determined by the position of the lesion within the breast. In an upright stereo device, clients with lesions within the upper half of the breast should be positioned in the cranio-caudal position. Lesions in the lower inner quadrant are positioned medio-laterally and lesions identified in the lower outer quadrant positioned latero-medially (Fig. 36.3).

Technique

Following client positioning a scout image is taken. This will aid positioning of the lesion within the digital window and provide a visual reference throughout the procedure; the stereo pair is then acquired. The X-ray tube is moved in the horizontal plane to different positions either side of the vertical axis, this generates two images forming the stereo pair. In most cases the fixed angulation is ±15° [2] and is determined by the manufacturer. The combination of the degree of tube angulation and the position of the lesion within the breast will influence the degree of shift seen in the resultant stereo pair. It is important that the practitioner is familiar with this concept,

Fig. 36.3 Illustration of lesion accessibility in relation to location within the breast

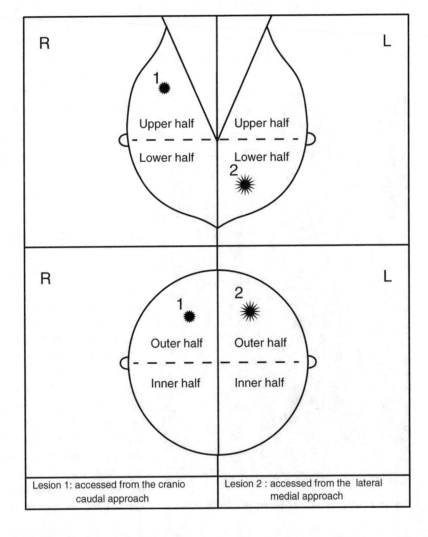

therefore it is advisable to study the characteristics associated with lesion shift by practice with a dedicated biopsy phantom.

Once the appropriate stereotactic images have been acquired, biopsy targets are set. The rationale for targeting small lesions, areas of distortion and clusters of calcification may differ from unit to unit and will usually be defined within local protocols. Following targeting the skin is prepared and local anaesthesia administered. Again, the choice of anaesthesia is decided locally, in many units a local anaesthesia combined with adrenaline is used. The addition of adrenaline acts locally as a vasoconstrictor reducing bleeding and systemic absorption. The lasting action of the anaesthetic is also prolonged with the addition of adrenaline.

Prior to the insertion of the biopsy needle, a small cut is made into the skin allowing access for the biopsy needle and minimise the possibility of skin tearing. Currently there are a number of spring-loaded automated core biopsy devices available for purchase. These comprise of either a fully or part disposable system available in a range of needle lengths, 10–16 cm and gauges 14–18, 14 gauge being the most commonly used in stereotactic biopsy. For the majority of lesions, the choice of a 10 cm biopsy needle is adequate (Fig. 36.4). However, when a large, compressed thickness is achieved and the lesion appears to be deep within the breast, it is advisable to use a 13 cm needle to reach the lesion [17].

It is usual for between 5 to 10 core samples to be taken. The exact number of samples retrieved will be guided by local sampling regimes, the type of lesion to be sampled, and in some cases client compliance. The optimum number of samples required to achieve a reliable histological diagnosis varies, with fewer samples required for mass lesions than areas of microcalcification [14]. For adequate sampling of microcalcification an optimum of either three or more cores containing calcium, or five or more flecks of calcium in total, should be retrieved [18]. As such, specimen imaging of the core samples is essential to demonstrate the removal of a representative sample of calcification [18]. During specimen imaging the breast should remain in compression

because if further sampling is required then the procedure can immediately recommence.

Once the required number of samples has been obtained, a gel-based marker clip may be placed into the biopsy site. Studies have shown the placement of gel-based markers following SCB can facilitate post-operative ultrasound localisation at a later date [19]; they can also assist the multidisciplinary team discussion in cases of non-concordant results. The placement of gel-based markers following biopsy may be routine practice in many units, however, the decision to deploy markers varies and may often be directed by a 'marker placement protocol' outlining to the practitioner the situations where a marker may be deployed.

Following the procedure, the application of a constant amount of pressure to the wound site for approximately 5 min is advised. This will achieve haemostasis and minimise the risk of haematoma formation. When bleeding has ceased, a simple pressure dressing should be placed to cover the wound. The client should be issued with appropriate after care instructions including a follow-up appointment to obtain results of the biopsy.

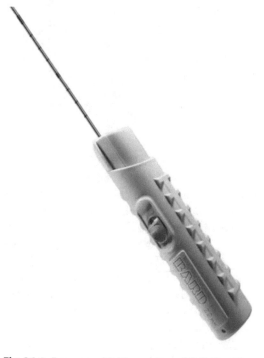

Fig. 36.4 Image provided by courtesy of C. R. Bard Inc

Vacuum Assisted Biopsy (VAB)

The development of VAB in the late 1990s provided an invaluable addition to achieving accurate pre-operative diagnosis. VAB rapidly overcame the limitations of SCB particularly in diagnosing small lesions and areas of microcalcification where under-sampling may have underestimated disease [20].

Currently, The UK National Institute for Clinical Health and Care Excellence (NICE) and the UK National Health Breast Screening Programme (NHSBSP) have validated the use of VAB in both the diagnostic and therapeutic setting.

The indications for use of VAB include:

- Failed conventional core biopsy
- Indeterminate pathology diagnosed at core biopsy
- Small clusters of calcification which may be difficult to sample with conventional 14g SBC
- Discordant imaging/pathological correlation
- Small lesions and clusters of calcification in areas of the breast difficult to access
- Complete excision of some benign breast lesions subject to specific criteria

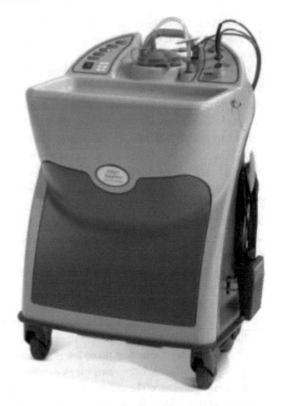

Fig. 36.5 Images ATEC® (Hologic®). Image provided courtesy of Hologic

There are many examples in the literature outlining the benefits for VAB, highlighting its association with increased rates of calcium retrieval and lower rates of under diagnosis in both in situ and invasive disease [21]. In 2018 the NHSBSP outlined the use of VAB in the management of lesions with uncertain malignant potential (B3 lesions). This publication gave guidance in both the use of VAB in the diagnosis and subsequent excision of B3 lesions avoiding surgical intervention in most cases [22].

Currently there are four VAB systems available commercially. Three of these comprise of a single-entry operating system while the fourth, Vacora® (BARD®), utilises a multiple entry approach. Two examples of the single-entry systems (i.e. the ATEC® (HOLOGIC®) and the EnCore Enspire® (BARD®)) are represented in Figs. 36.5 and 36.6, the third being Mammotome®, Breast Care, Ethicon Endo-Surgery®. A comprehensive comparative review of all four VAB systems has been undertaken by Wilson et al. and is recommended for reading [23].

VAB can be incorporated with both upright and prone stereotactic systems with initial imaging and client positioning being similar to that undertaken prior to SCB. It requires a single insertion of the biopsy probe and thereafter contiguous samples of tissue are acquired with vacuum assistance. VAB incorporates the use of a range of probes from 7–12 gauge, the larger gauge probes being mostly used for therapeutic excisions. Suction is applied to the sampling chamber to draw in the lesion to be sampled. The

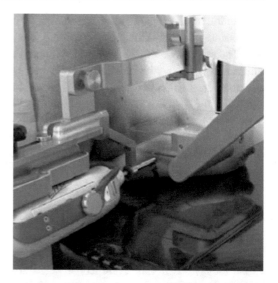

Fig. 36.7 VAB—upright stereotactic system incorporating the use of a 'Lateral Arm'. Image provided courtesy of C. R. Bard Inc

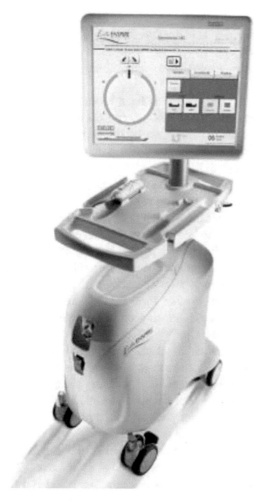

Fig. 36.6 EnCore Enspire® (BARD®). Image provided courtesy of Bard Inc

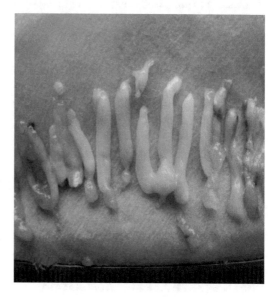

Fig. 36.8 VAB—biopsy sample Image provided courtesy of C. R. Bard Inc

integrated rotating cutter advances across the sampling chamber separating the breast tissue. The resultant specimen is then transported into the specimen collection area. The VAB also has the facility to wash out the biopsy site via an integrated saline flush, this aims to reduce and evacuate any haematoma formation.

A lateral arm available with some VAB systems (Fig. 36.7) allows for small previously inaccessible lesions close to the chest wall and lesions in clients with limited breast tissue to be adequately sampled in the upright position.

It is usual for a minimum of 12 samples to be taken throughout the procedure during which the probe is rotated through 360° [19]; an example of the sample size is demonstrated in Fig. 36.8. However, the number of samples required to optimally evaluate a lesion has initiated much debate and may be in part attributed to a number of variable parameters, including mammographic appearance and operator preference [19].

As the volume of tissue retrieved during the VAB is much larger than that sampled during conventional SCB it is necessary to administer a larger amount of local anaesthesia to the biopsy site. The amount of local anaesthesia required to adequately anaesthetise the site has been widely discussed in the literature [24]. However, within the UK, the administration of approximately 10–12 ml with infiltration of additional anaesthesia during the procedure if necessary is common practice. The strength of the anaesthesia used may vary and will usually be determined locally.

Once the required amount of tissue has been retrieved a biopsy marker clip is deployed into the biopsy site. VAB may remove the vast majority of the lesion and in some cases the entire lesion. Marker deployment facilitates correct localisation of the biopsy site if further surgery is necessary wherein the marker clip will be removed [25, 26]. However, migration of marker clips has been indicated in case reports and other studies [27–29]. It is advisable to image the client whilst the breast is still compressed, post clip insertion.

Overall VAB is well tolerated and popular with clients. It provides an alternative to surgical excision as it is carried out under local anaesthesia. Post procedural complications are low showing no significant differences to those attributed to SCB [20]. The use of VAB has become established in many UK breast units as part of the management pathway in clients who have previously required surgical excision biopsy, an example of such a pathway is well described by Rajan et al. [29]. VAB may also be utilised in conjunction with both ultrasound and magnetic resonance imaging modalities.

Pre-Operative Needle Localisation

Stereotactic pre-operative needle localisation is primarily used to localise impalpable lesions, areas of architectural distortion and clusters of microcalcification prior to surgery. The aim of the procedure is to facilitate the removal of the lesion at the first surgical operation [17]. It requires placement of the wire into, but no further than, 10 mm beyond the lesion [30]. The wire is housed within an introducing needle which is directed to the lesion via stereotactic or ultra-

sound guidance. A number of localisation wires are available in the marketplace, each with a varying shaped stabilising hook. The most common shapes being curved, single or multiple barbed.

The shape of the hook in some cases affects the stability of the wire, a double barbed localisation wire being described as the most commonly used in the UK whilst remaining stable in the breast [31]. The curved shaped hook is less stable but has the facility to be repositioned prior to wire deployment if required [17].

Client preparation prior to localisation is not dissimilar to that undertaken prior to SCB. Previous images must be evaluated to determine optimum positioning, this is especially important as the localisation wire and the mammogram together form the sole mechanism of guidance for the surgeon to undertake accurate excision [32].

Once the client has been positioned and the optimum scout image produced the stereo pair images are taken. It is generally accepted that a combination of the shortest route and the lesion visibility partly determine the most accurate approach to the lesion.

Following target acquisition, the skin is prepared and local anaesthesia is administered. The localising needle is placed in the breast and the central wire deployed into the target area. Once the needle has been withdrawn the residual wire can be seen protruding from the skin. It is necessary for this to be coiled, covered with a dressing and taped to the breast, the wire within the breast will not move as it is anchored by the localising barbs.

Final check images should be taken to aid the surgical team in theatre. The optimum position is achieved if the wire has transected the lesion and the tip lies within a distance of 10mms. This position will facilitate optimum surgical excision (Fig. 36.9).

When larger areas of microcalcification require localisation, the insertion of bracketing wires can be considered. This method was first described by Silverstein et al. in 1987 [33]. The insertion of bracketing wires has been attributed to a reduction in the need for re-excision when large areas of microcalcification are localised [34].

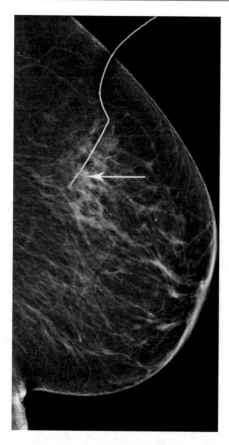

Fig. 36.9 Accurate positioning of Reidy localisation wire

Radio-Guided Occult Lesion Localisation (ROLL)

Introduced in 1996, the technique of ROLL offers an alternative to conventional wire guided stereotactic and/or ultrasound localisation. The technique involves a direct injection of Technetium 99m labelled colloid human albumin into the lesion via image guidance.

The procedure is performed up to 5 h prior to surgery whereupon the surgical excision is performed guided by a gamma probe. This facilitates a skin excision close to the site of greatest radioactivity, enabling the surgeon to excise the lesion achieving the best possible cosmesis. Once the lesion has been removed, the excision cavity can be checked for residual tumour [17].

As sentinel node biopsy (SNB) is the operation of choice in patients where normal axillary lymph nodes are identified, ROLL may be performed along with SNB. Firstly, the ROLL isotope is injected into the lesion, with the second injected around the areola, which will be absorbed by the lymphatic chain and directed to the sentinel lymph node.

The introduction of ROLL has been shown to be associated with a faster, more accurate technique, which provides better cosmetic results and a higher incidence of tumour free margins, ensuring complete excision [35, 36].

Magnetic Seed Localisation

Launched in 2016, localisation via Magseed® offers a further technique in the localisation of impalpable breast lesions prior to surgery. This new technique involves the image guided placement of a 1 × 5 mm medical grade stainless steel marker directly into the lesion to be localised. The marker can be placed into the lesion in the days prior to surgery which is hugely beneficial for patient scheduling.

At the time of surgery, the marker is detected by a sophisticated magnetometer, the Sentimag® Probe, which generates a magnetic field temporarily magnetising the Magseed®. The probe will then identify the magnetic signature generated by the seed allowing the surgeon to localise and subsequently remove the tumour.

A clinical evaluation of the effectiveness of magnetic seed localisation undertaken by Lamb et al. [36] concluded that the use of magnetic seed localisation is an effective method of localising breast lesions, having the potential to replace conventional wire and radioactive seed.

LOCalizer™: Tag Applicator System (Hologic©)

This method inserts a miniature radiofrequency tag into the impalpable lesion so that the surgeon can locate this area. The tag can be inserted any time in advance of the surgical date. The surgeon uses a small portable handheld reader and probe which works to a depth of 6 cm. Each tag has a unique identification number and is inserted with a needle that is guided by ultrasound or X-ray. Two areas can be marked if they are at least 2 cm apart [37].

> **Clinical Pearls**
>
> • Always review the mammograms to determine the shortest route to the abnormality
> • Consider the whole care pathway prior to biopsy
> • Always check the anticoagulant status of the client prior to commencing the biopsy

Chapter Review Questions
Review questions

1. What are the limitations of DBT stereotactic core biopsy?
2. Explain the 3 main indications where stereotactic procedures would be performed.
3. Describe your approach and best visualisation when sampling a distortion.
4. Describe the various outcomes with reference to the latest B3 guidelines from Q3.
5. Discuss the use of local anaesthesia for stereotactic procedures and why adrenaline may be used.
6. When is an area not suitable for a stereotactic vacuum assisted biopsy?

Answers

1. Faint calcifications maybe difficult to visualise.

   Artefacts e.g. surgical clips/macro calcifications/pacemaker/implants.

   Client cooperation is critical due to movement of machine.
2. Indeterminate calcifications not visualised on ultrasound.

   Lesions seen in only one mammographic view.

   Lesions located in the posterior aspect of the breast, or deep in the breast on ultrasound.

3. Although a distortion may be seen on ultrasound, stereotaxis approach is the ideal pathway due to the differentials being a radial scar/complex sclerosing lesion or malignancy.

   To correctly sample a distortion, guidelines advise sampling the centre as well as the periphery of the distortion to achieve concordancy and the best pathway for the patient.

   The centre of the distortion would determine a malignancy but not a radial scar/sclerosing lesion, however, sampling the periphery would determine if the latter lesion was present and also dictate if atypia or DCIS was present.

   If malignancy is excluded and a radial scar/sclerosing lesion is identified then the pathway would be to proceed to a therapeutic stereotactic vacuum assisted biopsy (VAB), ideally with a 7G needle for a therapeutic excision to yield 4g of tissue.
4. If the initial biopsy yielded no atypia/DCIS/malignancy, then the patient would be discharged back to the NHSBSP.

   If atypia only was present, follow up annual mammograms for 5 years is advised.

   DCIS/invasive disease present, proceed to surgery.
5. Ensure you are working safely and protected with regard to client wellbeing and within your professional scope of practice which is indemnified by your employer.

   Lidocaine—tend to be used for wire localisations or magnetic seed insertions/Tag applicator system. The area of insertion is sufficiently anaesthetized and usually only one insertion needed.

   Xylocaine, with the addition of adrenaline, acts locally as a vasoconstrictor reducing bleeding and systemic absorption. The adrenaline prolongs the lasting action of anaesthesia, therefore making the procedure more tolerable to the client. This is generally used for stereotactic biopsies and vacuum assisted biopsies.

   Points to consider: Caution should be exercised if client is allergic to Lidocaine/Xylocaine and appropriate steps should be taken during administration which are compliant with good practice and local requirements.

6. When the area is too superficial there is a potential risk of the skin being sucked in during the procedure. This is unsafe practice and can cause skin necrosis.

When the area is close to the nipple, again, there is a potential risk of causing damage to this area which is potentially not safe and should be avoided.

Appendix

Test your learning and check your understanding of this book's contents: use the "Springer Nature Flashcards" app to access questions using https://sn.pub/dcAnWL.

To use the app, please follow the instructions in Chap. 1.

Flashcard code:

48341-69945-ABCB1-2A8C7-CE9D2.

Short URL: https://sn.pub/dcAnWL.

References

1. Peart O. Mammography and breast imaging: just the facts. New York: McGraw-Hill Companies; 2005.
2. Willison KM. Fundamentals of stereotactic breast biopsy. In: Ed Fajardo LL, Willison KM, Pizzutiello RJ, editors. Comprehensive approach to stereotactic breast biopsy. Hoboken: Wiley; 1996.
3. Horvat JV, Keating DM, Rodrigues-Duarte H, Morris EA, Mango VL. Calcifications at digital breast tomosynthesis: imaging features and biopsy techniques. Radiographics. 2019;39(2):307–18.
4. Waldherr C, Berclaz G, Altermatt HJ, Cerny P, Keller P, Dietz U, Buser K, Ciriolo M, Sonnenschein MJ. Tomosynthesis-guided vacuum-assisted breast biopsy: a feasibility study. Eur Radiol. 2016;26(6):1582–9.
5. Shin K, Teichgraeber D, Martaindale S, Whitman GJ. Tomosynthesis-guided core biopsy of the breast: why and how to use it. J Clin Imag Sci. 2018;8:28.
6. Zuckerman SP, Maidment AD, Weinstein SP, McDonald ES, Conant EF. Imaging with synthesized 2D mammography: differences, advantages, and pitfalls compared with digital mammography. Am J Roentgenol. 2017;209(1):222–9.
7. Parker SH, Lovin JD, Jobe WE, Burke BJ, Hopper KD, Yakes WF. Non palpable breast lesions: ste-reotactic automated large core biopsies. Radiology. 1991;180:403–7.
8. Parker SH, Jobe WE, Dennis MA, Stavros AT, Johnson KK, Yakes WF, Truell JE, Price JG, Kortz AB, Clark DG. US-guided automated large-core breast biopsy. Radiology. 1993;187:506–11.
9. Brenner RJ, Bassett LW, Fajardo LL, Dershaw DD, Evans WP III, Hunt R, Lee C, Tocino I, Fisher P, McCombs M, Jackson VP. Stereotactic core needle breast biopsy; a multi institutional prospective trial. Radiology. 2001;218:866–72.
10. Rakha EA, Ellis IO. An overview of assessment of prognostic and predictive factors in breast cancer needle core biopsy specimens. J Clin Pathol. 2007;60(12):1300–6.
11. Gűműs H, Mills P, Fish D, Gűműs M, Devalia H, Jones S, Sever A, Diyarbakir TR, Kent UK. Underestimation rates of DCIS at stereotactic vacuum assisred biopsy and identifying factors leading underestimation. ECR 2012 Poster number C-0557. https://doi.org/10.1594/ecr2012/C-0557.
12. Brennan ME, Turner RM, Ciatto S, Marinovich ML, French JR, Macaskill P, Houssami N. Ductal carcinoma in situ at core-needle biopsy: meta-analysis of underestimation and predictors of invasive breast cancer. Radiology. 2011;260(1):119–28.
13. O'Flynn EAM, Wilson ARM, Michell MJ. Image guided breast biopsy: state of the art. Clin Radiol. 2010;65(4):259–70.
14. British Society of Breast Radiology. Protocol for breast biopsy in patients taking anticoagulants and antiplatelet therapy. London: British Society of Breast Radiology; 2012.
15. Chan T, Wong KW, Tsui KW, Lau HY, Au Yeung MC. Breast thickness and lesion depth measurement using conventional stereotactic biopsy systems. J Hong Kong Coll Radiol. 2003;6:28–9.
16. Evans A, Pinder S, Wilson R, Eliis I. Breast calcification, a diagnostic manual. London: Greenwich Medical Media; 2002.
17. Bagnall MJC, Evans AJ, Wilson ARM, Burrell H, Pinder SE, Ellis IO. When have mammographic calcifications been adequately sampled at needle core biopsy? Clin Radiol. 2000;55(7):548–53.
18. McMahon MA, James JJ, Cornford EJ, Hamilton LJ, Burrell HC. Does the insertion of a gel-based marker at stereotactic breast biopsy allow subsequent wire localisation to be carried out under ultrasound guidance? Clin Radiol. 2011;66(9):840–4.
19. Ramachandran N. Breast intervention: current and future roles. Imaging. 2008;20(3):176–84.
20. Wallis M, Tarvidon A, Helbich T, Schreer I. Guidelines from the European Society of Breast Imaging for diagnostic interventional breast procedures. Eur Radiol. 2007;17(2):581–8.
21. Pinder SE, Shaaban A, Deb R, Desai A, Gandhi A, Lee AH, Pain S, Wilkinson L, Sharma N. NHS Breast Screening multidisciplinary working group guidelines for the diagnosis and management of breast lesions

of uncertain malignant potential on core biopsy (B3 lesions). Clin Radiol. 2018;73(8):682–92.

22. Wilson R, Kavia S. Comparison of large-core vacuum assisted breast biopsy and excision systems. In: Del Re RB, editor. Minimally invasive breast biopsies. Recent results in breast cancer research, vol. 173. Berlin: Springer; 2009.

23. Lomoschitz FM, Helbich TH, Rudas M, Pfarl G, Linnau KF, Stadler A, Jackman RJ. Stereotactic 11-gauge vacuum-assisted breast biopsy: influence of number of specimens on diagnostic accuracy. Radiology. 2004;232(3):897–903.

24. Brem RF, Schoonjans JM. Local anaesthesia in stereotactic vacuum assisted breast biopsy. Breast. 2001;7:72–3.

25. Burbank F, Forcier N. Tissue marking clip for stereotactic breast biopsy; initial placement accuracy, long term stability, and usefulness as a guide for wire localisation. Radiology. 1997;205(2):407–15.

26. Burnside ES, Sohlich RE, Sickles EA. Movement of a biopsy –site marker clip after completion of stereotactic directional vacuum –assisted breast biopsy: case report 1. Radiology. 2001;221(2):504–7.

27. Parikh JR. Clip migration within 15 days of 11 gauge vacuum assisted stereotactic breast biopsy. Am J Roentgenol. 2005;184(3):43–6.

28. Rajan S, Shaaban AM, Dall BJG, Sharma N. New patient pathway using vacuum assisted biopsy reduces diagnostic surgery for B3 lesions. Clin Radiol. 2012;67(3):244–9.

29. ABS at BASO. The association of breast surgeons at the British Association of Surgical Oncology. Guidelines for the management of symptomatic breast disease. Eur J Surg Oncol. 2005;31(1):1–21.

30. Chaudary MA, Reidy JF, Chaudhuri R, Mills RR, Hayward JL, Fentiman IS. Localisation of impalpable breast lesions; a new device. Br J Surg. 1990;77(10):1191–2.

31. Saarela AO, Rissanen TJ, Lähteenmäki KM, Soini Y, Haukipuro K, Kaarela O, Kiviniemi HO. Wire-guided excision of non-palpable breast cancer: determinants and correlations between radiologic and histologic margins and residual disease in re-excisions. Breast. 2001;10(1):28–34.

32. Silverstein MJ, Gamagami P, Rosser RJ, Gierson ED, Colburn WJ, Handel N, Fingerhut AG, Lewinsky BS, Hoffman RS, Waisman JR. Hooked-wire-directed breast biopsy and overpenetrated mammography. Cancer. 1987;59(4):715–22.

33. Cordiner CM, Litherland JC, Young IE. Does the insertion of more than one wire allow successful excision of large clusters of malignant calcification. Clin Radiol. 2006;61(8):686–90.

34. Ramesh HS, Anguille S, Chagla LS, Harris O, Desmond S, Thind R, Audisio RA. Recurrence after ROLL lumpectomy for invasive breast cancer. Breast. 2008;17(6):637–9.

35. Van der Ploeg IM, Hobbelink M, Van Den Bosch MA, Mali WT, Rinkes IB, Van Hillegersberg R. 'Radioguided occult lesion localisation' (ROLL) for non-palpable breast lesions: a review of the relevant literature. Eur J Surg Oncol. 2008;34(1):1–5.

36. Lamb LR, Bahl M, Specht MC, D'Alessandro HA, Lehman CD. Evaluation of a nonradioactive magnetic marker wireless localization program. Am J Roentgenol. 2018;211(4):940–5.

37. Lowes S, Bell A, Milligan R, Amonkar S, Leaver A. Use of Hologic LOCalizer radiofrequency identification (RFID) tags to localise impalpable breast lesions and axillary nodes: experience of the first 150 cases in a UK breast unit. Clin Radiol. 2020;75(12):942–9.

Digital Breast Tomosynthesis

37

Cherish B. Parham

Learning Objectives
- Identify equipment specific to digital breast tomosynthesis
- Describe digital breast tomosynthesis image acquisition process and analyse image processing techniques
- Understand the effect of digital breast tomosynthesis on mean glandular dose
- Review screening and diagnostic recommendations
- Assess digital breast tomosynthesis procedure options and summarise quality control requirements

Introduction

The basic principle of Digital Breast Tomosynthesis (DBT) is the acquisition of a three-dimensional block of data comprising multiple images of the breast acquired at a range of angles above the image receptor. This is achieved by moving the X-ray tube and sometimes the detector in an arc over the compressed breast while making a series of exposures. This technology was developed to mitigate the challenges in breast imaging in the visualisation of structures in the breast due to summation artifact, or the overlapping of tissues, and the low subject contrast of the breast. Digital mammography (DM2D) improves contrast resolution but does not eliminate the issue of superimposition of structures within the breast on a DM2D image. Benign structures of the breast may still present with suspicious characteristics when superimposed upon the other. Likewise, malignant lesions may be obscured by benign features of the breast. DBT allows for the imaging of the breast in a series of reconstructed planes horizontal to the image receptor approximately 1 mm apart. By blurring planes above and below each section of the breast, DBT images are evaluated with minimal superimposition of tissue. This allows for more precise assessment of the breast, reducing false positive and false negative results, increasing the specificity and sensitivity of breast cancer detection (BCD) with DBT [1, 2].

Equipment

Like DM2D, the X-ray tube in DBT units is situated in the protective housing of the gantry, perpendicular to the chest wall of the client. The cathode side of the tube is positioned directly over the thickest part of the breast at the chest wall at a tube tilt of approximately 6° [3]. The anode is directed over the thinner

C. B. Parham (✉)
Department of Radiation Science, Virginia Commonwealth University, Richmond, VA, USA
e-mail: cbparham@vcu.edu

part of the breast toward the nipple, allowing for maximum utilisation of the anode heel effect. The angles of the anode range from 0° to 16° and focal spots range from 0.3 to 0.1 mm [4]. The breast is compressed using a radiolucent polycarbonate resin paddle, approximately 3 mm thick [4]. The materials that comprise the X-ray tube in a DBT unit are different than DM2D, and although DBT units are similar across manufactures, they are not identical.

DBT uses a higher X-ray energy photon beam than DM2D to acquire images because contrast is less crucial for image evaluation [5]. Each tomogram in the series blurs the noise above and below the plane of interest. This technique reduces the need for high contrast to visualise pathologies obstructed by superimposed tissues because a "stack" of images is acquired. Since higher energy X-ray photons are acceptable for DBT, the target material is typically tungsten (W), the exception being GE with a Rhodium (Rh) anode. Common filters are rhodium (Rh) or aluminum (Al), but silver (Ag) and molybdenum (Mo) are also used [6] (Table 37.1) [3–6].

Image Acquisition

The acquisition method of DBT images is based on the equipment manufacturer. The movement of the gantry is either a "step and shoot" method or a continuous method. "Step and shoot" systems come to a full stop in between each tomographic exposure [5, 6]. Although this increases the overall time the breast is under compression, it decreases focal spot motion blur from movement of the tube. Client motion is more likely to occur with "step and shoot" systems because of longer scan times compared with a tube using continuous motion [5]. A shorter over all scan time is achieved with the continuous image acquisition, but this method increases motion blur from focal spot blur and can occasionally obscure microcalcifications [5, 7]. However, multiple studies indicate DBT that includes the synthetic 2D image (SI) does not reduce rates of microcalcification detection [8–10]. Additionally, step and shoot methods cannot use grids due to the motion of the tube producing grid cutoff [11].

The tube and image receptor may have an isocentric geometry or partial isocentric geometry. Hologic is the only manufacturer employing an

Table 37.1 Parameters of DBT systems approved for use in both the United States and the EU

Manufacturer	Hologic	Siemens	GE	Giotto/IMS	Fuji
Image acquisition					
Tube motion	Continuous	Continuous	Step and shoot	Step and shoot	Continuous
Acquisition angle	15°	50°	25°	40°	15° or 40°ª
Number of projections	15	25	9	13	15
Scan time (s)	3.7	25	7	12	7 or 9ª
Image processing					
Pixel size	140 m (binned 2 × 2)	85 m	100 m	85 m	150 m (binned 2 × 1) or 100 mª
Pixel shape	Square	Square	Square	Square	Hexagonal
Space between reconstructed planes	1 mm	1 mm	0.5 mm	1 mm	1 mm
Reconstruction method	FBP	FBP	Iterative	Iterative	FBP
Equipment					
Detector type	Direct	Direct	Indirect	Direct	Direct
Detector material	a-Se	a-Se	CsI	a-Se	a-Se
Tube Target	W	W	Rh/Mo	W	W
Filtration	AL	Rh	Mo/Rh	Rh/Ag	AL/Rh
Grid	No	No	Yes	No	No

ª Fuji DBT systems operate in standard mode and high resolution mode (*)

isocentric design, with the image receptor moving in synchronisation with the angle of the tube [4–6]. Most DBT units have partial isocentric geometry. This means the image receptor is stationary as the tube rotates around the fulcrum, or pivot point [4]. [12].

The sweep angle, or the angle that arcs over the image receptor during exposure, ranges from 15° to 50°. A smaller scan angle will improve in-plane resolution. This is the resolution on the x–y axis and will improve the visualisation of smaller objects like microcalcifications [4, 6]. A larger scan angle will improve out-of-plane resolution, or z-axis resolution, allowing for enhanced visualisation of larger lesions that extend beyond one in-plane projection [4–6]. A larger angle will increase the total number of projections in the sweep. Systems range from 9 to 25 projections per sweep [5]. A larger number of projections will improve overall image quality, but increases scan time and increases the dose to the client [12]. Regardless of the number of projections, minimal dose is still required for each overall sweep. Dose is accumulated across all projections. A larger angle with an increased number of projections will require each projection to use less radiation. Thus, some of the image quality is lost due to noise from lower exposure rates distributed per projection [4] (Table 37.1).

DBT units are designed to operate in multiple clinical protocol modes selected by the technologist. These modes, selected at the control panel, include DM2D only, Combo (DM2D + DBT) and DBT only with the option for a SI. When DBT was first introduced on the market, combo mode was the recommended image acquisition mode [10]. Combo mode nearly doubles the radiation dose received by the client because a DM2D and a DBT sweep are executed by the unit. Radiation dose received from mammographic imaging is measured in mean glandular dose (MGD) [6]. When comparing MGD of DM2D with DBT alone, DBT produces a MGD 30–50% high than DM2D depending on breast thickness [1, 8]. When Combo mode is selected, MGD can approximately double, though this still remains within the dose limits set by EUREF and the FDA [13, 14].

Current DBT software has the ability to reconstruct an SI image from the DBT dataset. SI images eliminate the necessity of a DM2D view in the screening process, reducing the total exam exposure by half [2, 8]. Multiple studies comparing BCD rates with DBT plus DM2D and DBT only plus SI suggest that DBT plus SI has similar or superior sensitivities and specificities in detecting cancer compared to DBT plus DM2D, including the assessment of microcalcifications [7–10, 15]. Although this is a controversial topic in DBT, the FDA has approved mammography with SI images in lieu of an additional DM2D image for a screening mammogram and the UK National Health Service Breast Screening Programme (NHSBSP) updated DBT guidelines to include the SI image as a replacement for the DM2D image [14, 16].

Image Processing

DBT uses a digital method of converting exit radiation into an image with flat panel detectors using a scintillator (indirect) or a photoconductor (direct). The indirect systems use flat panel detectors with a scintillator made of cesium iodide to convert X-rays into visible light and then into an electronic signal. Direct systems use flat panel detectors made of selenium to convert X-rays directly to an electronic signal [6]. The electronic signal is converted to a digital signal in the analog to digital converter. Pixels range in size across manufactures from 50 to 150 μm which is comparable to DM2D [6]. Several manufacturers go through a process called 'rebinning' that allows the system to evaluate a block of pixels together in 2 × 2 or 2 × 1 block [4–6] (Table 37.1). The advantage of reconstruction using binning mode is an increase in effective pixel size, SNR and processing speed with a slight loss in x–y resolution [4]. Most DBT systems use a standard pixel shape, with the exception of Fuji. This system uses a hexagon pixel shape to increase effective pixel size [6].

DBT images are not a true 3D reconstruction of the breast like computed tomography (CT) because the sweep angle and number of projections are limited in DBT [17]. Some Z-plane resolution is lost in the reconstruction. Filtered back projection (FBP) and iterative mathematical algorithms are applied to the data set to reconstruct the DBT image [4, 17]. Both techniques are widely used in CT reconstruction processes [3]. During the FBP process, data is filtered through multiple equations spatially across tomographic angles which produces less optimal spatial resolution due to the limited sweep angle [6]. Iterative reconstruction applies algebraic and statistical equations to the data set, improving DBT image quality by increasing sharpness and reducing quantum mottle and streak artifact [3, 6], [17]. However, the algorithm is more complicated than FBP and requires additional processing time and computer capacity [3].

The in-focus images are viewed at planes parallel to the image receptor separated by 0.5–1 mm depths [4, 5], [11]. Out-of-focus planes are created solely from reconstruction [6]. Noise is removed above and below each depth to visualise the in-focus plane. DBT images are viewed as individual x–y planes or in a continuous loop through the stack of planes [5]. The number of reconstructed images is dependent on the compressed tissue thickness of the breast. A breast compressed to 45 mm will result in 45 reconstructed images [6], [18].

Screening

Early population based DBT screening studies indicate that DBT plus DM2D increases BCD rates up 9.5–40% [9, 19]. Continued evaluation of the effectiveness of DBT in BCD shows sustained higher rates of BCD (15–53%) with DBT [20–25]. Early studies of DBT and BCD rates were evaluated using DBT plus DM2D. More recently, research has compared DBT plus DM2D with DBT plus SI, excluding the DM2D. Screening using SI as a replacement for the DM2D results in similar or increased rates of BCD than with DBT plus DM2D [8–10]. This finding indicates screening DBT programs can eliminate the DM2D and reduce MGD by half [2–8]. Studies evaluating the incidence of interval cancers findings, or cancers detected after a negative result mammogram, suggest there may be increased sensitivity in detecting interval cancers with DBT screening programs [20, 23]. However, a meta-analysis of the literature on BCD with DBT plus SI did not detect a change in interval BCD, but it did find that overall BCD, recall rate and biopsy rates were reduced using DBT plus SI compared to DBT plus DM2D [21].

The literature solidly supports the use of DBT as a primary screening tool, but DM2D remains the standard of care for breast imaging [2]. The ACR appropriateness criteria for mammography screening still recognises DM2D an adequate screening tool, but includes DBT as an option [26]. NHSBSP recommends DBT screening only for those in the approved clinical trial, or as the first tool in diagnostic workups of masses, asymmetries and architectural distortions [16]. Considerations such as cost, interpretation time, digital storage space and IT connectivity issues make the conversion to DBT difficult in some cases, but may eventually be needed as a standard of care in breast imaging with evidence mounting that DBT performs better than DM2D overall [6].

The replacement or conversion of DM systems to units with DBT capability requires considerable capital investment in addition to the added cost of longer interpretation times and PACS storage. Because DBT requires the image reader to review both the 2D (synthetic or DM) and scroll through the DBT planes, interpretation time for DBT may increase by 15–53%, research has demonstrated that time is proportionally lower with increased years of experience [27, 28]. Although, with a reduction in call back rates and fewer views needed for diagnostic interpretation, overall workflow efficiency may not be significantly impacted [7–10, 15, 19, 24]. Sizable storage space is required for DBT images. DBT files range from 200 to 400 MG per view compared to DM at 8–24 MG [28]. Insufficient storage can lead to lag time in images sent from the acquisition station to the reporting workstation and issues with image retrieval for comparison, reducing workflow efficiency.

Diagnostic Evaluation

Mammography screening recall rates have decreased with the advent of DBT, reducing the need for additional diagnostic evaluations [29, 30]. Lesion localisation and mapping the extent of disease is clearer on DBT, eliminating the need for spot compression views in some cases [31, 32]. While, DBT improves the detection of some mammographic abnormalities, including architectural distortion, asymmetries and masses, diagnostic workups are still recommended for suspicions finding [33].

Architectural distortion is a subtle mammographic finding characterised by focal distortion of tissue without the presence of a mass. Architectural distortion is difficult to assess on DM2D due to summation artifact and may be an early sign of breast cancer. DBT improves upon DM2D in the identification of architectural distortion by minimising summation artifacts [31, 34]. Multiple studies have concluded that architectural distortions are identified more often with DBT and of the percentage of those representing positive findings are higher [29, 33, 35, 36]. Correlation with additional imaging modalities such as ultrasound and/or additional DBT images is recommended. However, spot views occasionally diffuse the appearance of potentially malignant architectural distortions [34].

Breast masses are evaluated based on their margins, shape and density [31, 34]. Studies indicate DBT improves the detection of moth malignant and benign masses [33, 37, 38]. Benign lesions are often visualised with a radiolucent halo appearance around the denser centre of the mass. The halo affect is more prominent on DBT, but sometimes DBT can depict a halo type appearance for malignant masses, so continued investigation with ultrasound and additional views may be needed [32, 37]. Further, small spiculations radiating from the centre of a mass, suggesting malignancy, may be more conspicuous on DBT images [32, 33].

An asymmetry describes an area of fibro glandular tissue that has a discordant appearance from the contralateral breast [31]. Asymmetries are resolved at higher rates on DBT without the need for a diagnostic workup, reducing false positive recall rates [32]. This is attributed to the removal of summation artifact resolving the suspicious area or the abnormality to be characterised as a mass [34].

Identification of calcifications remains consistent between DM2D, DBT plus 2D and DBT plus SI. However, there are some advantages of using DBT to recognise benign calcifications' characteristics and the distribution of calcifications in the breast [10, 32, 33]. Skin calcifications are sometimes eliminated from suspicion on DBT images without the need for a time consuming skin calcification workup, as the z-plane would help identify the plane location of the calcifications [32, 33]. In some cases, the distribution of calcifications can also aid in the mapping of the distribution of the abnormality in both suspicions and benign pathologies [10, 34]. Additionally, the removal of noise above and below each section of the tomogram allows for easier identification of vascular calcifications and rim calcifications [32]. However, it is still recommended that DM2D magnification views are used to characterise calcification findings when malignancy is a differential diagnosis [32–34].

Compression

Although client positioning has not changed in crossing over to DBT, studies indicate it is feasible to reduce compression force without impacting image quality or lesion detection performance [39–42]. Breast compression helps reduce the effect of superimposed breast tissue on the mammographic image, but DBT improves the visualisation of overlapping tissue and diminishes summation artifacts [42]. Compression decreases client dose by reducing tissue thickness, creating a more uniform breast thickness and immobilises the breast to prevent motion blur [43]. Compression should not be eliminated with the use of DBT, but a 45–50% reduction in compression force has been shown to reduce client discomfort without compromising image quality in DBT [39, 41, 42].

Quality Control (QC) Performed by the Practitioner

Maintaining consistent quality images using DBT acquisition is paramount in breast cancer detection. Because DBT equipment varies by manufacturer, each system has its own recommended protocol for DBT QC. Additionally, the NHS Cancer Screening Programme, European Reference Organization for Quality Assured Breast Screening and Diagnostic Services (EUREF) and the American College of Radiology (ACR) offer protocols specific to both Medical Physicists and Radiographers [17]. Because DBT units are also equipped to perform DM2D, all QC tests recommended for DM2D should be performed on DBT units in 2D mode. Additional Radiographer QC test are recommended for DBT evaluating image quality, the homogeneity of images and geometric accuracy in DBT systems on a suggested schedule [17].

Evaluation of image quality using a phantom evaluates the DBT system's ability to detect a range of simulated pathologies with varying characterisation [17, 44, 45]. The test can be done in conjunction with the DM2D phantom image evaluation in combination mode or independent of the DM2D in tomographic mode only [17, 46]. To ensure consistency, it is important to conduct the test using the same parameters each time the test is performed, using the same phantom, mode, technique, and compression. Quality is determined by comparing the acquired phantom image with the baseline standards established by the physicist. This should be conducted at the acquisition station computer and the computer used for image interpretation [44]. The PMMA phantom prominent in the United States is the ACR phantom consisting of an acrylic block with a wax insert. Masses, fibers and specks of various sizes are embedded in the wax. Image quality is measured by how many masses fibers and specks are seen on the phantom image in full resolution and scrolling through the resolution plane [46]. The Leeds Test Object TOR (MAS) or TOR (MAM) is an option in Europe and the UK using similar standards [45, 47].

Signal to noise ratio (SNR) and contrast to noise ratio (CNR) can be calculated automatically by the DBT system using a PMMA phantom to ensure consistency of the image receptor response [46, 48]. SNR measures intensity of exposure compared to noise on the DBT image and CNR measures contrast resolution compared with noise on the DBT image [49]. Both of these measurements are difficult to calculate accurately on DBT due to the reconstructed planes. However, using the SNR measurement to monitor signal consistency and CNR to measure fluctuations in noise is recommended [50].

Regular evaluation of the image receptor for homogeneity and artifacts is important to exclude ghosting and artifacts that could mimic pathologies on the DBT image [17]. Manufacturers recommend slightly different procedures to evaluate these factors. In some units such as Hologic, this is done by calibrating the system with a series of images using the flat-field phantom, a clear acrylic block phantom covering the entire detector and completing an artifact evaluation image using the same detector [46]. Other systems only require that the artifact image is taken using a flat-field phantom to evaluate inconsistencies with the detector [46, 51].

Geometric Accuracy testing is performed for DBT to assess distortion and assure the entire breast is included in each image [47]. This test should be done per the manufacturer's guideline using phantoms specific for the system or with the quality phantom. Hologic uses a phantom with radiopaque beads fixed at different locations in the z and $x–y$ planes. DBT system software is used to analyse the phantom [46]. Any discrepancy of more than 0.1 mm could result in excluded tissue, inaccurate image measurements and failed localisation efforts [45]. Geometric accuracy can also be assessed using an image quality phantom, by evaluating the consistency of dept for the specks, fibers, and masses [17].

Spatial resolution is measured in spatial frequency, or line pairs per mm (lp/mm). This is how many high contrast line pairs can be resolved on the image [43]. Bar test pattern phantoms used in evaluating spatial resolution for DM2D can also be used in DBT mode. High contrast bar patterns ranging from 3 lp/mm to 10 lp/mm are placed on top of or embedded in an acrylic phantom and an image is acquired in DBT mode [45, 46, 51]. Another method for testing spatial resolution is through the evaluation of modulation transfer function (MTF), or the ability of the imaging system to differentiate the contrast between objects of varying size and shape [49]. Some manufacturers such as GE have dedicated phantoms for this purpose. Regardless of method, requirements for spatial resolution range for 2–4 lp/mm for DBT to ensure image quality [17, 44, 46, 51].

DBT Procedures

As DBT has become more widely implemented in the past 10 years, so have biopsy methods to sample breast tissue using DBT guidance. Tomosynthesis-guided vacuum assisted breast biopsy (DBT-VB) and pre-operative needle wire localisation (DBT-WL) can be performed upright on a DBT unit with specialised equipment attached for the procedure or a dedicated DBT prone biopsy table [52–55].

DM2D vacuum assisted stereotactic biopsy (ST-VB) has been the standard biopsy technique for lesions seen on DM2D such as microcalcifications, masses and architectural distortions. It reduces the need for surgical excision biopsies [53]. ST-VB is typically performed on a dedicated prone biopsy table. It requires an initial scout image to visualise the lesion in the biopsy window, then two images are acquired (stereotactic pair) at ±15° angles to the scout image. The lesion is localised using triangulation with a cartesian coordinate system (x, y, z) [55]. Pre and post fire stereotactic images are captured to verify the location of the needle and lesion before sampling.

DBT-VB units function in a similar way, but improve upon this system by allowing the target to be localised in the z-depth scrolling through the DBT planes [53, 56]. This eliminates the need for stereotactic pair images throughout the procedure, because the z-depth of the lesion is identified on the DBT image [55, 56]. DBT-VB units have improved spatial resolution over ST-VB units because the entire detector and a radiolucent compression paddle are used to capture biopsy images, increasing field of view (18 × 24) and allowing for the visualisation of tissue landmarks in relation to the targeted lesion [56]. The DBT-VB biopsy needle and vacuum device is similar to that of ST-VB. Stroke margin, or the space between the fired needle and the detector, is calculated by the DBT-VB system once the needle is mounted and targeting coordinates are transmitted [56]. Care should be taken in evaluating the stroke margin to eliminate the possibility of firing the needle through the breast, piercing the skin on the opposite side, potentially damaging the detector with injury to the breast tissue. Biopsy samples are acquired in the same protocol as ST-VB [53].

DBT-VB visualises architectural distortions, subtle calcifications and masses not seen well on ST-VB, and thus has increased sensitivity in targeting difficult to see pathologies [52, 54, 55, 57]. In addition to increased technical performance, multiple studies report that biopsies on DBT-VB equipment reduce the overall procedure time, increase client comfort when done on an upright system and reduce client dose [54, 55, 57]. Dose is lessened by eliminating the need for stereotactic pairs throughout the procedure, reducing the total number of exposures [52, 53]. The more efficient targeting time observed in DBT-VB is attributed to the elimination of the stereotactic pairs, ease of positioning in the upright system, and ability to identify z-depth in the scout DBT image [55]. Additionally, the use of a transparent biopsy compression paddle that allows for a full view of the breast improves targeting time because the lesion and surrounding landmarks are visualised on the scout image, allowing for more efficient positioning adjustments [53]. ST-VB units have a smaller field of view and use a radi-opaque compression paddle, making adjustments more complicated.

Limited studies are available that compare the performance upright and prone DBT-VB methods. Research to date yields similar results in accuracy, but increased client comfort and ease of targeting was observed in upright DBT-VB systems [52, 55]. Additionally, prone units require dedicated clinical space that can only be utilised for procedures and have weight limits that restrict client access [56]. Some sites report the drawback of an upright DBT-VB is increased client vasovagal response because the procedure is done in a manner that the client can see [58].

Localising lesions for surgical excision has long been performed using DM2D guidance (DM-WL) and occasionally stereotactic guidance to aid the surgeon in excising a specimen not seen in other imaging modalities. The method improves cosmetic outcomes for clients by reducing the amount of tissue removed [43]. With the advent of DBT, some pathologies like architectural distortions, subtle masses and faint calcifications are only seen on DBT, requiring a localisation method guided by DBT [59]. The needle wire localisation method is used in DBT (DBT-WL) and yields similar results as DM-WL. The client is positioned with an open alphanumeric grid compression paddle with an orientation that allows for the shortest distance from skin to lesion [43, 59]. A DBT scout image is acquired and alphanumeric coordinates are selected for the initial placement of the needle. A depth measurement can be made from the scout to determine the depth of the needle [60]. The client remains in compression for the acquisition of images and placement of the needle to prevent any movement of the breast that would impact the placement of the wire. Additional images are obtained to ensure the proper placement of the needle before the wire is placed. Although depth of the lesion can be determined from the DBT image, it is recommended to obtain images in a plane perpendicular to that of the initial needle placement for inserting the wire [60].

Chapter Review Questions
Review Questions

1. How does DBT imaging improve the visualisation of superimposed structures in the breast?
2. How many mm apart are DBT images reconstructed in planes horizontal to the image receptor?
3. Why is tungsten an appropriate target material for DBT X-ray tubes?
4. Which method of DBT image acquisition comes to a full stop in between projections?
5. A DBT unit that arcs over a stationary image receptor employs what kind of geometry?
6. How does using combo mode on the control panel affect client MGD?
7. A compressed 50 cm breast will result in how many reconstructed images?
8. DBT improves the visualisation of?
   a. masses
   b. architectural distortions
   c. asymmetries
   d. all of these
9. What is the geometric accuracy QC test performed on DBT units used to evaluate?
10. In what image does a DBT guided breast biopsy target the lesion z-depth?

Answers

1. By removing summation artifact
2. 0.5–1 mm
3. It has reduced emphasis on contrast
4. Step and shoot
5. Partial isocentric design
6. It increases by approximately 50%
7. 50
8. Masses, architectural distortions and asymmetries
9. Distortion and tissue exclusion
10. Scout image

Acknowledgments The author would like to acknowledge the two previous authors of this chapter from the first edition Consultant Radiologists in the United Kingdom Dr Yit Y. Lim and Dr Anthony J. Maxwell.

Appendix

Test your learning and check your understanding of this book's contents: use the "Springer Nature Flashcards" app to access questions using https://sn.pub/dcAnWL.

To use the app, please follow the instructions in Chap. 1.

Flashcard code: 48341-69945-ABCB1-2A8C7-CE9D2.

Short URL: https://sn.pub/dcAnWL.

References

1. Feng SSJ, Sechopoulos I. Clinical digital breast tomosynthesis system: Dosimetric characterization. Radiology. 2012;263(1):35–42.
2. Gao Y, Moy L, Heller SL. Digital breast tomosynthesis: Update on technology, evidence, and clinical practice. Radiographics. 2021;41(2):321–37.
3. Bushong S. Radiologic Science for Technologists: Physics, Biology and Protection. 12th ed. Elsevier Health Sciences; 2021.
4. Bushberg JT, Seibert JA, Leidholdt EM, Boone JM, Abby C. The Essential Physics of Medical Imaging. 4th ed. Wolters Kluwer; 2021.
5. Yaffe MJ, Mainprize JG. Digital Tomosynthesis: Technique. Radiol Clin North Am. 2014;52(3):489–97.
6. Tagliafico A, Houssami N, Calabrese M. Digital Breast Tomosynthesis: A Practical Approach. Switzerland: Springer; 2016.
7. Horvat JV, Keating DM, Rodrigues-Duarte H, Morris EA, Mango VL. Calcifications at digital breast tomosynthesis: imaging features and biopsy techniques. Radiographics. 2019 Mar;39(2):307–18.
8. Garayoa J, Chevalier M, Castillo M, Mahillo-Fenandez I, Amallal EI, Ouahabi N, Estrada C, Tejerina A, Benitez O, Valverde J. Diagnostic value of the stand-alone synthetic image in digital breast tomosynthesis examinations. Eur Radiol. 2018;28(2):565–72.
9. Skaane P, Bandos AI, Eben EB, Jebsen IN, Krager M, Haakenaasen U, Ekseth U, Izadi M, Hofvind S, Gullien R. Two-view digital breast tomosynthesis screening with synthetically reconstructed projection images: comparison with digital breast tomosynthesis with full- field digital mammographic images. Radiology. 2014 Jun;271(3):655–63.
10. Choi JS, Han BK, Ko EY, Kim GR, Ko ES, Park KW. Comparison of synthetic and digital mammography with digital breast tomosynthesis or alone for the detection and classification of microcalcifications. Eur Radiol. 2019;29(1):319–29.
11. Sechopoulos I. A review of breast tomosynthesis. Part II. Image reconstruction, processing and analysis, and advanced applications. Med Phys. 2013;40(1):1–17.
12. Barkhausen J, Rody A, Schaefer F. Digital Breast Tomosynthesis: Technique and Cases. Thieme; 2015 Oct 20.
13. Maldera A, De Marco P, Colombo PE, Origgi D, Torresin A. Digital breast tomosynthesis: Dose and image quality assessment. Phys Medica. 2017;33:56–67.
14. U.S. Food and Drug Administration. Mammography. Available from: https://www.fda.gov/radiation-emitting-products/medical-x-ray-imaging/mammography [Accessed March 3rd 2022].
15. Zuley ML, Guo B, Catullo VJ, Chough DM, Kelly AE, Lu AH, Rathfon GY, Lee Spangler M, Sumkin JH, Wallace LP, Bandos AI. Comparison of two-dimensional synthesized mammograms versus original digital mammograms alone and in combination with tomosynthesis images. Radiology. 2014 Jun;271(3):664–71.
16. UK National Health Service. Guidance Breast screening: digital breast tomosynthesis. Available from: https://www.gov.uk/government/publications/breast-screening-digital-breast-tomosynthesis/breast-screening-digital-breast-tomosynthesis [Accessed March 3 rd 2022].
17. Tirada N, Li G, Dreizin D, Robinson L, Khorjekar G, Dromi S, Ernst T. Digital breast tomosynthesis: physics, artifacts, and quality control considerations. Radiographics. 2019 Mar;39(2):413–26.
18. Barkhausen J, Rody A, Schaefer F. Digital Breast Tomosynthesis : Technique and Cases. Incorporated: Thieme Medical Publishers; 2015.
19. Ciatto S, Houssami N, Bernardi D, Caumo F, Pellegrini M, Brunelli S, Tuttobene P, Bricolo P, Fantò C, Valentini M, Montemezzi S. Integration of 3D digital mammography with tomosynthesis for population breast-cancer screening (STORM): a prospective comparison study. The Lancet Oncology. 2013;14(7):583–9.
20. Johnson K, Lång K, Ikeda DM, Åkesson A, Andersson I, Zackrisson S. Interval breast cancer rates and tumor characteristics in the prospective population-based Malmö breast tomosynthesis screening trial. Radiology. 2021;299(3):559–67.
21. Zeng B, Yu K, Gao L, Zeng X, Zhou Q. Breast cancer screening using synthesized two- dimensional mammography: A systematic review and meta-analysis. Breast. 2021;59:270–8.
22. Bahl M, Mercaldo S, Dang PA, McCarthy AM, Lowry KP, Lehman CD. Breast cancer screening with digital breast tomosynthesis: Are initial benefits sustained? Radiology. 2020;295(3):529–39.
23. Houssami N, Bernardi D, Caumo F, Brunelli S, Fanto C, Valentini M, Romanucci G, Gentillini MA, Zorzi M, Macaskill P. Interval breast cancers in the 'screening with tomosynthesis or standard mam-

mography' (STORM) population-based trial. Breast. 2018;38:150–3.

24. Sharpe RE, Venkataraman S, Phillips J, Dialani V, Fein-Zachary VJ, Prakash S, Slanetz PJ, Mehta TS. Increased cancer detection rate and variations in the recall rate resulting from implementation of 3D digital breast tomosynthesis into a population-based screening program. Radiology. 2016;278(3):698–706.

25. Seth Broder J, Bhat R, Boyd JP, Ogloblin IA, Limakakeng A, Hocker MB, Drake WG, Miller T, Harringa JB, Repplinger MD. Who explicitly requests the ordering of computed tomography for emergency department patients? A multicenter prospective study. Emerg Radiol. 2016;23:221–7.

26. American College of Radiology. ACR Appropriatness Criteria Breast Cancer Screening. Available from: https://www.acr.org/Advocacy-and-Economics/ ACR-Position-Statements/Breast-Tomosynthesis [Accessed July 3 rd 2021].

27. Dang PA, Freer PE, Humphrey KL, Halpern EF, Rafferty EA. Addition of tomosynthesis to conventional digital mammography: Effect on image interpretation time of screening examinations. Radiology. 2014;270(1):49–56.

28. Hooley RJ, Durand MA, Philpotts LE. Advances in digital breast tomosynthesis. Am J Roentgenol. 2017;208(2):256–66.

29. Skaane P, Sebuødegård S, Bandos AI, Gur D, Østerås BH, Gullien R, Hofvind S. Performance of breast cancer screening using digital breast tomosynthesis: results from the prospective population-based Oslo Tomosynthesis Screening Trial. Breast Cancer Res Treat. 2018;169(3):489–96.

30. Alabousi M, Wadera A, Kashif Al-Ghita M, Kashef Al-Ghetaa R, Salameh JP, Pozdnyakov A, Zha N, Samoilov L, Dehmoobad Sharifabadi A, Sadeghirad B, Freitas V. Performance of Digital Breast Tomosynthesis, Synthetic Mammography, and Digital Mammography in Breast Cancer Screening: A Systematic Review and Meta-Analysis. J Natl Cancer Inst. 2021;113(6):680–90.

31. Peppard HR, Nicholson BE, Rochman CM, Merchant JK, Mayo RC III, Harvey JA. Digital breast tomosynthesis in the diagnostic setting: indications and clinical applications. Radiographics. 2015 Jul;35(4):975–90.

32. Kulkarni S, Freitas V, Muradali D. Digital Breast Tomosynthesis: Potential Benefits in Routine Clinical Practice. Can Assoc Radiol J. 2022;73(1):107–20.

33. Amir T, Ambinder EB, Harvey SC, Oluyemi ET, Jones MK, Honig E, Alvin MD, Mullen LA. Benefits of digital breast tomosynthesis: A lesion-level analysis. J Med Screen. 2021 Sep;28(3):311–7.

34. Chong A, Weinstein SP, McDonald ES, Conant EF. Digital breast tomosynthesis: Concepts and clinical practice. Radiology. 2019;292(1):1–14.

35. Dibble EH, Lourenco AP, Baird GL, Ward RC, Maynard AS, Mainiero MB. Comparison of digital mammography and digital breast tomosynthesis in

the detection of architectural distortion. Eur Radiol. 2018;28(1):3–10.

36. Suleiman WI, McEntee MF, Lewis SJ, Rawashdeh MA, Georgian-Smith D, Heard R, Tapia K, Brennan PC. In the digital era, architectural distortion remains a challenging radiological task. Clin Radiol. 2016;71(1):e35–40.

37. Nakashima K, Uematsu T, Itoh T, Takahashi K, Nishimura S, Hayashi T, Sugino T. Comparison of visibility of circumscribed masses on Digital Breast Tomosynthesis (DBT) and 2D mammography: are circumscribed masses better visualized and assured of being benign on DBT? Eur Radiol. 2017;27(2):570–7.

38. Bian T, Lin Q, Cui C, Li L, Qi C, Fei J, Su X. Digital Breast Tomosynthesis: A New Diagnostic Method for Mass-Like Lesions in Dense Breasts. Breast J. 2016;22(5):535–40.

39. Förnvik D, Andersson I, Svahn T, Timberg P, Zackrisson S, Tingberg A. The effect of reduced breast compression in breast tomosynthesis: Human observer study using clinical cases. Radiat Prot Dosimetry. 2010;139(1-3):118–23.

40. Abdullah Suhaimi SA, Mohamed A, Ahmad M, Chelliah KK. Effects of reduced compression in digital breast tomosynthesis on pain, anxiety, and image quality. Malaysian J Med Sci. 2015;22(6):40–6.

41. Agasthya GA, D'Orsi E, Kim YJ, Handa P, Ho CP, D'Orsi CJ, Sechopoulos I. Can breast compression be reduced in digital mammography and breast tomosynthesis? Am J Roentgenol. 2017;209(5):W322–32.

42. Moshina N, Larsen M, Holen ÅS, Waade GG, Aase HS, Hofvind S. Digital breast tomosynthesis in a population based mammographic screening program: Breast compression and early performance measures. Eur J Radiol. 2021;139:109665.

43. Andolina V. Mammographic Imaging : A Practical Guide. 3rd ed. Philadelphia: Wolters Kluwer/ Lippincott Williams & Wilkins Health; 2011.

44. ACR. Mammography Accreditation Program Requirements. Available from: https://www. acraccreditation.org//media/ACRAccreditation/ Documents/Mammography/Requirements. pdf?la=en [Accessed November 29 th 2021].

45. van Engen RE, Bosmans H, Bouwman RW, Dance DR, Heid P, Lazzari B. Protocol for the quality control of the physical and technical aspects of digital breast tomosynthesis systems. 2018;v1. 03:March.

46. Hologic. Quality Control Manual: Selenia Dimensions DM & BT. Vol 4. Hologic, Inc; 2016.

47. Burch A, Hay E, Loader R, Parkyn E, Phillips V, Rowberry B, Strudley C, Whitwam D. Routine quality control tests for breast tomosynthesis (Radiographers) NHSBSP Equipment Report 1406 About the NHS Cancer Screening Programmes About Public Health England. Public Health England; 2014.

48. Sage J, Fezzani KL, Fitton I, Hadid L, Moussier A, Pierrat N, Martineau A, Dreuil S, Heulers L, Etard C. Experimental evaluation of seven quality control

phantoms for digital breast tomosynthesis. Phys Medica. 2019;57(November 2018):137–44.

49. Fauber TL. Radiographic Imaging & Exposure. 5th ed. Missouri: Elsevier Health Sciences; 2018.

50. Strudley CJ, Young KC, Looney P, Gilbert FJ. Development and experience of quality control methods for digital breast tomosynthesis systems. Br J Radiol. 2015;88(1056):1–11.

51. Siemens. Quality Control Manual MAMMOMAT Inspiration. Published online. 2008;

52. Choudhery S, Johnson M, Fazzio RT. Prone versus upright digital tomosynthesis-guided biopsy. Am J Roentgenol. 2020;215(3):760–4.

53. Jonna AR, Sam KQ, Huynh PT. Stereotactic breast biopsies: An update in the era of digital tomosynthesis. Appl Radiol. 2018;47(9):17–20.

54. Schrading S, Distelmaier M, Dirrichs T, Detering S, Brolund L, Strobel K, Kuhl CK. Digital breast tomosynthesis- guided vacuum-assisted breast biopsy: Initial experiences and comparison with prone stereotactic vacuum-assisted biopsy. Radiology. 2015;274(3):654–62.

55. Bahl M, Maunglay M, D'Alessandro HA, Lehman CD. Comparison of Upright Digital Breast Tomosynthesis–guided versus Prone Stereotactic Vacuum-assisted Breast Biopsy. Radiology. 2019;290(3):298–304.

56. Vijapura CA, Wahab RA, Thakore AG, Mahoney MC. Upright tomosynthesis-guided breast biopsy: Tips, tricks, and troubleshooting. Radiographics. 2021;41(5):1265–82.

57. Weinfurtner RJ, Carter T. Transition to digital breast tomosynthesis-guided biopsies: Results and complications compared to stereotactic biopsies. Breast J. 2021;27(1):21–6.

58. Omofoye TS, Martaindale S, Teichgraeber DC, Parikh JR. Implementation of Upright Digital Breast Tomosynthesis-guided Stereotactic Biopsy. Acad Radiol. 2017;24(11):1451–55.

59. Freer PE, Niell B, Rafferty EA. Preoperative tomosynthesis-guided needle localization of mammographically and sonographically occult breast lesions. Radiology. 2015;275(2):377–83.

60. Friedewald SM, Young VA, Gupta D. Lesion localization using the scroll bar on tomosynthesis: Why doesn't it always work? Clin Imaging. 2018;47:57–64.

Contrast Enhanced Investigations

38

Eva Maria Fallenberg

Learning Objectives
- Understand and apply the examination protocols in regard to contrast enhanced mammography
- Describe and evaluate the indications for contrast enhanced digital mammography examinations
- Describe the complications and side effects of contrast agents

Introduction

The sensitivity of mammography is limited especially in dense breasts [1]. Additional imaging modalities have been developed to compensate for some of the technical limitations of conventional mammography, such as lack of contrast and superimposing tissue. Initial approaches assessing contrast uptake of the breast were made in the 1980s using CT scanning.

E. M. Fallenberg (✉)
Klinikum rechts der Isar, TU München, Institut für diagnostische und interventionelle Radiologie, München, Germany
e-mail: eva.fallenberg@tum.de

Whilst this technique was useful in the detection of breast cancer, it resulted in very high radiation doses to the breast, thyroid and the chest wall [2]. Presently, breast MRI with high spatial resolution using gadolinium containing contrast agents is considered the most sensitive imaging method overall, but there remains some concern regarding specificity, particularly with inexperienced readers and lack of widespread availability with biopsy facilities and costs.

The introduction of digital mammography enabled further developments such as contrast enhanced digital mammography and tomosynthesis [3, 4]. Contrast enhanced digital mammography (CEM) demonstrates contrast uptake of breast cancers. When a malignant tumour is still small, it is nourished and oxygenated by diffusion, but as the tumour grows the diffusion process becomes insufficient for its requirements. If the tumour grows larger than 2 mm, there will be a lack of oxygen and nutrients. By releasing vascular endothelial growth factor, the tumour induces vessel growth from the surrounding vessels towards the tumour. This is called neoangiogenesis. The new tumour feeding vessels are poor quality and have leaky walls which results in contrast material being deposited in the tumour interstitial spaces. This process enables contrast enhancement of the tumour.

Encouraging clinical results of examinations with CEM with different examination protocols have been published in the past few years, all of them acquired on a prototype of a commercially available full-field digital silicon based flat panel system [5–8]. The initial studies demonstrated that due to the contrast uptake of the lesion the technique is feasible. The resulting dynamic curves have been comparable to MRI [5, 6]. An increase in the detection rate of breast lesions up to 17.5% by using contrast enhanced mammography could be demonstrated [6–12].

The technique is commercially available and different vendors brought their CEM Systems on the market. A recent metanalysis of 60 studies reported a significant higher pooled sensitivity of 95% and specificity of 81% of reading results of the combination of low energy images and recombined images than reading the recombined images alone [13].

Basic Principle of Contrast Mammography Technique

In CEM the different X-ray attenuation characteristics of various composites of the breast, especially the glandular tissue, fat and iodine-based contrast agents are demonstrated. However, the exposure parameters used in conventional mammography are not optimal to visualise the low concentration contrast uptake. Consequently, the technique had to be adapted to enable visualisation [14, 15]. To demonstrate iodine uptake in the breast, it has to be imaged with an X-ray spectrum above and below the K-edge of iodine located at 33.2 kVp. If the breast is imaged after contrast injection with a kVp-spectrum below this value, (which is equivalent to the normal spectrum of about 26–32 kVp used in conventional digital mammography) the iodine in the breast does not cause a significant visible increased absorption of X-rays. The resulting image is comparable to a normal mammogram demonstrating the usual features being looked for when searching for possible breast cancer such as masses, densities, architectural distortions, and microcalcifications [14, 15].

If the kVp is increased to a higher energy level output above the k-edge of iodine at 33.2 kVp, it is possible to visualise low concentrations of Iodine without significantly increasing client dose. To do so, the energy level needs to be raised to 45–47 kVp combined with an additional filtering of the X-ray-spectrum with a copper or titanium filter to obtain an X-ray spectrum with a peak above the k-edge of iodine. This will be absorbed by iodine, if it is enriched in the tissue. The beam is filtered to reduce the lower energy parts of the spectrum

Table 38.1 Specifications of different CEM machines

Vendor	GE	Siemens	Hologic	Fuji
Detector	a-Si	a-Se	a-Se	a-Se
Pixel size (μm)	100	85	70	50
Tube	Molybdenum/rhodium	Tungsten	Tungsten	Tungsten
Filter	Copper	Titanium	Copper	Copper
Add. HE-dose (%)	20	30–50	50	50–80

and therefore avoid image noise induced by these photons. The resulting image is called a high energy image [14, 15].

These low and high energy images are then combined to produce an image demonstrating the iodine uptake only. The background tissue is removed. The low energy image with the anatomical information and the recombined image showing areas with increased iodine concentration are used together to obtain diagnostic information. Anatomical structures and mammographically demonstrated abnormalities such as masses, architectural distortions, microcalcifications, and densities maybe visualised. Additional contrast uptake is often an indication of malignant change [14, 15].

The adaption of the machines has been made differently by the different vendors. The resulting dose levels are dependent on breast composition and thickness as well as the number of images of the sequence. One high energy image requires approximately 20–80% of a normal mammography image depending on the machine used (Table 38.1).

Temporal Subtraction Technique

Due to the experiences with contrast enhanced breast MRI and technical limitations, a temporal subtraction approach was initially used in contrast enhanced mammography. In this procedure, the client is positioned seated in front of the mammography system, the breast is compressed either in the CC, the MLO or the ML view. First a standard high energy image is obtained. The breast remains compressed, and the contrast agent is injected intravenously. After the contrast

agent injection repeated exposures of the same breast are performed over a time of 2–10 min. This results in a series of one pre contrast and several post contrast high energy images of the same breast in one view only with some dynamic information. In most studies the CC view is preferred, as it is more tolerable for the client than other projections [16].

The advantage of this approach is the ability to obtain dynamic information comparable to breast MRI. Disadvantages of this approach are: there is no image containing anatomical information; it is very sensitive to movement artefact; it can be uncomfortable for the client due to the long breast compression time (up to 10 min depending on the chosen number of repetitions). Motion can result in artefacts and problems with orientation of the images due to slight differences in breast position. This might degrade the quality of the images and their diagnostic accuracy. Also, only one view of one breast is acquirable and no information of the contralateral breast is obtained [16].

Bilateral Dual-Energy Technique

Currently the most widely accepted approach is the bilateral two-view contrast enhanced spectral mammography. The contrast agent is injected through an intravenous line which is usually within the antecubital vein. During the injection the patient is comfortably seated in a chair in the mammography room. After injection the client is disconnected from the injector and lead to the mammography machine. 2 min after the start of the injection the client is positioned as for a normal two view mammogram. The system program results in a double exposure, with one high and one low kVp image per projection. The system switches automatically from the low to the high energy mode. Depending on the exposure time an additional time of 1–2 s for the switch from low to high energy mode is required. Within approximately 5 min CC and MLO bilateral images can be performed in the same way as conventional mammography. With this approach it is possible to acquire several bilateral images with a single contrast injection. Assessment of the locality and extent of the lesion is much more accurate with the two view approach [17].

The dose of CEM also depends on the breast thickness and composition and results in approxi-

mately 1.2–1.8 times of the conventional digital mammography dose. Nevertheless, the resulting dose of CEM is below the recommended dose levels of the EUREF guidelines for mammography screening [18].

Several studies have demonstrated the increased sensitivity of CEM compared to mammography without a decrease in specificity [7, 10, 18]. In addition, the experiences comparing bilateral CEM with MRI showed nearly equal results [8, 11, 18]. Figures 38.1 and 38.2 clearly demonstrate the presence of a 6 cm mucinous carcinoma in the recombined CEM image.

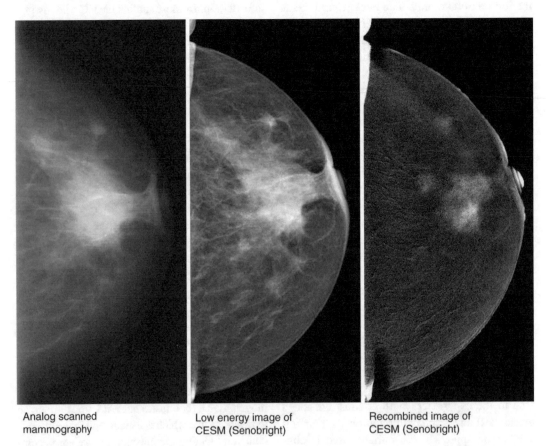

Analog scanned mammography

Low energy image of CESM (Senobright)

Recombined image of CESM (Senobright)

Fig. 38.1 Example of an analog mammography and the low energy and recombined CESM image (CC-view) showing a 6 cm mucinous carcinoma in a 75 years old woman with a palpable mass in the left breast. CESM images have been aquired on an a-Si based full field digi-tal mammography Prototype CESM (GE Senographe DS, Chalfont St. Giles, UK). Now a FDA approved product (Senobright) for additional workup of inconclusive MX and US

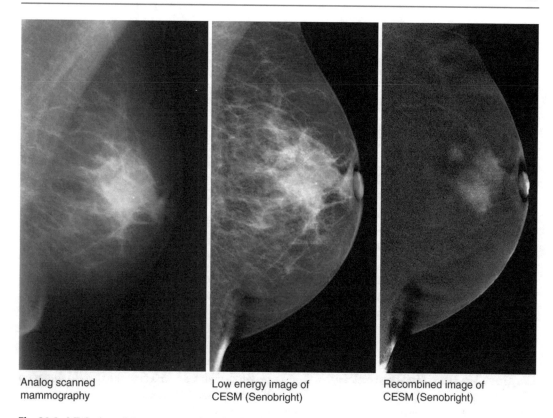

Analog scanned
mammography

Low energy image of
CESM (Senobright)

Recombined image of
CESM (Senobright)

Fig. 38.2 MLO view of the same example as in Fig. 38.1

Contrast Agent Administration

For contrast enhanced mammography iodinated X-ray contrast agents are used. Usually a concentration of 300 mg/ml Iodine and a dose of 1.5 ml/kg body weight (minimum 50 ml, maximum 120 ml) is sufficient. The client should be consented for the injection according to local protocols which include informing them about the possible side effects and asking about their medical history to identify possible contraindications. As so fare there are only a few companies with dedicated approval of the use of Iodine for CEM, an off-label-use should be declared to the patient as well. If there is no contraindication an intravenous line should be inserted, preferably into the antecubital vein. It is recommended to test this line with about 10 ml sodium chloride injected manually for confirming correct placement and flow. If the line is working well, this

cannula will be connected to an automatic injector ideally [19].

The contrast agent is injected with a flow rate of about 3 ml/s. If the vessel is noted to be very small or the injection is difficult when testing the venous access before the contrast injection, the injection speed may need to be adapted. A saline flush of 20–30 ml can be considered after contrast medium injection, but it is not mandatory. Iodinated contrast agents are used frequently in clinical practice and are generally considered safe. Nevertheless, there are some contraindications and side effects the client has to be informed about or they have to be ruled out before doing the examination. Low and iso-osmolar, non-ionic contrast agents are preferable as they tend to have fewer side effects [20]. There are several contrast agents with different iodine concentrations available on the market. An overview is displayed in Table 38.2.

Table 38.2 Commonly used iodinated contrast agents

Compound	Name	Type	Iodine content (mgI/ml)	Osmolality	
Ionic	Iothalamate Meglumine (Conray)-Guerbet	Monomer	325	1843	High
Ionic	Metrizoate (Isopaque 370) Nycomed	Monomer	370	2100	High
Ionic	Ioxaglate (Hexabrix) Guerbet	Dimer	320	580	Low
Non-ionic	Iopamidol (Isovue 300) Bracco	Monomer	300	616	Low
Non-ionic	Iohexol (Omnipaque 350) GE	Monomer	350	884	Low
Non-Ionic	Ioversol (Optiray) Guerbet	Monomer	300	651	Low
Non-ionic	Lobitridol (Xenetix 300) Guerbet	Monomer	300	695	Low
Non-ionic	Iomeprol (Iomeron 350) Bracco	Monomer	350	618	Low
Non-ionic	Iopromide (Ultravist 300-370)	Monomer	300–370	610–774	Low
Non-ionic	Iodixanol (Visipaque 320) GE	Dimer	320	290	Low

Contrast Agent Side Effects

It is important for all practicing contrast media injections to fully understand the current guidelines from the Contrast Media Safety Committee [20]:

Contrast Medium Nephrotoxicity

Administration of contrast agents to clients suffering from kidney dysfunction can result in kidney failure. The client should be asked about any known kidney disease and the kidney function should be tested with a blood test before doing the examination, especially if the client is elderly or has any history of kidney disease or elevated serum-creatinine levels especially related to diabetic nephropathy. In addition, dehydration, age over 70 years, congestive heart failure, and concurrent administration of nephrotoxic drugs like non-steroid anti-inflammatory medicine can increase the risk [20, 21]. If the creatinine levels are acceptable but the client has risk factors, the client should be well hydrated. Nephrotoxic drugs should be stopped for 24 h and alternative imaging modalities should be considered. If the kidney function is less than <45 ml/min/1.73 m^2 eGFR, clients are at elevated risk for contrast agent induced nephropathy and administration of contrast agent should be avoided.

Interaction with the Thyroid Gland

The iodine injection can also induce a severe hyperthyreosis with a thyrotoxic crisis in clients with occult hyper thyreosis or thyroid nodules. Also any radioiodine therapy of thyroid nodules is not possible for about 6 months after applying contrast agents, so this should be checked by a detailed client anamnesis and thyroid function blood test [20, 22].

Allergic Reactions

Like all contrast agents and pharmaceutical drugs acute mild, moderate or severe allergic reactions with a rush, itching, exanthema, urticaria, nausea, vomiting, difficulty to breathe, or shock including respiratory and cardiac arrest can occur. Some of these reactions are due to hypersensitivity/allergy, others are caused by chemotoxicity. The risk for these reactions is increased in clients with a previous history of reactions to iodine-based contrast agents, known asthma or allergy to some medicines. Also, anxiety of the clients can result in symptoms; not all of the experienced symptoms within an hour of the administration of the contrast mediums is caused by the agent itself. You should also be aware that mild reactions at the beginning can develop into more serious ones later [21].

To reduce the risk of any allergic reaction, nonionic contrast agents are preferable, and the client should be monitored for 30 min in the department. Drugs and equipment for resuscitation should be readily available. In clients with known reaction or elevated risk, an alternative test should be considered, if that is not possible, a suitable alternative contrast agent should be used, and a premedication considered [20, 22].

Extravasation

If the intravenous access is not placed correctly or at a less optimal injection side, like the lower limb or small distal veins, extravasation of the contrast agent can occur. It is important to ensure good intravenous access. This can be tested by injecting sodium chloride manually in order to observe correct placement. Adjust the flow rate if the injection is difficult or the vessel is small, provided there is no extravasation when testing [21].

Common Side Effects and Reactions

A feeling of ascending heat in the whole body, a feeling of needing to urinate and a metallic taste in the mouth are normal but can cause alarm, therefore, the client should be informed about these possibilities prior to commencing the examination. They may also feel the contrast agent flowing into the vein, as the agent is usually slightly colder than the human body. In general, warming of the contrast agent makes it more comfortable for the client, reduces viscosity and therefore may reduce risk for extravasation and general adverse events [21, 23].

Clinical Applications

As contrast enhanced digital mammography are invasive and require intravenous administration of contrast agents, they are mainly used in the non-screening setting, indications for CEM are mainly in the assessment of inconclusive findings in conventional mammography with work up of equivocal lesions in dense breasts and staging clients with newly diagnosed breast cancer. It may also have a role as a first line assessment tool in some symptomatic cases. Regarding diagnostic performance of CEM in assessment of suspicious findings detected on mammography, a higher pooled sensitivity of 92% and 84% specificity in dense breasts of 95% and 78% respectively were reported [24–26].

As the indications and also the sensitivity and specificity for CEM are similar to those for MRI, it may be considered as an alternative to MRI in women with contraindications to MRI such as metallic implants, cochlea implants or claustrophobia. Further indications include situations where MRI is unavailable or not reimbursed and a preoperative assessment of disease extent is required. In addition, it is more and more under discussion whether CEM would be a good and less costly alternative to MRI in screening people with dense breasts [24–26].

With the incoming evidence of the benefit of this technique in the above mentions, the CEM is included more and more in clinical guidelines, e.g. the AGO-recommendations and S3 guidelines of Germany [24–26].

Initially the possibility of doing a biopsy under CEM guidance was missing and had to be done under MRI guidance or assessed using anatomical landmarks. In the meantime, the vendors also developed solutions for contrast guided biopsy.

CEM is further helpful in monitoring treatment response as neoadjuvant treatment regimes are increasingly used and, due to side effects, it is important to have an easy, available tool for judging treatment effect [26, 27] (Fig. 38.3). Exclusion of recurrence in follow up cases and detection of mammographically occult cancers in women with proven axillary metastasis may also benefit from CEM, even if for this indication there are still good clinical studies missing (Fig. 38.4).

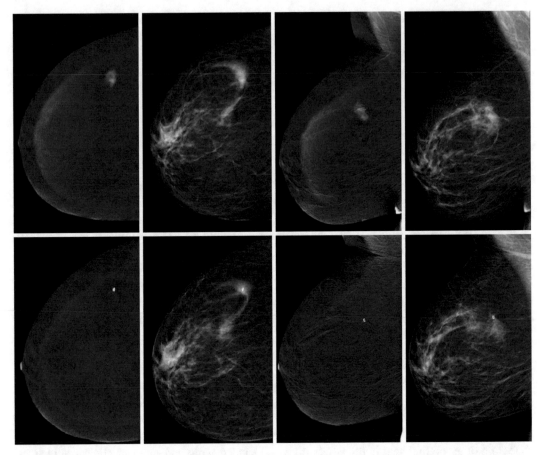

Fig. 38.3 Example of monitoring of a NST breast cancer before and after neoadjuvant treatment with combined chemotherapy with EC and paclitaxel, trastuzumab and pertuzumab. The enhancement of the clip marked tumour disappeared completely, the tissue is much more transparent and smaller in size, the final histology showed a clear decrease in size with only a few distributed tumour cells in a large sclerosing zone and some DCIS

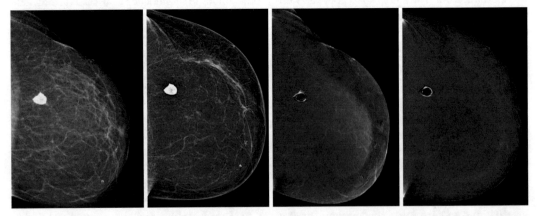

Fig. 38.4 CEM examinations in follow up of a 62 years BRCA1 positive high risk breast cancer patient, not able to underwent MRI due too panic attacks. This example shows the influence of different reconstruction algorithms and further improvement of processing of different vendors in regards to LE imaging appearance as well as artefact reduction in recombined images. GE Senograph Essential images on the left side, Siemens Mammomat Revelation images on the right side

Conclusion

Contrast enhanced mammography is a very promising, widely available technique, able to improve the diagnostic performance of mammography. It is important to combine both images, the anatomical low energy image and the recombined image for diagnosis. It is relatively simple to perform, widely available and highly acceptable technique.

Chapter Review Questions
Review Questions

1. Regarding contrast administration of contrast agent in bilateral CEM which answer is correct
   (a) The breast is compressed during injection.
   (b) Clients have to be informed about normal reactions
   (c) Contrast agent can only be injected if kidney function is completely normal
2. CEM
   (a) Exist of low and high energy images
   (b) Can be acquired with every mammography machine
   (c) Has significantly higher sensitivity and specificity than conventional mammography

Answers

1. Clients have to be informed about normal reactions
2. Exist of low and high energy images
   Has significantly higher sensitivity and specificity than conventional mammography

Appendix

Test your learning and check your understanding of this book's contents: use the "Springer Nature Flashcards" app to access questions using https://sn.pub/dcAnWL.

To use the app, please follow the instructions in Chap. 1.

Flashcard code: 48341-69945-ABCB1-2A8C7-CE9D2.

Short URL: https://sn.pub/dcAnWL.

References

1. Pisano ED, Gatsonis C, Hendrick E, Yaffe M, Baum JK, Acharyya S, Conant EF, Fajardo LL, Bassett L, D'Orsi C, Jong R. Diagnostic performance of digital versus film mammography for breast-cancer screening. N Engl J Med. 2005;353(17):1773–83.
2. Chang CH, Nesbit DE, Fisher DR, Fritz SL, Dwyer SJ 3rd, Templeton AW, Lin F, Jewell WR. Computed tomographic mammography using a conventional body scanner. Am J Roentgenol. 1982;138(3):553–8.
3. Diekmann F, Diekmann S, Taupitz M, Bick U, Winzer KJ, Hüttner C, Muller S, Jeunehomme F, Hamm B. Use of iodine-based contrast media in digital full-field mammography-initial experience. RöFo. 2003;175(3):342–5.
4. Smith JA, Andreopoulou E. An overview of the status of imaging screening technology for breast cancer. Ann Oncol. 2004;15:18–26.
5. Diekmann F, Diekmann S, Jeunehomme F, Muller S, Hamm B, Bick U. Digital mammography using iodine-based contrast media: initial clinical experience with dynamic contrast medium enhancement. Investig Radiol. 2005;40(7):397–404.
6. Dromain C, Balleyguier C, Muller S, Mathieu MC, Rochard F, Opolon P, Sigal R. Evaluation of tumor angiogenesis of breast carcinoma using contrast-enhanced digital mammography. Am J Roentgenol. 2006;187(5):528–37.
7. Dromain C, Thibault F, Diekmann F, Fallenberg EM, Jong RA, Koomen M, Hendrick RE, Tardivon A, Toledano A. Dual-energy contrast-enhanced digital mammography: initial clinical results of a multireader, multicase study. Breast Cancer Res. 2012;14(3):1–8.
8. Fallenberg EM, Dromain C, Diekmann F, Engelken F, Krohn M, Singh JM, Ingold-Heppner B, Winzer KJ, Bick U, Renz AD. Contrast-enhanced spectral mammography versus MRI: initial results in the detection of breast cancer and assessment of tumour size. Eur Radiol. 2014;24(1):256–64.
9. Dromain C, Thibault F, Muller S, Rimareix F, Delaloge S, Tardivon A, Balleyguier C. Dual-energy contrast-enhanced digital mammography: initial clinical results. Eur Radiol. 2011;21(3):565–74.
10. Dromain C, Vietti-Violi N, Meuwly JY. Angiomammography: a review of current evidences. Diagn Interv Imaging. 2019;100(10):593–605.
11. Jochelson MS, Dershaw DD, Sung JS, Heerdt AS, Thornton C, Moskowitz CS, Ferrara J, Morris EA. Bilateral contrast-enhanced dual-energy digi-

tal mammography: feasibility and comparison with conventional digital mammography and MR imaging in women with known breast carcinoma. Radiology. 2013;266(3):743–51.

12. Lobbes MB, Lalji U, Houwers J, Nijssen EC, Nelemans PJ, van Roozendaal L, Smidt ML, Heuts E, Wildberger JE. Contrast-enhanced spectral mammography in patients referred from the breast cancer screening programme. Eur Radiol. 2014;24(7):1668–76.

13. Cozzi A, Schiaffino S, Sardanelli F. The emerging role of contrast-enhanced mammography. Quant Imaging Med Surg. 2019;9(12):2012.

14. Lewin JM, Isaacs PK, Vance V, Larke FJ. Dual-energy contrast-enhanced digital subtraction mammography: feasibility. Radiology. 2003;229(1):261–8.

15. Puong S, Bouchevreau X, Patoureaux F, Iordache R, Muller S. Dual-energy contrast enhanced digital mammography using a new approach for breast tissue canceling. Phys Med Imag. 2007;65(1):65102.

16. Dromain C, Balleyguier C. Contrast-enhanced digital mammography. In: Bick U, Diekmann F, editors. Digital mammography. Berlin: Springer; 2010. p. 187–98.

17. Daniaux M, De Zordo T, Santner W, Amort B, Koppelstätter F, Jaschke W, Dromain C, Oberaigner W, Hubalek M, Marth C. Dual-energy contrast-enhanced spectral mammography (CESM). Arch Gynecol Obstet. 2015;292(4):739–47.

18. EUREF. European guidelines, 5th ed. Available from: https://www.euref.org/european-guidelines/5th-edition. Accessed 20 February 2022.

19. Fallenberg EM, Schmitzberger FF, Amer H, Ingold-Heppner B, Balleyguier C, Diekmann F, Engelken F, Mann RM, Renz DM, Bick U, Hamm B. Contrast-enhanced spectral mammography vs. mammography and MRI–clinical performance in a multi-reader evaluation. Eur Radiol. 2017;27(7):2752–64.

20. ESUR. ESUR guidelines on contrast agents. Available from: https://www.esur.org/fileadmin/content/2019/ESUR_Guidelines_10.0_Final_Version.pdf. Accessed 20 February 2022.

21. Zanardo M, Cozzi A, Trimboli RM, Labaj O, Monti CB, Schiaffino S, Carbonaro LA, Sardanelli F. Technique, protocols and adverse reactions for contrast-enhanced spectral mammography (CESM): a systematic review. Insights Imaging. 2019;10(1):1–5.

22. van der Molen AJ, Thomsen HS, Morcos SK. Effect of iodinated contrast media on thyroid function in adults. Eur Radiol. 2004;14(5):902–7.

23. Bellin MF, Stacul F, Webb JA, Thomsen HS, Morcos SK, Almén T, Aspelin P, Clement O, Heinz-Peer G, Reimer P, van der Molen A. Late adverse reactions to intravascular iodine based contrast media: an update. Eur Radiol. 2011;21(11):2305–10.

24. Ditsch N, Kolberg-Liedtke C, Friedrich M, Jackisch C, Albert US, Banys-Paluchowski M, Bauerfeind I, Blohmer JU, Budach W, Dall P, Fallenberg EM. AGO recommendations for the diagnosis and treatment of patients with early breast cancer: update 2021. Breast Care. 2021;16(3):214–27.

25. Woeckel A, Festl J, Stueber T, Brust K, Krockenberger M, Heuschmann PU, Jírů-Hillmann S, Albert US, Budach W, Follmann M, Janni W. Interdisciplinary screening, diagnosis, therapy and follow-up of breast cancer. Guideline of the DGGG and the DKG (S3-Level, AWMF Registry Number 032/045OL, December 2017)–Part 2 with recommendations for the therapy of primary, recurrent and advanced breast cancer. Geburtshilfe Frauenheilkd. 2018;78(11):1056–88.

26. Wockel A, Festl J, Stuber T, Brust K, Stangl S, Heuschmann PU, et al. Interdisciplinary screening, diagnosis, therapy and follow-up of breast cancer. Guideline of the DGGG and the DKG (S3-Level, AWMF Registry Number 032/045OL, December 2017) - part 1 with recommendations for the screening, diagnosis and therapy of breast cancer. Geburtshilfe Frauenheilkd. 2018;78(10):927–48.

27. Iotti V, Ravaioli S, Vacondio R, Coriani C, Caffarri S, Sghedoni R, Nitrosi A, Ragazzi M, Gasparini E, Masini C, Bisagni G. Contrast-enhanced spectral mammography in neoadjuvant chemotherapy monitoring: a comparison with breast magnetic resonance imaging. Breast Cancer Res. 2017;19(1):1–3.

Index

A

Abnormal area, 328–331
Advanced practice, 161
Anxiety, 14, 95, 122, 129–131, 137–151, 158–160, 162, 181, 187, 278, 352, 359, 367
Artificial intelligence (AI), 3, 6, 7, 41, 43–45, 213, 217–221
Asymmetrical density, 327, 329, 331, 334
Atypical hyperplasia, 24, 87, 102
Automated, 41–45, 213, 248, 250–255, 314

B

Benign breast disease (BBD), 24, 54, 55, 60, 61, 86, 89
Best practice, 140, 172, 190, 236, 250, 255, 292, 293, 369
Breast anatomy, 21–28, 31, 345
Breast augmentation, 278, 343, 345, 348
Breast cancer, 3–7, 11–18, 28, 33, 34, 36, 37, 41–43, 45, 51–61, 80, 81, 85, 87, 89, 93–97, 102–105, 107, 113, 114, 117, 120, 123–132, 138, 156, 158, 159, 161, 170, 179, 221, 224, 229, 247, 248, 259, 278, 279, 314, 343, 351–353, 355, 361, 365, 393, 394, 402, 407
Breast cancer screening, 3–5, 11–14, 18, 51, 60, 125, 132, 138, 167, 187, 229, 247, 310, 348
Breast compression, 200, 204, 214, 226, 247, 291, 296, 306, 310, 314, 393, 403
Breast conserving surgery (BCS), 180, 181, 339, 357
Breast diagnosis, 94, 97
Breast dimpling, 93, 94
Breast health promotion, 129, 166–170
Breast imaging, 5, 12, 21, 95, 161, 162, 167, 171, 172, 187, 188, 190, 199, 200, 212, 278, 284, 286, 292, 320, 321, 330, 343, 349, 365, 367, 377, 389, 392
Breast lesion, 33, 71, 77, 78, 81, 85, 86, 93, 94, 96, 278, 279, 402
Breast mass, 79, 80, 393
Breast screening, 4, 7, 12, 18, 33, 34, 41, 53, 59, 60, 89, 96, 105, 107, 108, 125, 127, 131, 155, 156, 158, 159, 161, 162, 165–167, 169, 172, 177, 179, 185, 187, 188, 217, 221, 255, 281, 282, 286, 289, 296, 367, 370

Breast screening experience, 156, 157, 172
Breast screening programme (BSP), 18, 42, 53, 127, 172, 262, 357
Breast size, 94, 180, 225, 226, 296, 305, 313, 353
Breast structure, 5, 31, 34, 296
Breast symptoms, 93, 155, 277, 279
Breast tissue, 17, 21–23, 27, 28, 32–37, 41–43, 53, 71, 78, 80–82, 89, 90, 94, 103, 158, 199, 201, 203, 213, 225, 228, 229, 238, 242, 247, 249, 251, 259, 262, 263, 266–269, 278, 295, 296, 298–301, 304–306, 317, 319–322, 343–345, 347, 348, 353, 356, 357, 383, 395

C

Cancer, 4–6, 12–15, 17, 24, 26, 51–54, 59, 60, 81, 84, 93, 94, 99–103, 105, 107, 108, 127, 130, 131, 169, 217–220, 224, 229, 248, 348, 351, 353, 356
Cancer development, 15, 99, 224
Cancer mechanisms, 104, 107
Cell mutation, 104
COM-B Model, 126, 128, 132
Communication, 25, 26, 95, 96, 99, 100, 113, 127, 130–133, 138–141, 155, 156, 159–162, 165, 168–170, 172, 278, 279, 292, 295, 330, 355, 366–368
Compression force, 156–158, 180, 188, 189, 201–204, 238–240, 242, 296, 297, 299–302, 304, 305, 310–313, 318, 321, 331, 343, 344, 348, 352, 356, 357, 359, 362, 393–394
Compression paddle, 200–204, 208, 226, 238–240, 291, 296, 297, 300, 303, 304, 314, 320, 323, 329–331, 333, 337, 339, 357, 395, 396
Compression pressure, 204, 255, 296, 306, 314
Computer aided detection (CAD), 6, 7, 218, 220
Contact area, 297, 299, 301, 305, 310–312
Continuous professional development (CPD), 237, 262
Contrast agent, 119, 199, 215, 402, 403, 405–407
Contrast enhanced digital mammography, 402
Contrast enhanced mammography, 41, 220, 402, 403, 405
Conversion factor, 226–228

C. Mercer et al. (eds.), *Digital Mammography*, https://doi.org/10.1007/978-3-031-10898-3

Printed in the United States
by Baker & Taylor Publisher Services